Second Supplement to

GLOSSARY OF INDIAN MEDICINAL PLANTS WITH ACTIVE PRINCIPLES

SECOND SUPPLEMENT TO

GLOSSARY OF INDIAN MEDICINAL PLANTS WITH ACTIVE PRINCIPLES

PART - I (A — K)

(1965 – 1981)

by

L.V. ASOLKAR
K. K. KAKKAR
O.J. CHAKRE

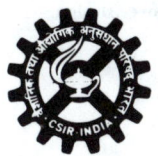

PUBLICATIONS & INFORMATION DIRECTORATE (CSIR)
DR. K.S. KRISHNAN MARG
NEW DELHI-110 012

1992

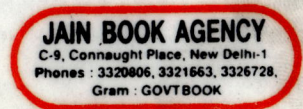

© 1992
Publications & Information Directorate (CSIR)
Dr. K.S. Krishnan Marg, New Delhi - 110 012

ISBN 81-7236-048-7

Production

S.N. Saxena
Supriya Gupta, Pamila Khanna

Computer & DTP Processing

Vinod Sharma	S. Ramalingam
R.K. Kaushik	M.S. Saluja
S. Vardarajan	C.P.S. Khari

Cover Design: Mohan Singh Meena

Printed and Published by   **Publications & Information Directorate,**
Dr. K.S. Krishnan Marg, New Delhi-110 012

Dedicated to

Late COL. R.N. CHOPRA

Whose researches paved the way for further surveys of Indian medicinal plants and whose works such as "Indigenous Drugs of India", "Poisonous Plants of India" and "Drug Addiction with Special Reference to India" in general, and "Glossary of Indian Medicinal Plants" & (First) "Supplement to Glossary" in particular gave impetus to further researches on active principles.

FOREWORD

The Second Supplement to Glossary of Indian Medicinal Plants with Active Principles, covers information by and large from 1965 to 1981. Part I (A-K) of this
supplement runs into 414 pages covering 841 genera with 689 new species. The number
of periodicals referred to for this volume were 1245.

The credit for completing the Part I (A-K) of the Second Supplement goes primarily
to Miss L.V. Asolkar, who along with her colleagues Dr. O.J. Chakre and Dr. K.K.
Kakkar, have done a commendable job of not only up-dating this Glossary Supplement
from 1965 onwards, but also incorporating other relevant earlier information thereby
making it comprehensive. Further information on active principles in some detail, albeit
Glossary style, is also included.

This Part I of Second Supplement to Glossary would complement the two volumes
of Compendium of Indian Medicinal Plants by Rastogi and Mehrotra published by us.
Whereas the former gives plant- partwise information on medicinal uses/properties and
chemical constituents followed by information on active principles with standard
chemical names for important ones and structure-activity correlationship, the later
enlists chemical constituents, new compounds with graphic structures, and biological
activities.

We hope to publish early, Part II of this Supplement which will cover the remaining
plants with names starting with alphabets L to Z. In the mean time, research workers in
chemistry and pharmacology and even industrialists can derive benefits from the
information covered in Part I (A-K), which is bound to prove an asset to them as was
Chopra's Glossary of Indian Medicinal Plants.

Dated: 10 Aug. 1992   Dr. G.P.Phondke

PREFACE

This long-awaited "Second Supplement to Glossary of Indian Medicinal Plants with Active Principles, Part I (A-K)" covers as many as 841 medicinal genera of which 219 are new; 1780 species of which 689 are carved for the first time. As before, the information on plants is arranged alphabetically according to their botanical names. Those that appear for the fist time in this volume are marked with an asterix.

The Second Supplement to Glossary is designated to cater to the needs of economic botanists, research chemists and pharmacologists, drugs and pharmaceutical industrialists, and those involved in the production of perfumes and cosmetics. Even health conscious individuals could derive some benefit from the coverage of food plants many of which have some medicinal property or other.

Primarily, this volume has put together information that became available from 1965 to 1981. However, even earlier information has been included if the article so demanded. In *Acorus*, biosystematics have been covered in some details. Confusing information on *Abrus* lectins, abrins and agglutinins has been sorted out for the benefit of users.

This volume covers information upto 1981 which coincides with the last coverage year of the 10th Collective Indexes of *Chem Abstr*. This can make it convenient for the users to up-date the article(s) by scanning subsequent collective indexes wherever available.

This Supplement uses up-dated nomenclature, mainly through the efforts of Dr. O.J.Chakre, who also gave new medicinal species in both existing as well as new genera, their Indian names, medicinal properties and/or uses and distribution through a number of floras and other standard works. It also gives names of transferred genera as per the international convention and not their species.

The spadework for medicinal and chemical information for all the existing and new species has been done by Dr. K.K. Kakkar; new species were also added by him through original papers. More than 25,000 references have been scanned for the purpose.

Standardization of the chemical compound names was beyond the realm of this Supplement. However, in the case of important medicinal compounds, this exercise has been done. Compounds of economic importance and of topical interest have been covered in some details.

Asarones or rather β-asarone may require some more information. Hederagenin, as saponin has been retained because of the residual sugar moiety in the genin. β-Sitosterol is a mixture of β-sitosterol and campesterol, as per Thomson et al., *Steroids*, 1963, **2**, 505. Double spellings of compounds prevalent in literature have been included, in fact both English and American spellings have been used for compounds as well as activities, however, 'e' has been added for German spellings for names of alkaloids ending with 'n'. Radicals rather than their full names have been used in the compounds; some liberties such as di-OH for dihydroxy in place of -(OH)$_2$ have been taken, while full compound names have been included in the index; readers finding any difficulty should consult the reference incorporated in the text.

International standards for periodical abbreviations have been used with some modifications. Wherever periodicals and *CA* years happen to be the same, only volume number is mentioned for *CA*. In this Supplement, *natl* stands for *Natural* and *Nat* for *National* whereas the international standards demand *vice versa*. Our apology to the users for interchanging of abbreviations.

Coloured photo of *Catharanthus roseus* or *sadabahar* on the jacket is by Dr. Ramesh Bedi of New Delhi on the left side of *sadabahar* are line drawings of *Digitalis lanata* (top); and sclerotia of *Claviceps purpurea* (below); on the back side is *Cannabis sativa*.

I take this opportunity of expressing my gratitude to those who rendered their co-operation in Glossary work at one time or other.

Thanks are due to Miss Rohini Kaul, for her efficient typing as also for computerizing of some portions of the manuscript, and to Mrs. Indu Sanhotra and Mrs. Renu Manchanda for giving a helpful hand in typing some of the major articles for making them press- ready.

I am grateful to Shri Y.R. Chadha, ex-Editor-in-Chief for his encouragement.

Miss L.V. Asolkar

BOOKS REFERRED TO

Allen, O.N. & Allen, E.K.—The Leguminosae: A Source Book of Characteristics, Uses and Nodulation (Macmillan Publishers, Ltd., London, UK), 1981.

Arctander, S.— Perfume and Flavour Materials of Natural Origin (Elizabeth, New Jersey), 1960.

Asolkar, L.V. (Miss) & Chadha, Y.R. — Diosgenin and Other Steroid Drug Precursors (Publications & Information Directorate, CSIR, New Delhi), 1979; reprinted, 1982.

Atal, C.K. & Kapur, B.M. (editors), Med. Plants—Cultivation and Utilization of Medicinal & Aromatic Plants (Regional Research Laboratory, CSIR, Jammu-Tawi), 1982.

Atlas of Poisonous Plants—A Colour Atlas of Poisonous Plants, by Frohne, D & Pfänder, H.J. (Wolfe Publishing Ltd., Stuttgart), 1984.

Babu, C.R.—Herbaceous Flora of Dehra Dun (Publications & Information Directorate, CSIR, New Delhi), 1977.

Beal, J.L. & Reinhard, E.(editors)—Natural Products as Medicinal Agents (Hippokrates Verlag, Stuttgart), 1981.

Behl, P.N., Captain,R.M., Bedi, B.M.S. & Gupta,S.—Skin-Irritant and Sensitizing Plants Found in India (Asian Printers Pvt. Ltd., Bombay), 1966.

Benthall, A.P.—The Trees of Calcutta and its Neighbourhood (Thacker, Spink & Co. Ltd., Calcutta), 1946.

Bressers, J.—The botany of Ranchi District, Bihar, India (The Govt. of Bihar, Catholic Press, Ranchi), 1951.

Brossi, A. (editor)—The Alkaloids, Vol. 38 (in continuation with Manske Series), (Academic Press Inc., California), 1990.

Brossi, A. & Suffness, M. (editors)—The Alkaloids, Vol. 37 (in continuation of Manske Series), (Academic Press, Inc., California), 1990.

Burkill, I.H.—A Dictionary of the Economic Products of the Malay Peninsula (The Crown Agents for the Colonies, London), 2 Vols., 1935.

Chopra, R.N., Badhwar, R.L. & Ghosh, S.— Poisonous Plants of India (Indian Council of Agricultural Research, New Delhi), 2 Vols., 2nd edn, 1965.

Chopra, R.N., Chopra, I.C., Handa K.L. & Kapur, L.D.—Indigenous Drugs of India (U.N. Dhur & Sons Pvt. Ltd., Calcutta) 2nd edn, 1958.

Chopra, R.N. et al—Glossary of Indian Medicinal Plants (Council of Scientific & Industrial Research, New Delhi), 1956. Reprinted, 1974, 1980. Supplement, 1969.

Companion to Chopra's Glossary of Indian Medicinal Plants, by Mehrotra, B.N., Aswal, B.S. & Bisht, B.S. (Bishen Singh Mahendra Pal Singh, Dehra Dun, India), 1987.

Cowan, A.M. & Cowan, J.M.—The Trees of Northern Bengal (Govt. of Bengal, Calcutta), 1929.

Dictionary Org. Compds—Dictionary of Organic Compounds (Chapman and Hall, New York) 5 Vols., 5th edn, 1982. Supplements 1 & 2, 1983, 1984.

Fl Bashahr Himal—Flora of Bashahr Himalayas, by Nair, N.C. (International

Bioscience Publishers, Hissar, Haryana), 1977.

Fl Bhagalpur—Flora of Bhagalpur (Dicotyledons), by Verma, S.K. (Today & Tomorrow's Printers & Publishers, New Delhi), 1981.

Fl Bhopal—The Flora of Bhopal (Angiosperms), by Oommachan, M. (J.K. Jain Brothers, Bhopal), 1977.

Fl Br Ind—Flora of British India, by Hooker, J.D. (Secretary of State for India, London), 7 Vols., 1872-1897.

Fl Delhi— The Flora of Delhi, by Maheshwari, J.K. (Council of Scientific & Industrial Research, New Delhi), 1963.

Fl East Himal—The Flora of Eastern Himalaya: Second and Third Reports, by Hara, H. & Ohasi, H. (The University of Tokyo Press, Japan), 1966.

Fl Gorakhpur—Flora Gorakhpurensis, by Srivastava, T.N. (Today & Tomorrow's Printers & Publishers, New Delhi), 1976.

Fl Hassan—Flora of Hassan District, Karnataka, India, by Saldanha, C.J & Nicolson, D.H. (Amerind Publishing Co. Pvt. Ltd., New Delhi), 1976.

Fl Howrah District—Flora of Howrah District, by Bennet, S.S.R. (Published by C.R.P.S. Gahlot, International Book Distributors, Dehra Dun, India), 1979.

Fl Indian Desert—Flora of the Indian Desert, by Bhandari, M.M. (Scientific Publishers, Jodhpur), 1978.

Fl Iraq—Flora of Iraq, by Townsend, C.C. & Evan Guest (Ministry of Agriculture, Baghdad, Iraq), 9 Vols., 1966-68.

Fl Med.—Flora Medica, by Lindley, J. (Ajay Book Service, New Delhi), Indian Reprint, 1981, 2nd Impression, 1985.

Fl Missouri—Flora of Missouri, by Steyermark, J.A.(The Iowa State University Press, Ames, USA).

Fl Murshidabad—Flora of Murshidabad District, West Bengal, India, by Guha Bakshi, D.N.(Scientific Publishers Jodhpur, India), 1984.

Fl N-E Rajasthan—Flora of North-East Rajasthan, by Sharma,S.& Tiagi, B. (Kalyani Publishers, New Delhi), 1979.

Fl Punjab Plains—Flora of Punjab Plains: Haryana and Punjab State, by Nair, N.C. [Rec Bot Surv India, 1978, 21(1)] (Botanical Survey of India, IBG, Howrah), 1978.

Fl Tripura—The Flora of Tripura State, by Deb, D.B. (Today & Tomorrow's Printers & Publishers, New Delhi),2 Vols., 1981-1983.

Fl W Pakistan—Flora of West Pakistan, by Nasir, E. and Ali, S.I. (editors) (Fakhri Printing Press, Karachi), 1972-76.

Goodman, L.S. & Gilman, A. (editors)—The Pharmacological Basis of Therapeutics (The Macmillan Co., New York), 1966.

Herbal Med.—Herbal Medicine: the natural way to get well and stay well, by Buchman, D.D. (Gramercy Publishing Co., New York), 1979.

Hocking, G.M.—A Dictionary of Terms in Pharmacognosy and Other Divisions of Economic Botany (Charles C. Thomas, Illinois), 1955.

Hoppe, H.A.—Drogenkunde: Handbuch der Pflanzlichen Und Tierischen Rohstoffe (Cram, De Gruyter & Co., Hamburg), 1958.

Hortus Third—Concise Dictionary of Plants Cultivated in the United States and Canada, by Bailey, L.H.F & Bailey, E.Z. (Macmillan Publishing Co., Inc., New York; Collier Macmillan Publishers, London), revised, 1978.

IP, 1966—Pharmacopoeia of India (Ministry of Health, Govt. of India), 2nd edn, 1966.

Jacobs, M.L. & Burlage, H.M.—Index of Plants of North Carolina with Reputed Medicinal Uses (Texas), 1958.

Jacobson, M.—Insecticides from Plants:A Review of Literature, 1941-53(US Department of Agriculture, Washington DC), Agriculture Handbook No. 154, 1958.

Jacobson, M. & Crosby, D.G. (editors)— Naturally Occurring Insecticides (Marcel Dekker, Inc., New York), 1971.

Jain, S.K. (editor)—Glimpses of Indian Ethnobotany (Oxford & IBH Publishing Co., New Delhi), 1981.

Jeffrey, C.—Biological Nomenclature (Oxford & IBH Publishing Co., New Delhi), 1977.

Keeler, R.F., Van Kampen, K.R. & James, L.F. (editors)—Effects of Poisonous Plants on Livestock (Academic Press, New York), 1978.

Ketkar, C.M.—Utilization of Neem (*Azadirachta indica* A. Juss.) and its By-products (KVIC, Bombay), 1976.

Kingsbury, J.M.—Poisonous Plants of the United States and Canada (Prentice-Hall Inc., Englewood Cliffs, New Jersey), 1964.

Liener, I.E. (editor)—Toxic Constituents of Plant Foodstuffs (Academic Press, New York), 1980.

Mabberley—The Plant-Book: A Portable Dictionary of the Higher Plants, by Mabberley, D.J. (Cambridge University Press, Cambridge), 1987, Reprint 1990.

Manske, R.H.F. (editor)—The Alkaloids(Academic Press, New York), Vols. V-XX, 1955-1981, Vols. 37 & 38, 1990.

Markets Selected Med. Plants—Markets for Selected Medicinal Plants and their Derivatives (International Trade Centre UNCTAD/GATT, Geneva), 1982.

Martindale—The Extra Pharmacopoeia Martindale, edited by Wade, A. & Reynolds, J.E.F. (The Pharmaceutical Press, London), 1977; reprinted, 1979.

Med. Bot.—Medicinal Botany. Plants affecting man's health, by Lewis, W.H. & Elvin-Lewis, M.P.F. (John Wiley & Sons, New York), 1977.

Med. Plants—Medicinal Plants and their Uses, by Hans Flück, translated by Rowson, J.M. (W. Foulsham & Co. Ltd., England), 1976.

Merck Index— An Encyclopaedia of Chemicals and Drugs, edited by Stecher, P.C. *et al* (Merck & Co., Inc., Rohway), 8th edn, 1968.

Miller, L.P.—Phytochemistry (Van Nostrand Reinhold Co., New York), 3 Vols., 1973.

Murti, K.S. & Achaya, K.T.—Cottonseed Chemistry & Technology: in its setting in India (Publications & Information Directorate, CSIR, New Delhi), 1978.

Parry, J.W.—Spices (Chemical Publishing Co., Inc., New York), 1969.

Plant and Fungal Toxins—Handbook of Natural Toxins; Vol.1, edited by Keeler, R.F. & Tu Anthony, T. (Marcel Dekker, Inc., New York), 1983.

Purseglove, J.W., Brown, E.G., Green, C.L. & Robbins, S.R.J.— Spices (Longman, Inc., New York), 2 Vols., 1981.

Quisumbing, E.—Medicinal Plants of the Philippines (Dep. of Agriculture and Natural Resources, Manila), *Tech Bull*, No. 16, 1951.

Rodrigo, R.G.A. (editor)—The Alkaloids: Vol.XX (in continuation of Manske series), (Academic Press, New York), 1981.

Santapau, H. & Henry, A.N.—A Dictionary of the Flowering Plants in India (Publications & Information Directorate, CSIR, New Delhi), 1973.

SEPASAT—Survey of Economic Plants for Arid & Semi-Arid Tropics (Royal Botanic Gardens, Kew, Economic Botany Division, Computer printout), 1985.

Sim, S.K.—Medicinal Plant Alkaloids (University of Toronto Press, Toronto), 2nd edn, 1965.

Standley, P.C.—Trees and Shrubs of Mexico (Smithsonian Press, Washington, DC.), 2 Vols., 1920-26.

Sturtevant's Notes on Edible Plants, by Hedrick, U.P.(J.B. Lyon Co., Albany), 1919.

Suppl. Gloss. Indian Med. Plants—Supplement to Glossary of Indian Medicinal Plants by Chopra, R.N. *et al* (Publications & Information Directorate, CSIR, New Delhi), 1969.

Swain, T.(editor)—Chemical Plant Taxonomy(Academic Press, London), 1963.

Swern, D.(editor)—Bailey's Industrial Oil & Fat Products (John Wiley & Sons, New York), Vol.1, 4th edn, 1979.

Taylor, I. & Farnsworth, N.R.(editor)—The Catharanthus Alkaloids (Marcel Dekker, Inc., New York), 1975.

Thomson, R.H.—Naturally Occurring Quinones (Academic Press, London), 2nd edn, 1971.

Uphof, J.C.Th.—Dictionary of Economic Plants (Verlag Von J. Cramer), 2nd edn, 1968.

USD—The Dispensatory of the United States of America (J.B. Lippincott Co., Philadelphia), 25th edn, 1955; Supplement, 1960.

Wagner, H. & Wolff, P. (editors)—New Natural Products and Plant Drugs with Pharmacological, Biological or Therapeutical Activity (Springer-Verlag, Berlin, New York), 1977.

Watt, J.M. & Breyer-Brandwijk, M.G.—The Medicinal & Poisonous Plants of Southern & Eastern Africa (E & S Livingstone Ltd., Edinburgh), 2nd edn, 1962.

White, F.—Forest Flora of Northern Rhodesia (Oxford University Press, London), 1962.

Willis, J.C.—A Dictionary of the Flowering Plants & Ferns, revised by Airy Shaw, H.K. (Cambridge University Press, London), 7th edn. 1966; 8th edn., 1973.

Wlth India—The Wealth of India, Raw Materials (Publications & Information Directorate, CSIR, New Delhi), Vols. I-XI, 1948-76; revised & enlarged Vols. IA, 1985; 2B, 1988.

JOURNALS REFERRED TO

Abh Dtsch Akad Wiss Berlin Kl Chem Geol Biol— Abhandlungen der Deutschen Akademie der Wissenschaften zu Berlin, Klasse fuer Chemie, Geologie und Biologie. Berlin.

ACS Symp Ser—ACS Symposium Series. Washington, DC.

Acta Agric Scand—Acta Agriculture Scandinavia. Stockholm.

Acta Allergol—Acta Allergologica. Copenhagen.

Acta Biochim Pol—Acta Biochimica Polanica. Warsaw.

Acta Bot Indica—Acta Botanica Indica. Meerut.

Acta Chem Scand—Acta Chemica Scandinavica. Copenhagen.

Acta Chim Sin—Acta Chimica Sinica. Beijing.

Acta Chim Acad Sci Hung—Acta Chimica Academiae Scientiarum Hungaricae. Budapest.

Acta Cient Compostelana—Acta Cientifica Compostelana. Spain.

Acta Crystallogr—Acta Crystallographica. Copenhagen.

Acta Endocrinol—Acta Endocrinologica. Copenhagen.

Acta Histochem—Acta Histochemica et Cytochemica. Kyoto.

Acta Histochem—Acta Histochemica. Jena.

Acta Manilana Ser A—Acta Manilana, Series A. Manila.

Acta Med Philipp—Acta Medica Philippina. Manila.

Acta Med Port—Acta Medica Portuguesa. Lisbon.

Acta Med Scand—Acta Medica Scandinavica. Stockholm.

Acta Microbiol Acad Sci Hung—Acta Microbiologica Academiae Scientiarum Hungaricae. Budapest.

Acta Microbiol Pol Ser B—Acta Microbiologica Polonica, Series B. Warsaw.

Acta Pharm—Acta Pharmaceutica Hungaricae. Budapest.

Acta Pharm Hung—Acta Pharmaceutica Hungaricae. Budapest.

Acta Pharm Jugosl—Acta Pharmaceutica Jugoslavica. Zagreb.

Acta Pharm Pol—Acta Pharmaceutica Polaniae. Warsaw

Acta Pharm Sin—Acta Pharmaceutica Sinica. Beijing.

Acta Pharm Suec—Acta Pharmaceutica Suecica. Stockholm.

Acta Pharmacol Toxicol—Acta Pharmacologica et Toxicologica. Copenhagen.

Acta Physiol Pol—Acta Physiologica Polonica. Warsaw.

Acta Phytother—Acta Phytotherapeutica. Amsterdam.

Acta Pol Pharm—Acta Poloniae Pharmaceutica. Warsaw.

Acta Soc Bot Pol—Acta Societatis Botanicorum Polaniae. Warsaw.

Acta Unio Int Contra Cancrum—Acta Unio Internationalis Contra Cancrum. Geneva.

Acta Univ Palacki Olomuc Fac Med—Acta Universitatis Palackianae Olomucensis, Facultatis Medicae. Olomous, Czechoslovakia.

Acta Univ Szeged Acta Phys Chem—Acta Universitatis Szegediensis de Attila Jozsef Nominatae. Acta Physica et Chemica. Hungary.

Adv Cereal Sci Technol—Advances in Cereal Sciences and Technology. St. Paul, Minn.

Adv Chem Ser—Advances in Chemistry Series. Washington, DC.

Adv Exp Med Biol—Advances in Experimental Medicine and Biology. New York.

Adv Mass Spectrom—Advances in Mass Spectrometry. New York.

Adv Mod Toxicol—Advances in Modern Toxicology. Washington, DC.

Afinidad—Afinidad. Barcelona.

Agents Actions—Agents and Actions. Basel.

Agra Univ J Res—Agra University Journal of Research: Science. Agra.

Agressologie—Agressologie. Paris.

Agric Louvain—Agricultura. Louvain.

Agric Biol Chem—Agricultural and Biological Chemistry. Tokyo.

Agric Res Delhi—Agricultural Research. Delhi.

Agric Res USDA—Agricultural Research. US Department of Agriculture. Washington, DC.

Agroplantae—Agroplantae. Pretoria.

Aktual Vopr Farm—Aktual'nye Voprosy Farmatsii.

Aliment Vie—Alimentation et la Vie. Paris.

Alkaloids—Alkaloids. London/New York.

Allerg Asthma—Allergie und Asthma. Leipzig, Germany.

Am J Anat—American Journal of Anatomy. New York.

Am J Bot—American Journal of Botany. Columbus.

Am J Clin Nutr—American Journal of Clinical Nutrition. Bethesda.

Am J Hosp Pharm—American Journal of Hospital Pharmacy. Bethesda.

Am J Pathol—American Journal of Pathology. Philadelphia, Pa.

Am J Pharm—American Journal of Pharmacy and the Sciences Supporting Public Health. Philadelphia, Pa.

Am J Vet Res—American Journal of Veterinary Research. Schaumburg.

Am Pharm—American Pharmacy. Washington, DC.

Am Soc Brew Chem Proc—American Society of Brewing Chemists, Proceedings. St. Paul.

An Acad Bras Cienc—Anais da Academia Brasileira de Ciencias. Rio De Janeiro.

An Assoc Bras Quim—Anais da Associacao Brasileira de Quimica. Sao Paulo.

An Asoc Quim Argent—Anales de la Asociacion Quimica Argentina.

An Bromatol—Anales de Bromatologia. Lisbon

An Fac Farm Porto—Anais da Faculdade de Farmacia do Porto. Porto.

An Fac Farm Univ Fed Pernambuco—Anais da Faculdade de Farmacia, Universidade Federal de Pernambuco. Brazil.

An Fac Quim Farm Univ Chile—Anales de la Facultad de Quimica y Farmacia, Universidad de Chile. Santiago.

An Farm Quim Sao Paulo—Anais de Farmacia e Quimica de Sao Paulo. Sao Paulo.

An Inst Bot A J Cavanilles—Anales del Instituto Botanico A.J. Cavanilles. Madrid.

An Quim—Anales de Quimica. Madrid.

An R Acad Farm—Anales de la Real Academia de Farmacia. Madrid.

An R Soc Esp Fis Quim Ser B—Anales de la Real Sociedad Espanola de Fisica y Quimica, Serie B: Quimica. Madrid.

An Soc Cient Argent—Anales de la Sociedad Cientifica Argentina. Buenos Aires.

Anal Biochem—Analytical Biochemistry. San Diego.

Anal Chem—Analytical Chemistry. Washington, DC.

Anal Chim Acta—Analytica Chimica Acta. Amsterdam.

Analyst Lond—Analyst. London.

Ancient Sci Life—Ancient Science of Life. Coimbatore.

Andhra Agric J—Andhra Agricultural Journal. Guntur.

Anesthesiology—Anesthesiology. Philadelphia. Pa.

Angew Bot—Angewandte Botanik. Berlin.

Angiology—Angiology. Roslyn, New York.

Ankara Univ Eczacilik Fak Mecm—Ankara Universitesi Eczacilik Fakultesi Mecmuasi. Ankara.

Ankara Univ Tip Fak Mecm—Ankara Universitesi Tip Fakultesi Mecmuasi. Ankara.

Ann—Ann.

Ann Acad Bras Cienc—Annaes da Academia Brasileira de Ciencias.

Ann Appl Biol—Annals of Applied Biology. Warwick.

Ann Biochem Exp Med—Annals of Biochemistry and Experimental Medicine. Calcutta.

Ann Biol Anim Biochim Biophys—Annales de Biologie Animale, Biochimie, Biophysique. Jouy-en-Josas, France.

Ann Bot Lond—Annals of Botany. London.

Ann Chem Warsaw—Annals of Chemistry. Warsaw.

Ann Chim Paris—Annales de Chimie. Paris.

Ann Chim Rome—Annali di Chimica. Rome.

Ann Fac Med Chir Univ Studi Perugia—Annali della Facolta di Medicina e Chirurgia della Universita degli, Studi di Perugia.

Ann Fac Sci Univ Saigon—Annales of Faculty of Science, University of Saigon.

Ann Gembloux—Annales de Gembloux. Gembloux.

Ann Intern Med—Annals of Internal Medicine. Philadelphia. Pa.

Ann Ist Super Sanita—Annali dell'Istituto Superiore di Sanita. Rome.

Ann Med Exp Biol Fenn—Annales Medicinae Experimentalis et Biologiae Fenniae. Helsinki.

Ann Med Nancy—Anales Medicales de Nancy. Paris.

Ann N Y Acad Sci—Annals of the New York Academy of Sciences. New York.

Ann Nutr Aliment—Annales de la Nutrition et de l'Alimentation. Paris.

Ann Pharm Fr—Annales Pharmaceutiques Francaises. Paris.

Ann Pharm Poznom—Annales Pharmaceutici Poznan. Warsaw.

Ann Sci Univ Besancon Bot—Annales Scientifiques de l'Universite de Besancon, Botanique. Besancon.

Ann Univ Mariae Cueie-Skladowska Sect D—Annales Universitatis Mariae Curie-Sklodowska, Sectio D Medicina. Lublin, Poland.

Annu Confr Indian Pharmacol Soc—Annual Conference of Indian Pharmacological Society. 1980.

Annu Rep CDRI Lucknow—Annual Report Central Drug Research Institute. Lucknow.

Annu Rep DRI Jammu—Annual Report Drug Research Institute. Jammu.

Annu Rep ICMR—Annual Report Indian Council of Medical Research. New Delhi.

Annu Rep Nat Inst Nutr Tokyo—Annual Report National Institute of Nutrition. Tokyo.

Annu Rep RRL Jammu—Annual Report Regional Research Laboratory. Jammu.

Annu Rep RRL Jorhat—Annual Report Regional Research Laboratory. Jorhat.

Antibiotiki Moscow—Antibiotiki. Moscow.

Antiseptic—Antiseptic. Madras.

Appl Environ Microbiol—Applied and Environmental Microbiology. Washington, DC.

Appl Microbiol—Applied and Environmental Microbiology. Washington, DC.

Appl Polym Symp—Applied Polymer Symposia. New York.

Aptechn Delo—Aptechnoe Delo. Moscow.

ARC Res Rev—ARC Research Reviews. U.K.

Arch Biochem—Archives of Biochemistry. New York.

Arch Biochem Biophys—Archives of Biochemistry and Biophysics. New York.

Arch Exp Pathol Pharmacol—Archiv fuer Experimentelle Pathologie and Pharmakologie. Leipzig.

Arch Farm—Archivos Farmaceuticos. Bago.

Arch Farmacol Toxicol—Archives de Farmacologiya y Toxicologia. Madrid.

Arch Immunol Ther Exp—Archivum Immunologiae et Therapiae Experimentalis (English Translation). Wroclaw. Poland.

Arch Int Pharmacodyn Ther—Archieves Internationales de Pharmacodynamie et de Therapie. Ghent, Belgium.

Arch Int Physiol Biochim—Archives Internationales de Physiologie et al Biochimie. Liege, Belgium.

Arch Invest Med—Archivos de Investigacion Medica. Mexico.

Arch Ital Sci Farmacol—Archivio Italiano di Scienze Farmacologiche. Florence.

Arch Kriminol—Archiv fuer kriminologie. Luebeck, Germany.

Arch Microbiol—Archives of Microbiology. Chicago.

Arch Oral Biol—Archives of Oral Biology. London.

Arch Pathol—Archives of Pathology and Laboratory Medicine. Chicago.

Arch Pharm Ber Dtsch Pharm Ges—Archiv der Pharmazie und Berichte der Deutschen Pharmazeutischen Gesellschaft. Weinheim.

Arch Pharm Wein—Archiv der Pharmazie Weinheim.

Arerugi—Arerugi. Tokyo.

Arh Farm—Arhiv za Farmaciju. Belgrade/Tokyo.

Arogya—Arogya. Gorakhpur.

Arogya J Hlth Sci—Arogya Journal of Health Science. Gorakhpur.

Arq Biol Technol—Arquivos de Biologia e Technologia . Parana, Brazil.

Arzneim Forsch—Arzneimittel-Forschung. Aulendorft. Germany.

Asian J Med—Asian Journal of Medicine. Hongkong.

Asian J Pharm—Asian Journal of Pharmacy. Philippines.

Asian Symp Med Plants and Spices—Asian Symposium on Medicinal Plants and Spices. 4th, 1980.

Atherosclerosis—Atherosclerosis. Amsterdam.

Atherosclerosis Berlin—Atherosclerosis. Berlin.

Atti Acad Nazl Lincei Rend Cl Sci Fis Mat Nat—Atti della Academia Nazionale dei Lincei Rendiconti della Classe de Scienze Fisiche, Matematiche e Naturali. Rome.

Aust J Biol Sci—Australian Journal of Biological Sciences. Melbourne.

Aust J Chem—Australian Journal of Chemistry. Melbourne.

Aust J Dairy Technol—Australian Journal of Dairy Technology. Melbourne.

Aust J Exp Biol Med Sci—Australian Journal of Experimental Biology and Medical Science. Adelaide.

Aust J Pharm—Australian Journal of Pharmacy. Melbourne.

Aust J Plant Physiol—Australian Journal of Plant Physiology. Melbourne.

Aust Vet J—Australian Veterinary Journal. Sydney.

Azerb Med Zh—Azerbaidzhanskii Meditsinskii Zhurnal. Baku. Azerbaijan S.S.R. USSR.

Bacteriol Rev—Bacteriological Reviews. Washington, DC.

Background Migraine Symp—Background Migraine, Migraine Symposium, 2nd, 1967 (Pub.1969), New York.

Bangladesh Counc Sci Ind Res—Bangladesh Council of Scientific & Industrial Research. Dhaka.

Bangladesh J Agric—Bangladesh Journal of Agriculture. Dhaka.

Bangladesh J Sci Ind Res—Bangladesh Journal of Scientific and Industrial Research. Dhaka.

Bangladesh Med J—Bangladesh Medical Journal. Dhaka.

Bangladesh Med Res Counc Bull—Bangladesh Medical Research Council Bulletin. Dhaka.

Beitr Biochem Physiol Naturstotten Festschr—Beitring Biochemie und Physiologie der Naturstoffen Festschrift.

Bibl Haematol Basel—Bibliotheca Haematologica. Basel.

Berufs-Dermatosen—Berufs-Dermatosen. Aulendorf, Germany.

Biochem J—Biochemical Journal. Essex, England.

Biochem Biophys Res Commun—Biochemical and Biophysical Research Communications. San Diego.

Biochem Physiol Pflanz—Biochemie und Physiologie der Pflanzen. Jena.

Biochem Physiol Plant Growth Subst Proc Int Conf Plant Growth Subst—Biochemistry and Physiology of Plant Growth Substance, Proceedings International Conference on Plant Growth Substances, 6th, 1967.

Biochem Prep—Biochemical Preparations. New York.

Biochem Soc Trans—Biochemical Society Transactions. London.

Biochem Syst Ecol—Biochemical Systematics and Ecology. Elmsford.

Biochemistry—Biochemistry. Washington, DC.

Biochem Biophys Acta—Biochimica et Biophysica Acta. Amsterdam.

Biochimie—Biochimie. Paris.

Biokhimiya—Biokhimiya. Moscow.

Biol of Cancer Cell Proc Fifth Meet Eur Assoc for Cancer Res—Biology of Cancer Cell, Proceedidngs, Fifth Meet,European Association for Cancer Research. Vienna.

Biol Nauki—Biologicheskie Nauki. Alma-Ata.

Biol Plant—Biologia Plantarum. Prague.

Biol Plant Acad Sci Bohemoslov—via *CA*.

Biol Psychiatry—Biological Psychiatry. New York.

Biol Rundsch—Biologische Rundschau.Jena, Germany.

Biol Zentralbl—Biologisches Zentralblatt. Leipzig.

Biovigyanam—Biovigyanam. Pune.

Bitamin Kyoto—Bitamin. Kyoto.

Biul Inst Rosl Leczn—Biuletyn Instytutu Roslin Leczniczych. Poznam, Poland.

Blumea—Blumea. Leiden.

Bol Fac Farm Univ Coimbra Ed Cient—Boletim da Faculdade de Farmacia, Universidade de Coimbra, Edicao Cientifica.

Bol Soc Quim Peru—Boletin de La Sociedad Quimica del Peru.

Boll Chim Farm—Bollettino Chimico Farmaceutico. Milan.

Boll Lab Chim Prov—Bollettino dei Laboratori Chimici Provinciali. Italy.

Boll Soc Ital Biol Sper—Bollettino della Societa Italiana di Biologia Sperimentale. Naples.

Boll Soc Ital Farm Osp—Bollettino della Societa Italiana di Farmacia Ospedaliera. Turin.

Boll Soc Med Chir Catania—Bollettino della Societa Medico-Chirurgica di Catania. Cremona.

Bombay Technol—Bombay Technologist. Bombay.

Bor'ba Poteryami Zhivotnovodstv Sb—Bor'ba s Poteryami v Zhivotnovodstve Sbornik.

Bordeaux Med—Bordeaux Medical. Bordeaux, France.

Borgyogy Venerol Sz—Borgyogyaszaties Venerologiai Szemle.

Bot Bull Acad Sin—Botanical Bulletin of Academia Sinica. Taipei, Taiwan.

Bot J Linn Soc—Botanical Journal of the Linnean Society. New York.

Bot Mag—Botanical Magazine. London.

Bot Mus Leafl Harv Univ—Botanical Museum Leaflets, Harvard University. Cambridge. Mass.

Bot Sady Pribaltiki—via *CA*

Bot Zh Leningrad—Botanicheskii Zhurnal.Leningrad.

Br J Cancer—British Journal of Cancer. London.

Br J Exp Pathol—British Journal of Experimental Pathology. London.

Br J Ind Med—British Journal of Industrial Medicine. London.

Br J Nutr—British Journal of Nutrition. Cambridge.

Br J Pharmacol—British Journal of Pharmacology. London.

Br Med J—British Medical Journal. London.

Br Poult Sci—British Poultry Science. Edinburgh, Scotland.

Br Vet J—British Veterinary Journal. London

Brasserie—Brasserie. Belgium.

Bratisl Lek Listy—Bratislavske Lekarske Listy. Bratislava.

Brew Sci—Brew Science. London.

Brittonia—Brittonia. New York.

Bul Kebun Raya—Buletin Kebun Raya. Bogor, Indonesia.

Bul Univ Shteteror Tiranes Ser Shkencat Mjekesore—Buletin i Universitetit Shteteror te Tiranes, Seria Shkeneat Mjekesore.

Bull Acad Nat Med Paris—Bulletin de l' Academie Nationale de Medecine. Paris.

Bull Acad Pol Sci Cl D Ser Sci Biol—Bulletin de l'Academie Polonaise des Sciences, Classe II. Serie des Sciences Biologiques. Varsovie, Warsaw.

Bull Acad Pol Sci Ser Sci Chim—Bulletin de L'Academie Polonaise des Sciences, Serie des Sciences Chimiques.

Bull Acad Serbe Sci Arts Cl Sci Math Nat Sci Nat—Bulletin Academie Serbedes Sciences et des Arts, Classe Sciences Mathematiques et Naturelles, Sciences Naturelles.

Bull Bot Soc Bengal—Bulletin of the Botanical Society of Bengal. Calcutta.

Bull Bot Soc Univ Saugar—Bulletin of the Botanical Society University of Saugar. Sagar.

Bull Bot Surv India—Bulletin of the Botanical Survey of India. Calcutta.

Bull Brew Sci—Bulletin of Brewing Science. Tokyo.

Bull Calcutta Sch Trop Med—Bulletin of the Calcutta School of Tropical Medicine. Calcutta.

Bull Chem Soc Jpn—Bulletin of the Chemical Society of Japan. Tokyo.

Bull Chiang Mai Assoc Med Sci—Bulletin of Chiang Mai Associated Medical Sciences. Chiang Mai, Thailand.

Bull Environ Contam Toxicol—Bulletin of Environmental Contamination and Toxicology. Heidelberg.

Bull Fac Pharm Cairo Univ—Bulletin of the Faculty of Pharmacy, Cairo University. Cairo.

Bull Fac Sci Riyadh Univ—Bulletin of the Faculty of Science, Riyadh University. Riyadh.

Bull Haffkine Inst—Bulletin of Haffkine Institute. Bombay.

Bull Inst Chem Res Kyoto Univ—Bulletin of the Institute for Chemical Research, Kyoto University. Kyoto.

Bull Med Ethno Bot Res—Bulletin of Medico Ethno Botanical Research. New Delhi.

Bull Narc—Bulletin of Narcotics. Geneva.

Bull Nat Inst Sci India—Bulletin of National Institute of Science of India. New Delhi.

Bull RRL Jammu—Bulletin of Regional Research Laboratory Jammu.

Bull RRL Hyderabad—Bulletin of Regional Research Laboratory. Hyderabad.

Bull Sci Res Counc Jamaica—Bulletin of the Scientific Research Council of Jamaica. Jamaica.

Bull Soc Chim Belg—Bulletin de la Societe Chimique de Belgique. Gent, Belgium.

Bull Soc Chim Fr—Bulletin de la Societe Chimique de France. Paris.

Bull Soc Pharm Bordeaux—Bulletin de la Societe de Pharmacie de Bordeaux. Bordeaux.

Bull Soc Pharm Lille—Bulletin de la Societe de Pharmacie de Lille. Lille.

Bull Soc Pharm Marseille—Bulletin de la Societe de Pharmacie de Marseille. Marseille.

Bull Soc R Sci Liege—Bulletin de la Societe Royale des Sciences de Liege. Liege.

Bull Tech, Gattefosse SFPA—Bulletin Technique Gattefosse SFPA.

Bull Trav Soc Pharm Lyon—Bulletin des Travaux de la Societe de Pharmacie de Lyon.

Bull Torrey Bot Club—Bulletin of the Torrey Botanical Club. New York.

Byull Eksp Biol Med—Byulleten Eksperimental'noi Biologii i Meditsiny. Moscow.

CA—Chemical Abstracts. Philadelphia, Pa.

Cafe Cacao The—Cafe Cacao The. Paris.

Cancer Philadelphia—Cancer. Philadelphia.

Can Inst Food Sci Technol J—Canadian Institute of Food Science and Technology Journal. Ottawa.

Can J Anim Sci—Canadian Journal of Animal Science. Ottawa.

Can J Chem—Canadian Journal of Chemistry. Ottawa.

Can J Comp Med—Canadian Journal of Comparative Medicine. Ottawa.

Can J Microbiol—Canadian Journal of Microbiology. Ottawa.

Can J Pharm Sci—Canadian Journal of Pharmaceutical Sciences. Ottawa.

Can J Physiol Pharmacol—Canadian Journal of Physiology and Pharmacology. Ottawa.

Can J Zool—Canadian Journal of Zoology. Ottawa.

Cancer Chemother Proc Takeda Int Conf Osaka—Cancer Chemotherapy, Proceedings, Takeda International Conference. Osaka.

Cancer Chemother Rep—Cancer Chemotherapy Reports. Washington, DC.

Cancer Res—Cancer Research. Baltimore.

Cannabis Hlth—Cannabis Health.

Carbohydr Res—Carbohydrate Research. Amsterdam.

C R Acad Bulg Sci—Comptes Rendus de l'-Academie Bulgare des Sciences. Sofia.

C R Acad Sci Ser A B C & D—Comptes Rendus, Hebdomadaires des Seances de l'Academie des Sciences. Series A, B, C & D. Paris.

C R Congr Nat Soc Savantes Sect Sci—Comptes Rendus du Congres National des Societes Savantes, Section des Sciences.

C R Seances Soc Biol—Comptes Rendus des Seances de la Societe de Biologie. Paris.

Cah Nutr Diet—Cahiers de Nutrition et de Dietetique. Paris.

Cellul Carta—Cellulosa e Carta. Rome.

Cereal Chem—Cereal Chemistry. St. Paul.

Cervisia—Cervisia. Belgium.

Cesk Farm—Ceskoslovenska Farmacie. Prague.

Cesk Mykol—Ceska Mykologie. Prague.

Cesk Oftamol—Ceskoslovenska Oftalmologie. Prague.

Ceylon Coconut Q—Ceylone Coconut Quarterly. Lunuwila.

Ceylon J Med Sci—Ceylone Journal of Medical Science. Colombo.

Chagyo Kenkyu Hokoku—Chagyo Kenkyu Hokoku. Japan.

Chanyonmul Hwahak Yonguso Yongu Pogo—Chanyonmul Hwahak Yonguso Yongu Pogo.

Cheiron Madras—Cheiron. Madras.

Chem Age India—Chemical Age of India. Bombay.

Chem Alkaloids—Chemistry of Alkaloids. New York.

Chem Ber—Chemische Berichte. Weinheim.

Chem Can—Chemistry in Canada. Ottawa.

Chem Commun—see *J Chem Soc, Chem, Commun.*

Chem Commun Univ Stockholm—Chemical Communications, Unversity of Stockholm. Stockholm.

Chem Era—Chemical Era. Calcutta .

Chem Ind Lond—Chemistry and Industry. London.

Chem Ind News—Chemical Industrial News. Bombay.

Chem Lett—Chemistry Letters. Tokyo.

Chem Mikrobiol Technol Lebensm—Chemie, Mikrobiologie, Technologie der Lebensmittel. Nuernberg.

Chem Petrochem J—Chemical and Petrochemical Journal. Bombay.

Chem Pharm Bull—Chemical and Pharmaceutical Bulletin. Tokyo.

Chem Phys Lipids—Chemistry and Physics of Lipids. Limerick.

Chem Rev—Chemical Reviews. Washington, DC.

Chem Scr—Chemica Scripta. Stockholm.

Chem Ztg Chem Appar—Chemiker-Zeitung, Chemische Apparatur. Heidelberg.

Chem Zvesti—Chemicke Zvesti. Bratislava.

Chemosphere — Chemosphere. Oxford.

Chemtech—Chemtech. Washington, DC.

Chemotherapy Cancer Proc Int Symp Lugano Switz— Chemotherapy of Cancer, Proceedings of International Symposium. Lugano, Switzerland.

Chest—Chest. Illinois.

Chih Wu Hsueh Pao—Chih Wu Hsueh Pao. Beijing.

Chim Acta Turc—Chimica Acta Turcica.

Chim Ind Milan—Chimica e l' Industria. Milan.

Chim Ther—Chimica Therapeutica. Arcueil.

Chin Chem Soc J Taipei—Chinese Chemical Socity Journal Taipei. Taiwan.

Chin J Microbiol—Chinese Journal of Microbiolcgy. Beijing.

Chin Med J—Chinese Medical Journal. Beijing.

Chromatographia—Chromatographia. Wiesbaden.

Chung-Hua I Hsueh Tsa Chih—Chung Hua I Hsueh Tsa Chih. Beijing.

Chung Ts'ao Yao—Chung Ts'ao Yao.

Chung Yao T'ung Pao—Chung Yao T'ung Pao.

Chungang Uihak—Chungang Uihak. Seoul.

Ciencia—Cienica. Brazil/Mexico

Cienc Cult Sao Paulo—Cienica e Cultura. Sao Paulo.

Circ Res—Circulation Research. Taxas.

Clin Chem N Y—Clinical Chemist. New York.

Clin Chim Acta—Clinica Chimica Acta. Amsterdam.

Clin Pharmacol Ther—Clinical Pharmacology and Therapeutics. St. Louis, Mo.

Clin Term—Clinica Termale.

Clin Toxicol—Clinical Toxicology. New York.

Clujul Med—Clujul Medical. Bucharest.

CNS Drugs Symp CSIR India—CNS Drugs Symposium CSIR India. 1966.

Coffee Tea Ind—Coffee and Tea Industries.

Coll Czech Chem Commun—Collection of Czechoslovak Chemical Communications. Prague.

Colloq Int C N R S—Colloques Internationaux du Center National de la Recherche Scientifique. Paris.

Colloq Int Chim Cafes C R—Colloque International sur la Chimie des cafes, Comptas Rendus.

Commun Fac Sci Univ Ankara Ser B—Communications de la Faculte des Sciences de l'Universite d'Ankara. Ankara.

Comp Biochem Physio—Comparative Biochemistry and Physiology. New York.

Comp Gen Pharmacol—Comparative and General Pharmacology. Elmsford, New York.

Comp Physiol Ecol—Comparative Physiology and Ecology. Jodhpur.

Compt Rend—Competes Rendus. Paris.

Contact Dermatitis—Contact Dermatitis. Copenhagen.

Cornell Univ Agric Expt Sta Mem—Cornell University, Agriculture Experimental Station Memoriers.

Cornell Vet—Cornell Veterinarian. Ithaca, New York.

Corr Farm—Corriere del Farmacista. Naplas, Italy.

Corsi Semin Chim—Corsi e Seminari di Chimica. F. Giordani.

Cosmet Toiletries—Cosmetics and Toiletries. Oak Park, Illinois.

CRC Crit Rev Food Sci Nutr—C R C Critical Reviews in Food Science and Nutrition. Boca Raton.

Crop Sci—Crop Science. Madison, Wis.

Cruciferae Newsl—Cruciferae Newsletter. Scotland.

CSIR News—Council of Scientific and Industrial Research News. New Delhi.

Cuoio Pelli Mater Concianti—Cuoio, Pelli, Materie Concianti. Naples.

Curr Chem Pap—Current Chemical Papers. London.

Curr Med Pract—Current Medical Practice. Bombay.

Curr Sci—Current Science. Bangalore.

Curr Topics Plant Sci—Current Topics in Plant Science.

Curr Trends Life Sci—Current Trends in Life Sciences. New Delhi.

Dacca Univ Stud—Dacca University Studies. Dhaka.

Dakar Med—Dakar Medical. Dakar, Senegal.

Dan Med Bull—Danish Medical Bulletin. Copenhagen.

Dan Tidsskr Farm—Dansk Tidsskrift for Farmaci. Copenhagen.

Dev Plant Biol—Developments in Plant Biology. Amsterdam.

Diabetes—Diabetes. New York.

Diabetologia—Diabetologia. Berlin.

Diss Abstr—Dissertation Abstracts. Ann Arbor.

Diss Abstr Int B—Dissertation Abstracts International Section B. Ann Arbor.

Diss Pharm—Dissertationes Pharmaceuticae. Warsaw.

Diss Pharm Pharmacol—Dissertationes Pharmaceuticae et Pharmacologicae. Wroclow, Poland.

Dokl Akad Nauk SSSR—Doklady Akademii Nauk SSSR. Moscow.

Dokl Akad Nauk Tadzh SSR—Doklady Akademii Nauk Tadzhikskoi SSR.

Dokl Akad Nauk Uzb SSR—Doklady Akademii Nauk Uzbekskoi SSR.

Dokl Bolg Akad Nauk—Doklady Bolgarskoi Academii Nauk. Sofia.

Dokl Vses Akad Skh Nauk im V I Lenina—Doklady Vsesoyuznoi Akademii Sel'skokhozyaistvennykh Nauk im V I Lenina.

Dragoco Rep—Dragoco Report. Holzminden.

Drug Cosmet Ind—Drug & Cosmetic Industry. New York.

Drug Pharm Patent Awareness Bull—Drug Pharmaceutical Patent Awareness Bulletin. Lucknow.

Drug Res—Drug Research. Aulendorf, Germany.

Drug Pharm Ind Highlights—Drugs and Pharmaceutie Industry Highlights. Lucknow.

Drugs Exp Clin Res—Drugs under Experimental and Clinical Research. Barcelona.

Dtsche Apth—Deutsche Apotheker. Stuttgart.

Dtsch Apoth Ztg—Deutsche Apothekar-Zeitung. Stuttgart.

Dtsch Gesundheitswes—Deutsche Gesundheitswessen. Berlin.

Dtsch Lebensm Rundsch—Deutsche Lebensmittal Rundschau. Stuttgart.

Dtsch Z Gesamte Gerichtl Med—Deutsche Zeitschrift fuer die Gesampte Gerichtliche Medizin. Berlin.

Duoc Hoc—Douc Hoc.

East Afr Agric For J—East African Agricultural and Forestry Journal. Nairobi.

East Pharm—Eastern Pharmacist. Delhi.

Ecol Food Nutr—Ecology of Food and Nutrition. New York.

Econ Bot—Economic Botany. New York.

Egypt J Chem—Egyptian Journal of Chemistry. Cairo.

Egypt J Hortic—Egyptian Journal of Horticulture. Cairo.

Egypt J Pharm Sci—Egyptian Journal of Pharmaceutical Sciences. Cairo.

Egypt Pharm Bull—Egyptian Pharmaceutical Bulletin. Cairo.

Eisei Dobutsu—Eisei Dobutsu. Tokyo.

Eisei Kagaku—Eisei Kagaku. Tokyo.

Eiyo To Shokuryo—Eiyo To Shokuryo. Tokyo.

Eiyogaku Zassh—Eiyogaku Zasshi. Tokyo.

Ekologiya—Ekologiya. Sofia.

Eksp Med Morfol—Eksperimentalna Medisina i Morfologiya. Sofia.

Elelmiszervizsgalati Kozl—Elelmiszervizsgalati Kozlemenyek. Budapest.

Endocrinol Exp—Endocrinologia Experimentalis. Bratislava.

Endocrinology—Endocrinology. Baltimore.

Entomon—Entomon. Trivandrum.

Environ India—Environment India. Gorakhpur.

Enzymologia—Enzymologia. Hague.

Epidemiol Mikrob Infektsiozni Bolesti—Epidemiologiya, Mikrobiologiya i Infektsiozni Bolesti. Sofia.

Erfahrungsheilkunde—Erfahrungsheilkunde. Heidelberg, Germany.

Ernaehr Umsch—Ernaehrungs - Umschau. Frankfurt.

Ernaehrungsforschung— Ernaehrungsforschung. Berlin.

Esc Farm—Escuela de Farmacia. Guatemala.

Essenze Deriv Agrum—Essenze e Derivati Agrumari. Italy.

Ethnomedicine—Ethnomedicine. Humburg.

Eur J Biochem—European Journal of Biochemistry. Berlin.

Exp Eye Res—Experimental Eye Research. New York.

Exp Med Surg—Experimental Medicine and Surgery. Brooklyn, New York.

Exp Mol Pathol—Experimental and Molecular Pathology. New York.

Experientia—Experientia. Basel.

Excerpta Bot—Excerpta Botanica. Stuttgart.

Farm Aikak—Farmaseuttinen Aikakauslehti. Finland.

Farm Bull CIMAP—Farm Bulletin of Central Institute of Medicinal and Aromatic Plants. Lucknow.

Farm Ed Sci—Farmaco, Edizione Scientifica. Milan.

Farm Glas—Farmaceutski Glasnik. Zagreb, Yugoslavia.

Farm Obz—Farmaceuticky Obzor. Bratislava, Czechoslovakia.

Farm Pol—Farmacja Polska. Warsaw.

Farm Tijdschr Belg—Farmaceutisch Tijdschrift voor Belgie.

Farm Vestn Ljubljana—Farmacevtski Vestnik Ljubljana. Yugoslavia.

Farm Zh Kiev—Farmatsevtichnii Zhurnal. Kiev.

Farmacia Buc—Farmacia. Bucharest.

Farmaco Ed Prat—Farmaco, Edizione Pratica. Milan.

Farmakol Alkaloidov Glikozidov—Farmakologiya Alkaloidov Glikozidov. Tashkent. 1967.

Farmakol Alkaloidov Serdech Glikozidov—Farmakologiya Alkaloidov Serdech. Glikozidov. 1971.

Farmakol Toksikol Kiev & Moscow—Farmakologiya i Toksikologiya. Kiev & Moscow.

Farmatsia Sof—Farmatsia. Sofia.

Farmatsiya Moscow—Farmatsiya. Moscow.

Farumashia—Farumashia. Tokyo.

Fats Oils Relat Food Prod their Persp Symp—Fats and Oils related Food Products and their Perspective Symposium. Mysore.

FEBS Lett—Federation of European Biochemical Societies Letters. Amsterdam.

Fed Prod Fed Am Soc Exp Biol—Federation Proceedings, Federation of American Societies for Experimental Biology. Baltimore.

Fed Regist—Federal Register. Washington.

Fert News—Fertilizer News.Delhi.

Fette Seifen Anstrichm—Fette, Seifen, Anstrichmittel. Leinfelden, Germany.

Field Crop Abstr—Field Crop Abstracts. Oxon, England.

Fitoterapia—Fitoterapia. Milan.

Fiziol Aktiv Soedin Rast Kirg—Via Ca

Fiziol Akt Veschestva Respub Mezhvedom Sb—Fiziologicheski Aktivnye Veschestva Respublikanskii Mezhvedomstvennyi Sbornik Nauchnykh Trudov. Ukrainian.

Fiziol Zh Kiev—Fiziologichnii Zhurnal. Kiev.

Fiziol Zh SSSR—Fiziologicheskii Zhurnal SSR. Leningrad.

Flavour Ind—Flavour Industry. London.

Fleischwirtschaft—Die Fleischwirtschaft. Frankfurt.

Flora Jena—Flora Jena.

Folia Med Plovdiv—Folia Medica. Plovdiv.

Folia Med Bialosto—Folia Medica Bialostocensia. Warsaw.

Folia Microbiol Prague—Folia Microbiologica. Prague.

Folia Pharm—Folia Pharmaceutica. Italy.

Food Chem—Food Chemistry. Barking.

Food Cosmet Toxicol—Food and Cosmetics Toxicology. Oxford.

Food Technol N Z—Food Technology in New Zealand. Auckland.

For Abstr—Forestry Abstracts. Oxford.

Forensic Sci Soc J—Forensic Science Society Journal. North Yorkshire, England.

Fortschr Chem Forsch—Fortschritte der Chemischen Forschung.New York.

Forotschr Chem Org Naturst—Fortschritte der Chemie Organische Naturstoffe. Berlin.

Fortschr Veterinaermed—Fortschritte der Veterinaermedizin. Berlin.

Gann—Gann. Amsterdam.

Garcia de Orta—Garcia de Orta. Lisbon.

Gard J—Garden Journal. Bronx.

Gazz Chim Ital—Gazzetta Chimica Italiana. Rome.

Gdansk Tow Nauk Rozpr Wydz—via *CA*

Gen Pharmacol—General Pharmacology. Elmsford.

Gendai Toyo Igaku—Gendai Toyo Igaku. Japan.

Geobios—Geobios. Jodhpur.

Gerontology—Gerontology. Basel.

Ghana J Sci—Ghana Journal of Science. Legon.

Gidroliz Lesokhim Promst—Gidroliznaya i Lesokhimicheskaya Promyshlennost. Moscow.

Gifu Daigaku Igakubu Kiyo—Gifu Daigaku Igakubu Kiyo. Gifu.

Gig Sanit—Gigiena i Sanitariya. Moscow.

Glas Hem Drug Beograd—Glasnik Hemijskog Drustva, Beograd. Belgrade.

Glas Hem Tehnol Bosne Hercegovine—Glasnik Hemicara i Tehnologa Bosne i Hercegovine. Sarajevo.

God Vissh Khimikotekhnol Inst Sofia—Godishnik na Visshiya Khimikotekhnologicheski Institut. Sofia.

Gujarat Agric Univ Res J—Gujarat Agricultural University Research Journal. Ahmedabad.

Gunma J Med Sci—Gunma Journal of Medical Sciences. Maebasji, Japan.

Gut—Gut. London.

Gyogyszereszet—Gyogyszereszet. Budapest.

Hahnemannian Gleanings—Hahnemannian Gleanings. Calcutta.

Hakko Kogaku Zashi—Hakko Kogaku Zasshi. Osaka.

Hakko Kyokaishi—Hakko Kyokaishi. Tokyo.

Haksurwon Nonmunjip Cha'yon Kwahak P'yon—Haksurwon Nonmunjip, Cha'yon Kwahak P'yon. Korea.

Hamdard—Hamdard. Karachi.

Hanguk Yongyang Hakhoe Chi—Hanguk Yongyang Hakhoe Chi. Seoul.

Harokeach Haivri—Harokeach Ha-ivri. Tel Aviv.

Hautarzt—Der Hautarzt. Berlin.

Helv Chim Acta—Helvetica Chimica Acta. Basel.

Hem Ind—Hemijska Industrija. Belgrade.

Herba Hung—Herba Hungarica. Budapest.

Herba Pol—Herba Polonica. Warsaw.

Heterocycles—Heterocycles. Tokyo.

Hind Antibiot Bull—Hindustan Antibiotics Bulletin. Pimpri, Pune.

Holzforschung—Holzforschung. Berlin.

Hoshi Yakka Daigaku Kiyo—Hoshi Yakka Daigaku Kiyo. Tokyo.

Hrana Ishrana—Hrana i Ishrana. Belgrade.

Hua Hsueh Hsueh Pao—Hua Hsueh Hsueh Pao.

Huan Ching Pao Hu—Huan Ching Pao Hu.

IDMA Bull—Indian Drug Manufacturers Association Bulletin. Bombay.

Ind Bull Bombay—Industrial Bulletin. Bombay.

Ind Chim Belge—Industrie Chimique Belge.

Indian Agric—Indian Agriculturist. Calcutta.

Indian Cashew J—Indian Cashew Journal. Ernakulam.

Indian Chem J—Indian Chemical Journal. Bombay.

Indian Coffee—Indian Coffee. Bangalore.

Indian Drugs—Indian Drugs. Bombay.

Indian Drugs Pharmac Ind—Indian Drugs and Pharmaceuticals Industry. Bombay.

Indian Farming N S—Indian Farming, New Series. New Delhi.

Indian For—Indian Forester. Dehra Dun.

Indian Fmrs' Dig—Indian Farmer's Digest. Pantnagar.

Indian Heart J—Indian Heart Journal. Calcutta.

Indian J Agric Sci—Indian Journal of Agricultural Science. New Delhi.

Indian J Anim Hlth—Indian Journal of Animal Health. Calcutta.

Indian J Anim Res—Indian Journal of Animal Research. Karnal.

Indian J Anim Sci—Indian Journal of Animal Science. New Delhi.

Indian J Appl Chem—Indian Journal of Applied Chemistry. Calcutta.

Indian J Biochem—Indian Journal of Biochemistry. New Delhi.

Indian J Biochem Biophys—Indian Journal of Biochemistry & Biophysics. New Delhi.

Indian J Cancer—Indian Journal of Cancer. Bombay.

Indian J Chem—Indian Journal of Chemistry. New Delhi.

Indian J Dermatol Vernereol —Indian Journal of Dermatology and Venereology. Bombay.

Indian J Entomol—Indian Journal of Entomology. New Delhi.

Indian J Exp Biol—Indian Journal of Experimental Biology. New Delhi.

Indian J For—Indian Journal of Forestory. Dehra Dun.

Indian J Genet Plant Breeding—Indian Journal of Genetics and Plant Breeding. New Delhi.

Indian J Hist Sci—Indian Journal of History of Science. New Delhi.

Indian J Hosp Pharm—Indian Journal of Hospital Pharmacy. New Delhi.

Indian J Med Res—Indian Journal of Medical Research. New Delhi.

Indian J Med Sci—Indian Journal of Medical Sciences. Bombay.

Indian J Microbiol—Indian Journal of Microbiology. Pune.

Indian J Mycol Plant Pathol—Indian Journal of Mycology and Plant Pathology. Udaipur.

Indian J Nutr Diet—Indian Journal of Nutrition and Dietetics. Coimbatore.

Indian J Pharm—Indian Journal of Pharmacy. Bombay.

Indian J Pharmacol—Indian Journal of Pharmacology. Bombay.

Indian J Pharm Sci—Indian Journal of Pharmaceutical Sciences. Bombay.

Indian J Physiol Allied Sci—Indian Journal of Physiology and Allied Sciences. Calcutta.

Indian J Physiol Pharmacol—Indian Journal of Physiology and Pharmacology. Bombay.

Indian J Psychiatry—Indian Journal of Psychiatry. Pune.

Indian J Technol—Indian Journal of Technology. New Delhi.

Indian J Vet Sci Anim Husb—Indian Journal of Veterinary Science and Animal Husbandry. New Delhi.

Indian Livestk—Indian Livestock. Delhi.

Indian Med Gaz—Indian Medical Gazette. Calcutta.

Indian Med J—Indian Medical Journal. Calcutta.

Indian Oilseeds J—Indian Oilseeds Journal. Hyderabad.

Indian Oil & Soap J—Indian Oil and Soap Journal. Calcutta.

Indian Phytopathol—Indian Phytopathology. New Delhi.

Indian Pulp Pap—Indian Pulp and Paper. Calcutta.

Indian Sci Abstr—Indian Science Abstracts. New Delhi.

Indian Soap J—Indian Soap Journal. Calcutta.

Indian Spices—Indian Spices. Ernakulam.

Indian Vet J—Indian Veterinary Journal. Madras.

Indo-Soviet Symp on Chem of Natl prod—Indo-Soviet Symposium on the Chemistry of Natural Products.

Inf Grasas Aceites—Informaciones sobre Grasas y Aceites.

Insect Sci Appl—Insect Science and its Application. Elmsford.

Inst Nac Pesqui Amazonia Publ Quim—Instituto Nacional de Pesquisas da Amazonia, Publicacao, Quimica.

Int Arch Allergy Appl Immunol—International Archives of Allergy and Applied Immunology. Basel.

Int Congr Essent Oils—International Congress on Essential Oils. 1977.

Int Congr Ser Excerpta Med—International Congress Series on Excerpta Medica. 1980.

Int Flavours Food Addit—International Flavours and Food Aditives. London.

Int J Cancer—International Journal of Cancer. Geneva.

Int J Neurosci—International Journal of Neuroscience. London.

Int J Pept Protein Res—International Journal of Peptide and Protein Research. Copenhagen.

Int J Vitam Nutr Res—International Journal for Vitamin and Nutrition Research. Berne.

Int Pharm Abstr—International Pharmaceutical Abstracts. Hamilton.

Int Symp Hepatotoxic—International Symposium on Hepatotoxicity. 1973.

Int Symp Med Plants—International Symposium on Medicinal Plants.

Int Z Vitaminforsch—Internationale Zeitschrift fuer Vitaminforschung. Berne.

Invest Clin—Investigacion Clinica. Maracaibo.

ISI Bull—Indian Standard Institute Bulletin. New Delhi.

Isr J Chem—Israel Journal of Medical Scinces. Jerusalem.

Ital J Biochem—Italian Journal of Biochemistry. Rome.

IUPAC Int Symp Chem Nat Prod—International Union of Pure and Applied Chemistry, International Symposium on the Chemistry of Natural Products. 1978.

Izv Akad Nauk Az SSR Ser Biol Nauk—Izvestiya Akademii Nauk Azerbaidzhanskoi SSR, Seriya Biologicheskikh Nauk. Baku.

Izv Akad Nauk Gruz SSR Ser Khim—Izvestiya Akademii Nauk Gruzinskai SSR. Seriya Khimicheskaya. Tiflis.

Izv Akad Nauk Kaz SSR Ser Biol—Izvestiya Akademii Nauk Kazakhskoi SSR, Seriya Biologicheskaya. Alma-Ata.

Izv Akad Nauk Kirg SSR—Izvestiya Akademii Nauk Kirgizskoi SSR. Frunze.

Izv Akad Nauk SSSR, Ser Khim—Izvestiya Akademii Nauk SSSR, Seriya Khimicheskaya. Moscow.

Izv Akad Nauk Tadzh SSR Otd Biol Nauk—Izvestiya Akademii Nauk Tadzhikskoi SSR, Otdelenie Biologicheskikh Nauk. Dushanbe.

Izv Akad Nauk Turkm SSR, Ser Biol Nauk—Izvestiya Akademiya Nauk Turkmenskoi SSR, Seriya Biologicheskikh Nauk. Ashkhabad.

Izv Akad Nauk SSSR Ser Biol—Izvestiya Akademii Nauk SSSR, Seriya Biologicheskaya. Moscow.

Izv Akad Nauk Turkm SSR Ser Fiz Tekh Khim Gel Nauk— Izvestiya Akademiya Nauk Turkmenskoi SSR, Seriya Fiziko-Tekhnicheskikh, Khimicheskikh i Geologicheskikh Nauk. Ashkhabad.

Izv Durzh Inst Kontrol Lek Sredstva—via CA

Izv Inst Fiziol Bulg Acad Nauk—Izvestiya na Instituta po Fiziologiya, Bulgarska Akademiya na Naukite. Sofia.

Izv Sib Otd Akad Nauk SSSR Ser Biol Nauk— Izvestiya Sibirskogo Otdelaniya Akademii Nauk SSSR, Seriya Biologicheskikh Nauk. Novosibirsk.

Izv Sib Otd Akad Nauk SSSR Ser Khim Nauk—Izvestiya Sibirskogo Otdeleniya Akademii Nauk SSSR, Seriya Khimicheskikh Nauk. Novosibirsk.

J Anim Sci—Journal of Animal Science. Champaign, Illinois.

J Appl Crystallogr—Journal of Applied Crystallography. Copenhagen.

J Assoc Off Agric Chem—Journal of the Association of Official Agricultural Chemists. Baltimore.

J Assoc Off Anal Chem—Journal of the Association of Official Analytical Chemists. Arlington, Va.

J Assoc Physicians India—Journal of the Association of Physicians of India. Bombay.

J Atheroscler Res—Journal of Atherosclerosis Research. Amsterdam.

J Bangladesh Acad Sci—Journal of Bangladesh Academy of Sciences. Dhaka.

J Biol Chem—Journal of Biological Chemistry. Baltimore, Md.

J Biosci—Journal of Biosciences. Bangalore.

J Bombay Natl Hist Soc—Journal of the Bombay Natural History Society. Bombay.

J Cancer Chemother Rep—Journal of Cancer Chemotherapeutic Reports.

J Chem Ecol—Journal of Chemical Ecology. New York.

J Chem Res Synop—Journal of Chemical Research Synopsis. Nottinghsm.

J Chem Soc—Journal of the Chemical Society. London.

J Chem Soc Chem Commun—Journal of the Chemical Society, Chemical Communication. London.

J Chem Soc Perkin Trans I—Journal of the Chemical Society, Parkin Transactions. London.

J Chem Soc Pak—Journal of the Chemical Society of Pakistan. Karachi.

J Chem UAR—Journal of Chemistry of the United Arab Republic. Cairo.

J Chin Chem Soc Taipei—Journal of the Chinese Chemical Society. Taipei.

J Chromatogr—Journal of Chromatography. Amsterdam.

J Clin Pharmacol—Journal of Clinical Pharmacology. New York.

J Commun Dis—Journal of Communicable Diseases. Delhi.

J Dent Res—Journal of Dental Research. St. louis.

J Drug Res—Journal of Drug Research. Cairo.

J Econ Entomol—Journal of Economic Entomology. Lanham.

J Econ Tax Bot—Journal of Economic and Taxonomic Botany. Jodhpur.

J Egypt Med Assoc—Journal of the Egyptian Medical Association. Cairo.

J Endocrinol—Journal of Endocrinology. London.

J Entomol Res—Journal of Entomological Research. New Delhi.

J Ethnopharmacol—Journal of Ethnopharmacology. Lausanne.

J Exp Bot—Journal of Experimental Botany. Oxford, England.

J Exp Med—Journal of Experimental Medicine. New York.

J Food Prot—Journal of Food Protection. Iowa.

J Food Sci—Journal of Food Science. Champaign, Illinois.

J Food Sci Technol—Journal of Food Science and Technology. Mysore.

J Food Technol—Journal of Food Technology. Oxford, England.

J Formosan Med Assoc—Journal of the Formosan Medical Journal Association. Taipei.

J Immunol—Journal of Immunology. New York.

J Indian Acad Wood Sci—Journal of the Indian Academy of Wood Science. Bangalore.

J Indian Chem Soc—Journal of the Indian Chemical Society. Calcutta.

J Indian Dent Assoc—Journal of the Indian Dental Association. Bombay.

J Indian Inst Sci—Journal of the Indian Institute of Sciences. Bangalore.

J Indian Leather Technol Assoc—Journal of the Indian Leather Technologists' Association. Calcutta.

J Indian Med Assoc—Journal of the Medical Association. Calcutta.

J Insect Physio—Journal of Insect Physiology. London.

J Inst Brew—Journal of the Institute of Brewing. London.

J Inst Chem—Journal of the Institutions of Chemists, India. Calcutta.

J Invest Dermatol—Journal of Investigative Dermatology. Baltimore.

J Karnatak Univ—Journal of the Karnatak University. Dharwar.

J Lipid Res—Journal of Lipid Research. Memphis, Tenn.

J Liq Chromatogr—Journal of Liquid Chromtography. New York.

J Med Assoc Thailand—Journal of the Medical Association of Thailand. Bangkok.

J Med Chem—Journal of Medicinal Chemistry. Easton, Pa.

J Med NY—Journal of Medicine. New York.

J Mol Biol—Journal of Molecular Biology. London.

J Nat Cancer Inst—Journal of the National Cancer Institute. Washington.

J Nat Integ Med Assoc—Journal of the National Integrated Medical Association. Mysore.

J Natl Prod—Journal of Natural Products. Ohio.

J Natl Res Counc Thailand—Journal of the National Research Council of Thailand. Bangkok.

J Nutr—Journal of Nutrition. Philadelphia.

J Nutr Diet—Journal of Nutrition and Dietetics. Coimbatore.

J Nutr Sci Vitaminol—Journal of Nutritional Science and Vitaminology. Tokyo.

J Occup Med—Journal of Occupational Medicine. Chicago.

J Oil Technol Assoc India—Journal of the Oil Technologists Association of India. Kanpur.

J Org Chem—Journal of Organic Chemistry. Easton, Pa.

J Oslo City Hosp—Journal of the Oslo City Hospitals. Oslo.

J Pathol—Journal of Pathology. London.

J Pharm Chim—Journal de Pharmacie et de Chimie. Paris.

J Pharm Pharmacol—Journal of Pharmacy and Pharmacology. London.

J Pharm Sci—Journal of Pharmaceutical Sciences. Washington.

J Pharm Sci UAR—Journal of Pharmaceutical Sciences of the United Arab Republic. Cairo.

J Pharmacol Exp Ther—Journal of Pharmacology and Experimental Therapeutics. Baltimore.

J Philipp Med Assoc—Journal of the Philippine Medical Association. Manila.

J Physiol Paris—Journal de Physiologie. Paris.

J Plant Crops—Journal of Plantation Crops. Kasaragod.

J Postgrad Med Bombay—Journal of Postgraduate Medicine. Bombay.

J Radioanal Chem—Journal of Radioanalytical Chemistry. Amsterdam.

J Res Ayur Sidha—Journal of Research in Ayurveda and Sidha. New Delhi.

J Res Indian Med—Journal of Research in Indian Medicine, Yoga and Homoeopathy. New Delhi.

J Res Orissa Univ Agric Technol—Journal of Research, Orissa University of Agriculture and Technology. Bhubaneshwar.

J Res Punjab Agric Univ—Journal of Research, Punjab Agricultural University. Ludhiana.

J S Afr Chem Inst—Journal of the South African Chemical Institute. Pretoria.

J S Carolina Med Assoc—Journal of the South Carolina Medical Association. Charleston.

J Sci Food Agric—Journal of the Science of Food and Agriculture. London.

J Sci Food Technol—Journal of Science and Food Technology. Mysore.

J Sci Ind Res—Journal of Scientific & Industrial Research. New Delhi.

J Sci Res Bhopal—Journal of Scientific Research. Bhopal.

J Sci Res BHU—Journal of Scientific Research of the Banaras Hindu University. Varanasi.

J Sci Res Counc Jam—Journal of the Scientific Research Council of Jamaica. Kingston.

J Sci Res Plants Med—Journal of Scientific Research in Plants and Medicines. Hardwar.

J Shivaji Univ—Journal of Shivaji University. Kolhapur.

J Soc Cosmet Chem—Journal of the Society of Cosmetic Chemist. New York.

J Toxicol Env Hlth—Journal of Toxicology and Environmental Health. Washington, DC.

J Univ Poona Sci Technol—Journal of the University of Poona, Science and Technology. Pune.

Jpn Heart J—Japanese Heart Journal. Tokyo.

Jpn J Antibiot—Japanese Journal of Antibiotics. Tokyo.

Jpn J Exp Med—Japanese Journal of Experimental Medicine. Tokyo.

Jpn J Pharmacol—Japanese Journal of Pharmacology. Kyoto.

Justus Liebigs Ann Chem—Justus Liebigs Annalen der Chimie. Weinheim.

Kagaku Keisatsu Kenkyusho Hokoku—Kagaku Keisatsu Kenkyusho Hokoku. Tokyo.

Kagaku To Kogyo—Kagaku To Kogyo. Tokyo.

Kagaku To Seibutsu—Kagaku To Seibutsu. Japan.

Kagoshima Daigaku Igaku Zasshi— Kagoshima Daigaku Igaku Zasshi. Kagoshima.

Kagoshima Daigaku Nogakubu Gakujutsu Hokoku—Kagoshima Daigaku Nogakubu Gakujutsu Hokoku.

Kansai Ika Daigaku Zasshi—Kansai Ika Daigaku Zasshi. Moriguchi.

Kardiologiya—Kardiologiya. Moscow.

Kaseigaku Zasshi—Kaseigaku Zasshi. Japan.

Kem Ind—Kemija u Industriji. Zagreb.

Kert Egy Kozl— Kerteszeti Egyptem Kozlemenyei. Budapest.

Ketsueki to Myakkan—Ketsueki To Myakkan.

Kexue Tongbao—Kexue Tongbao. Beijing.

Khadi Gramodyog—Khadi Gramodyog. Bombay.

Khim Farm Zh—Khimiko-Farmatsevticheskii Zhurnal. Moscow.

Khim Khim Tekhnol Alma-Ata—Khimiya i Khimicheskaya Tekhnologiya. Alma-Ata.

Khim Prir Soedin—Khimiya Prirodnykh Soedinenii. Tashkent.

Khim Prir Soedin Akad Nauk Uz SSR—via CA.

Kinki Daigaku Rikogakubu Kenkyu Hokoku—Kinki Daigaku Rikogakubu Kenkyu Hokoku.

Klin Med—Klinicheskaya Meditsina Moscow or Klinische Medizin Vienna.

Klin Wochenschr—Klinische Wochenschrift. Berlin.

Koen Yoshishu-Koryo, Terupen Oyobi Seiyu Kagaku ni Kansuru Toronkai— Koen Yoshishu-Koryo, Terupen Oyobi Seiyu Kagaku ni Kansuru Toronkai. 1979.

Kogyo Kagakku Zasshi—Kogyo Kagaku Zasshi. Tokyo.

K'o Hsueh Fa Chan Yuch K'an—K'o Hsueh Fa Chan Yuch K'an.

K'o Hsueh Nung Yeh Taipei—K'o Hsueh Nung Yeh. Taipei.

K'o Hsueh T'ung Pao—K'o Hsueh T'ung Pao. Beijing.

Konservn Ovoshchesush Promst— Konservnaya i Ovoshchesushil'naya Promyshlennost. Moscow.

Koryo—Koryo. Tokyo.

Kumamoto Pharm Bull—Kumamoto Pharmaceutical Bulletin. Kumamoto.

Kuo Li Taiwan Ta Hsueh I Hsueh Yuan Yen Chiu Pao Kao—Kuo Li Taiwan Ta Hsueh I Hsueh Yuan Yen Chiu Pao Kao. Taipei.

Kvasny Prum—Kvasny Prumysl. Prague.

Kyoto-fu Eisei Kogai Kenkyusho Nempo— Kyoto-fu Eisei Kogai Kenkyusho Nempo.

Kyoto Yakka Daigaku Gakuho—Kyoto Yakka Daigaku Gakuho.

Kyushu Daigaku Nogakubu Gakugei Zasshi—Kyushu Daigaku Nogakubu Gakugei Zasshi. Fukuoka.

Lab Invest—Laboratory Investigation. New York.

Labdev—Labdev Journal of Science and Technology. Kanpur.

Lakartidningen—Lakartidningen. Stockholm.

Lancet—Lancet. London.

Latv PSR Zinat Acad Vestis—Latvijas PSR Zinatnu Akademijas Vestis. Riga.

Leandra—Leandra. Riga.

Leandra—Leandra. Rio de Janeiro.

Leather—Leather. London.

Leath Sci—Leather Science. Madras.

Leban Pharm J—Lebanese Pharmaceutical Journal. Beyruth.

Lebensm Wiss Technol—Lebensmittel-Wissenschaft Technologie. London.

Leder—Leder. Darmstadt.

Lek Sirovine—Lekovite Sirovine. Yugoslavia.

Lekarstv Rast—Lekarstvennye Rasteniya.

Lepr India—Leprosy in India. Delhi.

Leprosy Rev—Leprosy Review. London.

Liebigs Ann Chem—Liebigs Annalen der Chemie. Leipzig.

Liet TSR Aukst Mokyklu Mokslo Darb Med—Lietuvos TSR Aukstuju Mokyklu Mokslo Darbai Medicina.

Liet TSR Moslu Akad Darb, Ser—Lietuvos TSR Mokslu Akademijos Darbai, Serija. Vilnius.

Life Sci—Life Sciences. England.

Life Sci Res Rep—Life Sciences Research Report. Elmsford.

Lipids—Lipids. Champaign, Illinois.

Liver Proc Int Gstaad Symp—Liver, Proceedings of International Gstaad Symposium, 1975.

Lloydia—Lloydia. Ohio.

Lucr Stiint Inst Agron Bucuresti Ser B—Lucrasi Stiintifice, Institutul Agronomic "N. Balcoscu" Seria B: Horticultura. Bucuresti.

Lyon Pharm—Lyon Pharmaceutique. Lyon.

Macco Agric Digest—Macco Agricultural Digest. Manglore.

Madras Agric J—Madras Agricultural Journal. Coimbatore.

Magy Tud Akad Kem Tud Oszt Kozl—Magyar Tudomanyos Akademia, Kemiai Tudomanyok Osztalyanak Kozlemenyei. Budapest.

Maharashtra Med J—Maharashtra Medical Journal. Pune.

Malay Agric J—Malayan Agricultural Journal. Kaula Lumpur.

MARDI Res Bull—Mardi Research Bulletin. Selangor.

Maslo-Zh Promst—Masloboino Zhirovaya Promyshlennost. Moscow.

Med Anthropol—Medical Anthropology. Washington, DC.

Med Chem Academic—Medicinal Chemistry (Academic). 1980.

Med Clin North Am—Medical Clinics of North America. Philadelphia, Pa.

Med Exp—Medicina Experimentalis. Basel.

Med J Aust—Medical Journal of Australia. Sydney.

Med J Malays—Medical Journal of Malaysia. Kuala Lumpur.

Med Leg Toxicol—via CA

Med Promst SSSR—Meditsinskaya Promyshlennost SSSR. Moscow.

Med Parazitol Parazit Bolezni—Meditsinskaya Parazitologiya i Parazitarnye Bolezni. Moscow.

Med Pharmacol Exp—Medicina et Pharmacologia Experimentalis. Basel.

Med Surg—Medicine and Surgery. Baroda.

Med Welt—Die Medizinische Welt. Stuttgart.

Med Zh Uzb—Meditsinskii Zhurnal Uzbekistana. Tashkent.

Medicamenta, Ed Farm—Medicamenta, Edicion para et Farmaceutico. Madrid.

Medd Not Farm Selsk—Meddelelser fra Norsk Farmaceutisk Selskap. Oslo.

Meded Fac Landbouwwet Rijksuniv Gent—Mededelingen van de Faculteit

Landbouwwetenschappen, Rijksuniversiteit Gent. Ghent.

Medikon—Medikon. Belgium.

Mediscope—Mediscope. Madras.

Meiji Daigaku Nogakubu Kenkyu Hokoku— Meiji Daigaku Nagakubu Kenkyu Hokoku. Kanagawa-Ken.

Meijo Daigaku Nogakubu Gakujutsu Hokoku—Meijo Daigaku Nogakubu Gakujutsu Hokoku. Nagoya.

Mem Fac Agric Kagoshima Univ—Memoirs of the Faculty of Agriculture. Kagoshima.

Met Miner Rev—Metals and Minerals Review. Calcutta.

Methods Carbohydr Chem—Method in Carbohydrate Chemistry. New York.

Methods Enzymol—Methods in Enzymology. San Diego.

Microbios Lett—Microbios Letters. Cambridge.

Mie Daigaku Nogakubu Gakujutsu Hokoku— Mie Daigaku Nogakubu Gakujus;u Hokoku. Mie, Japan.

Mikrobiol Zh Kiev—Mikrobiologichnii Zhurnal. Kiev.

Mikrobiologiya—Mikrobiologiya. Moscow.

Miles Int Symp Ser—Miles International Symposium Series. New York.

Minerva Pediatr—Minerva Pediatrica. Turin.

Mitt Dtsch Pharm Ges—Mitteilungen der Deutschen Pharmazeutischen Gesellschaft. Weinheim.

Mitt Geb Lebensmittelunters Hyg—Mitteilungen aus dem Gebiete der Lebensmitteluntersuchung und Hygiene. Berne.

Mitt Versuchsstn Gaerungsgewerbe Wien— Mitteilungen der Versuchsstation fuer das Gaerungsgewerbe in Wien. Vienna.

Mod Kemi—Modern Kemi. Sweden.

Mod Med Jpn—Modern Medicine. Japan.

Mod Pharmacol Toxicol—Modern Pharmacology. Toxicology Series. New York.

Mokuzai Gakkaishi—Mokuzai Gakkaishi. Tokyo.

Monatash Chem—Monatshefte fuer Chemie. Vienna.

Monatsschr Brau—Monatsschrift fuer Brauerei. Jena.

Mycologia—Mycologia. Bronx.

N A SNRC Publ—National Academy of Sciences. National Research Council, Publication. Washington, DC.

N Engl J Med—New England Journal of Medicine. London.

N Z J Agric Bot—New Zealand Journal of Agricultural Botany.

NZ J Sci—New Zealand Journal of Science. Wellington.

Nagarjun—Nagarjun. Calcutta.

Nagasaki Igakkai Zasshi—Nagasaki Igakkai Zasshi. Nagasaki.

Nagoya Shiritsu Daigaku Yakugakubu Kenkyu Nempo. —Nagoya Shiritsu Daigaku Yakugakubu Kenkyu Nempo. Nagoya.

Nagpur Vet Coll Mag—Nagpur Veterinery College Magazine. Nagpur.

Nahrung—Nahrung. Berlin.

Nat Acad Sci Lett—National Academy of Sciences Letter. Allahabad.

Natl Appl Sci Bull—Natural and Applied Science Bulletin. Quezon.

Nature, Lond—Nature. London.

Naturwissenschaften—Die Naturwissenschaften. Berlin.

Nauchn Dokl Vyssh Shk Biol Nauki—Nauchnye Doklady Vysshei Shkoly Biologischeskie Nauki.

Nauchn Tr Aspir Ordinatorov Pervogo Mosk Med Inst— Nauchnye Trudy Aspirantov i Ordinatorov Pervogo Moskovskogo Meditsinskogo Instituta.

Nauchn Tr Permsk Farm Inst—Nauchnye Trudy Permskogo Farmatsevticheskogo Instituta.

Nauchn Tr Tashk Gos Univ— Nauchnye Trudy, Tashkentskii Gosudarstvennyi Universitet.

Nauchni Tr Vissh Inst Khranit Vkusova Prom St Plovdiv—Nauchni Trudove, Vissh Institut po Khranitelna i Vkusova Promishlenost, Plovdiv. Bulgaria.

Nauchni Tr Vissh Med Inst, Sofia—Nauchni Trudove na Visshiya Medjtsinski Institut. Sofia.

Neoplasma—Neoplasma. Bratislava.

New Bot—New Botanist. New Delhi.

New Sci—New Scientist. London.

NIDA Res Monogr—NIDA Research Monograph. Rockville.

Nihon Daigaku Yakugaku Kenkyu Hokoku—Nihon Daigaku Yakugaku Kenkyu. Tokyo.

Nippon Kagaku Zasshi—Nippon Kagaku Zasshi. Tokyo.

Nippon Kingakkai Kaiho—Nippon Kingakkai Kaiho. Japan.

Nippon Mokuzai Gakkaishi—Nioppon Mokuzai Gakkaishi. Tokyo.

Nippon Nogei Kagaku Kaishi—Nippon Nogei Kagaku Kaishi. Tokyo.

Nippon Shokuhin Kogyo Gakkaishi—Nippon Shokuhin Kogyo Gakkaishi. Ibaraaki-ken, Japan.

Nippon Suisan Gakkaishi—Nippon Suisan Gakkaishi. Tokyo.

Nor Apotekerforen Tidsskr—Norges Apotekerforenings Tidsskrift. Oslo, Norway.

Nord Veterinaermed—Nordisk Veterinaermedicin. Copenhagen.

Nouv J Chim—Nouveau Journal de Chimie. Paris.

Nutr Abstr Rev—Nutrition Abstracts and Reviews. Aberdeen, Scotland.

Nutr Dieta—Nutritio et Dieta. Basel.

Nutr Metab—Nutrition and Metabolism. Basel.

Nutr Rep Int—Nutrition Reports International. Los Altos, California.

Oftal'mol Zh—Oftal'mologicheskii Zhurnal. Kiev.

Oils Oilseeds J—Oils and Oilseeds Journal. Bombay.

Oleagineux—Oleagineux. Paris.

Oncology—Oncology. Basel.

Onkologiya Kiev—Onkologiya. Kiev.

Org Geochem—Organic Geochemistry. Elmsford.

Orissa Vet J—Orissa Veterinary Journal. Bhubaneswar.

Orv Szemle—Orvosi Szemle. Hungary.

Osaka Kogyo Daigaku Kiyo, Rikohen—Osaka Kogyo Daigaku Kiyo Rikohen. Osaka.

Otolaryngol Pol—Otolaryngologia Polska. Warsaw.

Oyo Yakuri—Oyo Yakuri Kenkyukai. Sendai.

Pafai J—Pafai Journal. Bombay.

Pahlavi Med J—Pahlavi Medical Journal. Shiraz.

Pak J Biochem—Pakistan Journal of Biochemistry. Lahore.

Pak J Biol Agric Sci—Pakistan Journal of Biological and Agricultural Sciences. Dhaka.

Pak J For—Pakistan Journal of Forestry. Peshawar.

Pak J Sci—Pakistan Journal of Science. Lahore.

Pak J Sci Ind Res—Pakistan Journal of Scientific and Industrial Research. Karachi.

Pak J Sci Res—Pakistan Journal of Scientific Research. Lahore.

Pan-Am Assoc Biochem Soc Symp—Pan American Association of Biochemical Societies Symposium. San Diego.

Parfuem Kosmet—Parfumerie und Kosmetik. Heidelberg.

Parfum Cosmet Aromes—Parfums, Cosmetiques, Aromes. Paris.

Parfums Cosmet Savons Fr—Parfums, Cosmetiques, Savons de France. Paris.

Patol Fiziol Eksp Ter—Patologicheskaya Fiziologiya i Eksperimentalnaya Terapiya. Moscow.

Pazhoohandeh Tehran—Pazhoohandeh. Tehran.

Pei I Hsueh Pao—Pei I Hsueh Pao.

Pei-Ching I Hsueh Yuan Hsueh Pao—Pei-Ching I Hsueh Yuan Hsueh Pao.

Perfum Essent Oil Rec—Perfumery and Essential Oil Record. London.

Perfum Flav—Perfumer and Flavourist. Oak Park, Illinois.

Perfum Flav Int—Perfumer and Flavourist International. Illinois.

Period Polytech Chem Eng—Periodica Polytechnica, Chemical Engineering. Budapest.

Pestic Sci—Pesticide Science. Oxford, England.

Pesticides—Pesticides. Bombay.

Pestology—Pestology. Bombay.

Pharm Acta Helv—Pharmaceutica Acta Helvetiae. Berne.

Pharm J—Pharmacutical Journal. London.

Pharm Tijdschr Belg—Pharmaceutisch Tijdschrift Voor Belgie. Belgium.

Pharm Weekbl—Pharmaceutisch Weekblad. Amsterdam.

Pharm Zentralhalle—Pharmazeutische Zentralhalle. Dresden.

Pharm Zentralhalle Dtschl—Pharmazeutische Zentralhalle fuer Deutschland. Dresden.

Pharm Ztg—Pharmazeutische Zeitung. Frankfurt.

Pharmaceutist—Pharmaceutist. Bombay.

Pharmacol Res Commun—Pharmacological Research Communication. London.

Pharmacol Rev—Pharmacological Reviews. Baltimore.

Pharmacology—Pharmacology. Basel.

Pharmatimes—Pharmatimes. Bombay.

Pharmazie—Die Pharmazie. Berlin.

Philipp Abstr—Philippine Abstract. Manila.

Philipp Agric—Philippine Agriculturist. Los Banos.

Philipp J Sci—Philippine Journal of Science. Manila.

Physiol Bohemosla—Physiologia Bohemoslovaca. Prague.

Physiol Veg—Physiologie Vegetale. Paris.

Phytochemistry—Phytochemistry. Oxford.

Phyton Buenos Aires—Phyton. Vicente Lopez, Argentina.

Phytoparasitica—Phytoparasitica. Det Dagan.

Phytopathol Z—Phytopathologische Zeitschrift. Berlin.

Phytopathology—Phytopathology. St. Paul.

Plant Biochem J—Plant Biochemical Journal. New Delhi.

Plant Cell Physiol—Plant and Cell Physiology. Kyoto.

Plant Med Phytother—Plantes Medicinales et Phytotherapie. Angers, France.

Plant Foods Hum Nutr—Plant Foods for Human Nutrition. Netherlands.

Plant Physiol—Plant Physiology. Bethesda.

Plant Syst Evol—Plant Systematics and Evolution. Vienna.

Planta—Planta. Berlin.

Planta Med—Planta Medica. Stuttgart.

Pol J Chem—Polish Journal of Chemistry. Warsaw.

Pol J Pharmacol Pharm—Polish Journal of Pharmacology and Pharmacy. Warsaw.

Politecnica—Politecnica.

Postepy Biochem—Postepy Biochemii. Warsaw.

Postepy Hig Med Dosw—Postepy Higieny i Medycyny Doswiadczalnej. Wroclaw.

Poult Sci—Poultry Science. Champaign, Illinois.

Poznan Tow Przyj Nauk Wyd Lek Pr Kom Farm—Poznanskie Towanzystwo Przyjaciol Nauk Wydzial Lekarski Prace Komisji Farmaceutycznej. Warsaw.

Pr Inst Przem Org—Prace Instytutu Przemyslu Organicznego.

Prakt Lek—. Prakticky Lekar. Prague.

Prikl Biokhim Mikrobiol—Prikladnaya Biokhimiya i Mikrobiologiya. Moscow.

Probe—Probe. Bombay.

Probl Farm—Problemi na Farmaciyata. Bulgaria.

Probl Gematol Pereliv Krovi—Problemy Gematologii i Perelivaniya Krovi. Moscow.

Proc Am Soc Hort Sci—Proceedings of the American Society for Horticultural Science. Alexandra.

Proc Asian-Pacific congr Cardiol 3rd Kyoto—Proceedings of Asian-Pacific Congress on Cardiology, 1964. New York.

Proc Chem Soc London—Proceedings of the Chemical Society. London.

Proc Fla State Hortic Soc—Proceedings of the Florida State Horticultural Society. Lake Alfred.

Proc Hung Annu Meed Biochem—Proceedings of the Hungarian Annual Meeting for Biochemistry. Budapest.

Proc Indian Acad Sci—Proceedings of the Indian Academy of Sciences. Bangalore.

Proc Indian Sci Congr—Proceedings of Indian Science Congress. Calcutta.

Proc Int Pharmacol Meet—Proceedings of the International Pharmacological Meeting. Oxford, England.

Proc K Ned Akad Wet—Proceedings, Koninklijkc Nederlandse Academie van Wetenschappen. Series A; B or C. Amsterdam.

Proc Nat Acad Sci India—Proceedings of National Academy of Sciences, India. Allahabad.

Proc Nat Inst Sci India Part A & B—Proceedings of the National Institute of Sciences of India. New Delhi.

Proc Nat Sci Counc Taiwan—Proceedings of National Science Council of Taiwan.

Proc Nat Sci Counc Repub China—Proceedings of National Science Council, Republic of China. Taipei.

Proc Okla Acad Sci—Procedings of the Oklahoma Academy of Science. Oklahoma.

Proc Pak Sci Conf—Proceedings of Pakistan Science Conference. Lahore.

Proc Sci Program Joint Meet American Soc Pharmacog Soc Econ Bot—Proceedings of the Scientific Program for the Joint Meeting of the American Society for Pharmacognosy and the Society for Economic Botany. Boston. 1981.

Proc Soc Exp Biol Med—Proceedings of the Society of Experimental Biology and Medicine. New York.

Proc W Va Acad Sci—Proceedings of the West Virginia Academy of Science. Morgantown.

Prog Biochem Pharmacol—Progress in Biochemical Pharmacology. Basel.

Prog Flavour Res (Proc Weurman Flavour Res Symp)—Progress in Flavour Research. Proceedings of Weurman Flavour Research Symposium. 1978.

Prog Org Chem—Progress in Organic Chemistry. London.

Prostaglandins Med—Prostaglandins and Medicine. Los Altos, California.

Przem Ferment Rolny—Przemysl Fermentacyjny i Rolny. Warsaw.

Prezem Spozyw—Przemysl Spozywczy. Warsaw.

Psychopharmacologia— Psychopharmacologia. Berlin.

Psychopharmacology— Psychopharmacology. New York.

Psychosomatics—Psychosomatics. Washington, DC.

Pure Appl Chem—Pure and Applied Chemistry. Oxford, England.

Pyrethrum Post—Pyrethrum Post. Nakuru, Kenya.

Q J Crude Drug Res—Quarterly Journal of Crude Drug Research. Amsterdam.

Q J Surg Sci—Quarterly Journal of Surgical Sciences. Varanasi.

Quad Merceol—Quaderni di Merceologia. Italy.

Qual Plant Mater Veg—Qualitas Plantarum et Materiae Vegetabiles. The Hague.

Qual Plant-Plant Foods Hum Nutr-—Qualitas Plantarum-Plant Foods for Human Nutrition. The Hague.

Queensl J Agric Anim Sci—Queensland Journal of Agricultural and Animal Sciences. Brisbane.

Rajasthan Med J—Rajasthan Medical Journal. Jaipur

Rakuno Kagi u Shokuhin No Kenkyu— Rakuno K ُaku Shokuhin No Kenkyu. Sendai-Shi.

Ras Chim—Rassegna Chimica. Rome.

Rastenievud Nauki—Rastenievudni Nauki. Sofia.

Rastit Resur—Rastenievudni Nauki. Sofia.

Rastit Resur—Rastitel'nuie Resursui. Moscow.

Recent Adv Phytochem—Recent Advances in Phytochemistry. New Nork.

Recent Adv Stud Car Struct Metab—Recent Advances in Studies on Cardiac Structure and Metabolism. London.

Recent Dev Chem Nat Carbon Compd— Recent Development in the Chemistry of Natural Carbon Comppounds. Budapest.

Recherche—Recherche. Paris.

Recl Trav Chim Pays-Bas—Recueil des Travaux Chimiques des Pays-Bas. Amsterdam.

Rend Acad Sci Fis Mat Naples—Rendiconti dell' Accademia delle Scienze Fisiche e Matematiche. Naples, Italy.

Rep Res Lab Kirin Brew Co—Report of the Research Laboratories of Kirin Brewery Company. Gumma.

Reproduction—Reproduction. England.

Res Bull Panjab Univ Sci—Research Bulletin of the Punjab University, Science. Chandigarh.

Res Commun Chem Pathol Pharmacol—Research Communications in Chemical Pathology and Pharmacology. Westbury.

Res Ind—Research and Industry. New Delhi.

Res Vet Sci—Research in Veterinary Sciences. London.

Rev Agroquim Technol Aliment—Revista de Agroquimica y Technologia de Alimentos. Valencia.

Rev Asoc Bioquim Argent—Revista de la Asociacion Bioquimica Argentina. Buenos Aires.

Rev Biol Trop Univ Costa Rica—Revista de Biologia Tropicale Universidad Nacional de Costa Rica. San Jose.

Rev Bras Farm—Revista Brasileira de Farmacia. Rio de Janeiro, Brazil.

Rev Bras Frutic—via *CA.*

Rev Cent Cienc Biomed—Revista do Centro de Ciencias Biomedicas, Universidade Federal de Santa Maria.

Rev Chim Bucharest—Revista de Chimie. Bucharest.

Rev Colomb Quim—Revista Colombiana de Quimica.

Rev Col Quim Ing Quim Costa Rica—via *CA.*

Rev Cubana Farm—Revista Cubana de Farmacia. Havana.

Rev Esp Fisiol—Revista Espanola de Fisiologia. Pamplona, Spain.

Rev Fac Agron, Univ Nac La Plata—Revista de la Facultad de Agronomia, Universidad Nacional de La Plata. Buenos Aires.

Rev Fac Farm Bioquim Univ Sao Paulo—Revista da Faculdade de Farmacia e Bioquimicada Universidade de Sao Paulo. Sao Paulo.

Rev Fac Farm, Univ Los Andes—Revista de la Facultad de Farmacia, Universidad de Los Andes.

Rev Farm Buenos Aires—Revista Farmaceutica. Buenos Aires.

Rev Fiz Chim Ser A or *B*—Revista de Fizica si Chimie. Seria. Bucharest.

Rev Fr Corps Gras—Revue Francaise des Corps Gras. Paris.

Rev IBPT Curitiba—Revista IBPT, Curitiba.

Rev Immunol—Revue d'Immunologie. Paris.

Rev Latinoam Quim—Revista Latinoamericana de Quimica. Nuero Leon, Mexico.

Rev Med Tirgu-Mures—Revista Medicala. Tirgu-Mures, Romania.

Rev Med Hanoi—Revue Medicale. Hanoi.

Rev Med Univ Fed Ceara—Revista de Medicina da Universidade Federal do Ceara. Ceara.

Rev Microbiol—Revista de Microbiologia. Sao Paulo, Brazil.

Rev Peru Bioquim—Revista Peruana de Bioquim.

Rev Port Farm—Revista Portuguesa de Farmacia. Lisbon.

Rev R Acad Farm Barcelona—Revista de la Real Academia de Farmacia de Barcelona.

Rev Soc Quim Mex—Revista de la Sociedad Quimica de Mexico.

Rev Univ Ind Santander—Revista de la Universidad Industrial de Santander. Bucaramanga.

Rev Zooteh Med Vet—Revista de Zootehnie si Medicina Veterinara. Bucharest.

Rheumatism—Rheumatism. New Delhi.

Riechst Aromen—Riechstoffe und Aromen. Hannover.

Riechst Aromen Kosmet—Riechstoffe, Aromen, Kosmetica. SE Peter-Ording.

Riv Ital EPPOS—Rivista Italiana Essenze Profumi Piante Officinali Saponi. Milan.

Riv Ital Essenze Profumi Piante Off—Rivista Italiana Delle Essenze Die Profumi e delle Piante Officinali. Milan.

Riv Ital Essenze Profumi Piante Off Saponi Cosmet Aerosol— Rivista Italiana Essenze Profumi Piante Officinali Arom Saponi Cosmetici Aerosol. Milan.

Riv Ital Essenze Profumi Piante Off Arom Saponi Cosmet Aerosol—Rivista Italiana Essenze Profumi Piante Officinali Aromi Saponi Cosmetici Aerosol. Milan.

Riv Ital Sostanze Grasse—Rivista Italiana delle Sostanze Grasse. Milan.

Rocz Akad Roln Poznaniu—Roczniki Akademii Rolniczej w Poznaniu.

Rocz Chem—Roczniki Chemii. Poland.

Rocz Inst Przem Mlecz—Roczniki Instytutu Przemyslu Mleczarskiego. Warsaw.

Rocz Nauk Roln Ser A,B,....H—Roczniki Nauk Rolniczych, Seria. Warsaw.

Rocz Panstw Zakl Hig—Roczniki Panstwowego Zakladu Higieny. Warsaw.

Rocz Technol Chem Zywn—Roczniki Technologii i Chemii Zywnosci. Warsaw.

Rozpr Wydz 3:Nauk Mat Mat Przyr Gdansk Tow Nauk—Rozprawy Wydzialu 3:Nauk Matematyczno-Przyrodniczych, Gdanskie Towarzysstwo Naukowe.

Ryukyu Daigaku Nogakubu Gakujustu Hokoku—Ryukyu Daigaku Nogakubu Gakujustu Hokoku. Okinawa.

S Afr Med J—South African Medical Journal. Captown.

Sachitra Ayurveda—Sachitra Ayurveda. Calcutta.

Sankyo Kenkyusho Nempo—Sankyo Kenkyusho Nempo. Tokyo.

Sb Nauch Rab Vses Nauch Issled Inst Lek Rast—Sbornik Nauchnykh Rabot, Vsesoyuznyi Nauchno-Issledovatel'skii Institut Lekarstvennykh Rastenii.

Sb Nauchn Tr Ryazan Med Inst—Sbornik Nauchnykh Trudov, Ryzanskii Meditsinskii Institut.

Scand J Gastroenterol—Scandinavian Journal of Gastroenterology. Oslo.

Schweiz Apoth Ztg—Schweizerische Apotheker-Zeitung. Berne.

Schweiz Brau Rundsch—Schweizer Brauerei-Rundschau. Zurich.

Schweiz Med Wochanschr—Schweizerische Medizinische Wochenschrift. Basel.

Sci Hortic—Scientific Horticulture. Kent.

Science—Science. Washington, DC.

Sci Cult—Science and Culture. Calcutta.

Sci Ind Karachi—Science and Industry. Karachi.

Sci Pharm—Scientia Pharmaceutica. Vienna.

Sci Res Dacca—Scientific Researches Dacca. Dhaka.

Sci Sin—Scientia Sinica. Beijing.

Sci Tecnol Alimenti—Scienza e Tecnologia degli Alimenti.

Seifen Oele Fette Wachse—Seifen, Oele, Fette, Wachse. Augsburg.

Sem Rep—Seminar Reporteur. Delhi.

Settim Med—Settimana Medica. Rome.

Shizuoka Daigaku Kogakubu Kenkyu Hokoku—Shizuoka Daigaku Kogakubu Kenkyu Hokoku. Shizuoka-shi.

Shokubutsu Boeki—Shokubutsu Boeki. Tokyo.

Shokubutsugaku Zasshi—Shokubutsugaku Zasshi. Tokyo.

Shokuhin Eiseigaku Zasshi—Shokuhin Eiseigaku Zasshi. Tokyo.

Shoyakugaku Zasshi—Shoyakugaku Zasshi. Tokyo.

Soap Perfum Cosmet—Soap, Perfumery & Cosmetics. London.

Soobshch Acad Nauk Gruz SSR—Soobshcheniya Akademii Nauk Gruzinskoi SSR.

Soul Uidae Chapchi—Soul Uidae Chapchi. Seoul.

South Pac Bull—South Pacific Bulletin. New South Wales.

Southwest Vet—Southwestern Veterinarian. Texas.

Sri Lanka For—Sri Lanka Forester. Colombo.

Ssu Ch'uan I Hsueh Yuan Hsueh Pao—Ssu Ch'uan I Hsueh Yuan Hsueh Pao.

Staerke—Staerke. Weinheim.

Steroids—Steroids. San Francisco.

Steroids Lipids Res—Steroids and Lipids Research. Basel.

Stud Cercet Biochim—Studii si Cercetari de Biochimie. Bucharest.

Stud Cercet Med Interna—Studii si Cercetari de Medicina Interna. Bucharest.

Subtrop Kul't—Subtropicheskie Kul'tury.

Sudan J Food Sci Technol—Sudan Journal of Food Science and Technology. Khartoum.

Surg Forum—Surgical Forum. Chicago.

Sven Farm Tidskr—Svensk Farmaceutisk Tidskrift. Stockholm.

Symp Pap IUPAC Int Symp Chem Natl Prod—Symposia Papers of IUPAC International Symposium on Chemistry of Natural Products. 1978.

Symp Phytochem Proc Meeting Univ Hongkong—Symposia on Phytochemistry, Proceedings of Meeting, University of Hongkong, 1961.

Taehan Yakrihak Chapchi—Taehan Yakrihak Chapchi. Seoul.

Taisha—Taisha. Japan.

T'ai-wan I Hsueh Hui Tsa Chih—Taiwan I Hsueh Hui Tsa Chih. Taipei.

T'ai-wan K'o Hsueh—Taiwan K'o Hsueh.

T'ai-wan Yao Hsueh Tsa Chih—Taiwan Yao Hsueh Tsa Chih.

Taiwania—Taiwania. Taipei, Taiwan.

Takeda Kenkyusho Ho—Takeda Kenkyusho Ho. Osaka-Shi.

Tampakushitsu Kakusan Koso—Tampakushitsu Kokusan Koso. Japan.

Tap Chi Hoa Hoc—Tap Chi Hoa Hoc.

Tartu Riikliku Ulik Toim—Tartu Rikkliku Ulikooli Toimetised. Tartu.

Tea Q—Tea Quarterly. Talawakele, Sri Lanka.

Tec Molitoria—Tecnica Molitoria. Pinerolo, Italy.

Technology Sindri—Technology. Sindri.

Tech Memo Niger Fed Inst Ind Res—Technical Memoiers of Nigerian Federal Institute of Industrial Research.

Tech Q Master Brew Assoc Am—Technical Quarterly, Master Brewers Association of America.

Tehnika—Tehnika. Beograd.

Tetrehedron—Tetrahedron. Oxford, England.

Tetrahedron Lett—Tetrahedron Letters. Oxford, England.

Ther Hung—Therapia Hungarica. Budapest.

Ther Potential Marihuana Proc Conf—Therapeutic Potential of Marihuana, Proceedings of Conference. 1975.

Therapie—Therapie. Paris.

Thromb Diath Haemorrh—Thrombosis et Diathesis Haemorrhagica. Stuttgart.

Tluszeze Srodki Piorace, Kosmet—Tluszeze, Srodki Piorace, Kosmetyki. Poland.

Tob Res—Tobacco Research. Rajahmundry.

Toho Igakkai Zasshi—Toho Igakkai Zasshi. Tokyo.

Top Enzyme Ferment Biotechnol—Topics in Enzyme and Fermentation Biotechnology. West Sussex, England.

Tottori Nogakkaiho—Tottori Nogakkaiho. Tokyo.

Toxicol Annu—Toxicology Annuals. New York.

Toxicol Appl Pharmacol—Toxicology and Applied Pharmacology. Sa Diego.

Toxicol Eur Res—Toxicological European Research. Paris.

Toxicology—Toxicology. Limerick, Ireland.

Toxicon—Toxicon. Elmsford.

Tr Alma-At Zoovetekh Vet Inst—Trudy Alma-Atinskogo Zooveterinarnogo Instituta.

Tr Bot Inst Akad Nauk SSSR Ser 5—Trudy Botanicheskogo Instituta, Akademiya Nauk SSSR, Seriya 5.

Tr Khim Prir Soedin—via CA.

Tr Leningr Khim Farm Inst—Trudy Leningradskogo Khimiko Farmatsev-ticheskogo Instituta.

Tr Nauchnoizsled Inst Farm—Trudove na Nauchnoizsledovatelskiya Khimiko - Farmatsevtichen Institut.

Tr Permsk Farm Inst—Trudy Permskogo Farmatsevticheskogo Instituta.

Tr Permsk Gos Med Inst—Trudy Permskogo Gosudarstvennogo Meditsinskogo Instituta.

Tr Prikl Bot Genet Sel—Trudy po Prikladnoi Botanike, Genetike i Salektsii. Leningrad.

Tr Vses Nauchno-Issled Inst Lek Rast—Trudy Vsesoyuznogo Nauchno-Issledovatel'skogo Instituta Lekarstvennykh Rastenii.

Trans Bose Res Inst, Calcutta—Transactions of the Bose Research Institute. Calcutta.

Trans Ill State Acad Sci—Transactions of the Illinois State Academy of Science. Illinois.

Trav Soc Pharm Montpellier—Travaux de la Societe de Pharmacie de Montpellier.

Trends Biochem Sci—Trends in Biochemical Sciences. Amsterdam.

Trop Sci—Tropical Science. Oxford, England.

Turk Hij Tecr Biyol Derg—Turk Hijiyen ve Tecrubi Biyoloji Dergisi. Ankara.

Tydskr Natuurwet—Tydskrif vir Natuur-wetenskappe. Pretoria.

Tzu Jan Tsa Chih—Tzu Jan Tsa Chih.

Uch Zap Yakutsk Gos Univ—Uchenye Zapis-ki Yakutskogo Gosudarstvennogo Universiteta.

Ukr Biokhem Zh—Ukrains'kii Biokhemichnii Zhurnal. Kiev.

Union Burma J Sci Tech—Union of Burma Journal of Science and Technology. Rangoon.

Univ Indore Res J Sci—University of Indore Research Journal, Science. Indore.

Univ Wyoming Agric Exp Sta (Laramie) Sci Monograph— University of Wyoming, Agricultural Experiment Station, Science Monograph. Laramie.

Urol Nefrol—Urologiya i Nefrologiya. Moscow.

Uzb Biol Zh—Uzbekskii Biologicheskii Zhurnal. Tashkent.

Var Foeda—Var Foeda. Uppsala, Sweden.

Varasarn Paesachasarthara—Varasarn Paesachasarthara. Thailand.

Vestn Mosk Univ—Vestnik Moskovskogo Universiteta. Moscow.

Vet Ital—Veterinaria Italiana. Teramo.

Vet Rec—Veterinary Record. London.

Viata Med Rev Inf Prof Stiint Med—Viata Medicala. Revista de Informare Profesionala si Stiintifica a Medicilor. Bucharest.

Vijnana Parishad Anusandhan Patrika—Vijnana Parishad Anusandhan Patrika. Allahabad.

Vishva Bharti J Res Sci—Vishva Bharti Journal of Scientific Research. Calcutta.

Voeding—Voeding. The Hague.

Vopr Izuch Ispol'z Solodki SSSR, Akad Nauk SSSR—via CA.

Vopr Med Khim—Voprosy Meditsinskoi Khimii. Moscow.

Vopr Onkol—Voprosy Onkologii. Moscow.

Vopr Pitan—Voprosy Pitaniya. Moscow.

Vox Sang—Vox Sanguinis. Basel.

Vrach Delo—Vrachebnoe Delo. Kiev.

Weed Sci—Weed Science. Champaign, Ill.

West Afri Pharm—West African Pharmacist. London.

West Indian Med J—West Indian Medical Journal. Jamaica.

Xenobiotica—Xenobiotica. England.

Yakhak Hoeji—Yakhak Hoeji. Seoul.

Yakhak Hoe Chi—Yakhak Hoe Chi.

Yakugaku Zasshi—Yakugaku Zasshi. Tokyo.

Yamaguchi Joshi Daigaku Kenkyu Hokoku Dai-2-bu—Yamaguchi Joshi Daigaku Kenkyu Hokoku Dai-2-bu. Yamaguchi.

Yao Hsueh Hsueh Pao—Yao Hsueh Hsueh Pao. Beijing.

Yao Hsueh T'ung Pao—Yao Hsueh Tung Pao. Beijing.

Yukagaku—Yukagaku. Tokyo.

Yunnan Chih Wu Yen Chiu—Yunnan Chih Wu Yen Chiu.

Z Allg Mikribiol—Zietschrift fuer Allgemeine Mikrobiologie. Berlin.

Z Anal Chem—Zeitschrift fuer Analytische Chemie. New York.

Z Chem—Zeitschrift fuer Chemie. New York.

Z Ernaehrungswiss—Zeitschrift fuer Ernaehrungswissenschaft. Darmstadt.

Z Gastroenterol—Zeitschrift fuer Gastroenterologie. Graefelfing.

Z Lebensm Unters Forsch—Zeitschrift fuer Lebensmittel- Untersuchung und-Forschung. Berlin.

Z Naturforsch Teil A, B, C—Zeitschrift fur Nautrforschung. Wiesbaden, Tubingen.

Z Pflanzenkr Pflanzenschutz—Zeitschrift fuer Pflanzenkrankheiten und Pflanzenschutz. Stutlgart.

Z Pflanzenphysiol—Zeitschrift fuer Pflanzenphysiologie. Stuttgart.

Z Pflanzenenzuecht— Zeitschrift fuer Pflanzenzuechtung. Berlin.

Z Physiol Chem—Zeitschrift fuer Physiologische Chemie.Berlin.

Z Urol Nephrol—Zeitschrift fuer Urologie und Nephrologie. Leipzig.

Zashch Rast Vred Bolez—Zashchita Rastenii ot Vreditelei i Boleznei. Moscow.

Zasso Kenkyu—Zasso Kenkyu.

Zdravookhr Beloruss—Zdravookhranenie Belorussii. Minsk.

Zemled Zhivotnovod Mold—Zemledelie i Zhivotnovodstvo Moldavii.

Zentralbl Veterinaermed Reihe—Zentralblatt fuer Veterinaermedizin, Reihe. Berlin.

Zesz Nauk Acad Ekon Poznaniu, Ser 1—Z-Eszyty Naukowe- Akademia Economiczna w Poznaniu. Poland.

Zh Nevropatol Psikhiatr im S.S. Korsakova—Zhurnal Nevropatologii Psikhiatrii imeni S.S. Korsakova. Moscow.

Zh Obshch Khim—Zhurnal Obshchei Khimii. Moscow.

Zh Prikl Khim—Zhurnal Prikladnoi Khimii. Moscow.

Zhivotnovud Nauki—Zhivotnovudni Nauki. Sofia.

Zucker—Zucker. Berlin.

ABBREVIATIONS USED

Abortif.	abortifacient	Chemotaxon.	chemotaxonomy
Addn.	addition	Cholag.	cholagogue
Alc.	alcohol	Chromatogr.	chromatographic
Alk(s).	alkaloid(s)	Chr.	chronic
Alter.	alterative	Clin.	clinical
Amenor.	amenorrhoea	CN	cyanogenic
Amt(s).	amount(s)	CNS	Central nervous system
Analg.	analgesic	Colorim.	colorimetric
Anal.	analysis	Compn.	composition
Anthelm.	anthelmintic	Compd(s).	compound(s)
Antibact.	antibacterial	Constip.	constipation
Antibil.	antibilious	Contracep.	contraceptive
Antibiot.	antibiotic	Convuls.	convulsant/convulsions
Antid.	antidote		
Antidiar.	antidiarrial	Decoct.	decoction
Antidysen.	antidysenteric	Demulc.	demulcent
Antifert.	antifertility	Depress.	depressant
Antifung.	antifungal	Deriv(s).	derivative(s)
Antiinflam.	antiflammatory	Detn.	determination
Antimicrob.	antimicrobiol	Diaphor.	diaphoretic
Antiper.	antiperiodic	Diar.	diarrhoea
Antiphl.	antiphlogistic	Dil(s).	dilution(s)
Antiphlegm.	antiphlegmatic	Diur.	diuretic
Antiprot.	antiprotozoal	Dysen.	dysentery
Antipyr.	antipyretic	DOPA/Dopa	dihydroxyphenylalanine
Antiscor.	antiscorbutic	Dysmenor.	dysmenorrhoea
Antisep.	antiseptic	Dyspep.	dyspepsia
Antisp.	antispasmodic		
Antivir.	antiviral	Emmen.	emmenagogue
A.P.	Andhra Pradesh	Emol.	emollient
Aper.	aperient	Eng.	English
Aphrodis.	aphrodisiac	Esp.	especially
Aq.	aqueous	Essent.	essential
Arom.	aromatic	Estn.	estimation
Ass.	Assamese	Exp.	experiment/al
Astrin.	astringent	Expect.	expectorant
		Ext.	extract
B.	Bengali	Extn.	extraction
Biol.	biological		
B.P.	blood pressure	Febge.	febrifuge
Bronch.	bronchial	Flavon(s).	flavanoid(s)
Broncht.	bronchitis	Flourim.	flourimetric
Biosynth.	biosynthesis		
		G.	Gujarati
Carmin.	carminative	GABA	gamma aminobustyric acid
Catar.	catarrhal	Galact.	galactagogue
Cath.	cathartic	GLC	gas-liquid chromatography
Chem.	chemical	Glucd(s).	glucoside(s)

Glycd(s).	glycoside(s)	Powd.	powder/powdered
Gonor.	gonorrhoea	PPM	per part million
		Purg.	purgative
H.	Hindi		
Haemat.	haematuria	Quant.	quantity/quantitative
Haemor.	haemorrhage		
H.P.	Himachal Pradesh	Refs.	references
Hr(s)	hours(s)	Refrig.	refrigerant
Hypoglyc.	hypoglycaemic	Resolv.	resolvant
Hyperten.	hypertensive	Resp.	respectively
Hypoten.	hypotensive	Restor.	restorative
Identn.	identification	Rev.	review
im/i.m.	intramuscular	Rheum.	rheumatic/rheumatism
Indign.	indigestion	Rubft.	rubefacient
Inflam.	inflammation/inflammatory	Sans.	Sanskrit
Insectic.	insecticidal/insecticide	sc/s.c.	subcutaneous
ip/i.p.	intra perritoneal	Sed.	sedative
Irrit.	irritant/irritation	Sepn.	separation
IU	international units	Sik.	Sikkim/Sikkimese
iv/i.v.	intravenous	Sp./Spp.	(one)/(several) species
J. & K.	Jammu & Kashmir	Spasmol.	spasmolytic
		Spasmog.	spasmogenic
Kan.	Kannada	Spectrophotom.	spectrophotometric
Kash.	Kashmir/Kashmiri	Spermator.	spermatorrhoea
		Spermic.	spermicidal
Lactag.	lactagogue	Stim.	stimulant
Laxt.	laxative	Stomch.	stomachic
Leucor.	leucorrhoea	Str(s).	structure(s)
Liq.	liquid	Tam.	Tamil
		T.B.	tuberculosis
Mal.	Malayalam	Tel.	Telugu
Mar.	Marathi	Temp.	temperature
Mech.	mechanism	T.N.	Tamil Nadu
Menor.	menorrhagia	Terp(s).	terpenoid(s)/terpene(s)
mg	malligram		
Mixt.	mixture	Unsap.	unsaponifiable
ml	millilitre	U.P.	Uttar Pradesh
M.P.	Madhya Pradesh	UV	ultraviolet
NMR	nuclear magnetic resonance	V.D.	veneral diseases
No.	number	Vesic.	vesicant
		Vet.	veterinary
P.	Punjab/Punjabi	Vit.	vitamin
Pet.	petroleum	Volat.	volatile
Pharmacol.	pharmacological/ogy		
Phlegm.	phlegmative	W.B.	West Bengal
Photom.	photometric	w.-insol./sol.	water insoluble/soluble
Piscic.	piscicidal/piscicide	wt.	weight
Pleur.	pleurisy	w.r.t.	with respect to
Pneum.	pneumonia		

PART I (A – K)
(1965 - 1981)

ENGLISH AND VERNACULAR NAMES, MEDICINAL USES, CHEMICAL
COMPOSITION, ACTIVE PRINCIPLES AND DISTRIBUTION

(Asterisks denote plants which were not included in the Glossary & its Supplement)

ABELMOSCHUS (*Malvaceae*)

*A. crinitis Wall.

B.–*Bankapas, birkapas.*

Santals use plant against gravel and dysen. (*Econ Bot*, 1970, **24**, 255).

N-W Himalayas, Bihar, W. Bengal and hills of Andhra Pradesh at *c.* 1,000 m.

A. esculentus (Linn.) Moench syn. *Hibiscus esculentus* Linn.

Eng.– *Lady's finger, okra, gumbo.*

Fatty ext. from fresh watery ext. of seeds inhibits cancerous cell growth *in vitro (Indian J Med Res*, 1968, **56**, 445). Used to treat bites of venomous animals and to settle stomach (*Econ Bot*, 1970, **24**, 344). Fruit useful as aphrodis. and in chr. dysen. Tender pods eaten in spermator. [*Indian Fmrs Dig*, 1978, **11**(6 & 7), 73].

Seed ext. fungitoxic against *Helminthosporium oryzae (Nat Acad Sci Lett*, 1978, **1**, 287).

Petals yield 13 flavon. glycds. (*Am J Bot*, 1968, **55**, 431); gossypetin & hibiscetin glucds. (*Phytochemistry*, 1969, **8**, 177).

Oxalate content of lady's finger, commonly used in Kashmir, 455.3 mg fresh or 880.7 mg/100g dry wt (*Indian J Med Res*, 1967, **55**, 278). F content of uncooked (0.2 - 0.9 ppm); and fried (0.4- 0.6 ppm) from Lucknow (*ibid*, 1972, **60**, 1470; 1472); that from Calcutta, 0.4 ppm (*Indian J Nutr Diet*, 1971, **8**, 66). Oxalic acid content of a sample from Udaipur 26.2 mg/100g (dry wt) with Ca (578 mg) and Ca/P ratio of 1:1 (*Qual Plant Mater Veg*, 1972-73, **22**, 335).

I, 0.5 ppm and F, 4.0 ppm (dry edible matter) (*Indian J Nutr Diet*, 1971, **8**, 66). F, Ca, Mg and P of cooked vegetable (*Indian J Med Res*, 1972, **60**, 1470).

Volat. oils from Egyptian okra pods and seeds contain aliphatic alcohols, cyclohexanol, *p*-tolualdehyde (in fruits),α-terpenyl-OAc (in seeds) and citral; nonvolat. neutral part, β-sitosterol & its 3β-galactoside (in seeds). Leaves, more or less same constituents (*Indian J Chem*, 1974, **12**, 1019).

Compn. of okra-mucilage (*J Sci Food Agric*, 1977, **28**, 519). Okra-mucilage from fruits has been used as a plasma replacement or blood volume expander and i.v. circulation agent and is composed of partially acetylated acidic polysaccharide and protein, in a ratio of 8:1:10 (Wlth India, IA, 8; *Chem Pharm Bull*, 1980, **28**, 2933)

A. ficulneus Wight & Arn. syn. *Hibiscus ficulneus* Linn.

Eng.–*White wild musk mallow.*

Seeds used in asthma (*J Econ Tax Bot*, 1980, **1**, 139).

Green stem and roots, mucilage, str. (*Indian J Chem*, 1966, **4**, 545; 1969, 7, 780).

A. manihot(Linn.) Medic. syn. *Hibiscus manihot* Linn.

Ass.–*Usipag*; G.–*Kantali*; Mar.–*Jangli bhendi.*

Chinese, as also Miris in Assam, smash leaves and roots into a plaster and use it as a poultice for boils, sprains and sores.

1

In China, flowers used in chr. broncht. and toothache. Flowers contain flavons. (*Chih Wu Hsueh Pao*, 1981, **23**, 222; *CA*, **95**, 156426 r).

Crushed roots on extn. with water yield mucin; compn. of purified mucin (*Mokuzai Gakkoishi*, 1970, **16**, 173; *CA*, 1971, **79**, 94495t). Roots contain mucilage named "Abelmoschus- mucilage M" composed of 82% polysaccharide and 17% protein (*Chem Pharm Bull*, 1977, **25**, 3061). Flowers, cyanidin-3-glycd. & -3-sambubioside (*Phytochemistry*, 1976, **15**, 1395).

A. moschatus Medic. syn. *Hibiscus abelmoschus* Linn.

Eng.–*Ambrette plant, musk mallow.*

Seeds — as diur. and demulc. (Wlth India, IA, 12). A decoct. or infusion or tincture, useful in nervous debility, hysteria, and other nervous disorders (*Indian J Pharm*, 1974, **36**, 102). Powd. seeds dusted over woollen and other garments as insect-repellent (*Nagarjun*, 1979-80, **23**, 177).

Fatty fraction of fresh aq. ext. of seeds, antitumour *in vitro* (*Indian J Med Res*, 1968, **56**, 445).

Seed oil may be used as a substitute for cotton seed oil in pharmaceutical formulation (*J Sci Food Agric*, 1974, **25**, 401).

Juice of fresh plant used as febge. and expect., and poultice made of whole plant, reduced to pulp, applied to chest in broncht.

Mucilage made from root and leaves in V.D. (*Acta Phytother*, 1971, **18**, 134), in urinary discharges, painful micturition and as aphrodis. Flower infusion used as contracep.

Fruits and leaves may cause skin irritation (*Planta Med*, 1973, **23**, 381; 167; *Indian J Med Res*, 1978, **68**, 650). Root paste, in T.B. (*Bull Med Ethno Bot Res*, 1980, **1**, 8).

Seeds, macrocyclic musk compds. (*Perfum Essent Oil Rec*, 1966, **57**, 64). Phospholipids (*Planta Med*, 1969, **17**, 190). Standardization of an arom. concentrate from ambrette seeds using the method of Indian pat., 1962, 72408, for extn. of seeds, lower mol. wt fraction retained. This fraction gives the ext. its floral note and prevents deterioration on storage (*Riechst Aromen Koerperpflegem*, 1970, **20**, 303; *CA*, **73**, 80401b).

Flowers, flavons. (*Curr Sci*, 1964, **33**, 431). Leaves, β-sitosterol and other common compds. (*Khim Prir Soedin*, 1971, **7**, 215; *CA*, **75**, 31318n). Leaves, β-sitosterol & its glucd.; petals, β-sitosterol, myricetin & its glucd.; fruit husk, β-sitosterol (*Acta Phytother*, 1971, **18**, 134). Farnesol and lactone of ambrettolic acid from plant of Ecuador (*Politecnica*, 1973, **3**, 163; *CA*, 1976, **84**, 102302b).

ABIES (*Pinaceae*)

A. pindrow Royle syn. *A. pindrow* Spach.; *A. webbiana* Lindl. var. *pindrow* Brandis; *Pinus pindrow* Royle

Eng.–*West-Himalayan low-level fir, pindrow* or *silver fir*; H.–*Morinda, ragha*; Kash.–*Badar*; P.–*Paludar, rai.*

EtOH(50%) ext. of aerial parts, hypoglyc. and spasmol. (*Indian J Exp Biol*, 1971, **9**, 91).

Some aspects of chem. of the order Pinales; the genus *Abies* [*Indian Pulp Paper*, 1973, **27**(8), 5].

Leaves (needles) contain, an essent. oil with balsamic odour (yield, 0.25% from Jubbal, H.P.); oil constituents, α-pinene, *l*-limonene, Δ^3- carene, dipentene, *l*-cadinene, and *l*-bornyl-OAc (Wlth India, IA, 16). Essent. oil of Indian plants, rev.(*Perfum Essent Oil Rec*, 1967, **58**, 437).

Stems, okanin, butein & their glucds., tri-OH-flavanone, and a new chalcone glycd. (*Phytochemistry*, 1980, **19**, 2501).

Temperate Himalayas from Kashmir to Nepal at 2,100 - 3,600 m.

A. spectabilis (D. Don) Spach. syn. *A. webbiana* Lindl. Incl. *A. densa* Griff.

Eng.–*West-Himalayan high-level fir; East-Himalayan* or *Indian silver-fir.*

Powd. leaves used alongwith juice of *Adhatoda zeylanica* and honey, in haemoptysis, phthisis and in catarrh of bladder. Infusion of leaves given to infants suffering from fever and chest infections; also in hoarseness and during dentition. In West Bengal, given as tonic after parturition. They form an ingredient of a no. of Ayurvedic formulations; *Thalisyaadichoornam* for pulmonary T.B. and broncht.; *Yogaraajaguggulu* for rheum. and chr. nervous diseases; *Nowshadhara* and *Gorojanam* pills (Wlth India, IA, 17). In Ayurveda, plant mentioned as contracep. (*ISI Bull*, 1967, **19**, 393). One of the constituents of indigenous drug *Mezhugu* used against rheum. (*Rheumatism*, 1976-77, **12**, 38).

Tree yields a toxic resin which is mixed with oil of roses and applied in neuralgia (Wlth India, IA, 17).

Leaves [could be of var. *brevifolia* (Henry) Rehder syn. *A. webbiana* Lindl. var. *brevifolia*, Ed.] contain an alk. (0.16% dry wt) (*Pak J Sci Ind Res*, 1963, **6**, 53); and an essent. oil (*Q J Crude Drug Res*, 1971, **11**, 1742).

Throughout inner Himalayas from Kashmir to Assam; in Western Himalayas, above the level of *A. pindrow* up to 4,500m; in Eastern Himalayas, from 1,600 to 4,500m.

ABROMA (*Sterculiaceae*)

See **AMBROMA**

ABRUS (*Fabaceae*)

*A. fruticulosus Wall. ex Wight & Arn. syn. *A. pulchellus* Wall.

Used for same med. purposes as *A. precatorius* (Wlth India, IA, 20).

Found throughout India.

A. precatorius Linn.

Eng.–*Crab's eye, Indian liquorice, jequirity.*

Seeds—Paste applied locally in sciatica, stiffness of shoulder joint and paralysis; said to be useful in diar. and dysen. (Wlth India, IA, 19); paste used against skin diseases (*Bull Bot Surv India*, 1973, **15**, 15). Ext., fungistatic against *Cryptococcus neoformans* [*Hind Antibiot Bull*, 1963, **6**(2), 39]. Used as abortif. [*J Res Indian Med*, 1978, **13**(2), 104]. Half-boiled seeds taken as tonic. Crushed roots to cure white eyes of cattle (*J Econ Tax Bot*, 1980, **1**, 140).

Seed exts. anticancer against Ehrlich ascites tumour cells (*Philipp J Sci*, 1967, **96**,393). Aq. ext., antibact. [*Indian J Pharm*, 1973, **35**, 203; *J Res Indian Med*, 1974, **9**(2), 65]; Seeds, poor anthelm; ext., CNS depress., analg., anti-muscarinic, antisp. and uterine stim. [*ibid*, 1975, **10**(3), 138; 1976, **11**(3), 94]; ext., showed antifert. activity in female albino rats; pharmacol. of seeds (*Indian J Exp Biol*, 1976, **14**, 623; 1971, **9**, 369).

Leaves—sweetish taste. Used as a substitute for liquorice. Considered useful in biliousness and in leucoderma, itching and other skin diseases (Wlth India, IA, 19). Decoct. widely used for cough, cold and colic. Juice employed as a cure for hoarseness; mixed with oil, applied to painful swellings. Dried leaves, refrig. (*Econ Bot*, 1978, **32**, 281). Paste as a germicide to wounds in cattle (*J Econ Tax Bot*, 1981, **2**, 177).

Roots—diur. Used in preparations prescribed for gonor., jaundice and haemoglobinuric bile. Also substitute for liquorice (Wlth India, IA, 18), but not suitable (*Indian J Pharm*, 1973, **35**, 102). Exts. showed antifert. activity in rats (*Pharmacol Res Commun*, 1970, **2**, 159; *CA*, 1971, **74**, 746a). Roots, emmen. (*Q J Crude Drug Res*, 1972, **12**, 1922); in Sudan, as purg., in eye infections and as antifert. agent (*Fitoterapia*, 1981, **52**, 243).

Various plant parts used in night blindness, inflam. of gums, muscular pain, convuls., pain in loins, mucus in urine, gravel, diar. and bone fracture in cattle (*Econ Bot*, 1970, **24**, 241; *Sri Lanka For*, 1980, **14**, 145).

Seed contains abrine, hypaphorine and an unknown alk.; seed coat devoid of these compds., gallic acid (*Taiwan I Hsueh Hui Tsa Chih*, 1960, **59**, 868; *CA*, 1964, **61**, 9777c). Antimicrob. activity of seeds (scarlet). EtOH ext. inhibits growth of *Staphylococcus aureus*, enteric and dysenteric group of micro-organisms and some pathogenic fungi. Pigments (anthocyanins) active only on *Staphylococcus aureus*, while other fraction showed wider spectrum of inhibition; gallic acid and two other phenolic compds. present in the ether fraction; also chem. and pharmacol. (*Indian J Pharm*, 1966, **28**, 164; 340). Roots, leaves, stem and seeds, alks., hypaphorine and trigonelline; seeds, hypaphorine, Me ester of N, N-di-Me-tryptophan metho cation, precatorine; compds. from leaves, stems and roots also identified (*Phytochemistry*, 1971, **10**, 195). Seed alks., trigonelline, choline, hypaphorine and abrine [*Herba Hung*, 1980, **19**(3), 21]. Seeds, new flavons., abrectorin and aknone (*Phytochemistry*, 1980, **19**, 2040). Chem. investigation of red and white seeds, with other coloured seeds mentioned [*J Res Indian Med*, 1978, **13**(4), 34].

Seeds, keto steroid P-sterone (*Pak J Biol Agric Sci*, 1965, **8**, 218; *CA*, 1966, **64**, 13052g). Two steroids; one, oily and other crystalline, former tested for its antifert. activity on albino rats and swiss mice; steroidal oil fraction from seeds showed antifert. activity in mice (*Indian J Pharm*, 1966, **28**, 344; 1967, **29**, 235). Seeds contain β-sitosterol and stigmasterol; 5 β-cholanic acid (*Phytochemistry*, 1969, **8**, 791; *Steroids*, 1974, **23**, 357). New steroids, abricin and abridin alongwith known ones, cholesterol, stigmasterol, β-sitosterol, terps., and squalene (*Pak J Sci Ind Res*, 1978, **21**, 158; *CA*, 1980, **92**, 194420e).

Roots contain precol, abrol; alks. abrasine and precasine (*Sci Res Dacca*, 1966, **3**, 203; *CA*, 1967, **67**, 90987n). Roots and leaves, glycyrhizin (*Q J Crude Drug Res*, 1972, **12**, 1922). Isoflavanquinones, abrusquinone A, B & C (*Gazz Chim Ital*, 1979, **109**, 9).

Plant ext., one of the constituents of long-acting oral contracep. preventing implantation of fertilized ovum; see also *Embelia ribes* (Brit. Pat., 1976, 1445599; *CA*, 1977, **86**, 21786b).

Seed toxicity to cattle [*Indian Farming*, 1966-67, **16**(9), 43]; toxicol. studies (*Lloydia*, 1970, **33**, 493); toxicity in animals (*Arzneim Forsch*, 1971, **21**, 888; *CA*, **75**, 107849y); elevation of enzyme levels in serum due to poisoning (*Toxicon*, 1977 **15**, 577).

Seed kernel contains toxin and an inhibitor of toxin (*Toxicon*, 1969, **7**, 211); protease inhibitors (*Indian J Biochem Biophys*, 1976, **13**, 52).

Seeds contain lectins and toxic proteins having a strong inhibitory effect on growth of Ehrlich ascites tumour cells, in mice (*Nature Lond*, 1970, **227**, 292).

Abrin(s)—chief poisonous constituent of seeds is abrin, a toxalbumin similar to ricin of caster seed. Abrin, powerful irritant; produces oedema and ecchymosis at the site of inoculation. Abrin resolved into a globulin and an albuminose, both of which are poisonous and are inactivated by heat (Wlth India, IA, 19).

Inflam. caused by sc injection of abrin in paws of Swiss mice diminished with 2 ip of abrin (*Rev Immunol*, 1967, **31**, 389; *CA*, 1968, **68**, 85733t). Useful in inflam. (*FEBS Lett*, 1980, **139**, 297).

Iodinated abrin less toxic in rat (*Toxicon*, 1970, **8**, 193). Toxicity, distribution and elimination of abrin and ricin in mice (*Br J Cancer*, 1976, **34**, 418).

Toxic and nontoxic lectins—seeds contain toxic protein(s), abrin(s), and nontoxic protein, *Abrus* agglutinin. Both the toxin and the agglutinin are referred to as lectins. More than one variety of abrin with hemagglutinating activity and binding affinity for D-galactose with or without such properties have been obtained. Highly purified agglutinin (i.e. without any contamination of toxin) is nontoxic. The toxins as well as the agglutinin consist of polypeptide chains of nearly the same size, while abrins consist of two polypeptide chains one of which is involved in the binding to cells; the agglutinin consists of four chains only two of which appear to be involved in binding to cell surface, however, agglutinins with two chains have also been obtained. Within one kind of seed, the polypeptide chains involved in binding of agglutinin and toxins to cell surface are very similar to identical. Variation of properties of different abrins, from different laboratories may be due to different sources or varieties of seeds, or seeds from different plant strains (*Arch Biochem Biophys*, 1976, **174**, 359; *Int J Pept Protein Res*, 1978, **12**, 311; *J Biol Chem*, 1974, **249**, 803; *Toxicòn*, 1981, **19**, 41; *Biochim Biophys Acta*, 1981, **667**, 397).

Str. and mechanism of action of toxins consisting of two polypeptide chains joined by a disulphide bond. The two chains — larger B-chains (Mol. wt, c 35,000) and shorter A-chains (32,000). Binding of toxic and nontoxic lectins on Ehrlich ascites tumour cells, is similar and they probably use the same receptors [*Trends Biochem Sci*, 1978, **3**(1), 7].

Abrins are named as abrin a, b, c & d, however, capital letters A & C have also been used, causing confusion, especially when capital letters are also used for two polypeptide chains of individual abrin (*J Biol Chem*, 1974, **249**, 3061; *Int J Pept Protein Res*, 1978, **12**, 311; *Toxicon*, 1981, **19**, 41).

Detection of abrins by biological method in the absence of chem. method (*Forensic Sci Soc J*, 1971, **11**, 109; *CA*, 1972, 76, 10804y).

Abrin varieties, studies on isolation, purification, crystal data, some properties, etc.(*Taiwan I Hsueh Hui Tsa Chih*, 1969, **68**, 518; *CA*, **72**, 98695q; *FEBS Lett*, 1972, **28**, 48; 1973, **35**, 257; *Eur J Biochem*, 1973, **35**, 179; *J Biol Chem*, 1973, **248**, 3745; 1974, **249**, 3061; *Arch Biochem Biophys*, 1976, **174**, 359; *Proc Fifth Int Symp Toxins: Animal, Plant and Microbial*, 1978, 837; *Int J Pept Protein Res*, 1978, **12**, 311; *Toxicon*, 1981, **19**, 41).

Red seeds from Calcutta contain an abrin and an agglutinin; abrin was non-haemagglutinating and did not bind D-galactose (*Arch Biochem Biophys*, 1976, **174**, 359). Chem. modification of abrin and ricin (*Eur J Biochem*, 1978, **84**, 323).

Abrin and ricin show higher toxicity for certain tumour cells than for normal cells; a protein ext. (10% NaCl ext. of cotyledon) showed antitumour activity on Yoshida sarcoma (solid & ascites forms) in rats and fibrosarcoma in mice; ip route more effective than sc (*Cancer Res*, 1969, **29**, 1447; *Nature Lond*, 1970, **227**, 292). Purification of proteins and their biological properties; A_1, A_{4a}, A_{4b}, A_{5a} & A_{5b} with their agglutinating activity (A_{5a} does not agglutinate); toxicity with MTD, and effect on Yoshida ascites sarcoma in rats (*Indian J Biochem Biophys*, 1971, **8**, 321). Use of abrin and ricin against various forms of gynaecological cancers in China (*J Formosan Med Assoc*, 1974, **73**, 526). Abrin and ricin inhibit protein synthesis by inactivating ribosome-dependent GTP-ase (*Biochem Biophys Res Commun*, 1977, **75**, 845). A discussion with 18 ref. on binding, entry and action of abrin, ricin and modeccin (*Life Sci Res Rep*, 1978, **11**, 103; *CA*, 1980, **92**, 141268e). Pharmacol. studies sufficiently encouraging to warrant clin. studies in humans (*J Toxicol Env Hlth*, 1979, **5**, 1073). Effects of abrin and ricin observed on murine tumours and on human xenografts, promising; the finding that abrin and ricin in contrast to most cytostatic agents have little or no bone marrow suppressing effect seems to make them interesting candidate for combination therapy. Rev., 22 refs. [*Biol Cancer Cell Proc Fifth Meet Eur Assoc Cancer Res Vienna*, 1979, 261(Kugler Pub. Amsterdam), 1980; *CA*, 1981, **94**, 114030f]. An immuno-potentiator comprising abrin (Eur. Pat. Appl, 1981, 28814; *CA*, **95**, 68062p); effective combination with synth. antitumour drugs (*J Nat Cancer Inst*, 1981, **66**, 523; *Experientia*, 1981, **37**, 256).

Formulation containing abrin as neoplasm inhibitors; also in anticancer compn. (Ger Offen, 1974, 2319472; 1975, 2518529; *CA*, 1975, **82**, 103161a; 1976, **84**, 35349g). Proteins with tumour-inhibiting properties (Brit. Pat., 1978, 1522620; *CA*, 1979, **90**, 192540d).

Abrus agglutinin—nontoxic protein or lectin; purification (*Experientia*, 1972, **28**, 84). Isolation of agglutinin (Oslo sample), its mol. wt, subunit str. and sugar-binding specificity, and comparison of properties with toxic lectin abrin (*J Biol Chem*, 1974, **249**, 803; 4790).

From Indian seed (red), agglutinin (0.05%) isolation, purification and some properties; mol. wt 132,000 giving noncovalent bound subunits of mol. wt 64,000; crystalline lectin showing presence of 3 isolectins; different in amino acid compn. from their counterparts elsewhere, probably arising out of different seed source (*Arch Biochem Biophys*, 1976, **174**, 359).

Abrin, ricin and their associated agglutinin, rev., 185 refs [Receptors and Recognition Ser. B, 1977, I (Specificity and Plant Toxins), 129; *CA*, 1978, **88**, 69828k]. Different nontoxic lectins along with toxic ones (*Proc Fifth Int Symp Toxins: Animal, Plant and Microbial*, 1978, 837). Isolation of 4 isotoxic protein and one agglutinin from Taiwan sample probably of different plant, str.; agglutinin (mol. wt, 67,000 with 2 subunits AB only), and their properties (*Toxicon*, 1981, **19**, 41).

Haemagglutinin, a heat-labile protein located in cotyledons (*Indian J Exp Biol*, 1968, **6**, 108). Interaction of erythrocytes of various animal spp. with seed agglutinin (*Indian Vet J*, 1970, **47**, 648).

Highly purified agglutinin initiates DNA synthesis in lymphocytes (*J Biol Chem*, 1974, **249**, 810). Abrus agglutinin as also ricinus agglutinin, both mitogenic, as shown by their ability to stimulate thymidine incorporation in human lymphocytes (*J Immunol*, 1975, **115**, 1045).

Lectins, immunochem. relation between toxins and agglutinin (*J Immunol*, 1974, **113**, 835). Abrus as also ricinus agglutinin, biological properties and application in immunoglobin subfractions, rev. with many refs. [*J Oslo City Hosp*, 1977, **27**(5), 53; *CA*, **87**, 131988x]. Different precipitin reactions of highly purified lectin (*Experientia*, 1978, **34**, 531).

Seed agglutinin, tumour-immunizing in mice (*J Formosan Med Assoc*, 1979, **78**, 605). Seed lectin, isolation and leucoagglutinin activity (*Yamaguchi Joshi Daigaku Kenkyu Hokoku Dai-2-bu*, 1979, **4-5**, 35; *CA*, 1981, **94**, 137603j). Growth inhibition of S-180 sarcoma cells by agglutinin, in mice (*Taiwan I Hsueh Hui Tsa Chih*, 1981, **80**, 1; *CA*, **95**, 78309p).

ABUTILON (*Malvaceae*)

A. indicum(Linn.) Sweet syn. *A. indicum* G. Don

Eng.–*Country mallow.*

Plant—drug in Ayurvedic and Unani med.; useful as febge., anthelm., antiinflam., in urinary and uterine discharges, piles and lumbago. Juice as emol. to relieve soreness of nates in young children (Wlth India, IA, 21). Various plant parts used in convuls., cramps, colic pain, spermator., dysen., consumption, broncht., menor., and bone fracture in cattle (*Econ Bot*, 1970, **24**, 241). EtOH(50%) ext. of plant, CNS depress. (*Indian J Exp Biol*, 1971, **9**, 91).

Leaves—cooked and eaten in bleeding piles. Leaf ext., diur. and as emol.; given in diar. Decoct. as mouth wash in toothache; also useful in gonor., inflam. of bladder, as wash for wounds and ulcers, and for enema and vaginal infections (Wlth India, IA, 21).

Leaf paste applied in fever and headache (*Bull Bot Surv India*, 1980, **22**, 161).

Flowers — applied to boils and ulcers. Powd. eaten in ghee in blood vomiting and cough (Wlth India, IA, 21).

Seeds—used in cough, gonor., gleet and chr. cystitis.

Roots—nervine tonic, used in piles and leucoderma. Also used in strangury, haemat., stones in bladder and as wash in eye diseases (Wlth India, IA, 21); powd. roots in cough and leprosy (*J Econ Tax Bot*, 1980, **1**, 139).

Plant contains flavons. gossypetin 8- & 7-glucds., and cyanidin-3-rutinoside (*Phytochemistry*, 1972, **11**, 1518). Aerial parts contain alkanol, β-sitosterol, etc. (*Planta Med*, 1976, **30**, 174). Essent. oil, antibact. to human pathogenic bacteria (*Acta Ciencia Indica*, 1978, **4**, 248); antifung. (*Indian Drugs*, 1978-79, **16**, 122); drug augments antibody in animals showing immunological value [*J Res Indian Med*, 1978, **13**(3), 50]. Leaves yield β-sitosterol and tocopherol oil (0.3%) (*Bull Med Ethno Bot Res*, 1980, **1**, 534).

A. indicum ssp. **guineense** Borssum syn. *A. asiaticum* (Linn.) Sweet

Rajasthan–*Itawari*.

EtOH(50%) ext. of plant, anticancer (*Indian J Exp Biol*, 1971, **9**, 91).

A. pannosum Schlecht. syn. *A. glaucum* Sweet

H.–*Kakrai*; Mar.–*Karnadi, kasili*.

Leaves used as cure for piles (Wlth India, IA, 20).

*A. ramosum Guill. & Perr.

EtOH(50%) ext. of plant, spasmol. and CNS depress. (*Indian J Exp Biol*, 1973, **11**, 43).

Found in Chitorgarh, Rajasthan.

A. theophrastii Medic. syn. *A. avicennae* Gaertn.

Eng.–*American jute, Indian mallow*.

Seed decoct. in dysen., fistulae and eye sores (Wlth India, IA, 22).

ACACIA (*Mimosaceae*)

*A. auriculaeformis A. Cunn. ex Benth.

EtOH(50%) ext. of aerial parts, CNS depress. and hypoten. (*Indian J Exp Biol*, 1980, **18**, 594) ext., α-spinasterol and flavan glycd., auriculoside which is CNS depress. (*Phytochemistry*, 1980, **19**, 1560).

Heartwood and bark flavons. (*Chem Ind Lond*, 1965, 1342; *Biochem J*, 1966, **98**, 493).

Native to Australia, introduced into semi-arid zones of Bihar, Orissa and W. Bengal.

A. catechu Willd.

Eng.–*Cutch tree*.

Ayurvedic drug for leprosy (*ISI Bull*, 1967, **19**, 393). Various plant parts used in sore mouth, pain in chest, cancer, colic pain, gravel, dysen., phthisis, broncht., asthma, consumption and strangulation of intestine (*Econ Bot*, 1970, **24**, 241). Bark useful in skin diseases [*J Res Indian Med* 1973, **8**(2), 67]. Bark juice alongwith asafoetida used in haemoptysis. Mixt. of flower tops, cumins, etc. given in gonor. (*J Econ Tax Bot*, 1980, **1**, 140).

EtOH(50%) ext. of stem, antivir. and spasmol. (*Indian J Exp Biol*, 1968, **6**, 232). Heartwood ext., antifung. (*Geobios*, 1976, **5**, 49).

Katha—pale catechu (different from cutch, the dark catechu) obtained from heartwood of 20-30 yr. old trees. Astrin., cooling and digest. Used in relaxed conditions of throat, mouth, gums and in cough and diar. Also enters into a no. of compd. preparations. Reported to be antileprotic. Associated with oral cancer as a result of *pan*-chewing.

Kheersal— a product met with in some older trees in the form of white crystalline deposit of catechin; used for treatment of cough and sore throat.

Gum—a good substitute for true gum arabic. Gum-resin used in masticatories.

Seed ext., hypoglyc. to normal albino rats but not effective in diabetic rats (*Indian J Med Res*, 1976, **64**, 754).

Heartwood, 8 flavons. (*Indian J Chem*, 1981, **20B**, 628).

*A. chundra Willd. syn. *A. sundra* DC.

Kan.–*Kempu jali or kagli*; Mal.–*Kannali*; Mar.–*Lal khair*; Tam.–*Karangali*; Tel.–*Sandra;* Trade–*Red cutch.*

EtOH(50%) ext. of aerial parts, spermic. and spasmol. (*Indian J Exp Biol*, 1980, **18**, 594). Stem bark paste and leaves applied to abscesses (*Bull Med Ethno Bot Res*, 1980, **1**, 8). Bark, astrin., applied to boils and ulcers as antisep.; yields tannin (*J Econ Tax Bot*, 1981, **2**, 178).

Tree yields a gum; heartwood, red cutch and *Katha.* Gum compn.; a tentative str. suggested (Wlth India, **IA**, 30); aldotriuronic acid (0.35g) (*Indian J Chem*, 1970, **8**, 48).

Rajasthan, Gujarat, Maharashtra, Andhra Pradesh and Tamil Nadu.

*A. dealbata Link syn. *A. decurrens* Willd. var. *dealbata* F. Muell. ex. Maiden

Eng.–*Silver wattle.*

Gum—viscous, high quality, resembling gum arabic but with strongly astrin. taste. Suitable for pharmaceutical use, has been used as a remedy in bronch. diseases and as an antid. to alc. and ammonia poisoning.

Flowers—used for preparation of Mimosa perfume. Flower concrete, constituents (*Soap Perfum Cosmet*, 1969, **42**, 511). Pigment (*Chem Ind Lond*, 1980, 786).

Pollen, rutin. Seeds, rich in α-tocopherol; γ- & δ- also present (*Plant Med Phytother*, 1979, **13**, 1278). Plant, rutin and quercetin (*Anales Fac Quim Farm Univ Chile*, 1964, **16**, 133; *CA*, 1966, **64**, 13034f).

Native to Australia and Tasmania, naturalized in the Nilgiri and Palni hills.

*A. decurrens Willd.

Eng.–*Common or green wattle*; Tam.–*Seemai velam pattai.*

Bark, astrin., decoct. used in cases of severe dysen. Rich in tannins (30-40%)

(Wlth India, IA, 31). Dimeric and higher polymeric flavonols, antitumour (*Ann Acad Bras Cienc*, 1972, **44**, 41; *CA*, 1973, **78**, 119383c).

Native to Australia and Tasmania. Cultivated in Kodaikanal and Palni hills, T.N., and in Uttar Pradesh.

A. farnesiana Willd.

Eng.–*Cassie flower.*

Various plant parts used in madness, carbuncle, epilepsy, rabies, convuls., delirium, sores, cholera, sterility in women, snakebite and rinderpest (*Econ Bot*, 1970, **24**, 241). Bruised tender leaves given in gonor. (*J Econ Tax Bot*, 1980, **1**, 140).

Pharmacol. of essent. oil from pods; essent. oil, direct plain-muscle relaxant, cardiac depress. and sed. (*Indian J Physiol Pharmacol*, 1978, **22**, 234).

Isolation and characterisation of compds. from absolute prepared from flower concrete. Absolute re-investigated by using several combined chromatogr.; 38 new constituents including three C_{11} compds. with characteristic fragrance of cassie oil. A homoterpene lactone, dihydroactinidiolide also present (*Helv Chim Acta*, 1969, **52**, 24). Flowers, *d*-pinitol (*Ciencie*, 1967, **25**, 107; *CA*, **67**, 18532t); and pigment, isorhamnetin-3,7-glucorhamnoside (*J Indian Chem Soc*, 1970, **47**, 183).

Pod phenolics (*Phytochemistry*, 1973, **12**, 2303).

Leaves, tannin and alks. (*Esc Farm*, 1965, **26**, 1; *BA*, 1966, **47**, 54264); also rutin and apigenin-6,8-bis-C- glucd.(0.4%) (*Pharmazie*, 1974, **29**, 352; *CA*, 1975, **82**, 28475a); cyanogens; linamarin, lotaustralin and an unidentified one; amt. of cyanide from 0 to 1.4% dry matter (*Phytochemistry*, 1976, **15**, 1703; 1979, **18**, 1389).

A. ferruginea DC.

EtOH(50%) ext. of stem bark, hypoten. and spasmol. (*Indian J Exp Biol*, 1968, **6**, 232).

A. jacquemontii Benth.

Roots contain two cassane diterps. having unique 7-membered hemiacetal ring B (*Tetrahedron*, 1979, **35**, 1449).

A. leucophloea Willd.

Bark—bitter and cooling. Used in broncht. and biliousness. Acts as clarifying and flavouring agents (Wlth India, IA, 34). Bark, demulc., aphrodis.; leaves used in syphilis [*J Res Indian Med*, 1973, **8**(2), 67]. EtOH(50%) ext. of aerial parts, hypoten. and CNS depress. (*Indian J Exp Biol*, 1971, **9**, 91).

Gum, demulc. (*J Agric Trop Bot Appl*, 1966, **13**, 275).

Variation of HCN in different plant parts (*Curr Sci*, 1981, **50**, 689).

Stem bark, *n*-hexacosanol, β-amyrin and β-sitosterol; heartwood, *n*-octacosanol and β-sitosterol (*J Indian Chem Soc*, 1977, **54**, 649).

Grazing of shrub causes HCN-poisoning (*Indian Vet J*, 1977, **54**, 748). HCN-content (in ppm); leaves, 242.2 (in May) and 19 (in Sept.); buds and flowers, 513 and 478.8 (in Oct.); pods,400.7 (in April) and 987 (in Nov.). HCN content of leaves gradually increases thereafter (*Curr Sci*, 1981, **50**, 689).

Root bark, pimarene diterp., leucophleol and leucophleoxol, their str. (*Phytochemistry*, 1980, **19**, 1979); leucoxol, its str. (*Tetrahedron Lett*, 1980, **21**, 2843).

*A. mearnsii De Wild. syn. *A. mollissima* sensu auct. mult., non Willd.; *A. decurrens* Willd. var. *mollis* Lindl.

Eng.–*Black wattle*; Tam.–*Chavakku*.

EtOH(50%) ext. of stem bark, hypoten. and diur. (*Indian J Exp Biol*, 1974, **12**, 512).

Gum, compn. (*Carbohydr Res*, 1968, **7**, 421). Condensed tannins (*J Chem Soc Chem Commun*, 1978, 700); studies on gum mucilage [*East Pharm*, 1981, **24**(281), 119]

Resorcinol which finds use as a lotion in certain skin diseases from heartwood in greater yield; difficulties attending extn. from waste fines of wood clippings discussed (*Appl Polym Symp*, 1976, **28**, 1365; *CA* 1977, **86**, 108226t).

Young leaves (before flowering time), a good source of 1-*trans*-4-OH-pipecolic acid (*Yakugaku Zasshi*, 1969, **89**, 1723; *CA*, 1970, **72**, 136340e). Leaf flavon., mearnsitrin (8%) (*Phytochemistry*, 1969, **8**, 435; 1813).

Native to Tasmania, introduced near Kodaikanal, cultivated on large scale in Nilgiris, Palnis and Kerala and also in Assam.

*A. melanoxylon R. Br.

Eng.–*Australian blackwood*.

Seeds—hyperglyc. and hypercholesteremic in normal young rats (*Indian J Med Sci*, 1972, **26**, 729). Contradictory findings in albino rats [*Med Surg*, 1976, **16**(4), 5]. Seed protein isolates, hypoglyc., and hypocholesteremic in rats (*J Indian Med Assoc*, 1977, **68**, 201).

Blackwood causes allergic contact dermatitis and bronch. asthma in wood workers; allergens: 2 or 3 benzoquinones; one of them acamelin; their strs. (*Naturwissenschaften*,1977, **64**, 534;*Tetrahedron Lett*, 1980, **21**, 149; *Br J Ind Med*, 1981, **38**, 105).

Flowers contain hyperoside (*Naturwissenschaften*, 1964, **51**, 462).

Native to Tasmania and S. Australia; introduced and naturalised in Nilgiris, and grown in Kodaikanal.

A. modesta Wall.

Seeds hypoglyc.; stimulate insulin-secretion in normal rats (*Indian J Physiol Pharmacol*, 1975, **19**, 167). Stembark, octacosanol, α-amyrin, betulin and ψ-sitosterol; heartwood, γ-sitosterol and pinitol; leaves, octacosane, hentriacontane, octacosanol and hentriacontanol (*Planta Med*, 1975, **27**, 281).

A. nilotica Delile ssp. **indica** (Benth.) Brenan syn.*A. arabica* Willd. var. *indica* Benth.

Gum—substitute for true gum arabic. Used in sore throat (Wlth India, IA, 37); alongwith latex of *Calotropis procera* given to cure asthma (*J Agric Trop Bot Appl*, 1966, **13**, 274); stops bleeding and urinary and vaginal discharges; also useful in diabetes; bark, cooling and anthelm.; cures skin diseases, bleeding piles, etc. (*Indian Drugs*, 1977-78, **15**, 145).

Bark—EtOH (50%) ext., antiprot., hypoten. and spasmol. (*Indian J Exp Biol*, 1969, **7**, 250); used in asthma and broncht. (*J Econ Tax Bot*, 1980, **2**, 141); med. value, methods of administration, etc.; decoct., in leucor. (*Sachitra Ayurveda*, 1980-81, **33**, 210). Used as substitute for soap. In Sudan, in pneum., meningitis, etc. (*Fitoterapia*, 1981, **52**, 243). Decoct., hypoglyc. in alloxan diabetic rabbits; max. reduction after 2 hrs of drug administration (*Cheiron*, 1981, **10**, 1); for gargling. Antivir. (Wlth India, IA, 41).

Pods—used in impotency and effective in urinogenital disorders (*J Agric Trop Bot Appl*, 1966, **13**, 274).

Flowers—cause allergy. Flowers, pods and gum-resin used as tonic in diar. and dysen. (*J Econ Tax Bot*, 1980, **1**, 141).

Seeds—hypoglyc. in normal rats; no such effect in diabetic rats; some seed component stimulates insulin secretion by β-cells (*Indian J Physiol Pharmacol*, 1975, **19**, 167; actually this ref. mentions *A. benthamii* which is *A. nilotica* ssp. *subulata* this probably is same as ssp. *indica*). Seed oil and unsap. matter, antifung. (*Indian Drugs*, 1979-80, **17**, 12).

Leaves—bruised leaves applied to sore eyes in children (*J Agric Trop Bot Appl*, 1966, **13**, 274); eaten in throat infection and poultice used in sore eyes. Paste of burnt leaves effective ointment in itch (*J Econ Tax Bot*, 1980, **1**, 141).

Various plant parts used in hair-fall, earache, syphilis, cholera, dysen., leprosy and rinderpest (*Econ Bot*, 1970, **24**, 241);

roots and trunk paste to heal wounds [*J Res Indian Med*, 1978, **13**(4), 92].

Gum slightly dextrorotatory, unlike the true gum arabic from *A. senegal*. Gum constituents: galactose; *l*-arabinose, *l*-rhamnose, and 4 aldobiouronic acids (*J Chem Soc C*, 1967, 1476); arabinobioses (*Can J Chem*, 1968, **46**, 2311). Emulsifying properties (*J Indian Chem Soc*, 1981, **58**, 620).

Bark, several polyphenols (*J Chem UAR*, 1962, **5**, 155). Bark from Egypt, higher tannin content (27%) than that from India; 30 phenolics from tanning exts. (*Leder*, 1967, **18**, 32; *CA*, **67**, 3716g).

Pods contain gallic acid & its Me-ester, *n*-digallic acid and 2 condensed tannins (*Fitoterapia*, 1979, **50**, 115).

Med. uses, chem. constituents and pharmacol., a rev., 11 refs. (*J Nat Integ Med Assoc*, 1980, **22**, 112). Present status of plants used in traditional med. in W. Africa, a med. approach and a chem. evaluation; work done on chem. screening of *A. nilotica* among others reviewed (*J Ethnopharmacol*, 1980, **2**, 109).

Root bark, octacosanol, betulin, β-amyrin and β-sitosterol; heartwood, last 2 compds. (*J Indian Chem Soc*, 1981, **58**, 96).

A. pennata (Linn.) Willd.

Bark used as substitute for soap in M.P. (Wlth India, IA, 41). Decoct. of young leaves given in body pain, headache and fever in Bastar, M.P. (*Econ Bot*, 1965, **19**, 241). Fruit pulp, piscic. (*ibid*, 1970, **24**, 134). EtOH(50%) ext. of aerial parts, hypoten. (*Indian J Exp Biol*, 1969, **7**, 250).

Bark contains lupeol and α-spinasterol (*J Indian Chem Soc*, 1966, **43**, 191); stem, β-sitosterol (*Indian J Chem*, 1976, **14B**, 473).

*A. planifrons Wight & Arn.

Tam.—*Kodaivelom*; Tel.—*Gadugu thumma*.

EtOH(50%) ext. of aerial parts, diur. (*Indian J Exp Biol*, 1974, **12**, 512).

Wood and bark, *d*-catechin (1.0-1.5%) (*Leath Sci*, 1965, **12**, 162); pods, tannin (Wlth India, IA, 42).

Occurs in Kerala and Tamil Nadu.

A. polyacantha Willd. syn. *A. suma* Buch.-Ham. ex Voigt; *A. suma* Kurz; *Mimosa suma* Roxb.

Plant reported to have anticancer activity (*Annu Rep CDRI Lucknow*, 1970, 76). Seeds, marked hypoglyc. effect on normal albino rats (*Indian J Med Res*, 1976, **64**, 754).

Cutch prepared from heartwood; quercetin and 3′,7-di-MeO-hyperin in heartwood (*Curr Sci*, 1976, **45**, 294). Seed protein essent. amino acids including methionine, 2.0 g/16g N (*ibid*, 1974, **43**, 235).

A. pycnantha Benth.

Eng.–*Golden wattle.*

Gum, an arabogalactan (Wlth India, IA, 46).

Seeds, β-lectin: alteration in compn., caused by chem. and enzymic attack. Very high content of serine and hydroxyproline of β-lectin is of interest (*Aust J Plant Physiol*, 1979, **6**, 25). Anal. of methylated polysaccharides (*J S Afr Chem Inst*, 1973, **26**, 106; *CA*, 1974, **80**, 48275g).

A. senegal Willd.

Eng.–*Gum arabic tree.*

Roots used for dysen., gonor. and nodular leprosy.

EtOH(50%) ext. of stem bark, antiinflam. and spasmol. (*Indian J Exp Biol*, 1977, **15**, 208).

Gum called 'gum arabic', *l*-rotatory. Gum, an acid polysaccharide containing sugars, *d*-galactose, *l*-arabinose, *l*-rhamnose and *d*-glucoronic acid. Studies on uronic acid materials; compn. of gum exudates; constituents of partial hydrolysis of gum (*J Chem Soc*, 1966, 762; 1959).

Roots, ceryl alcohol, betulin and sitosterol; bark, uvaol, octacosanol, β-amyrin and sitosterol; heartwood, sitosterol; leaves, nonacosane, hentriacontane, hentriacontanol, octacosanol and

d-pinitol; flowers *n*-octacosanol, sitosterol, β-sitosterol- glucd. and ceryl alc. (*Indian J Chem*, 1975, **13**, 638). Leaves contain an alk., di-Me-tryptamine (*Lloydia*, 1975, **38**, 176). Stembark (another anal.), erythrodiol, sucrose, β-amyrin, β-sitosterol & its glucd. (*Indian J For*, 1981, **4**, 63).

Pod polyphenols (*J Indian Leather Technol Assoc*, 1974, **22**, 151). Pods yield kaempferol, quercetin, β-amyrin, β-sitosterol & its glucd. (*Indian J For*, 1981, **4**, 63).

A. sinuata (Lour.) Merrill syn. *A. concinna* DC.

Leaves—infusion given in malarial fever. Leaves acidic; a chutney made of tender leaves, salt, tamarind and chillies given in bilious affections, such as jaundice.

Pods and seeds—in N. Bengal as fish-poison. An ointment prepared from ground pods, used for skin diseases. A decoct. used to remove dandruff. Known as *shi(ka)kai*, extensively used as a detergent; seeds reported to be roasted and eaten. Pod decoct. used to kill lice (*Nagarjun*, 1979-80, **23**, 177); and in skin diseases (*J Econ Tax Bot*, 1980, **1**, 140).

Bark ext., in leprosy (*J Nat Integ Med Assoc*, 1981, **23**, 43).

EtOH(50%) ext. of aerial parts, hypoten., spasmol. and diur. (*Indian J Exp Biol*, 1971, **9**, 91). Used as domestic germicidal [*J Res Indian Med*, 1973, **8**(2), 67].

Leaves contain alks., nicotine and colycotomine; a triterp. saponin; ascorbic acid, rutin, tannin and also oxalic, tartaric, citric and succinic acids; tartaric racimase. Constituents similar to *Tamarindus indicus* and some other indigenous plant used for jaundice (Wlth India, IA, 45; *Planta Med*, 1970-71, **19**, 55).

Seeds yield acacinin-A & B, and free sugar, concinnin (*J Indian Chem Soc*, 1973, **50**, 544). Partial str. of acacinnin-A (*Indian J Chem*, 1976, **14B**, 228).

Pods yield saponins (20.8%) (*Indian J Technol*, 1963, **1**, 97); 3 saponins (acacinin-C, -D & -E), oligo- and polysaccharides (*J Indian Chem Soc*, 1976, **53**, 153). Aq. ext. of pods, machaerinic acid & its lactone, sapogenin B,and a new ester of acacic acid (*Indian J Chem*, 1977, **16B**, 1, 7). Str. of acacigenin-B. Neutral fraction of acid hydrolysate of saponins of pods, acacic acid lactone-3-OAc and a new nortriterpenene, acacidiol (28-norolean-15, 18-diene-3, 21-diol) (*Phytochemistry*, 1979, **18**, 463; 1199).

Bark contains hexacosanol, lupeol, α-spinasterol, α-spinasterone, acacic acid lactone, and an amorphous saponin; the saponin spermic. with max. activity at 0.004% dilution (*J Indian Chem Soc*, 1980, **57**, 1043). An acacic acid saponin from bark, spermic.; bark saponin also haemolytic (*Indian Drugs*, 1979-80, **17**, 6; 1980-81, **18**, 121).

A. torta (Roxb.) Craib. syn. *A. caesia* Wight & Arn. non Willd.; *A. intesia* Wight & Arn.

Bark used by the Lepchas for washing hair; shredded bark as a substitute for soap in the West Coast.

Plant used in Ayurvedic treatment on menstrual disorders; decoct. given in cattle murrain (Wlth India, IA, 46).

EtOH(50%) ext. of aerial parts, hypoten. (*Indian J Exp Biol*, 1973, **11**, 43). Used in fracture (*Sri Lanka For*, 1980, **14**, 145).

Various plant parts used in tubercular fistula, measles, consumption, cough and broncht. (*Econ Bot*, 1970, **24**, 241).

Bark contains triterp. saponins of acacic acid, lupeol and a steroid, acaciol (α-spinasterol); another sample, lupeol, α-spinasterol and stigmasterol but no saponin (*Indian J Chem*, 1969, **7**, 446; *J Indian Chem Soc*, 1966, **43**, 191; 1980, **57**, 1043); lactones of acacic and machaerinic acids (*Curr Sci*, 1972, **41**, 600); tryptamine, also in roots (*Planta Med*, 1972, **21**, 200).

Seeds, acacic acid saponin (*Indian J Chem*, 1969, **7**, 446).

ACALYPHA (*Euphorbiaceae*)

*A. alnifolia Klein ex Willd.

Leaves used in dysen. (*J Econ Tax Bot*, 1981, **2**, 189).

Palamalai, in Coimbatore district.

*A. ciliata Forsk.

G.–*Dandaro, inchane.*

Herb, laxt. and vermifuge (Wlth India, IA, 48).

Kashmir to Kumaun, and in Bihar.

A. fruticosa Forsk.

Eng.–*Birch-leaved acalypha.*

Leaf juice used in opthalmia. Leaf infusion as vulnerary to wash pustules. Root used in gonor. (Wlth India, IA, 47).

A. indica Linn.

Eng.–*Indian acalypha.*

Leaf—paste applied on burns; with lime juice, useful in early cases of ringworm. Fresh leaf juice useful in rheum. arthritis and skin affections. Powd. leaves for bedsores and maggot-infested wounds (Wlth India, IA, 47). Leaf ext. useful in wheezing, cough, desponoea, etc., clin. study [*J Res Indian Med*, 1979, **14**(3-4), 81]; juice with salt applied on eczema (*J Res Ayur Siddha*, 1981, **2**,109). Leaf ext., antifung. (*Indian Phytopathol*, 1981, **34**, 385).

Plant — eating raw plant caused death in human (*S Afr Med J*, 1965, **39**, 344). In homoeopathy, used in severe cough associated with bleeding from lungs, haemoptysis and incipient phthisis (*Bull Bot Soc Bengal*, 1972, **26**, 25); in gastrointestinal and respiratory affections (*Bull Bot Surv India*, 1976, **18**, 161). Plant used in fractures (*Sri Lanka For*, 1980, **14**, 145); used in toothache and earache (Wlth India, IA, 47).

Plant contains kaempferol [*J Res Indian Med*, 1973, **8**(3), 50]. Leaves and twigs, acalyphamide and other amides, quinone, sterols, etc. (*Indian J Chem*, 1981, **20B**, 974); cyanogenic glycd. (*Planta Med*, 1981, **42**, 102).

A. racemosa Wall. ex Baill. syn. *A. paniculata* Miq.

Mal.–*Valiakuppameni.*

Herb substitute for *A. indica.* Juice in erysipelas and haemor. (Wlth India, IA, 48).

A. sanderi N.E. Br. syn. *A. hispida* Burm. f.

Eng.–*Red hot cat-tail, chenille plant;* Mal.– *Vattattali;* Tel. – *Moorukonda.*

Leaves applied to ulcers. Flowers in diar.; other uses similar to *A. indica* (Wlth India, IA, 48).

ACAMPE (*Orchidaceae*)

A. praemorsa Blatter & McCann syn. *A. wightiana* Lindl.

Kan.–*Marabale;* Mar.–*Kanbher.*

Plant credited with anti-typhoid properties; active against *Salmonella typhosa.* Paste of pounded leaves applied to fractures (Wlth India, IA, 48).

ACANTHOPANAX (*Araliaceae*)

*A. trifoliatum Voss syn. *A. aculeatum* Seem.

Khasi–*Shiah-tyngkhwari;* Miri–*Chobol-aksinriube.*

In Taiwan, plant used in paralysis (Wlth India, IA, 49).

Hills of Assam up to 1,200 m.

ACANTHOSPERMUM (*Asteraceae*)

*A. hispidum DC.

Essent. oil from leaves, antibact.; and antifung. (*Planta Med,* 1971, 20, 118; 1972, 22, 136); plant paste, in skin diseases (*Bull Med Ethno Bot Res,* 1980, 1, 8; Wlth India, IA, 49). Leaf juice, in fever (*J Econ Tax Bot,* 1981, 2, 186).

Plant, terp. glycd., acanthospermol-β-galactosidopyranoside; melampolide and *cis-cis-* germacranolides (*Phytochemistry,* 1976, 15, 1776; 1979, 18, 625).

Native to Brazil, found as a weed throughout greater parts of India.

ACANTHUS (*Acanthaceae*)

A. ilicifolius Linn.

Mar.–*Maraneli;* Oriya–*Harkamcli.*

Plant decoct., diur. and a cure for dropsy. Leaves used as expect. and in bilious swellings. Roots useful in asthma, paralysis, leucor. and debility; decoct. for gargling in sore mouth and toothache (Wlth India, IA, 50). EtOH(50%) ext. of aerial parts, diur.; that from leaves graded analg. in albino mice and antiinflam. in carrageenin-induced oedema in rats (*Indian J Exp Biol,* 1974, 12, 512; 1979, 17, 1257).

Plant contains alk., acanthicifoline (*Pol J Chem,* 1980, 54, 857); oleanolic acid, β-sitosterol, lupeol, quercetin, its glucopyranoside and trigonellin (*ibid,* 1980, 54, 2089). Roots, new triterp. saponin, glycd. of 3β-OH-lup-20(29)-ene (*Phytochemistry,* 1981, 20, 135).

*A. leucostachyus Wall.

EtOH(50%) ext. of plant, CNS depress. (*Indian J Exp Biol,* 1971, 9, 91).

Reported from Mongpoh, Meghalaya.

ACCA (*Myrtaceae*)

*A. sellowiana Berg syn. *Feijoa sellowiana* Berg

Eng.–*Feijoa, pineapple guava, New Zealand banana.*

Fruits—galenicals from various I-containing plants in Azerbaidzhan: fresh fruits contain I, 72.3 mg/100 g; beneficial in mild cases of thyrotoxicosis, but less effective in more serious ones (*Pharmazie,* 1966, 21, 175; *CA,* 65, 3667e; *Arh Farm,* 1965, 15, 23; *CA,* 1967, 66, 68868g).

Fruits, iodine and vit. C; contain essent. oil. I content varies according to locality and fluctuates from year to year, usual range 1.65-3.9mg/kg. All parts except thin skin edible (Wlth India, IV, 13-14). Biochem. characteristics of different forms of feijoa; I levels in fruits grown in different ecological conditions in W. Georgia; accumulation of I found near sea in some cases [*Subtrop Kul' t,* 1971, (6), 122; 1972,

(4), 124; *CA*, 1972, **77**, 46947g; 1973, **78**, 41786q]. Vit. P-active polyphenols [*Tr Vses Semin Biol Aktiv Lech Veshchestvam Plodov Yagod*, 4th, 1970, (Pub. 1972), 82; *CA*, 1974, **81**, 90059a].

Essent. oil from fruits from Russia, Australia and Japan, constituents [*Subtrop Kul't*, 1969, (3), 82; *CA*, 1970, **72**, 2298p; *Phytochemistry*, 1970, **9**, 1355; *Koryo*, 1980, **128**, 35; *CA*, **93**, 184539g].

Native to S. America; introduced into India, grown mainly in hill gardens of S. India.

ACER *(Aceraceae)*

*A. campbellii Hook.f. & Thoms. ex Hiern emend. Banerji

Eng.–*Himalayan maple*; B.–*Kabashi*; Lepcha–*Daom, dom, yali, yatli kung.*

EtOH(50%) ext. of aerial parts, hypoten. (*Indian J Exp Biol*, 1974, **12**, 512).

Himalayas in Sikkim, W. Bengal up to 3,600 m.

*A. caudatum Wall.

Jaunsar–*Kainjli.*

Seed coat ext., antifung. (*Geobios*, 1978, **5**, 49).

Kashmir to Nepal at 3,300 m.

*A. hookeri Miq.

EtOH(50%) ext. of aerial parts, CNS depress., hypoten. and spasmol. (*Indian J Exp Biol*, 1974, **12**, 512).

Bomdila, N–E India.

*A. negundo Linn.

Eng.–*Ash-leaved maple, box elder.*

Bark, vulnerary (Wlth India, IA, 52). Leaves and stem ext., inhibitory to sarcoma 180 in mice.

Ext. contained two active acidic saponins, one of which, also inhibitory to Walker carcinosarcoma 256 tumour in rats (*J Pharm Sci*, 1967, **56**, 603). Vegetable drug for cancer, rev. (*Q J Crude Drug Res*, 1971, **11**, 1665). Hydrolysis of tumour-inhibiting saponin P yielded triterp. ester aglycones, acerotin and acerocin (*J Chem Soc D*, 1970, 969); and their strs. (*J Org Chem*, 1971, **36**, 1972).

Leaves flavon. pigments (*C R Acad Sci Ser D*, 1968, **267**, 317; *CA*, 1968, **68**, 74462y).

Native to America, introduced into Jammu & Kashmir and Dehra Dun; grown at Ootacamund in Nilgiri hills.

ACHILLEA *(Asteraceae)*

A. millefolium Linn.

Eng.–*Milfoil, yarrow.*

Herb—astrin., antisp., vulnerary and styptic; used in flatulent colic, heat burn, hysteria, epilepsy and rheum. Herb administered to suppress haemor. and profuse mucous discharge; its tincture in small and dilute doses, stops bleeding from lungs, kidneys or nose, but in larger doses aggravates bleeding. Decoct. or fresh juice applied to cuts, bruises, piles, varicose veins and ulcer (Wlth India, IA, 54); poultice of boiled plant, to whitlow (*Econ Bot*, 1970, **24**, 320); anticonvuls. (*C R Acad Bulg Sci*, 1965, **18**, 691; *BA*, 1967, **48**, 2517); infusion, constituent of facial cream to prevent premature aging of skin (USSR Pat., 1967, 191060; *CA*, 1968, **68**, 24513z); ext. in liquid CO_2, antihistamine, antibact., soothing and sed. [*Maslo-Zhir Promst*, 1969, **35**(5), 25; *CA*, **71**, 42162 a]. Carbonate ext. of herb increased antiphl. properties of tooth paste (USSR Pat., 1971, 290756; *CA*, **74**, 146419t); ext. in liniment for treating serious burns (Rom. Pat., 1971, 52874; *CA*, 1972, **77**, 66207u; Brit. Pat., 1976, 1456276; *CA*, 1977, **86**, 161296s). Infusion in earache and swollen tissues; herb chewed in toothache (*Econ Bot*, 1974, **28**, 316). Ext. in compn. for breast improvement (Fr. Demande, 1976, 2296425; *CA*, 1977, **87**, 172722z).

One of the constituents of Liv-52(*Indian J Med Res*, 1976, **64**, 738); also of indigenous drug "Geriforte" useful in anxiety neurosis, senile pruritus and fatigue (*Probe*, 1979-80, **19**, 99; *Rajasthan Med J*, 1980, **19**, 23; *Indian Drugs*, 1980-81, **18**, 346).

Herb, antiinflam., stimulates gastric secretion; regulatory and antisp. for menstrual troubles; resolutive. In large doses, it produces headache and vertigo (Med. Plants, 157).

EtOH(50%) ext. of herb, CNS-depress. and hypotens. (*Indian J Exp Biol*, 1980, **18**, 594); choline is said to be responsible for hypotens. effect of drug (Suppl. Gloss. Indian Med. Plants, 1).

Inflorescence—use rare (Med. Plants, 157). Aq. ext. of dried flower heads, antiinflam. in mouse paw oedema; active fraction a protein-carbohydrate mixt. (*J Pharm Sci*, 1969, **58**, 938); extn. of antiinflam. and antiirrit. principle from herb (US Pat., 1970, 3522350; *CA*, **73**, 102048w). Decoct, as a stim. and as lotion to sore eyes, piles and cold (*Econ Bot*, 1970, **24**, 320; Wlth India, IA, 55). Flower ext., inhibitory against β-haemolytic *Streptococci, Staphylococcus aureus* and *Candida albicans* (*Pharm Ztg*, 1981, **126**, 1140; *CA*, **95**, 36307f).

Powd. leaves and floral heads, carmin. and tonic; leaves, sternutatory.Roots used as stim. and emmen. (Wlth India, IA, 55).

Essent. oil—from aerial parts of flowering herb known as "Milfoil oil" has strong arom., but somewhat narcotic odour; used as haemostatic (Wlth India, IA, 55).

Herb contains alk. achilleine, reported to be active haemostatic, reducing blood-clot time in rabbits (Wlth India, IA, 54); dry plant collected from Ponitri contains no achilleine or any other alk., contains choline (Suppl. Gloss. Indian Med. Plants, 1). Herb, azulene (*Gesk Farm*, 1965, **14**, 423; *CA*, 1966, **64**, 13073h); germakranolides (*Naturwissenschaften*, 1965, **52**, 209); herb, betaine, choline, trigonelline, betonicine and stachydrine; hydrocarbons, ceryl alc., β-sitosterol & its -OAc [*God Vissh Khimikotekhnol Inst Sofia*, 1967, **14**(3), 195; **14**(4), 73; *CA*, 1972, **77**, 111471p; 111474s]; achillin and leukodin (*Rev Soc Quim Mex*, 1968, **12**, 212A; *CA*, 1969, **71**, 3493q).

Essent. oil from aerial parts of flowering herb, yield, 0.3-0.6% (Wlth India, IA, 55). Content of essent. oil, azulene and bitter principles in clones (*Planta Med*, 1969, **17**, 226). Constituent of essent. oil from flowers and flowering herb (*Lloydia*, 1974, **37**, 598; *Planta Med*, 1975, **27**, 361). Preparation of biologically active concentrate from aerial parts containing chiefly antiphl. substance, proazulenes (*Rastit Resur*, 1981, **17**, 105).

Inflorescence contains max. essent. oil and azulenes (*Liet TSR Mokslu Akad Darb Ser C*, 1971, 81; *CA*, **75**, 72509u); 3 lactones including millefin and de-Ac-matricarine (*Khim Prir Soedin*, 1972, 246; *CA*, **77**, 85556y). Oil located in anthodia and max. at the beginning of anthesis (Wlth India, IA, 55). Flowering head ext., 5-OH-tetra-MeO-flavone, artemetin and casticin (*J Pharm Sci*, 1975, **64**, 1838); proazulene, achillicin (*Phytochemistry*, 1979, **18**, 331). Inflorescence, essent. oil constituents (*Clujul Med*, 1980, **53**, 74).

Leaves contain rutin; also apigenin, cosmosin, luteolin & its glucd. (*Khim Prir Soedin*, 1972, 676; 1973, 273; *CA*, 1973, **78**, 94818h; **79**, 40007v).

A. santolina Linn.

Used in vet. med. and as insectic.

Bitter principle, santolin; possesses digitalis-like action and stimulates cardiac output (*Acta Pharm Suec*, 1965, **2**, 403; *CA*, 1966, **64**, 9997c); de-OAc-matricarin, its stereochem. (*Helv Chim Acta*, 1967, **50**, 1961). 4 Flavons., including tetra- and tri-MeO- derivs. (*Pharmazie*, 1976, **31**, 894; *CA*, 1977, **86**, 68401n). Aerial parts, lactones (*Khim Prir Soedin*, 1978, 530, 718; 1979, 580; *CA*, **89**, 193848b; 1979, **90**, 204284p; 1980, **92**, 124880f); and 2 triterp. diols, β-sitosterol & its glucd. (*Egypt J Pharm Sci*, 1978, **19**, 163).

Arid and semi-arid regions.

ACHRAS (*Sapotaceae*)

See **MANILKARA**

ACHYRANTHES (*Amaranthaceae*)

A. aspera Linn.
Eng.–*Prickly-chaff flower.*

Herb—with woody base; decoct. useful in pneum., cough, kidney stone; in large doses, acts as ecbolic (*J Agric Trop Bot Appl*, 1966, **13**, 250). EtOH(50%) ext., hypoglyc. (*Indian J Exp Biol*, 1968, **6**, 232). Used for Zn processing in Ayurvedic preparation [*J Res Indian Med*, 1971, **6**(4), 222]. Med. uses and pharmacognosy [*Indian Drugs Pharmac Ind*, 1976, **11**(5), 35]. Ext., antifung. (*Indian J Microbiol*, 1976, **16**, 78); ash given in haemorroids (*Nagarjun*, 1979-80, **23**, 11).

One of the constituents of indigenous drug 'Cystone' useful in urinary tract infections, clin. trials (*Probe*, 1979-80, **19**, 270). Ext., antimicrob. (*Fitoterapia*, 1980, **51**, 231). Tablet made from herb paste with fruits of *Piper longum* reported to cure effects of bite of mad dog (Wlth India, IA, 57).

Leaf—ext. called 'Achyrol' useful in leprosy; juice in eczema and leprosy [*East Pharm*, 1966, **9**(100), 107; *Bull Bot Surv India*, 1976, **18**, 161]. In Philippines, as diur. and sap for treating cataracts; heated sap, valued in tetanus. In Tonga, used in wounds; juice, antid. to insect bite (*Econ Bot*, 1971, **25**, 436; 1978, **32**, 283); used in ear and eye trouble (*Bull Med Ethno Bot Res*, 1980, **1**, 318). Alc. and aq. exts., antibiot. against *Micrococcus pyogenes* var. *aureus* and *Escherichia coli* (Wlth India, IA, 57).

Roots—given in stomach pain (*Econ Bot*, 1965, **19**, 244). Paste applied to remove opacity of cornea; and to wounds as haemostatic (*Bull Bot Surv India*, 1966, **8**, 237; 1973, **15**, 13). Used in abdominal tumour (*Lloydia*, 1967, **30**, 389). In Tahiti, roots used in mouth sores, toothache and syphilitic sores (*Econ Bot*, 1971, **25**, 436). Powd. in leprosy (*ibid*, 1981, **35**, 4). Decoct. and paste as antifert. agent (*Bull Med Ethno Bot Res*, 1980, **1**, 318; *Q J Crude Drug Res*, 1972, **12**, 1922). Ext. in menstrual disorders (*Indian J For*, 1981, **4**, 155).

Stembark—benzene ext., antiimplantation activity in mice (*Indian J Med Res*, 1975, **63**, 378); abortif. in rabbit (*Indian J Exp Biol*, 1977, **15**, 856).

Seed—paste applied to insect-bite (*J Agric Trop Bot Appl*, 1966, **13**, 250); leaf, seed and twigs used in bronch. affections (*Bull Bot Surv India*, 1976, **18**, 161). Powd. seeds soaked in butter milk given in biliousness (*Econ Bot*, 1974, **28**, 73).

Flowers—ground and mixed with curds and sugar given in menor.; flower-tops reported to be employed in the treatment of rabies. Pollen suspected to cause allergy (Wlth India, IA, 57).

Various parts used in atrophy, cachexy, rheum., scabies, syphilis, labour complaints and blindness to cattle (*Econ Bot*, 1970, **24**, 241).

Achyranthine—alk. identified as betaine (*Indian J Chem*, 1966, **4**, 461); it lowered B.P., depressed heart rate, caused vasodilation, increased respiration in animals and is slightly antipyr.; it is spasmodic on rectus muscle of frog; has diur. and purg. action on albino rats (*Indian J Pharm*, 1970, **32**, 43). Alk. content of root and shoots, at different stages of growth (*Curr Trends Life Sci*, 1979, **4**, 81; CA, 1981, **94**, 27375d).

Plant ash, potash (large quant.) (Wlth India, IA, 57).

Root contains ecdysterone and inokosterone, insect moulting hormones (*Yakugaku Zasshi*, 1967, **87**, 1481). Leaves and stem, ecdysterone (*Indian J Med Res*, 1975, **63**, 378); stem ext. gave +ve test for alk., sterol and saponins (*Fitoterapia*, 1980, **51**, 145).

Seeds, saponin A & B (*Phytochemistry*, 1970, **9**, 409); saponin, effect on phosphorylase activity of rat heart [*Indian J Physiol Pharmacol*, 1971, **15**(3), 107]; seed saponins, cardiac stim. in animals (*Indian J Med Res*, 1972, **60**, 462). Unripe fruit, saponin C & D (*Indian J Chem*, 1981, **20B**, 773).

A. bidentata Blume

Lushai–*Vangvathus.*

EtOH(50%) ext. of plant, spasmol. (*Indian J Exp Biol*, 1967, **7**, 250). Plant effective in whooping cough; juice useful in scrofula; leaf juice in blisters of mouth and in cholera (*Bull Med Ethno Bot Res*, 1980, **1**, 1; 8). Uterotonic activity of saponins (*4th Asian Symp Med Plants & Spices*, 1980, 63).

Roots, ecdysterone and inokosterone (*Yakugaku Zasshi*, 1968, **88**, 1293); rubrosterone useful as metamorphosis hormone (Jpn Pat., 1971, 7127472; *CA*, 1972, **76**, 23177w). Alk. content of roots and shoots at different growth stages (*Curr Trends Life Sci*, 1979, **4**, 81; *CA*, 1981, **94**, 27375d).

ACOKANTHERA (*Apocynaceae*)

*A. spectabilis Hook. f.

Leaves, friedelin (*Lloydia*, 1964, **27**, 233). Plant cardenolide glycd., acospectoside A (*J Pharm Sci*, 1965, **54**, 1834); cardiotonic glucd. different from ouabain and g- & k- strophanthins (*Sci Pharm Proc 25th*, 1965, **1**, 289; *CA*, 1968, **69**, 80146q). Wood, leaves, fruit ext. yield spectabiline; can be used as heart tonic (Fr. Demande 2114996, 1972; *CA*, 1973, **78**, 82196r). Plant, cardenolides, β-amyrin, etc.; assay of cardenolides and ouabain in different organ by colorim. (*Planta Med*, 1973, **24**, 234; 1974, **25**, 7). Cardenolides from various parts included acovenoside A, B and C, acolongifloroside K and ouabain [*Plant Med Phytother*, 1974, **8**(2), 89; *CA*, 1975,**82**, 28495g]. 4 Glucds. (*Egypt J Pharm Sci*, 1974, **15**, 33).

Cultivated in Calcutta gardens and elsewhere.

ACONITUM (*Ranunculaceae*)

Indian Aconites, classification and med. importance, rev. (*J Nat Integ Med Assoc*, 1978, **20**, 383). Bot., chem. and pharmacol. of Chinese spp., rev. (*J Ethnopharmacol*, 1981, **4**, 247). Chem. of *Aconitum*, rev. covering toxicity and str.-toxicity relations of alks. (*Gendai Toyo Igaku*, 1981, **2**, 50; *CA*, **95**, 192267y).

A. bisma Rap. syn. *A. palmatum* D. Don

One of the constituents of indigenous drug 'Gasex', useful in gastro-intestinal disorders in post-operative gastro intestinal symptoms, clin. trials (*Probe*, 1979-80, **19**, 277).

Root alks., vakognavine, palmatisine, vakatisine, vakatisinine and vakatidine (*J Indian Chem Soc*, 1965, **42**, 49); vakognavine, str. (*Tetrahedron Lett*, 1968, 2219; *Indian J Chem*, 1974, **12**, 1219); vakatisine, str. (*ibid*, 1972, **10**, 953).

A. chasmanthum Stapf ex Holmes

Root alks., chasmaconitine and chasmanthinine, str. (*Can J Chem*, 1964, **42**, 154); chasmanine, str. (*ibid*, 1965, **43**, 825; *J Chem Soc Chem Commun*, 1976, 253).

A. deinorrhizum Stapf

Roots and leaves used in rheum. fever, rheum., and acute headache (*Nagarjun*, 1978-79, **22**, 190).

A. falconeri Stapf

Roots in diseases of nervous and digest. systems, rheum., tatorus and fever (*Khadi Gramodyog*, 1972-73, **19**, 277). In Ayurveda, used in fever and rheum. (*Nagarjun*, 1978-79, **22**, 190). Treatment with cow's milk reduced cardiotoxic effect (*Ancient Sci Life*, 1981-82, **1**, 106).

Root alks, bishatisine and bishaconitine (*Indian J Chem*, 1966, **4**, 39). Alks., falconitine and mithaconitine (*J Chem Soc Chem Commun*, 1977, 12); veratroyl-ψ-aconine, ψ-aconitine and indaconitine; no bishatisine and bishaconitine (*Phytochemistry*, 1977, **16**, 623).

A. ferox Wall. ex Ser.

Tubers—diaphor., diur., antiper., anodyne, antidiabetic, and antiphl. Used in cough, asthma and snake-bite. Paste useful in neuralgia, muscular rheum., nasal catarrh, tonsilitis, coryza, etc. In large doses powerful sed.

Root alks., picro-aconine, aconine, benzyl aconine and homo-napalline (*Khadi Gramodyog*, 1976-77, **23**,115); bikhaconitine, chasmaconitine, indaconitine and ψ-aconitine (*Lloydia*, 1972, **35**, 55);

17

veratroyl-ψ-aconine and di-Ac-ψ-aconitine (*Phytochemistry*, 1974, **13**, 1975).

A. heterophyllum Wall. ex Royle

Root as antifert. agent (*Q J Crude Drug Res,* 1972, **12**, 1922). Tubers, bitter, tonic, stomch., astrin., antiper., aphrodis., diar., dysen., acute inflam., dyspep., cough, hysteria, loss of memory, piles and throat diseases (*Khadi Gramodyog,* 1976-77, **23**, 115). Root powd. in splenic fever and gastric troubles (*Nagarjun,* 1978-79, **22**, 190). Root, one of the constituents of Ayurvedic drug for giardiasis (*Sachitra Ayurveda,* 1981-82, **34**, 401).

Chem. of alk. heteratisine (*Can J Chem,* 1964, **42**, 172). Root alks., heterophyllisine, heterophylline and heterophyllidine (*Tetrahedron Lett,* 1967, 557); heteratisine, atisine, atidine, F-dihydroatisine, isoatisine, hetisine, hetidine and hetisinone (*Phytochemistry,* 1968, 7, 625); heteratisine, str. (*Tetrahedron,* 1973, **29**, 3297).

A. laeve Royle

Tubers, alk. (4.1% dry basis), lappoconitine (*Planta Med,* 1964, **12**, 177).

A. napellus Linn.

Aconitine, active alk., large doses fatal to human (*Prakt Lek,* 1964, **44**, 367; *CA,* **61**, 9946c). Str. of alks., rev., 39 refs. (*Fitoterapia,* 1965, **36**, 2; *CA,* 1966, **65**, 2313c). Total alk. detn. (*Plant Med Phytother,* 1972, **6**, 232; *CA,* 1973, **78**, 26091r).

*A. rotundifolium Kar. & Kir.

Plant, weakly active against tumours (*J Agric Trop Bot Appl,* 1974, **21**, 239).

Aerial portions, 2 unnamed alks. (mp 251-5°; and 173-74°) (Manske, XII, 121).

N-W Himalayas in alpine regions.

A. spicatum Stapf

Major alks. ψ-aconitine and bikhaconitine (*Can J Chem,* 1963, **41**, 3055). Plant, antipyr. and analg. (*Arch Int Pharmacodyn Ther,* 1965, **152**, 22; *BA,* 1966, **47**, 102612). Tuber, toxic; alks. 1.2%

(*Plant Med Phytother,* 1973, **7**, 151; *CA,* 79, 133509a).

A. violaceum Jacq. ex Stapf

In Pakistan, roots eaten by hillmen of Kunwar as tonic; they contain alk. indaconitine (*Phytochemistry,* 1971, **10**, 3320); alk. bikhaconitine (*J Indian Chem Soc,* 1977, **54**, 924).

ACONOGONUM (*Polygonaceae*)

*A. molle Hara var. frondosum syn. *Polygonum frondosum* DC.

Properties same as *A. molle* var. *molle.*

A. molle Hara var. molle syn. *Polygonum molle* D. Don; *P. paniculatum* Blume

Ass.–*Kochomah*; Lepcha–*Kandyeopam.*

Herb, pleasantly acidic; astrin. and prescribed in diar. [Wlth India, VIII, 199; *Rec Bot Surv India,* 1973, **20**, 175).

Both varieties distributed in Central and Eastern Himalayas and in Mishmi hills at 1,200-2,800 m and also wild in Nilgiris.

ACORUS (*Araceae*)

Biosystematics (*Proc K Ned Acad Wet,* 1978, **81C**, 428; 1979, **82C**, 113; *Planta Med,* 1979, **36**, 350); proposed classification for *Acorus* Linn. accepts only 2 spp.; *A. calamus* and *A. gramineus,* both polytypic (*Ibid,* 1979, **37**, 289).

A. calamus Linn.

Eng.–*Calamus, sweet flag/root/sedge.*

Biosystematics—several chromosomal races. *A. calamus,* aggregate sp.: a) var. *americanus* (Raf.) Wulff, diploid (2n = 24) and ecotypes (at the same time topotypes) and 2 chemotypes w.r.t. essent. oils; b) var. *calamus* Linn. (= var. *vulgaris* Linn.), triploid (2n = 36)) and totally sterile; Europe and also Himalayan region, spread to USA; morphological & chem. homogen.; and c) var. *angustus* Boss., tetraploid (2n = 48), variable in many respects, partly fertile; subtrop. & trop. S.E. Asia, far E. Asia and Japan; 2 chief ecotypes, a (sub)tropical and a temperate;

several chemotypes; a (sub)tropical ecotype, if desirable for practical purposes can be called var. *verus* Linn. (*Planta Med*, 1979, **37**, 289). Classification of commercial calamus: different drug types with varying content of Ph-propane deriv., β-asarone were obtained from *A. calamus*. The Ph-propane deriv. proved to be carcinogenic in several tested animals. Diploid drug did not contain β-asarone; triploids contained 0.3%; and tetraploid yielded two races with (a) 2%; and (b) between 4 and 8% β-asarone (*Planta Med*, 1981, **43**, 128).

Polyploidy in Indian *A. calamus* — Jammu plants, tetraploid (2n = 36); Kashmir plants, hexaploid (2n = 54). Asarone content higher but calamine and camphor contents lower in tetraploids than those in hexaploids confined to higher altitude and there seems to be correlation between chromosome no., altitude and chem. compn. (*Curr Sci*, 1964, **33**, 500). Chemotypes among arom. plants: case of polyploidal calamus. Root morphology, level and chem. compn. of essent. oil with physico- chem. properties and organoleptic characteristics of an aq.-alc. ext. of *A. calamus* Jammu. var. had the highest essent. oil content with a large amt. of β-asarone; in contrast European var. contained a large no. of arom. substances; characteristics of aq.-alc. ext. were significantly different in two varieties. Polyploidal characteristics discussed w.r.t. toxicol. of β-asarone (*Ann Falsif Expert Chim*, 1976, **69**, 833; *CA*, 1977, **87**, 19017d).

Rhizome—aq.(10%) ext. and alc. ext., hypothermic and hypoten. but not analg. and anticonvuls. up to 1g/k dose; latter potentiated action of narcotics and diminished toxicity of amphetamines (*Diss Pharm*, 1965, **17**, 157; *CA*, 63, 18890g); EtOH(50%) ext., spasmol. and CNS depress. (*Indian J Exp Biol*, 1969, 7, 250).

Roots and rhizomes used in various kinds of cancers (*Lloydia*, 1967, **30**, 412). Rhizome, official drug for flatulent colic

and chr. dyspep. Primitives use it as carmin., in catar., haemor. and burns; also as CNS stim., bitter tonic and anthelm. (*Econ Bot*, 1969, **23**, 97). Root for fever, cough and toothache (*ibid*, 1974, **28**, 311). Rhizomes used in headache and for teeth strengthening (*Khadi Gramodyog*, 1972-73, **19**, 271; *Ethnomedicine*, 1980, **6**, 139). Root ext, one of the constituents of tooth paste (USSR Pat., 1972, 353721; *CA*, 1973, **78**, 62202m).

Minor constituent of drug for treating flatulence and diar. in animals (Ger. Offen., 1979, 2611979; *CA*,**87**, 206532e). Rhizome useful in bronch. asthma, clin. trials (*J Res Ayur Siddha*, 1980, **1**, 329); fresh root, useful drug in asthma, clin. trials [*J Res Indian Med*, 1977, **12**(4), 92]. Usefulness of drug in mental disorders (*Sachitra Ayurveda*, 1979-80, **32**, 443).

Rhizomes, nauseant, expect., antisp. and nervine sed. Beneficial in diar. Powd. rhizome, insectic., useful against bed bugs, moths, flies; ext., insectic. against *Dysdercus cingulatus*; rhizome, insect repellent and anthelm. [*Khadi Gramodyog*, 1980-81, **27**, 401; *Indian J Entomol*, 1979, **41**, 91; 1976, **38**, 110; *Indian J Agric Sci*, 1979, **49**, 295; *J Res Indian Med*, 1977, **12**(4), 53].

One of the constituents of Ayurvedic and/or indigenous drugs 'Myostal' useful in puerperal patients, clin. trials; 'Vitafix' useful in premature ejaculation, clin. trials; 'Chandrodayawarti' useful in nebular corneal opacity and pterigium of recent origin [*Maharashtra Med J*, 1979, **26**, 433; *Indian Pract*, 1980, **33**, 81; *J Sci Res Plants Med*, 1981, 2(1&2), 35].

Herb—alc. ext. of plant, anticonvuls. in albino rats (*C R Acad Bulg Sci*, 1965, **18**, 691; *BA*, 1967, **48**, 2517). In epilepsy, indign. and consumption (*Econ Bot*, 1970, **24**, 241); in haemor. (*Nagarjun*, 1979-80, **23**, 11); against alopecia areata [*Farm Zh Kiev*, 1972, **27**(6), 78; *BA*, 1973, **56**, 56516].

Essent. oil from rhizome — calamus oil. with β-asarone as major constituent, carcinogenic in rats (*Proc Am Assoc Cancer*

Res, 1967, **8**, 24; *in* Plant and Fungal Toxins, 252). Neuropharmacol. action of oil from Indian origin (*Arch Int Pharmacodyn Ther*, 1968, **172**, 356; *CA*, **69**, 17829z). Calamus oil, and ext. prohibited from use in human food [*Fed Regist*, 1974, **39**(185), 34172; *CA*, 1975, **82**, 15379x]; antimicrob. [*Indian Perfum*, 1981, **25**(3 & 4), 4]; anthelm. against *Ascaris lumbricoides* (*Ancient Sci Life*, 1981-82, **1**, 103).

Choline content of rhizome, 0.26% [*Aptechn Delo*, 1966, **15**(4), 36; *CA*, **65**, 4091g]. Flavone from rhizomes produced sed. and calming effect on rhesus monkey (*Sci Cult*, 1977, **43**, 218); acoradin, 2,4,5-tri-MeO-benzaldehyde, 2, 5-di-MeO-benzoquinone, galangin and sitosterol (*Indian J Chem*, 1979, **17B**, 412).

Five new sesquiterps. in addn. to calameone (or calamendiol; with revised str.); their strs. (*Tetrahedron*, 1971, **27**, 5419); selinane-type sesquiterps., acolamone & isoacolamone (*Chem Lett*, 1972, 823; *CA*, **77**, 137400q); epoxyisoacoragermacrone (*Bull Chem Soc Jpn*, 1980, **53**, 1263).

Plant, choline, 124mg% (*Farm Pol*, 1966, **22**, 181; *CA*, **65**, 9341c). Chem. compn. of various plant parts (*Bot Sady Pribaltiki*, 1971, 445; *CA*, 1972, **76**, 138157g).

Aerial parts, luteolin-6,8-C-diglucd.; spectrophotom. detn. [*Khim Prir Soedin*, 1974, 94; *Farm Zh Kiev*, 1974, **29**(2), 92; *CA*, **80**, 121271z; **81**, 165718e].

Essent. oil, constituents of calamus oil from rhizomes of Bangladesh; Japan var.; E. Europe (*Sci Res Dacca*, 1967, **4**, 234; *Tetrahedron Lett*, 1968, 5315; 1969, 3729; 1970, 855; *Phytochemistry*, 1979, **18**, 279). Essent. oil, a rev., 299 refs.; insectic. and med. properties; uses and cultivation practices of *A. calamus* reviewed; extn. of oil, physicochem. properties and economics discussed (*Indian Perfum*, 1977, **21**, 103); review part in previous ref. criticized; details of biosystematics along with essent. oil compn. of various regions given.

Diploid *A. calamus* rhizome oil, no β-asarone; leaf top oil, geranyl acetate and/or β-farnesene as main constituents. Triploid *A. calamus* rhizome oil, 8-19% β-asarone; leaf top oils, 31-44% β-asarone but deviated in several constituents from Kashmir, which is reported to be hexaploid but most probably represent triploid populations. Tetraploid Indian type–rhizome oil, more than 90% β-asarone; leaf top oil, 60-70% β-asarone; some more chemotypes discussed (*Planta Med*, 1979, **37**, 289; **36**, 350). Six Ph-propane derivs. including asarones and acoramone & its str. (*J Natl Prod*, 1981, **44**, 668).

Chem. races of med. plants containing essent. oils from roots, compn. varies with ploidy [*Mezhdunar Kongr Efirnym Maslam Mater*, 4th, 1968, (Pub., 1972), **2**, 245; *CA*, 1974, **81**, 74886n].

Asarones—Ph-propane derivs.; one of the active constituents from essent. oil, asarone, *trans*-2,4,5-tri-MeO-1-propenylbenzene [E-1,2,4-tri-MeO-5-(1-propenyl) benzene], CNS depress. in rats; action resembled other CNS-depress. drugs like reserpine, and produced no undesirable side effects such as ataxia or muscle incoordination (*Indian J Exp Biol*, 1965, **3**, 252; Dictionary Org. Compds., 2nd Suppl., 456). Mech. of tranquillizing action (*J Pharm Pharmacol*, 1967, **19**, 170). Synth. and pharmacol.; prolong hypnosis, and hypoten. in dog (*Indian J Appl Chem*, 1969, **32**, 237); also anticonvuls. (*Q J Crude Drug Res*, 1970, **10**, 1555). β-Asarone (Z-form of above-mentioned asarone), chemosterilant (*Nature Lond*, 1977, **270**, 512); its estn.; by reversed-phase HPLC of this suspected carcinogenic principle of essent. oil (*J Chromatogr*, 1965, **17**, 195; 1980, **194**, 245); content in commercial drug (*Pharmazie*, 1981, **36**, 53).

A. gramineus Soland. ex Ait.

Diploid, mostly fertile (*Planta Med*, 1979, **37**, 289). Pet. ether ext. of rhizomes, significant insectic. activity on painted bug (*Bagroda cruciferum*) (*Indian J Entomol*, 1980, **42**, 775).

A. *gramineus* and tetraploid A. *calamus* proved to be very variable w.r.t. essent. oil compn.; in former, variation much more striking for leaf top oils (7 accessions) than for their rhizome oils. If rhizomes alone considered, two chemotypes, β-asarone type (84-92%) (from Japan and Thailand) and a *cis*-Me-isoeugenol (52-55%) + shyobunone-like sesquiterps. (12-24%) type can be distinguished (from Hong Kong). With leaf top oils, five chemotypes discussed. (*Planta Med*, 1979, **36**, 250).

ACROCARPUS (*Caesalpiniaceae*)

*A. fraxinifolius Wight & Arn.

B. & H.–*Mandania, mundani*; Eng.–*Pink* or *red cedar shingla-tree*; Kan.–*Hantige*; Mal.–*Kurunfan*; Tam.–*Kurungan, malaikonnei.*

Various plant exts., antimicrob. (*Indian Drugs*, 1977-78, **15**, 130).

Found in Eastern Himalayas extending to Nagaland and Manipur, and in evergreen forests of S. India.

ACRONYCHIA (*Rutaceae*)

A. pedunculata (Linn.) Miq. syn. *A. laurifolia* Blume

Plant used in fracture (*Sri Lanka For*, 1980, **14**, 145).

Stem bark, alk. bauerenol & K-oxalate (*Phytochemistry*, 1966, **5**, 379). Bark, acrovestone; wood, β-sitosterol (*Indian J Chem*, 1969, **7**, 873; 308); a new phenolic compd. acronylin (*Chem Ind Lond*, 1970, 654); 6-de Me-acronylin (*Indian J Chem*, 1973, **11**, 693).

Leaves of Sri Lanka plant, alk. kokusginine and wood, alk. evolitrine; both not present in Indian plant (*Phytochemistry*, 1979, **18**, 1255).

ACROSTICHUM (*Pteridaceae*)

*A. aureum Linn.

Young fronds edible. Old form an ingredient of med. for syphillitic ulcers. Rhizomes as paste applied on wounds and boils; fronds and rhizomes yield β-

sitosterol, an unknown compd. (mp.94°), flavon., tannin, etc. (Wlth India, IA, 67).

Fern, no. of known compds., as also new ones and their strs. (*Chem Pharm Bull*, 1981, **29**, 3455).

Found in tidal backwaters throughout India.

ACTAEA (*Ranunculaceae*)

A. spicata Linn.

Kan.–*Vishaphale.*

Contains *trans*-aconitic acid, cytostatic; its Me ether active against Ehrlich's ascites tumours (*Aptechn Delo*, 1963, **12**, 36; *CA*, 1964, **61**, 10535b).

ACTINDIA (*Actinidiaceae*)

*A. chinensis Planch.

Eng.–*Chinese gooseberry; kiwi fruit.*

EtOH ext. of leaves, active against Gram +ve bacteria (Wlth India, IA, 69).

Fresh fruit (Indian sample), vit. C, up to 300 mg/100 g; a proteolytic enzyme also present [*Indian Hort*, 1971-72, **16**(2), 13]. Str. of actinidin, a SH protease from fruit (*J Mol Biol*, 1976, **101**, 185).

Native to China, introduced at Lal Bagh Garden, Bangalore.

ACTINIOPTERIS (*Actinopteridaceae*)

A. australis (Linn. f.) Link syn. *A. radiata* Link; *A. dichotoma* Kuhn

Eng.–*Peacock's tail*; Mar.–*Bhui tad.*

Plant used as styptic and anthelm. [*J Res Indian Med*, 1973, **8**(2), 67]. Powd. along with seed of *Ocimum americanum*, antifert. [*ibid*, 1975, **10**(3), 77].

Mature sporophytes contain rutin; and fronds, hentriacontane, hentriacontol, β-sitosterol, its palmitate & also glucd. (*Curr Sci*, 1972, **41**, 788; 1974, **43**, 749).

ACTINODAPHNE (*Lauraceae*)

A. angustifolia Nees syn. *A. hookeri* Meissn.

EtOH(50%) ext. of leaf, spasmol. (*Indian J Exp Biol*, 1968, **6**, 232).

Fruit kernel, monoflaurin, lauric acid, n-hexacosanol, β-sitosterol & its glucd. (*Indian Oilseeds J*, 1964, **8**, 196). Leaves contain β-sitosterol, quercetin 3-rhamnoside and hydrocarbons (*Phytochemistry*, 1971, **10**, 2247).

ACTINORHYTIS (*Aracaceae*)

*A. calapparia Wendl. & Drude
Eng.–*Galappa palm.*
Seeds used as antiscor.; much in demand by native druggists of Java; chewed like betel in Sumatra (Uphof, 11).
Cultivated in IBG, Calcutta.

ADANSONIA (*Bombacaceae*)

A. digitata Linn.
Eng.–*Baobab tree, monkey bread tree.*
Stem bark, β-sitosterol (*Indian J Chem*, 1970, **8**, 851). Plant, promising amt. of pectin (23%) (*Indian J Pharm Sci*, 1978, **40**, 228).
Seed oil (34.4%), characteristics & fatty acid compn. (*Sudan J Food Sci Technol*, 1979, **11**, 15); β-sitosterol, stigmasterol, cholesterol, etc. (*Rev Fr Crops Gras*, 1979, **26**, 447; *CA*, 1980, **92**, 90895x).

ADELOCARYUM (*Boraginaceae*)

*A. coelestinum (Lindl.) Brandis
EtOH(50%) ext. of plant, diur. (*Indian J Exp Biol*, 1974, **12**, 512).
Found in Western Peninsula.

ADENANTHERA (*Mimosaceae*)

A. pavonina Linn.
Eng.–*Coral or red wood, red bead tree.*
Seeds used for treatment of cholera and general paralysis. Decoct. of seeds, in pulmonary affections, and externally applied in chr. ophthalmia. Bark used for washing hair and clothes (Wlth India, IA, 74).
Plant, robinetin, chalcone, butein, ampelopsin(dihydromyricetin) and dihydrorobinetin; ether ext. of wood contains 2,4-di-OH-benzoic acid as major compd. (*Phytochemistry*, 1972, **11**, 1515).

Seeds, dulcitol and stigmasterol (free and as glucd.); leaves, octacosanol; alc. ext. of bark contains saponins which on hydrolysis and methylation yield Me-odeanolate and Me- echynocystate (*Planta Med*, 1973, **23**, 145). Bark, stigmasterol glucd., a saponin, oleanoic and echinocystic acids (*ibid*, 1976, **29**, 176). Seeds, trypsin and chymotrypsin inhibitor; activity lost after heat-treatment for 30 min. at 95° (*Indian J Biochem Biophys*, 1976, **13**, 52; *J Sci Food Agric*, 1980, **31**, 967).

ADENIA (*Passifloraceae*)

*A. heterophylla Koord.
Plant, esp. fruit, poisonous; used as arrow poison. In Philippines, decoct. of roots prescribed for stomach trouble (Wlth India, IA, 75).
Found in Andamans.

ADENIUM (*Apocynaceae*)

*A. obesum Roem. & Schult.
Eng.–*Desert rose*; Mar.–*Aden-cha-kan-her.*
Roots and branches, source of poison used by the natives as arrow poison and to stupefy fish.
EtOH ext. of plant, cytotoxic against human epidermoid carcinoma of the nasopharynx test system. Active ext. contains cardenolides, somalin, hongheloside A, 16-Ac-strospeside, and honghelina and flavonol 3,3'-bis(OMe)-quercetin. Also contains inactive triterp., dehydroifflaionic acid and 3-OMe-kaempferol (*J Pharm Sci*, 1977, **66**, 1336).
Grown in S. India.

ADENOCALYMNA (*Bignoniaceae*)

A. alliaceum Miers.; see **Bignonia capreolata**

ADENOSMA (*Scrophulariaceae*)

*A. indianum Merrill syn. *A. capitatum* Hance
Eng.–*Camphor plant.*

In Ayurvedic system of med., used in preparation of *rasa bhasma* (HgO); also used as febge.

Plant, essent. oil(1%), odour resembling eucalyptus oil; essent. oil possesses flouring effect on Hg (Wlth India, IA, 75).

Outer Himalayas from Kumaun to Sikkim, Assam, Orissa and in Western Ghats.

ADENOSTEMMA (*Asteraceae*)

A. lavenia Kuntze syn. *A. viscosum* J.R. & G. Forst.

EtOH(50%) ext. of plant, diur. (*Indian J Exp Biol*, 1977, **15**, 208). Crushed leaves applied to cuts and wounds; and also to treat bites of poisonous insects and caterpillars (*Econ Bot*, 1981, **35**, 4).

Plant contains *ent*-11-hydroxylated kauranic acids (*Lloydia*, 1979, **42**, 183).

ADHATODA (*Acanthaceae*)

*A. beddomei C.B. Clarke

Mal.–*Cheria astalotakam*; Tam.–*Cinna aatatotai.*

Plant, more powerful and active than *A. zeylanica* and used in mėd. preparations in Kerala as antiemetic, antibechic, haemostatic, particularly in haemorrhages. Fresh leaf juice, beneficial in haemoptysis and menor. (Wlth India, IA, 79).

Found in Kerala up to 900 m; also cultivated.

A. zeylanica Medic. syn. *A. vasica* Nees

Eng.–*Malabarnut, vasaka.*

Leaves—preparation in clarified butter used for glandular tumours (*Lloydia*, 1967, **30**, 379). One of the constituents of drug 'Geriforte' used against senile pruritus and as antifatigue, clin. trial (*Rajasthan Med J*, 1980, **19**, 23; *Indian Drugs*, 1980-81, **18**, 346). Alc. ext., hypoten., bronchodilator, respiratory stim., hypoglyc. and antisp. Crude ext. more useful for respiratory ailments than pure alks., as latter exhibit uterine stim. and bronchoconstrictor as the undesirable side-effects (*Indian Vet J*, 1981, **58**, 107). Shoots in liver-enlargement (*Nagarjun*, 1980-81, **24**, 240). Fresh leaves used in homoeopathy for colds, coryza, coughs, pneum., spitting of blood, fever, jaundice, chixilly, catarrh, whooping cough and broncht. (*Bull Bot Soc Bengal*, 1972, **26**, 25). Leaves and roots, hypoglyc.; leaves antivir. against *Ranikhet disease* virus (*Indian J Exp Biol*, 1968, **6**, 232). Leaves and wood ashes mixed with honey used for coughs and asthma (*Econ Bot*, 1971, **25**, 414). Juice mixed with juice of *Feronia limonia* cures nose bleeding [*J Res Indian Med*, 1978, **13**(4), 92].

Essent. oil of leaves—bronchodilator, also vasicinone and ephedrine, potentiated (*Indian J Pharm Sci*, 1979, **41**, 247); anti-insect and juvenile hormone mimicking activity (*4th Asian Symp Med Plants and Spices*, 1980, 154).

Roots—expect. and mild bronch., antisep., antisp., given in intermittent fever, pulmonary and catar. affections (*Q J Crude Drus Res*, 1970, **10**, 1444). Aq. alc. and other exts., antibact. (Wlth India, IA, 79).

Bot., chem., pharmacol., etc. rev., 11 refs. (*J Nat Integ Med Assoc*, 1980, **23**, 257). *A. vasica*, a source of quinozoline alks., pharmacol., rev., 48 refs. (*Indian Drugs*, 1977-78, **15**, 62).

Ether ext. of alc. ext. of leaves on mild saponification yields a substance vasakin. Exogenous and endogenous Ac-choline and epinephrine are blocked by vasakin which has strong local anaesthetic effect. Vasakin inhibits salivary secretion induced by pilocarpine and is non-toxic in doses up to 1g/kg. In cholinergic-blocking activity it is less potent than atropine (*Planta Med*, 1965, **13**, 194). A non-nitrogenous principle from leaves, feeble hypoglyc. of short duration in male rabbits (*Indian J Pharm*, 1966, **28**, 105).

Plant used against various chest ailments, contains betaine, vasicinone and new alk. vasicinine (1%); in addn., β-sitosterol and tritriacontane in different parts (*Pak J Sci Ind Res*, 1965, **8**, 76; 1967, **10**, 224). Leaves, visicine (0.79%); and flowering tops, 0.47% (*Pak J Sci Res*, 1966, **18**, 109). Mass spectrum of alks., vasicine and vasicinol (*Indian J Chem*, 1966, **4**, 291). Plant from Jammu, alks. in leaves, 0.22%; roots, 0.14%; and seeds, 0.025% (*Indian Drugs*, 1978-79, **16**, 160).

Peganine (vasicine)—the chief active principle is a quinazoline alk.; yield from different leaf samples in India, 0.54 to 1.11% dry wt basis; that from foreign sample as high as 2.18% dry wt basis, consisting of more than half as *l*-form and remaining the *dl*-form; it is accompanied by *l*- vasicinone (Dictionary Org. Compds, IV, 4499; Wlth India, IA, 77). Biosynth. (*Helv Chim Acta*, 1971, **54**, 826). Bitter, bronchodilator, respiratory stim., hypoten., cardiac depress., uterotonic and abortif.; uterotonic action comparable to oxytocin and methergin (*Indian J Pharm*, 1976, **38**, 169; 1977, **39**, 162; *Indian J Med Res*, 1977, **66**, 680, 856; *Indian J Exp Biol*, 1978, **16**, 1075). Absorption and distribution, as novel uterotonic (*Planta Med*, 1980, **40**, 373). Potentiation of prostaglandins-evoked contractions of isolated rat uterus by vasicine-HCl (*Indian J Med Res*, 1981, **73**, 641). Chem. and pharmacol. of Vasicine - a New Oxytocic and Abortif. - a monograph [Atal CK, 1980, pp. 155; *CA*, 1981, **95**, 198090g].

Vasicinone—naturally occurs in *l*-form; racemizes to *dl*-form. *l*-Form more active bronchodilator, β-potentiating and antianaphylactic; useful in extrinsic asthma [Dictionary Org. Compds., V, 5686; *Bull Haffkin's Inst*, 1974, **2**(1), 6; 1976, **4**(2), 43]. Bronchodilatory *in vitro* but bronchoconstrictory *in vivo*; probably biotransformed *in vivo* and *in vitro*. When their mixt. was used, cardiac depress. effect significantly reduced, probably *l*-form is a weak cardiac stim. (*dl*-form has no such effect) (Wlth India, IA, 78); antiasthmatic potentiality (*4th Asian Symp Med Plants and Spices*, 1980, 137). Selective extn. (*Indian J Pharm Sci*, 1981, **43**, 221). Insignificant anthelm. (*Indian Drugs*, 1979-80, **17**, 99).

Flowers, tritriacontane, kaempferol & its glycds., quercetin, β-sitosterol & its glucd. (*Curr Sci*, 1971, **40**, 84). Inflorescence, vasicinone (*Naturwissenschaften*, 1979, **66**, 205); alk., *dl*-vasicinone & *l*-vasicinone (*Indian Agric*, 1977, **21**, 225).

Pharmacol. of alk. vasicinol, isolated from roots (*Indian J Exp Biol*, 1964, **2**, 219). Roots, a galactoside, sitosterol- β-D-glucd., D-galactose and deoxyvasicinone; a novel non-hormonal indole alk., vasicol (*Phytochemistry*, 1980, **19**, 1980; 1981, **20**, 319).

ADIANTUM (*Adiantaceae*)

A. capillus-veneris Linn.

Eng.–*Maidenhair fern*.

Fern—used in cold imposthumes of uterus, hard swellings and hard tumours of spleen (*Lloydia*, 1971, **33**, 385); antibiot. (*Econ Bot*, 1980, **34**, 284).

Fronds—for seasonal cold fever (*J Sci Res BHU*, 1969-70, **20**, 227); sores (*Econ Bot*, 1971, **25**, 245); with honey in catar. affections (*Indian Drugs*, 1977-78, **15**, 87).

Fern, 21-OH-adiantone (*Corsi Semin Chim*, 1968, **1**, 65; *CA*, 1970, **72**, 129386w); triterp., 3,4-epoxyfilicare (*Tetrahedron*, 1969, **25**, 2939); flavons. (*Planta Med Phytother*, 1971, **5**, 177; *CA*, 1972, **76**, 56579g).

A. incisum Forsk. syn. *A. caudatum* Linn.

EtOH(50%) ext. of plant, hypoglyc. and spasmog. (*Indian J Exp Biol*, 1968, **6**, 232). Fern, antibiot.; property varies with season (*Econ Bot*, 1980, **34**, 284). Distribution and local uses (*Sachitra Ayurveda*, 1980-81, **33**, 494).

Fern, hentriacontane, 16-hentriacontanone, adiantone, isoadiantone and β-sitosterol (*Indian J Pharm*, 1975, **37**, 64); femene (*Curr Sci*, 1978, **47**, 624).

A. pedatum Linn.

Eng.–*American maidenhair fern*.

Fronds, femene, isofemene, 7-femene; filicene; filicenal, adiantone and adipedatol (*Tetrahedron Lett*, 1966, 6069).

A. philippense Linn. syn. *A. lunulatum* Burm.

Eng.–*Walking maidenhair fern*.

Roots, in fever; plant in dysen., ulcers, febrile affections (*Indian Drugs*, 1977-78, **15**, 87). Plant alongwith *Asparagus racemosus* in gonor. [*J Res Indian Med*, 1978, **13**(4), 92]. Used for atrophy, emaciation or cachexy, muscular pain, diar., and rabies (*Econ Bot*, 1970, **24**, 241).

A. venustum D. Don

Eng.–*Black maidenhair, venus hair.*

Fronds—used in biliousness, diseases of chest, cold, headache, opthalmia, hydrophobia, inflam., and tumours (*Indian Drugs*, 1976-77, **14**, 136). Ext. inhibited formation of local lesions on *Chenopodium amaranticolor* by cucumber mosaic virus (*Indian J For*, 1980, **3**, 132).

ADINA (*Rubiaceae*)

A. cordifolia (Roxb.) Hook.f. ex Brandis

Used in night blindness, carbuncle, biliary colic, cholera and rinderpest (*Econ Bot*, 1970, **24**, 241). Plant ext., antibact. (*Bull Bot Soc Univ Saugar*, 1980, **27**, 57). Decoct. of stembark given internally in fever and to check yellow colour of urine (*Bull Med Ethno Bot Res*, 1980, **1**, 8).

Heartwood, 10-deoxyadifoline and 10-deoxycordifoline (*Gazz Chim Ital*, 1968, **98**, 974); str. of indole alk., cordifoline (*J Chem Soc Chem Commun*, 1967, 453).

Adifoline—revised str. of alk. from heartwood (*ibid*, 1968, 350); alk. obtained from acetone fraction of wood, CNS-depress. and hypoten. in exp. animals; another fraction, same activities and in addn. contractile activity in guinea pig ileum (*Indian J Pharm*, 1973, **35**, 203).

Oleo-resin from incision of trunk yields essent. oil (5.2-6.8%) (*Perfum Essent Oil Rec*, 1967, **58**, 437). Wood, umbelliferone (*Indian J Chem*, 1967, **5**, 523).

Yellow colouring matter, napthaquinone adinin (*Naturwissenschaften*, 1965, **52**, 2616); stem, di-OH-tetra-OMe flavone (*Indian J Chem*, 1981, **20**, 833); defatted heartwood, 2 flavanones, str. (*Indian J Pharm Sci*, 1981, **43**, 153).

ADONIS (*Ranunculaceae*)

A. aestivalis Linn.

Eng.–*Pheasant's eye.*

Flowers contain alk., 0.29% (*Pak J Sci Ind Res*, 1963, **6**, 53). Leaves and stems, a cardioactive glycd. cymarin (*Lloydia*, 1973, **36**, 426). Roots, sitosterol and ceryl alcohol (*Indian J Chem*, 1976, **14B**, 475).

*A. autumnalis Linn.

Eng.–*Flos adonis, pheasant's eye.*

Herb, bitter and astrin. (Wlth India, IA, 84).

Aerial parts, at flowering and fruiting contain 18 compds. including k-strophanthin-B, cymarin, adonin, adonitoxin, etc. (*J Pharm Sci UAR*, 1969, **10**, 81; *CA*, 1971, **74**, 1038r).

Grown in rockeries, and borders in gardens.

A. chrysocyathus Hook.f. & Thoms.

Kash.–*Marnil, nilmar.*

From whole plant, glycd., str. of sugoroside (*Khim Prir Soedin*, 1971, **7**, 846; *CA*, 1972, **76**, 113484y). Aerial parts, K-strophanthin-B and simarin, spectrophotom. detn. (*ibid*, 1972, **8**, 747; *CA*, 1973, **79**, 45887s).

Max. amt. of cardenolides in generative and at beginning of growth stages of aerial parts and other details (*Rastit Resur*, 1977, **13**, 632; *CA*, 1978, **88**, 19059q).

AEGICERAS (*Myrsinaceae*)

A. corniculatum (Linn.) Blanco syn. *A. majus* Gaertn.

Eng.–*Black mangrove, goat's horn mangrove.*

Bark contains rapanone, 4 triterp. alcs., and echinocystic acid (*Aust J Chem*, 1966, **19**, 169).

AEGINETIA (*Orobanchaceae*)

*A. indica Linn.

Pounded root given in snake-bite (*Nagarjun*, 1980-81, **24**, 1).

Plant, aeginetic acid, aeginetolide and β-sitosterol; 3 apocarotenoid polyenes D, E & F (*Indian J Chem*, 1977, **15B**, 546; 550). Found throughout India.

AEGLE (*Rutaceae*)

A. marmelos Correa ex Roxb.

Eng.–*Bael tree, Bengal quince.*

Fruit—EtOH(50%) ext. hypoglyc. and spasmog.

Root—EtOH(50%) ext., hypoglyc. and spasmog. (*Indian J Exp Biol*, 1968, **6**, 232); ingredient of 'Dasmula' (*Khadi Gramodyog*, 1972-73, **19**, 269); antiemetic (*Indian Drugs*, 1977-78, **15**, 145).

Root bark—useful in hypochondriasis, melancholia and palpitation of heart, and stomach pain (*Q J Crude Drug Res*, 1970, **10**, 1555).

Leaves—febge. (*Khadi Gramodyog*, 1972-73, **19**, 269). Leaf juice applied externally in abscess; ash used to kill worms and injuries caused by animals (*Bull Med Ethno Bot Res*, 1980, **1**, 8; 318).

Seed oil—yield, 32%, oil antibact. (*J Inst Chem India*, 1980, **52**, 59). *In vitro* screening of oil and its unsap. fraction against some bacteria and fungi; later more active (*Proc Indian Sci Congr*, 1980, Pt III, 102).

Plant—various parts used in night fever, convuls., cramps, nausea, constip., stomach-pain, diar., cholera, dysen., postnatal complications, puerperal fever, thirst, breast pain or suppuration, and snake-bite (*Econ Bot*, 1970, **24**, 241).

Plant, marmin, str. (*Tetrahedron Lett*, 1967, 471); minor phenolic alk.; similar to aegelinine (*Sci Cult*, 1967, **33**, 279); str. of two new alks. (*Phytochemistry*, 1978, **17**, 1814).

Alk. aegeline present in leaves efficacious in asthma (*Indian J Med Res*, 1968, **56**, 327).

Leaves, a minor alk., aegelenine, str. (*Indian J Chem*, 1971, **9**, 763); polyphenolic compds. (*J Inst Chem India*, 1975, **47**, 79); lupeol, sitosterol and aegelin; also rutin, marmesinin, β-sitosterol glucd. (*Indian J Chem*, 1979, **17B**, 385; 1980, **19B**, 162).

Essent. oil from leaves, constituents (*Indian Oil Soap J*, 1972, **37**, 301); oil, broad spectrum antifung., activity comparable to 0.5% hamycin [*Indian Drugs Pharmac Ind*, 1977, **12**(1), 55].

Fruit, psoralen, a powerful germination inhibitor and tamic acid (*Pak J For*, 1965, **15**, 250); gum, str. (*Carbohydr Res*, 1977, **54**, 115; *CA*, **87**, 23640u); minor lactonic constituent, aegelinol, str. (*Phytochemistry*, 1978, **17**, 328); furanocoumarin, marmelide (isomer of imperatorin) having tyrosinase-accelerating and tryptophan pyrrolase-inhibiting effect in *Bufo melanosticus* (*Chem Ind Lond*, 1978, 848). Ripe fruits, xanthotoxol; also scoparone, scopoletin, umbelliferone, marmesin, skimmin and β-sitosterol glucd. (*Indian J Chem*, 1980, **19B**, 162).

Bark, β-sitosterol, 2 unidentified alks. (mp 172- 73° and 136-37°) and 2 unknown compds. (*Sci Res Dacca*, 1970, **7**, 122; *CA*, 1973, **78**, 1973s); alc. ext., skimmianine; other constituents (*Bangladesh J Sci Ind Res*, 1978, **13**, 252; 1980, **15**, 16; *CA*, 1979, **90**, 183156s; 1981, **95**, 200604y). Bark, aurapten, marmin, umbelliferone and lupeol (*Indian J Chem*, 1979, **17B**, 385).

Root, xanthotoxin, 6,7-di-OMe-coumarin, scopoletin, tembamide, umbelliferone, marmesin, marmin, skimmianine, glycd. skimmin; non-basic portion of chloroform ext., decursinol and haplopine (*Phytochemistry*, 1973, **12**, 2971; 1974, **13**, 2329).

AEOLLANTHUS (*Lamiaceae*)

*A. myrianthus Baker syn. A. gamwelliae Taylor

Essent. oil-yielding plant; whole plant, 0.72 and flowers, 2.0% with geraniol 80.3 and 77.6% resp. [*Indian Drugs Pharmac Ind*, 1979, **14**(1), 25].

Introduced into India, cultivated in Jorhat, Assam.

AERVA (*Amaranthaceae*)

A. lanata Juss. ex Schult.

Flowers useful in kidney stone and in gonor. (*J Agric Trop Bot Appl*, 1966, **13**, 245).

Herb, diur.; used in haematemesis and diabetes (*Acta Phytother*, 1972, **19**, 141); also used against swelling and cutaneous affections (*J Econ Tax Bot*, 1980, **1**, 37). In white urine, diar., cholera, dysen. and snake-bite (*Econ Bot*, 1970, **24**, 241).

A. persica Merrill syn. *A. javanica* Juss. ex Schult.; *A. tomentosa* Forsk.

Eng.–*Javanese wool plant.*

Decoct. of flowers and seeds applied to inflammed parts of body against swelling. Woolly seeds when stuffed in pillows, relieve headache and protective against rheum. Plant, diur. and demulc. (*J Agric Trop Bot Appl*, 1966, **13**, 245). Seeds used in rheum. (*J Econ Tax Bot*, 1980, **1**, 137).

Plant, β-sitosterol, α-amyrin, fatty acids and kaempferol glycds. (*Egypt J Pharm Sci*, 1977, **18**, 377); β-sitosterol, β-amyrin and kaempferol-3-glycds.; roots, chrysin-7-O-galactoside (*Indian J Chem*, 1973, **11**, 83; 1979, **17B**, 416). Roots, a new flavanone, aervanone (*Phytochemistry*, 1980, **19**, 1265).

*A. pseudo-tomentosa Blatt. & Hall.

EtOH(50%) of plant, anticancer (*Indian J Exp Biol*, 1980, **18**, 594).

Ajmer, Rajasthan.

*A. sanguinolenta Blume syn. *A. scandens* Wall.

B.–*Naria, myriya;* Mundari–*Nauri lupu era.*

In Bihar, roots used in dysen. (Wlth India, IA, 92).

Found throughout India, ascending up to 1,800 m in Himalayas.

AESCHYNOMENE (*Fabaceae*)

*A. indica Linn.

Eng.–*Hard sola;* H.–*Shola.*

EtOH(50% ext. of plant, spermic. in rats and humans (*Indian J Exp Biol*, 1977, **15**, 208; 231).

Seeds, an unidentified alk., kernel, fatty oil (7%) with unsap. matter nujol, oleyl alc. and sterols (*Econ Bot*, 1966, **20**, 138; *Tokyo Gakugei Daigaku Kiyo Dai-4-Bu*, 1972, **24**, 125; *CA*, **77**, 137349e). Leaves contain flavon. reynoutrin (*Shoyakugaku Zasshi*, 1977, **31**, 172).

Found throughout India, ascending up to 1,500 m, and in the Andamans.

AESCULUS (*Hippocastanaceae*)

*A. assamica Griff. syn. *A. punduana* Wall. ex Hiern

Abor–*Sarlok-asing;* Ass.–*Ikuhia, raman-bih;* Khasi–*Dieng-chhang, dola, sangkenrop;* Lakhimpur–*Kaman-bi.*

Powd. bark, as fish poison (Wlth India, IA, 94).

EtOH ext. of aerial parts, diur. and antiamphetaminic (*Indian J Exp Biol*, 1971, **9**, 91).

EtOH ext. of seeds afforded a mixt. of saponins having oleanolic acid, barringrogenol C and protoescigenin-21-tiglate, β-sitosterol, kaempferol and quercetin (*Fitoterapia*, 1981, **52**, 285).

Tropical eastern parts of India ascending up to 1,400 m.

A. hippocastanum Linn.

Eng.–*Horse chestnut tree;* P.–*Pu.*

Seed—exts., antioedematic in various kinds of oedema in exp. animals; curative effect in brain oedema model (*Arzneim Forsch*, 1976, **26**, 402; *CA*, **85**, 391h). Exts. from unpeeled chestnuts meal for therapeutic and cosmetic uses (US Pat., 1965, 3170916; *CA*, **62**, 12997h; Ger. Offen, 1964, 1182385; 1965, 1194529; *CA*, 1965, **62**, 5499a; **63**, 5446a; Fr Demande, 1971, 2077708; *CA*, **77**, 118189m).

Leaves, in Europe, used in whooping cough; bark, astrin. and in fever; in India, antiper. (*Acta Phytother*, 1971, **18**, 21).

Oedema inhibiting action and lessening of vascular fragility by seed exts., due to saponin aescin; its str. (*Ann*, 1963, **669**, 171; *CA*, 1964, **60**, 5565g); seeds of same species show considerable difference in their aescin content (*Arch Pharm Wein*, 1971, **404**, 347; *CA*, **75**, 59808w). Seed flavonols (*Z Physiol Chem*, 1964, **335**, 232; *CA*, **60**, 15968g; *Arzneim Forsch*, 1967, **17**, 546; *CA*, **67**, 84793e).

(A)escin—oedema and varicose veins disappear after 20 days treatment with tablets taken 3 a day containing 250mg of Ca hydroquinonesulphinate and escin (Ger. Offen., 1970, 1966912; *CA*, **73**, 38576m). 100-Fold more effective than butadione in reducing formalin-induced inflam. oedema in mice. A combination of escin with a crystalline flavon. complex (1:10) isolated from horse chestnut had the strongest antiinflammatory action against anaphylactic oedema; flavon. increased intestinal absorption of escin 1.5 fold (*Farmakol Toksikol Moscow*, 1969, **32**, 174; *CA*, **71**, 1952q). Saponin mixt. initially hypoten. followed by a long-lasting hyperten. (*Herba Pol*, 1976, **22**, 154; *CA*, 1978, **88**, 31943f). Aescin (yield, 13%) is a mixt., though obtained in crystalline form; components of aescin given (*in* Wagner & Wolff, 185; *Tetrahedron*, 1969, **25**, 415).

A. indica Colebr. ex Camb.

Eng.–*Himalayan chestnut, Indian horse chestnut.*

Crushed seeds given to increase milk; roots in leucor. (*Econ Bot*, 1971, **25**, 414). Seed oil for healing of wounds; bark paste in dislocated joints [*J Res Indian Med*, 1973, **8**(1), 76]. Stembark, antifung. (*Labdev*, 1971, **9B**, 136). Crushed fruits used for washing clothes (Wlth India, IA, 96).

EtOH(50%) ext. of fruit, diur. (*Indian J Exp Biol*, 1974, **12**, 512; 1971, **9**, 91).

Leaves contain quercetih, β-sitosterol and aescin (*Planta Med*, 1978, **34**, 337); stems, rutin and astragalin (*Fitoterapia*, 1978, **49**, 247); leaves, *n*-hentriacontane, *n*-hentriacontanol, β-sitosterol and palmitone (*J Indian Chem Soc*, 1981, **58**, 1011).

AFRAMOMUM (*Zingiberaceae*)

A. melegueta (Rosc.) K. Schum. syn. *Amomum melegueta* Rosc.

Eng.–*Alligator pepper, grains of paradise, meleguetta pepper.*

Seeds, arom. and pungent. Used to relieve toothache and sometimes as an ingredient in fish poison. Crushed seeds rubbed on the body as counter-irrit. In W. Africa, fruit pulp around the seed, especially before maturity, chewed as stim. (Wlth India, IA, 97). High oxalic acid content in fruit, a serious health hazard as it causes reduced function of heart (*J Nutr Diet*, 1969, **6**, 1).

Grains, a series of pungent compds., 1-(4-OH-3-OMe-Ph)-alkan-3-ones; variation in constituents attributed to different sources of origin and climatic conditions (*Aust J Chem*, 1970, **23**, 369). Pungency due to paradol (*Phytochemistry*, 1975, **14**, 853).

Whole plant, arom. and its decoct. taken internally as a febge. Roots, cardamom-like taste, and given as a decoct. for constip. Root regarded as vermifuge for tapeworms. Juice of young leaves acts as styptic (Wlth India, IA, 97).

AGANOSMA (*Apocynaceae*)

A. dichotoma (Roth) K. Schum. syn. *A. caryophyllata* G. Don

Pet.ether ext. of leaves, anthelm. against earthworms (*Metaphire peguana*) (*Indian Drugs*, 1981-82, **19**, 310).

Leaves contain quercetin, kaempferol and phenolic acids (*Indian J Exp Biol*, 1978, **16**, 512).

A. wallichii G. Don syn. *A. calycina* DC. Oriya–*Maloti*; Tel.–*Paalamalle*.

Plant useful in diseases of bile and blood (Wlth India, IA, 98).

AGAPANTHUS (*Alliaceae*)

*A. africanus Hoffm. syn. *A. umbellatus* L' Herit. Eng.–*African blue lily.*

Plant—antimycotic (Wlth India, IA, 98).

EtOH ext. of air-dried rhizomes, β-sitosterol, yuccagenin and new spirostan sapogenins (*Indian J Pharm*, 1972, **34**, 90; *Phytochemistry*, 1974, **13**, 627; 1975, **14**, 2259).

Introduced into India as ornamental.

AGAPETES (*Ericaceaé*)

*A. saligna Hook. f.

EtOH(50%) ext. of aerial parts, diur. (*Indian J Exp Biol*, 1980, **18**, 594).

Found in Sikkim.

*A. sikkimensis Airy Shaw

Sik.–*Dhungaria phool.*

EtOH(50%) ext. of aerial parts, hypoglyc. (*Indian J Exp Biol*, 1980, **18**, 594).

Found in Sikkim.

AGATI (*Fabaceae*)

See **SESBANIA**

AGAVE (*Agavaceae*)

Agave yields hecogenin, a steroid drug precursor mainly used elsewhere, in the manufacture of corticosteroids, β-methasone and dexamethasone as antiinflammatories. Content of hecogenin in various species grown by Sisal Research Station, Bamra (Orissa) summarized (Asolkar & Chadha, 127, 130).

A. americana Linn.

Eng.–*American aloe, century plant.*

Leaf juice used for warts, cancerous ulcers, and putrid tumours (*Lloydia*, 1967, **30**, 390). Various plant parts used for ascites, dropsy, anasarca, venereal sores, syphilis and dysen. (*Econ Bot*, 1970, **24**, 241).

Leaves, hecogenin extn. (*Indian J Chem*, 1964, **2**, 297); piscidic acid (*Acta Chem Scand*, 1964, **18**, 1979); hecogenin (*Planta Med*, 1971, **19**, 87); TLC sepn. of 9 glycds. including agave-saponin C; steroid saponins (*Khim Prir Soedin*, 1975, **11**, 104;

CA, **83**, 75370t; *J Chromatogr*, 1976, **116**, 482); 9 steroid glycds., 'agave saponins' I-IX (*Pharmazie*, 1975, **30**, 396; *CA*, **83**, 144506f); 10 steroid glycds., 6 of them, spirostanolic and 4, furostanolic; common aglycone was hecogenin (*Dokl Akad Nauk SSSR Biochem*, 1975, **224**, 1442; *CA*, 1976, **84**, 102277x); new steroidal saponins, agavasaponin E & H (*Phytochemistry*, 1975, **14**, 2657). Eight 5 , 25 L - steroidal sapogenins (*Hua Hsueh Hsueh Pao*, 1975, **33**, 149; *CA*, 1976, **85**, 106664q); studies on the variation of sapogenin with geographical regions (*Chih Wu Hsueh Pao*, 1976, **18**, 156; *CA*, **85**, 198079d); hecogenin (*Farm Vestn Ljubljana*, 1981, **32**, 33; *CA*, **95**, 93818x).

Seeds contain steroid sapogenins including hecogenin (*Yao Hsueh Hsueh Pao*, 1965, **12**, 392; *CA*, 1966, **64**, 11553f); flowers, chlorogenin (0.5%) and kaempferol-3-glucd. & 3-rutinoside (*Phytochemistry*, 1970, **9**, 2582).

A. angustifolia Haw. syn. *A. wightii* Drum. & Prain

Eng.–*Dwarf aloe.*

Pharmacol. investigation with aq. ext.; B.P. depress. due to GABA (*J Pharm Pharmacol*, 1962, **14**, 556; 562). Tissue culture ext., antimicrob.; activity due to apigenin (*Indian J Pharm Sci*, 1980, **42**, 113).

Leaves, hecogenin (0.1%), tigogenin (0.44%) and gitogenin (in traces) (*Indian J Exp Biol*, 1979, **17**, 446). Steroidal sapogenins from tissue culture (*J Natl Prod*, 1980, **43**, 459).

A. cantala Roxb.

Eng.–*Bombay aloe, cantala.*

Leaves contain a new glycd. of hecogenin, cantalanin A (*J Natl Prod*, 1981, **44**, 662).

Diosgenin from yams of *A. cantala* (0.1%) and *A. sisalana* (1.0%) [*Bull Calcutta Sch Trop Med*, 1974, **22**(1-4), 8].

A. sisalana Perr. ex Engelm. syn. *A. rigida* Mill. var. *sisalana* Engelm.

Eng.–*Sisal.*

Leaf juice, pharmacol., uterine stim., emmen., laxt. and hypoten. (*Qual Plant Mater Veg*, 1967, **14**, 345).

Leaves, a source of hecogenin; small amts. of tigogenin also present [*Rev Fac Farm Univ Los Andes*, 1971, **8**(12), 51; *CA*, 1974, **80**, 124664j]. In bulbils tigogenin predominated, while in leaves hecogenin. Flowering pole, flower, rhizome and root contain tigogenin as predominant sapogenin; root, also $\Delta^{9(11)}$-hecogenin (*Lloydia*, 1974, **37**, 10). 10 Known steroidal compds. and 2 new tri-OH-sapogenins (*Hua Hsueh Hsueh Pao*, 1976, **34**, 179; *CA*, 1978, **88**, 117762h).

Hecogenin — (as its oxime) extn. from leaf juice (*Rev Soc Quim Mex*, 1974, **18**, 177; *CA*, 1975, **82**, 28508p); extn. method, better recovery (Ger. Offen., 1975, 2439883; *CA*, **83**, 48186f). Isolation of hecogenin, tigogenin and neotigogenin. GLC for estn. (*Steroids*, 1978, **31**, 661; *J Chromatogr*, 1979, **174**, 451); gas chromatogr. detn. (*Cesk Farm*, 1978, **27**, 136; *CA*, 1979, **90**, 12361q); extn. and purification (Span. Pat., 1980, 485514; *CA*, 1981, **94**, 145339t). See also hecogenin in Diosgenin and Other Steroid Drug Precursors (Asolkar & Chadha, 125-52).

A. vera-cruz Mill.

Hecogenin (0.1%) and $\Delta^{9(11)}$-dehydrohecogenin (0.01%) from pressed juice of mature leaves (*Indian J Chem*, 1974, **12**, 429).

Extn. procedure for hecogenin from leaves (0.1% yield); max. amt. in the sediment of juice (*J Indian Inst Sci*, 1981, **63A**, 227).

AGERATUM (*Asteraceae*)

A. conyzoides Linn.

Eng.–*Goat weed, white weed.*

Herb—used internally as a stim. tonic. Juice good remedy in *prolapsus ani*. Boiled with oil, applied externally in rheum. Decoct. or infusion in diar., dysen., colic, rheum. and fever; ash (9.72%), a good source of K (*c*. 28% sol. K salts) (Wlth

India, IA, 108). EtOH(50%) ext., insectic. (*Indian J Exp Biol*, 1978, **16**, 330]; plant, insectic. (*Nagarjun*, 1979-80, **23**, 177).

Leaves—useful in boils; used for fomentation in leprosy and skin diseases; said to prevent tetanus. Juice, as eye lotion (*Khadi Gramodyog*, 1972-73, **19**, 269; Wlth India, IA, 109). Crude ext., antibact. (*Planta Med*, 1977, **32**, 388). Powd. leaf of white-flowered form mixed with black pepper made into snuff, cures headache (*Bull Med Ethno Bot Res*, 1980, **1**, 318); juice used to kill the ticks of hen (*J Econ Tax Bot*, 1981, **2**, 183).

Flower—buds cure cancerous growth, active constituents; phenol, essent. oil (*Nagarjun*, 1980-81, **24**, 240).

Essent. oil—from twigs anthelm. against tapeworms and earthworms; overwhelmingly superior to piperazine citrate (*Indian Perfum*, 1979, **23**, 210); as well as herb, antibact. (*Sci Cult*, 1979, **45**, 327; *Indian Drugs*, 1979-80, **17**, 14); exhibits activity similar to Ac-choline chloride in isolated frog rectus abdominis [*Indian Drugs Pharmac Ind*, 1980, **15**(2), 21].

Herb, friedelin, β-sitosterol & stigmasterol (*Phytochemistry*, 1971, **10**, 899); hydrocarbons, 2 unidentified esters, stigmasterol and α-spinasterol (*Taiwan K'o Hsueh*, 1976, **30**, 101; *CA*, 1977, **86**, 52655n); coumarin and stigmasterol (*Indian J Chem*, 1973, **11**, 840); flavons. (*Acta Pharm Pol*, 1978, **35**, 241; *CA*, **89**, 176387h). Antigonadotropic hormones, precocenes 1 & 2 (*Insect Sci Appl*, 1981, **1**, 373; *CA*, **95**, 147186k).

Leaves as also stem, alks. (*Lloydia*, 1972, **35**, 7, 125). Leaves, stigmast-7-en-3-ol (major component), quercetin, kaempferol, fumaric and caffeic acids (*Indian J Pharm*, 1977, **39**, 108). A new chromone, conyzorigum from leaves of Nigerian plant and its str. (*J Chem Soc Chem Commun*, 1978, 152). In addn., β-sitosterol, stigmasterol, dotriacontene and 7-OMe-2,2-di-Me-chromen(e). New flavone, 5'-OMe-nobiletin from stem and leaves; herb oil, wound-dressing properties (*Phytochemistry*, 1979, **18**, 1863).

Leaves of fresh herb from Dehra Dun, essent. oil (yield, 0.2%); constituents by GLC agerotochromene, 75; its de-OMe-deriv., 10; caryophyllene, 7; γ-cadinene, 1.3%, and several trace constituents (*Perfum Essent Oil Rec*, 1969, **60**, 303). Essent. oil of semi-dried whole herb (yield, 0.16%) tetra-OMe- tetra-Me-3', (4)-dihydro-3', 4S-bichroman (*Indian J Chem*, 1973, **11**, 91); from flower similar to leaf, contains γ-cadinene, caryophyllene, de-OMe-ageratochromene and ageratochromene as main constituents (*Flavour Ind*, 1973, **4**, 77); from plant grown in N. Vietnam, ageratochromene (53-55%) and de-OMe-ageratochromene (30-32%) (*Tap Chi Hoa Hoc*, 1976, **14**, 29; *CA*, 1977, **86**, 2364w). 7-OMe-2, 2β-di-Me- ageratochromene (60%), major component [*Univ Indore Res J Sci*, 1980, **6**(2), 6].

*A. houstonianum Mill.

Herb yields an essential oil with ageratochromene as one of the constituents; also contains β-sitosterol, stigmasterol, friedelin & its -3 β-ol (Wlth India, IA, 109; *Phytochemistry*, 1971, **10**, 899).

Native of Mexico, common at hill-stations of India.

AGLAIA (*Meliaceae*)

A. diepenhorstii Miq. syn. *A. odoratissima* Blume *A. roxburghiana* Hiern non Miq.

Root and bark, acrid and bitter; in Ayurveda prescribed in dysen., fever and skin diseases. Leaves, emetic and used in abdominal pain.

Fruits and seeds, sweet, acrid and astrin.; given in biliousness and uterine complaints (Wlth India, IA, 110).

EtOH(50%) ext. of aerial parts, anticancer (*Indian J Exp Biol*, 1973, **11**, 43).

Roots, sitosterol (*Indian J Chem*, 1976, **14B**, 473).

A. elaegnoidea (A. Juss.) Benth. syn. *A. roxburghiana* Miq.

Seeds useful in painful micturition (Wlth India, IA, 110).

Leaves, a bis-amide of 2-aminopyrolidine, viz. roxburghilin & its 2-epimer (*J Chem Soc Perkin Trans I*, 1979, 3171).

A. odorata Lour.

Eng.–*Chinese rice-flower.*

Decoct. of roots and leaves used as tonic in China and Malaysia. Leaves, pectoral, stim. and antipyr.; also used in convuls. and menor. Infusion of flowers given in eruptive fevers and V.D. (Wlth India, IA, 110).

Leaves from Thai plant yield a compd., aglaiol (*Tetrahedron*, 1965, **21**, 917); Absolute configuration of aglaiol, an epoxytriterpene (*J Chem Soc Chem Commun*, 1973, 115); str. of aglaiondiol and 2 isomers of aglaitriol from Thai plant (*Tetrahedron*, 1974, **30**, 2211); str. of two dammarane triterp. (24*S*)- & (24*R*)-aglaitriol from plant (*J Chem Soc Perkin Trans I*, 1977, 519). Leaves of Thai plant, alks. odorine and odorinol (*Tetrahedron Lett*, 1979, 2247); odorine identical with roxburghiline (*Aust J Chem*, 1980, **33**, 1841).

AGLAONEMA (*Araceae*)

*A. commutatum Schott

Leaves used to reduce swellings (Wlth India, IA, 111). Leaves contain α- & β-carotenes; floral buds, carotenoids (small amts.); fruits, carotenoids and seeds, lutein (*Stud Cercet Biochem*, 1968, **11**, 287).

Cultivated as pot-herb.

*A. pictum Kunth

Roots anthelm. and tonic; leaves eaten as vegetable in Malaysia (Wlth India, IA, 111).

Cultivated as pot-herb.

AGRIMONIA (*Rosaceae*)

A. eupatoria Linn. syn. *A. pilosa* Hook.f. non Ledeb.; *A. pilosa*, Ledeb. var. *nepalensis* (D. Don) Nakai

Eng.–*Agrimony, cocklebur, stickle wort*.

Plant—dried flowering plant, astrin., antiinflam. and antibiot. Its actions on biliary secretion against calculi and as diur., doubtful (Med. Plants, 76); aq. ext. inhibited *Mycobacterium tuberculosis*; also those strains resistant to streptomycin and *p*-aminosalicylate (*Rev Med Targu-Mures*, 1964, **10**, 190; *CA*, 1965, **62**, 3150g). EtOH ext., antivir. against Columbia SK virus in mice (*Med Pharmacol Exp*, 1967, **16**, 407). Liquid preparation by mixing 80-90% EtOH exts. of plant among others for treating psoriasis and sebrrhoic eczemas (Czech. Pat., 1980, 185262; *CA*, 1981, **95**, 68027f).

Essent. oil, antibact.; active against *Bacillus subtilis* (*Indian Oil Soap J*, 1971-72, **37**, 230).

Dried flowering plant contains tannin, a little volat. oil and resin (Med. Plants, 76).

Agrimonolide—from plant reduced amplitude and tonus of an excised rabbit intestine and stopped movement of intestine at relaxation stage, also depressed peristalsis of mouse, *in vivo* (*Kumamoto Pharm Bull*, 1962, No.5, 58; *CA*, **60**, 992e). Str. of isocoumarin, *dl*-agrimonolide (*Chem Pharm Bull*, 1976, **24**, 200).

Plant flavons., hyperoside, luteolin and quercetin (*Izv Durzh Inst Kontrol Lek Sredstva*, 1977, **10**, 103; *CA*, 1978, **89**, 72948a); also glycds. of last two and apigenin 7-glucd. (*Diss Pharm Pharmacol*, 1972, **24**, 79; *CA*, **77**, 2772s). Str. of agrimols A, B, D & E from Chinese drug *A. pilosa* (*Hua Hsueh Hsueh Pao*, 1978, **36**, 35; *CA*, 1979, **90**, 19009q).

Rhizome, vanillic acid, *l*-taxifolin, ellagic acid and a triterp. compd. (*Kumamoto Pharm Bull*, 1962, No.5, 54; *CA*, 1964, **60**, 5891e). Taenifuge agrimophol from root sprout (*Hua Hsueh Hsueh Pao*, 1977, **35**, 87; *CA*, 1978, **89**, 20275j). TLC detn. of agrimophol in buds of *A. pilosa* (*Yao Hsueh T'ung Pao*, 1980, **15**, 6; *CA*, 1981, **95**, 49482j).

AGROPYRON (*Poaceae*)

A. repens Beauv. syn. *Triticum repens* Linn.

Eng.–*Couch grass, dog grass*.

Rhizome or root—juice used for scirrhous liver; its tea for cancer; decoct. for tumours on tonsils (*Lloydia*, 1969, **32**, 189); urinary antisep. Used in skin erruptions and rheum. complaints (Med. Plants, 31).

Aq. ext. orally to rats showed diur. effect; w. alc. ext. in parenteral administration showed max. efficiency (*Rev Med Tirgu-Mures*, 1971, **17**, 82; *CA*, **75**, 128341c). Infusion of rhizome showed pronounced sed. action on male albino mice, not central; sedation, a menifestation of toxicity (Wlth India, IA, 112). Phytoestrogenic and phototoxic effects on mouse (*Can J Zool*, 1980, **58**, 1575).

Rhizomes contain triticin, a carbohydrate allied to starch, K salts, essent. oil (small amts.) with antibiot. properties; possibly a saponin. Action not well defined (Med. Plants, 31). Antibiot. effect of agropyrene isolated from essent. oil of root-stock (*Cesk Mykol*, 1959, **13**, 183; *CA*, 1962, **56**, 5208e). Rhizome, (+)-abscisin II [(+)-dormin] (*Planta*, 1967, **76**, 93); (+)-abscisic acid [*Biochem Physiol Plant Growth Subst, Proc Int Conf Plant Growth Subst*, 6th, 1967 (Pub. 1968), 1531; *CA*, 1971, **74**, 28793n]; phytotoxin, growth inhibitor (*Weed Sci*, 1981, **29**, 155).

Aq. ext. contains 2 compds. capable of inhibiting growth of maize and lucerne seedlings (*Diss Abstr*, 1962, **22**, 3796).

Ergot sclerotia grown on grass contain ergothioneine (0.36%), ergotamine, etc. (Wlth India, IA, 112).

AGROSTEMMA (*Caryophyllaceae*)

A. githago Linn. syn. *Lychnis githago* Scop.

Eng.–*Corn cockle*.

Plant, toxic to both man and animals; seeds, most poisonous; intensity of poisoning depends on contamination of wheat or wheat-flour. Symptoms of poisoning given. Seeds, diur., emmen. and expect., prescribed in dropsy and jaundice. Root used for treating haemorrhoids and exanthema. Flower ext. inhibits growth of *Bacillus subtilis* (Chopra *et al*, I, 184; Wlth India, IA, 113).

Seed saponin had LD_{50} in rats 2.3 (mg/kg) (*Arzneim Forsch*, 1962, **12**, 815; *CA*, **57**, 15752e). Saponin, githagin (agrostenin, 4.7%) yielding githagenin probably identical with gypsogenin of *Gypsophilla* spp.; githagin responsible for poisoning among poultry, household animals and human beings (Wlth India, IA, 114; Chopra *et al.*, I, 184). Monodesmosidic triterp. glycd., githagoside as main glycd. of seeds, gave gypsogenin on hydrolysis; quillaic acid, as aglycon of minor saponins (*Chem Ber*, 1974, **107**, 2710). Protease inhibitor (trypsin inhibitor) from embryos (*Biol Rundsch*, 1975, **13**, 120; *CA*, **83**, 106775 y; *Biol Zentralbl*, 1975, **94**, 569; *CA*, 1976, **84**, 86753 s). Method for detn. of allantoin in seeds (*Anal Biochem*, 1978, **91**, 304). Seeds contain free and combined phenolic acids of benzoic and cinnamic series (*Plant Med Phytother*, 1979, **13**, 192).

Petal, flavons. & their glycds. (*ibid*, 1980, **14**, 148).

AIDIA (*Rubiaceae*)

*****A. tetrasperma**(Roxb.) Yamazaki syn. *Randia tetrasperma* Hook. f.

Jaunsar–*Bhedra, chhota gingaru, danwa*; Kumaun–*Bara garri, botya gingaru*; P.–*Kikra.*

Alc. ext. of plant, hypoten. accompanied by haemolysis due to saponins (Wlth India, IA, 115).

Roots, *d*-mannitol, scopoletin and saponin (Wlth India, VIII, 362); stems and leaves scopoletin (0.2%), *d*-mannitol (1%), β-sitosterol (0.1%), glucose, galactose and saponin; saponin gave 2 triterp. acid sapogenins, randialic acid A & B (*Planta Med*, 1977, **32**, 229).

Found in sub-tropical Himalayas from Kashmir to Sikkim and in Assam up to 2,000 m.

AILANTHUS (*Simaroubaceae*)

A. altissima (Mill.) Swingle syn. *A. glandulosa* Desf.

Eng.–*Ailanto, tree of heaven.*

In Africa, root and bark used in epilepsy (*Lloydia*, 1967, **30**, 4). Stem bark, antisp., active vermifuge and in powd. form, narcotic with strong nauseating odour. It exercises powerful depressing influence on nervous system similar to that of tobacco.

Plant ext., acoricide (*Zashch Rast Vred Bolez*, 1973, **2**, 167; *CA*, **81**, 146847 a). Leaves produce dermatitis, and their accumulation in well-water produces chr. gastritis (Wlth India, IA, 115-16).

Root bark, 4 indole alks., canthin-6-one & its 1-OMe-deriv., Me-4-OMe-β-carboline-1-carboxylate and an unidentified one (*Planta Med*, 1980, **40**, 337); 1-OH-canthin-6-one (*Fitoterapia*, 1981, **52**, 183); some more alks. (*Chem Pharm Bull*, 1981, **29**, 3900); shinjudilactone (*Chem Lett*, 1981, 597).

Stem bark (dried), quassin & neoquassin (*Boll Chim Farm*, 1965, **104**, 485; *CA*, **63**, 18646d). Defatted bark gave bitter compds., ailanthone and amarolide & Ac-amarolide (*Tetrahedron Lett*, 1965, 2273); a new bitter principle, shinjulactone B (*Chem Lett*, 1981, 1797).

Leaves contain quercetin, caffeic and gallic acids (*Blumea*, 1966, **14**, 309); unidentified alk. (*Qual Plant Mater Veg*, 1970-71, **20**, 311). Leaves, an antivir. phenolic protein [*Fitontsidy Mater Sovesch*, 6th, 1969 (Pub. 1972), 147; *CA*, 1973, **78**, 55310s]; 2-hexenal (*Phytochemistry*, 1972, **11**, 607).

Plant, 2,6-di-OMe-quinone and a compd., ailantone (*Atti Acad Nazl Lincei Rend Classe Sci Fis Mat Nat*, 1963, **35**, 348; *CA*, 1964, **61**, 10719b); str. of bitter ailant(h)one (*Tetrahedron Lett*, 1964,

3991). Plant, ailantone derivs., having antiamoebic properties (*Farm Ed Sci*, 1981, **36**, 116).

Wood alk., canthin-6-one, its 3-oxide & 1-OMe-derivs. (*Chem Pharm Bull*, 1976, **24**, 1532).

Seeds, 2,6-di-OMe-benzoquinone, chaparrinone, ailant(h)one, and ailantholide (*Tetrahedron Lett*, 1964, 3983).

A. excelsa Roxb.

Eng.–*Tree of heaven.*

Pharmacognosy of stem bark [*J Res Indian Med*, 1976, **11**(3), 61]. Bark decoct. for cure of wounds (*Econ Bot*, 1978, **32**, 278).

Leaves used as adulterant for *Adhatoda zeylanica* leaves (*Indian J Pharm*, 1970, **32**, 66). Leaves, ill-smelling; leaves and bark applied to skin irruptions (*J Econ Tax Bot*, 1980, **1**, 137). Leaf ext. contains a protein-like stable inhibitor which exhibited 100% inhibition of tobacco mosaic virus at 1:2 dilution (*Tob Res*, 1981, **7**, 192).

Root bark contains quassinoids, ailanthinone, glaucarbuninone, glaucarubol-15-isovalerate and 13, 18-dehydroglaucarubol-15-isovalerate; all compds., antitumour against P-388 lymphocytic leukaemia, and cytotoxic against KB test system. In addn., alks. canthin-6-one and its 1-OMe-, 5-OMe- & 8-OH-derivs. (*Lloydia*, 1977, **40**, 579; 1978, **41**, 166); a new triterp. (*Phytochemistry*, 1980, **19**, 1499).

Bark ext. yields five C_{20}-quassinoids, one identified as glaucarubin (*Indian J Chem*, 1978, **16B**, 1045); quassinoids, excelsin, 13, 18-dehydroexcelsin and glaucarubol (*ibid*, 1980, **19B**, 183; *Phytochemistry*, 1980, **19**, 2484).

*****A. integrifolia** Lamk ssp. **calycina**(Pierre) Nooteboom syn. *A. grandis* Prain

Ass.–*Borpat,* Khasi–*Diang-chao.*

Stem bark yields 2 antineoplastic quassinoids, 6-α-tigloyloxychaparrinone and 6-α-tigloyloxychaparrin; both inhibit growth of murine P 388 lympocytic leukaemia cell line *in vitro*, while only former active *in vivo* (*J Natl Prod*, 1980, **43**, 503).

Eastern Himalayas, and also in forests of W. Bengal, Meghalaya and Assam.

A. triphysa (Dennst.) Alston syn. *A. malabarica* DC.

Triterps. of trunk exudate, malabaricol, epoxymalabaricol and malabaricanediol; str. of malabaricol, chief triterp. of oleoresin (*Tetrahedron Lett*, 1967, 4837; 1979, 4153).

Roots, β-sitosterol (*Indian J Chem*, 1971, **9**, 611). Stem bark and roots contain eight β-carboline alks. (*Heterocycles*, 1977, **7**, 193; *CA*, 1978, **88**, 34493v).

AINSLIAEA (*Asteraceae*)

*****A. aptera** DC.

H.P.–*Kauri buti.*

Roots used in acute stomachache; a dose of 2g taken with lukewarm water relieves severe pain [*J Res Indian Med*, 1973, **8**(1), 76]. EtOH(50%) ext. of plant, diur. (*Indian J Exp Biol*, 1973, **11**, 43).

Found in Himalayas from Kashmir to Bhutan at 2,400-3,900 m, extending to Khasi hills of Meghalaya.

*****A. latifolia**·Sch.-Bip. syn. *A. pteropoda* DC.

EtOH(50%) ext. of plant, antiprot. and spasmog. (*Indian J Exp Biol*, 1968, **6**, 232). Herb flavon. (*Lloydia*, 1972, **35**, 288). Found in Himalayas.

AISANDRA (*Sapotaceae*)

A. butyracea (Roxb.) Baehni syn. *Diploknema butyracea* (Roxb.) Lamk; *Bassia butyracea* Roxb.; *Madhuca butyracea* (Roxb.) Macbr.

Eng.–*Hill mahua, Indian butter tree.*

Seed fat used in an ointment for rheum. (Wlth India, IA, 120). EtOH(50%) ext. of seeds, spasmog.; and antifert. in rats and human (*Indian J Exp Biol*, 1968, **6**, 232; *ibid*, 1977, **15**, 231). Oil cake used as fish poison, worm killer, applied over lawns and golf-greens for destroying earthworms and as insectic.

Bark used as fish poison; contains glucds., bassianin a, b & c (Wlth India, IA, 120; *Curr Sci*, 1966, **35**, 223).

Seed kernels yield fat called *Phulwa* or *Phulwara* butter, 55-66%; fat good source of pharmaceutical grade palmitic acid, which is suitable for manufacture of vitamin A-palmitate (*Indian Oil Seeds J*, 1963, **7**, 233; *Res Ind*, 1962, **7**, 63). EtOH Ext. of nut kernel contains flavon. mixt. of quercetin, 10; and dihydroquercetin, 90% (*J Org Chem*, 1962, **27**, 2636); also saponins, sterol glucd., and flavons. (*J Sci Ind Res*, 1962, **21D**, 102). Saponin fraction from seeds, spermic. against human spermatozoa (*Indian Drugs*, 1979-80, **17**, 6).

Leaves contain epiprotobassic acid (*Indian J Pharm Sci*, 1981, **43**, 67).

Flowers contain large amts. of nectar, easily collected by bees (Wlth India, IA, 119). Fruit pulp, edible; vit. C (27-36 mg/100g) (*Indian J Agric Sci*, 1971, **41**, 1084).

AJUGA (*Lamiaceae*)

A. bracteosa Wall. ex Benth.

EtOH(50%) ext. of plant, spasmog. and anticancer (*Indian J Exp Biol*, 1968, **6**, 232).

Leaf juice, blood purifier; powd., for burns and boils (*Econ Bot*, 1971, **25**, 414). Plant juice mixed with juice of *Centella asiatica* is given to women in gonor. and also in intermittent fever accompanied with shivering (*Bull Med Ethno Bot Res*, 1980, **1**, 1).

An alk. fraction of leaves had cardiostim. action on frog heart, rabbit auricle and rat ventricle (*Indian J Physiol Pharmacol*, 1962, **6**, 224).

Ecdysteroids from 6 genera including *Ajuga*, their occurrence, isolation, estn. and possible usefulness in new insecticides; rev., 80 refs. (*Khim Prir Soedin*, 1981, 685).

*A. macrosperma Wall. ex Benth.

Root used for colic and consumption (Bressers, 118).

Aka and Khasi hills and Upper Gangetic Plain, extending to Bihar and parts of Tamil Nadu.

ALANGIUM (*Alangiaceae*)

A. salviifolium (Linn.f.) Wang. syn. *A. lamarckii* Thw.

Fruit, preventive and a cure for eye ailments (*Econ Bot*, 1965, **19**, 236). EtOH(50%) ext. of leaves, spasmol., antiprot. and hypoglyc. (*Indian J Exp Biol*, 1968, **6**, 232). Various plant parts used in enlargement of spleen, dropsy, anasarca, colic pain, stomach-ache, *prolapsus ani* and *fistula ani*, cholera, phthisis, broncht. and snakebite (*Econ Bot*, 1970, **24**, 240). Powd. of root bark used in poisonous bites (*Bull Bot Surv India*, 1973, **15**, 13); Root paste or decoct. cures skin diseases (*Econ Bot*, 1978, **32**, 282). Bark ext. taken orally for lowering B.P. Ext. of flowers and fruits used externally to cure eye sores (*J Econ Tax Bot*, 1980, **1**, 137). Seeds, cooling and tonic; used in treatment of haemor. and as a cure for boil (Wlth India, IA, 123).

Root bark, alk. Al 64 (*Indian J Chem*, 1964, **2**, 468); alks. marckidine; and marckine & its str. (*Pak J Sci Ind Res*, 1965, **8**, 161; 166; *CA*, 1968, **68**, 899d; 29931u); tubulosine and cephaeline (*Lloydia*, 1965, **28**, 212); tubulosine & its Me deriv.; isotubulosine in roots (*Curr Sci*, 1966, **35**, 281; *Tetrahedron Lett*, 1966, 1081; 5077) also psychotrine, de-Me-psychotrine and a new alk. alangicine & its str. and stereochem. (*ibid*, 1967, 2143; 1976, 2553). Alc. ext. of root bark after sepn. of alks. yielded myricyl alc., wax and stigmasterol and β-sitosterol (*Vijanana Parishad Anusandhan Patrika*, 1966, **9**, 147).

Alkaloidal ext. of leaves, mild adrenolytic, antisp., hypoten. and anticholinesterase activity; pharmacol. of choline present in leaves (*Indian J Med Res*, 1965, **53**, 1055; 1966, **54**, 1060; *Ex-*

perientia, 1966, **22,** 287). Leaves of Indian plant yield alk., ankorine (*J Pharm Sci,* 1965, **54,** 481); str. revision of ankorine; its chem. correlation with *Cinchona* alks. (*Tetrahedron Lett,* 1974, 3725; 1975, 1527; 1965); also deoxytubulosine, alangimarckine, dehydroprotoemetine; str. of alangimarckine (*ibid,* 1966, 4965; 1978, 3111).

Constituents of leaves other than alks., steroids and triterps. (*Experientia,* 1966, **22,** 647); stigmasta-5,22,25-trien-3β-ol, myristic acid and 3 unidentified triterps; new D, E-*cis*-fused neohopane derivs., alangidiol & its isomer; their str.; also N-benzoyl-*L*-Ph-alaninol (*Tetrahedron Lett,* 1971, 365; 1975, 4275; *Indian J Chem,* 1974, **12,** 1218).

Alk., Al 60 from stem bark caused vasodepress. in atropinized and dibenamine-treated cats and also exhibited musculotropic activity on smooth muscle (*Ann Biochem Exp Med,* 1961, **21,** 109). Bark, alk. lamarchinine (*Pak J Biol Agric Sci,* 1965, **8,** 211; *CA,* 1966, **64,** 9782e); de-Me-cephaeline alongwith cephaeline, Al 60, tubulosine, psychotrine & its de-Me deriv.; Al 60, hypoten. (*Experientia,* 1970, **26,** 933).

Total alks. of seeds show a sustained and prolonged hyperten. effect at lower and hypoten. effect at higher doses in cat (*Ann Biochem,* 1962, **22,** 23; 1963, **23,** 285; Wlth India, IA, 123). Seed alks., include emetine, cephaeline, N-Me-cephaeline and psychotrine (*Tetrahedron,* 1964, **20,** 399); minor phenolic alks., alangamide (*Indian J Chem,* 1969, **7,** 635); novel quinolizine alks., alangimarine, alamarine, and alangimaridine (*Tetrahedron Lett,* 1980, **21,** 2667); deoxytubulosine (*Planta Med,* 1980, Suppl., 5). Constituents other than alks., betulin, betulinaldehyde, lupeol, betulinic acid & its hydroxy lactone A and β-sitosterol (*Phytochemistry,* 1968, **7,** 461).

Plant (root, leaves and fruit) yield monoterp. lactam, alangiside; its str., also isolation of loganic acid (*J Chem Soc D,* 1971, 904; *J Chem Soc Perkin Trans 1,* 1975, 1245). Plant yields venoterpine, *dl*-salsoline and isocephaeline (*Planta Med,* 1980, Suppl., 5).

ALBIZIA (*Mimosaceae*)

A. amara Boivin

Dried leaves, as substitute for soap (Santapau & Henry, 7); leaves toxic to rams (*J Res Punjab Agric Univ,* 1969, **6,** 388); paste used to kill worms in wounds of animals (*Indian J For,* 1981, **4,** 115).

EtOH(50%) ext. of aerial parts, spasmog. (*Indian J Exp Biol,* 1974, **12,** 512). EtOH ext. of seed, antibact. (*Indian Drugs,* 1979-80, **17,** 239).

Bark, β-sitosterol (*Indian J Pharm,* 1965, **27,** 231); leaves, flavon. glycd., 4'-O Me-quercetin-3-rutinoside (*Indian J Chem,* 1967, **5,** 613). Heartwood, melacacidin & its 3-Me-ether and melanoxetin & its 3'-Me ether (*ibid,* 1977, **15B,** 201).

A. chinensis (Osbeck) Merrill syn. A. stipulata Boivin

Aq. ext. of powd. bark, uterine constrictor; a process for extn. of active material (Brit. Pat., 1964, 952588; *CA,* **60,** 15686a). Leaves toxic to rams (*J Res Punjab Agric Univ,* 1969, **6,** 388). EtOH(50%) ext. of aerial parts, spasmog. and diur. (*Indian J Exp Biol,* 1974, **12,** 512).

A. julibrissin Durazz.

EtOH(50%) ext. of aerial parts, diur. (*Indian J Exp Biol,* 1977, **15,** 208).

Fresh tissues contain serotonin and norepinephirine (*Phytochemistry,* 1973, **12,** 191). Heartwood constituents (*Mokuzi Gakkaishi,* 1975, **21,** 577; *CA,* 1977, **84,** 102290w). EtOH ext. of bean valves yields a saponin, albiside (*Khim Prir Soedin,* 1977, 708; *CA,* 1978, **88,** 85989u). Flavons. (*Agric Biol Chem,* 1980, **44,** 1407).

A. lebbeck (Linn.) Willd.

Pods—EtOH(50%) ext., antiprot., hypoglyc. and anticancer; spermic. against rat and human spermatozoa at 2% conc.

(*Indian J Exp Biol*, 1968, **6**, 232; 1977, **15**, 231).

Seeds—hypoglyc., anticancer (*Indian J Exp Biol*, 1968, **6**, 232); abortif. (*Q J Crude Drug Res*, 1972, **12**, 1922).

Roots—same properties as pods except antiprot.

Bark—decoct., active on blood vessels of different animals; also pharmacol. studies [*J Res Indian Med*, 1976, **11**(3), 14; 1977, **12**(3), 37]. Aq. ext. decreased histamine-induced bronchospasm in guinea pigs; aq. ext. may prove protective in bronch. asthma and other allergic disorders (*Indian J Exp Biol*, 1979, **17**, 915); aq. ext. used against conception in women (*Indian J For*, 1981, **4**, 115). Bark, analg. (*J Sci Res Plants Med*, 1981, **2**, 110).

Pod saponin, labbekanin C (*Planta Med*, 1973, **24**, 183).

Seeds yield a mixt. of saponins lebbekanin A (major) & B (*J Indian Chem Soc*, 1970, **47**, 907); echinocystic and oleanolic acids as major sapogenins (*Bull Chem Soc Jpn*, 1970, **43**, 446); triterp. saponin, lebbekanin A from seeds; its partial str. (*Indian J Chem*, 1973, **11**, 1094); saponin prevented ovulation in 60% of the treated animals (*Indian J Pharm*, 1974, **36**, 77); saponin lebbekanin A; pharmacol. studies [*J Res Indian Med*, 1976, **11**(2), 113].

Heartwood, malanoxetin, *d*-pinitol, okanin and leucopelargonidin good source of first two compds.; melacacidin & its 3-Me ether and melanoxetin & its 3-Me ether also present (*Indian J Chem*, 1966, **4**, 139; 1977, **15B**, 201). Wood, saponin lebbekanin E, which exhibited spermic. activity (*J Indian Chem Soc*, 1976, **53**, 859; *Nat Acad Sci Lett India*, 1979, **2**, 135).

Bark contains 7-11% condensed tannin and also *d*-catechin and *d*-leucocyanidin (*Leath Sci*, 1965, **12**, 21). Bark yields 7 compds. including friedelan-3-one and γ-sitosterol (*Curr Sci*, 1974, **43**, 46; *Steroids*, 1963, **2**, 505).

Leaves, echinocystic acid and β-sitosterol (*Indian J Appl Chem*, 1969, **32**, 73). Leaves yield flavon., vicenin II (*Shoyakugaku Zasshi*, 1977, **31**, 172; *CA*, 1978, **88**, 148947b).

Flowers yield triterp. saponin labbekanin D (*J Indian Chem Soc*, 1975, **52**, 1202); 4 saponin glycds., lebbekanins D, F, G & H (*Indian J Chem*, 1978, **16B**, 131).

*A. moluccana Miq.

Seeds, hypoglyc. and hypocholesteromic in rats (*Indian J Med Sci*, 1972, **26**, 729).

Introduced into India from Java.

*A. myriophylla Benth.

Plant used in phthisis, broncht. and asthma (*Econ Bot*, 1970, **24**, 241).

Occurs in Eastern Himalayas, Assam and Khasi hills.

A. odoratissima Benth.

Seeds, hypoglyc. on normal albino rats (*Indian J Med Res*, 1976, **64**, 754). EtOH(50%) ext. of seeds, semen coagulant and diur. (*Indian J Exp Biol*, 1977, **15**, 208).

Heartwood, *d*-O-penta-Me-dihydromelanoxetin (*Tetrahedron*, 1963, **19**, 1371).

A. procera Benth.

Bark, piscic. (*Econ Bot*, 1970, **24**, 134). Paste of stem bark applied in backache (*Bull Med Ethno Bot Res*, 1980, **1**, 8).

EtOH(50%) ext. of aerial parts, anticancer (*Indian J Exp Biol*, 1971, **9**, 91).

Bark, β-sitosterol (*Indian J Pharm*, 1965, **27**, 231). Heartwood and bark, yielded 4 isoflavones viz., biochanin A; formononetin, genistein and daidzein, and heartwood, also a new pterocarpan (*Indian J Chem*, 1977, **15B**, 201).

A saponin from seeds (from Maharashtra); saponin on hydrolysis gave proceric acid (*J Pharm Sci*, 1964, **53**, 1532). Seeds from W. Bengal contain a triterp., procerogenin A also mechaerinic and proceric acids and 4 triterp. sapogenins (*Tetrahedron Lett*, 1966, 5743; *Experientia*, 1967, **23**, 182); str. of proceric acid (*Bull Nat Inst Gas*, 1972, **305**, 280; *CA*, **77**, 45522c); its partial str. (*Indian J Chem*,

1973, **11**, 1189); proceranin A, hypoten. in animals [*J Res Indian Med*, 1975, **10**(4), 45]. An oleanolic acid saponin and proceric acid saponin mixt. from seeds exhibited spermic. activity (*Indian Drugs*, 1979-80, **17**, 6).

α-Spinasterol, and oleanolic acid from roots, α-spinasterol, hentriacontane and hexacosanol from leaves. Root saponin, spermic. against human sperm (*Indian J Pharm Sci*, 1979, **41**, 115); also haemolytic (*Indian Drugs*, 1980-81, **18**, 121)

ALCEA (*Malvaceae*)

A. rosea Linn. syn. *Althaea rosea* (Linn.) Cav.

Eng.–*Hollyhock.*

Dried flowers either with or without calices, as antiinflam. and mild purg. (uncertain). Its action as a cure for coughs, doubtful (Med. Plants, 95).

Flowers contain kaempferol, its 3-glucd., quercetin, its 3-glucd., cyanidin-3-glucd. and -3-rutinoside (*Curr Sci*, 1964, **33**, 431). Deep yellow hollyhock a flavon. glycd., herbacin yielding on hydrolysis herbacetin (major pigment) (*Bull Nat Inst Sci India*, 1965, No.31, 100). Dark-coloured flowers, anthocyanins (*Med. Plants, 95; Stud Ceret Biochem*, 1976, **19**, 113; *CA*, **85**, 11958r).

Gibberellins A$_1$, A$_3$ & A$_8$; also A$_8$-glucd. (*Phytochemistry*, 1967, **6**, 1695; *Planta*, 1970, **92**, 100). Leaves, seeds and fruits of Egyptian plant contain sugars, lower alcs., *p*-tolualdehyde, β-sitosterol; limonene, phellandrene, citral and α-terpenyl-OAc (*Indian J Chem*, 1974, **12**, 1019). Lipid ext. of seeds, hydrocarbons, acids, esters, glycerides and alcs., their identn. and detn.; basic fraction of ext. gave +ve reactions for alk. (*Collect Czech Chem Commun*, 1978, **43**, 3087). Plant, ocimene (*J Econ Entomol*, 1980, **73**, 783). All parts of plant contain mucilage and are used in medicine (Wlth India, IA, 131).

ALCHEMILLA (*Rosaceae*)

*A. vulgaris Linn.

Eng.–*Lady's mantle, lion's foot.*

Leaves—dried leaves, also the dried flowering plant as a tisane for diar. and for excessive menstruation; also in menopause. Externally as an application to wounds. Also used in vet. med. for diar. (Med. Plants, 74). Flowers and leaves, flavons. (*Farmacia Buc*, 1977, **25**, 247; *CA*, 1978, **89**, 3170d). Fluid ext., antihaemor. preparation in obstetrics-gynaecology, clin. study; leaves, as also rhizomes, tannins; fluid ext. (containing flavone glycds. and tannins) non-toxic, and effective orally in juvenile menometrorrhagia (*Clujul Med*, 1978, **51**, 70; 1979, **52**, 78; 226).

Occurs in Kashmir at 2,400-2,700 m altitudes.

ALCHORNEA (*Euphorbiaceae*)

*A. rugosa Muell.-Arg.

Seeds used as purg. (*J Bombay Natl Hist Soc*, 1938, **40**, 269).

Found in Andamans.

ALECTRA (*Scrophulariaceae*)

*A. parasitica A. Rich. var. **chitrakutensis** M.A. Rau

Rhizome powd., effective drug in leprosy, clin. trial; not toxic (*Leprosy Rev*, 1962, **33**, 207).

Common in Banda district, U.P., Chitrakut, Jabalpur and Guna and also along Satna district borders, M.P.

ALEURITES (*Euphorbiaceae*)

*A. fordii Hemsl.

Eng.–*Tung oil tree.*

Fruit—kernel, toxic; min. fatal amt. for a human being not known. Fruit ext., antibact.

Seed oil—known as 'tung oil' finds use for treatment of boils, ulcers, swellings and burns. Acts as irrit. in gastrointestinal tract. Oil, probably heated one causes allergy to workers handling it in paints & varnish industry. Sufferer successfully desensitized by i.m. injection of a fresh distillate of oil dissolved in purified olive oil.

Seed meal—poisonous.

Leaves—poisonous to cattle; effects; profuse watery sanguinious diar., loss of appetite, atony of the rumen, listlessness, emaciation and death; symptoms and lesions, comparable to other spp. Also piscic. and nematic.

Leaf and flower contain toxic saponin (also present in fruit-kernel and oil cake) as well as another toxic ether-sol. principle deteriorating with aging of meal and not present in shell. Extn. or heating of meal with EtOH and hydrolysis with steam, decomposes the toxic substance or destroys enzyme necessary for its formation. Leaf and fruit contain tannins and sterols (Watt & Breyer-Brandwijk, 395-97; Kingsbury, 182-84).

Fruits, 2 toxic phorbol derivs. (*Chem Pharm Bull*, 1974, **22**, 971); stigmasterol, sitosterol and campesterol and their glycds. (*Phytochemistry*, 1975, **14**, 2513).

Leaves contain piscic. compds., of which 12-O-palmitoyl-16-OH- phorbol-13-OAc & its -4-deoxy-4 β-deriv. identified; both phorbol derivs. showed higher activity than rotenone (*Agric Biol Chem*, 1979, **43**, 2523; *Phytochemistry*, 1975, **14**, 509).

Cultivated in tea-estates of W. Bengal, Assam, Bihar and Karnataka.

A. moluccana (Linn.) Willd.

Eng.–*Candlenut tree.*

Leaves, toxic but less than *A. fordii* & *A. montana* (Kingsbury, 182).

Bark, antitumour (*Lloydia*, 1969, **32**, 153). Its decoct., to treat unconsciousness (*Econ Bot*, 1970, **24**, 279). In Hawaii, flowers, nuts and bark used in general debility, to treat asthma, sores, ulcers and swollen womb and as laxt. (*ibid*, 1971, **25**, 245). Bark or root, to treat wounds (*ibid*, 1974, **28**, 1). Fruit powd., as stomch. (*Nagarjun*, 1979-80, **23**, 242).

*A. montana Wils.

Eng.–*Wood oil tree.*

Leaves, toxic; *c.* half as toxic as *A. fordii*.

In E. Africa, commercial tung meal derived from this sp. as well as *A. fordii*, toxic to chick. An ext. of plant causes agglutination of chicken erythrocytes; a hydrolysate, detoxin inhibits the same.

A saponin and an unknown toxic principle present in leaf and oil-cake, which can be detoxicated by extn. with EtOH or by hydrolysis of saponin (Watt & Breyer-Brandwijk, 397; Wlth India, IA, 138).

EtOH(50%) ext. of aerial parts, antiprot. against *Entamoeba histolytica* and anticancer against P 388 lymphocytic leukaemia in mice (*Indian J Exp Biol*, 1973, **11**, 43).

Bark, a triterp. acid, aleuritolic acid (*J Indian Chem Soc*, 1969, **46**, 1063); also friedelin, betulinic acid and β-sitosterol; Str. detn. of aleuritolic acid (*Tetrahedron*, 1970, **26**, 3017).

Native to China and introduced into Assam, Himachal Pradesh, Uttar Pradesh and Karnataka.

ALHAGI(*Fabaceae*)

A. pseudalhagi (Bieb.) Desv. syn. *Hedysarum alhagi* Linn.

Eng.–*Camel thorn, Persian manna plant.*

EtOH(50%) ext. of plant, antiprot. and anticancer (*Indian J Exp Biol*, 1968, **6**, 232).

Stems and roots, β-Ph-Et-amine identified, and alks., hordenine, salsolidine and a tetrahydroisoquinoline alk.; preliminary pharmacol. of alks. (*J Pharm Sci*, 1973, **62**, 1555). Twigs contain 8 alks., detailed pharmacol. investigation; total alks., sympathomimetic (*Planta Med*, 1974, **26**, 318). Plant, seven 24-alkylsterols; their biogenesis (*Curr Sci*, 1981, **50**, 485).

ALISMA (*Alismataceae*)

*A. plantago-aquatica Linn. syn. *A. plantago* Linn.

Eng.–*Mad-dog weed, water-plantain.*

Rootstock—tonic, stim., laxt., diur. and galact. Prescribed in dropsy and in USSR it was used as a remedy for hydrophobia (Wlth India, IA, 160-61). Beneficial in inflam. and indurated tumours, leukemia and cancer of stomach (*Lloydia*, 1967, **30**, 389).

Rootstock, irritating if eaten fresh, but on drying its acrid principle lost and it becomes edible. Contains starch and a no. of sugars. Plant, a lipotropic substance different in biol. activity from choline and lecithin; a plant ext., lipotropic on rabbits and rats (Wlth India, IA, 160-61).

Marshy lands of Himalayas, up to 2,300m and also recorded in Karnataka.

ALLEMANDA (*Apocynaceae*)

*A. blanchettii DC.

Sap, emetic and cath.; large doses, poisonous (Uphof, 23).

Native to Brazil, introduced in IBG, Calcutta.

A. cathartica Linn.

Eng.–*Campanilla, golden trumpet.*

Alc. and aq. ext. of roots, hypoten. (*Bull Calcutta Sch Trop Med*, 1963, **11**, 91). Leaf ext., anticancer (*Philipp J Sci*, 1967, **96**, 393). Antifung. (*Acta Bot Indica*, 1979, **7**, 147). Flower ext., toxic; inhibits fungal growth (*Indian Biol J*, 1980, **2**, 109).

Leaves and stems yield ursolic acid, β-amyrin and β-sitosterol (*Phytochemistry*, 1969, **8**, 791). 2 Triterp. lactones, plumericin and isoplumericin from stem and rootbark (*Indian J Chem*, 1970, **8**, 851); also from leaves and roots, besides plumieride and long chain esters (*Asian J Pharm*, 1971, **2**, 5; *CA*, 1972, **76**, 89992q).

EtOH ext. of roots showed *in vivo* activity against P-388 leukaemia in mouse and *in vitro* against human carcinoma cells of nasopharynx (KB). Contains antileukaemic iridoid lactone, allamandin and

2 other iridoids, allamandicin and allamdin (*J Org Chem*, 1974, **39**, 2477). Plant contains antifung. sesquiterps. (*Pahlavi Med J*, 1975, **6**, 52; *CA*, **82**, 121741u).

Flowers, kaempferol, quercetin and hesperitin (*J Indian Chem Soc*, 1979, **56**, 944).

*A. violacea Gardn. & Field.

Root, powerful cath. Used in fevers. Aq. ext. of roots and stems, antiprot. (Wlth India, IA, 165).

Native of Brazil, cultivated in gardens.

ALLIARIA (*Brassicaceae*)

A. petiolata (Bieb.) Cavara & Grande syn. *A. officinalis* Andrzej. ex Bieb.; *Sisymbrium alliaria* Scop.

Eng.–*Garlic mustard, garlic wort, hedge garlic.*

Herb, lithontriptic. Herb and seeds, stim., antiscor. and vermifuge (Wlth India, IA, 165).

Herb yields a garlic-scented essent. oil with allyl and benzyl isothiocyanates (20-30:1); total amt. of isothiocyanates vary during vegetative period but ratio of allyl and benzyl-NCS remains constant. Allyl sulphide and rhodanallyl also present (just prior to flowering), rich source of vit. C and other vits. (*Econ Bot*, 1977, **31**, 76; Wlth India, IA, 165).

Seeds, fatty oil; fatty acid compn.; crucic acid (47%); in one sample as high as (77.7%), also yield essent. oil with allyl and benzyl mustard oils, the latter predominating (*J Am Chem Soc*, 1965, **42**, 817; Wlth India, IX, 361).

ALLIUM (*Alliaceae*)

A. ascalonicum Linn.

Eng.–*Shallot.*

Alc. ext. of bulb, anticoagulant, fibrinolytic and hypocholesteremic [*J Res Indian Med*, 1974, **9**(4), 1]. Shallot shows significant activity against P 388 lymphocytic leukaemia in mice.

Aq. ext. of bulb, fructose and other sugars, glucosamine and uronic acid, lysine, etc. (*Planta Med*, 1973, **23**, 99). Brown skin of bulbs, quercetol & its glucds. Fresh leaves, flavons. (*C R Acad Sci Ser D*, 1967, **265**, 2118).

A. cepa Linn.
Eng.–*Onion*.

Bulb—onion, antimal. and antirheum. (*Planta Med*, 1973, **23**, 381); antidiabetic; antiatherogenic, antihyperten. and antibact. effects of onion and garlic, rev., 73 refs. [*Medikon*, 1977, **6**(11), 5; *Nutr Abstr Rev*, 1980, **50A**, 7039]; hypocholesteremic and antihypercholesteremic; see also garlic (*Indian J Nutr Diet*, 1975, **12**, 288; *Indian J Med Res*, 1976, **64**, 1509; 1975, **63**, 1629); hypolipaemic, and increases clotting time and fibrinolytic activity in humans (*Indian Pract*, 1979, **32**, 337).

Regular use of onion (50g/day) reduces insulin requirement of a diabetic patient from 40 to 20 units a day (*Naturwissenschaften*, 1974, **61**, 172). Onion ext. also reduced blood sugar during i.v. glucose tolerance test and adrenalin-induced hyperglycaemia in man (*Indian J Med Res*, 1977, **65**, 422).

Continuous consumption of onion for 5 months (dose 80 g daily) decreased serum cholesterol below normal in healthy human (*Indian Med Gaz*, 1977, **111**, 378). Addn. of garlic or onion in breakfast of 5 male volunteers significantly reduced serum cholesterol; checked rise in serum triglycerides, β-lipoproteins and phospholipids; and increased clotting time and fibrinolytic activity (*J Assoc Physicians India*, 1979, **27**, 57).

Onion, med., chem., pharmacol., and clin. properties, rev., 35 refs. (*Pak J Sci Ind Res*, 1971, **14**, 395; *CA*, 1972, **77**, 85514h); as drug, rev., 33 refs. (*Indian Drugs*, 1976-77, **14**, 156); with salt, domestic remedy for colic and scurvy. In raw state, diur.; roasted or fresh, used as poultice to boils, bruises and wounds. Applied to navel in dysen. and in body heat. Eaten with black pepper, in malarial fever. Decoct., very useful in strangury and extreme heat sensation cases [*Indian Fmrs' Dig*, 1978, **11**(6 &

7), 73]. Onion and its preparations in various diseases (Herbal Med., 103-04; 121-22; 125; 127; 129; 131; 137-38; 146-47; 160; 175; 267).

Onion (without peel), remedy for circular alopecia (Ger. Offen, 1970, 1921148; *CA*, 1971, **74**, 6395g). Pharmaceuticals containing onion exts.; compns. useful as tonic, and in recovery of fatigue; exts. also useful for athelet's feet; contains allyl Pr-disulphide as active constituent (Jpn Kokai, 1978, 7809309; 7826314; *CA*, **88**, 141718u; **89**, 48914r).

Onion and garlic, trypsin inhibitor (*Indian J Biochem Biophys*, 1975, **12**, 383); onion ext., an inhibitor of microbiol. polygalacturonase (*in* Liener, 452).

Juice—testosterone-like effect, hypoglyc. action and a growth hormone-like activity in rats; juice of onion and garlic, antimicrob. (*Qual Plant Mater Veg*, 1967, **14**, 26; 1972, **22**, 29); used in faintness, convuls., headache, epileptic fits, hot juice relieves earache; sniffed in apistaxis and applied into eyes in dimness of vision, and locally to allay irritation of insect bites and scorpion stings. Good antid. for tobacco poisoning. With mustard oil (1:1), used against rheum. pain and inflam. swellings [*Indian Fmrs' Dig*, 1978, **11**(6 & 7), 73].

Effects of onion ext. on platelet aggregation and thromboxane synthesis (*Prostaglandins Med*, 1979, **2**, 413). A prostaglandin-like compd. from yellow onion; sepn. of prostaglandin A_1 (*Lipids*, 1973, **8**, 484; 1980, **15**, 292).

Crude exts. of onion and garlic, antimitotic on MTK-sarcoma III of albino rats (*Gann*, 1964, **55**, 325; *CA*, 1965, **63**, 1089d). Ether ext., cytotoxic to MFS-180 cells; lachrymatory factor also cytotoxic (*Indian J Exp Biol*, 1981, **19**, 598).

Aq. exts. of onion and garlic, antifung. (*New Bot*, 1979, **6**, 41); antimicrob. [*Indian Drugs Pharmac Ind*, 1980, **15**(2), 45; *Geobios*, 1980, **7**, 46].

Essent. oil—possibly active principle of onion, may find use in long term prophylaxis of individuals predisposed to atherosclerosis (*Indian Heart J*, 1974, **26**, 29). Onion and garlic oils inhibited toxin production by *Clostridium botulinum* type A in meat slurry (*J Food Prot*, 1979, **42**, 222).

Skin—ext. of onion and garlic skins, antibact. (*J Sci Food Agric*, 1970, **21**, 110); ether ext. inhibited gastric secretion in pylorus ligated rats; active substance, a phenol deriv. (*Shoyakugaku Zasshi*, 1977, **31**, 179; *CA*, 1978, **88**, 131005m). Ext. pronounced antioxidant; also copper-chelating properties and shows varying degrees of synergysm with ascorbic acid, due to flavons. present; also used in hair-dye and vit.P (Wlth India, IA, 167).

Leaves—of onion and seeds of garlic, ecbolic in mice and rats (*Qual Plant Mater Veg*, 1968-69, **17**, 153). Ext., as also its volat. fraction from garlic and onion, antifung. (*Acta Bot Indica*, 1977, **5**, suppl., 14; *Indian J Mycol Plant Pathol*, 1979, **9**, 250). Onion tops poisoning in bullocks (*Indian Vet J*, 1980, **57**, 690).

Seeds—chitinase and acetylglucosaminidase activity (*Comp Biochem Physiol*, 1965, **14**, 127); antimicrob. activities of seed oil and its unsap. matter (*Indian Drugs*, 1978-79, **16**, 207). Seeds with *Punica granatum* roots, *Cajanus cajan* and *Piper rubrum* juice taken with honey for abortion (*J Sci Res Plants Med*, 1981, **2**, 39).

Bulbs on steam distillation yield an essent. oil (0.005%), known as onion oil, with acrid taste and unpleasant odour (Wlth India, IA, 177); flavour components, rev. (*Coffee Tea Ind*, 1963, **86**, 30; *CA*, **60**, 6139e). Constituents; various mono-, di-, tri- & tetra-sulphides; thiols and thiophene derivs.; gas chromatogr. identn. of several flavour compds. (*Pharmazie*, 1965, **20**, 441; *CA*, **63**, 9744ds; *Symp Foods Oreg State Univ*, 1965, 390; *CA*, 1968, **68**, 38331a; *J Chromatogr*, 1970, **47**, 400; *J Agric Food Chem*, 1971, **19**, 984).

Allyl alc. and Me-disulphide, onion volat. compds. show antithyroid activity in female rats (*Aust J Biol Sci*, 1967, **20**, 683);

volat. aliphatic sulphides (*J Food Sci*, 1968, **33**, 298); allyl-Pr-disulfide caused fall in blood glucose level in human volunteers (*Clin Chim Acta*, 1975, **60**, 121). Cysteine sulphoxides and cycloalliin (*Curr Sci*, 1976, **45**, 863). Chem. and biol. properties of odoriferous substances of garlic and onion, rev., 6 refs. [*Indian Drugs Pharmac Ind*, 1978, **13**(2), 10]. Di-Me-2, 5-dioxo-2, 5-di-hydro-thiophene (*J Agric Food Chem*, 1980, **28**, 1037).

Lachrymatory factor—identn. of lachrymogenic compd. and other volat. components of onion (*Cornell Univ Agric Expt Sta Mem*, 1964, No. 385, 31; *CA*, **61**, 9771c); thiopropanal-S-oxide (*J Agric Food Chem*, 1971, **19**, 269). TLC of cysteine deriv., flavour and lacrimatory factor (*J Food Sci*, 1971, **36**, 662). TLC quant. detn. (*J Agric Food Chem*, 1975, **23**, 645); spectrophotom. detn. (*J Sci Food Agric*, 1975, **26**, 1529). Z-propanethial-S-oxide (*Tetrahedron Lett*, 1980, **21**, 1277; *J Am Chem Soc*, 1979, **101**, 2200); cytotoxic (*Indian J Exp Biol*, 1981, **19**, 598).

Bulb contains polyphenols, protocatechuic, caffeic, ferulic acids, etc. (*Curr Sci*, 1964, **33**, 471); quercetin & its derivs. (*Phytochemistry*, 1965, **4**, 107; *Ann Sci Univ Besancon Bot*, 1970, No. 10, 13; *CA*, 1973, **79**, 15824b). Comparative study of 3 vars. of onions, for quercetin content (*Indian J Appl Chem*, 1971, **34**, 142). Kaempferol and quercetin (*J Indian Chem Soc*, 1974, **51**, 975); method for quercetin extn. (USSR Pat., 1975, 438981; *CA*, **83**, 203536r); quercetin from bulbs [*Indian Drugs Pharmac Ind*, 1976, **11**(3), 30].

Bulb, carbohydrates (*C R Acad Sci Ser D*, 1970, **270**, 1583); sterols & sterol glycds. (*FEBS Lett*, 1970, **11**, 177). Hyper- and hypoglyc. agents from bulb juice (*Indian J Exp Biol*, 1973, **11**, 573). Onion contains a saponin, β-amyrin and β-sitosterol (*Zesz Nauk Akad Ekon Poznaniu, Ser 1*, 1978, **73**, 40; *CA*, 1979, **90**, 200256h).

Onion skins, kaempferol (*Naturwissenschaften*, 1966, **53**, 826). Dried skin, best source of quercetin (*Steroids Lipids Res*, 1970, **4**, 195; *CA*, 1972, **77**, 125003z). Sterols, 26% of unsap. lipids of pigmented skins; cholesterol, β-sitosterol & stigmasterol (*Qual Plant Food Hum Nutr*, 1974, **24**, 159).

Green onion tops solution, antioxidant; tops, quercetin derivs. and myricetin (*J Food Sci*, 1964, **29**, 27). Plant quercetin & its glycds. (*Zesz Nauk Akad Ekon Poznaniu Ser 1*, 1978, **73**, 35; *CA*, 1979, **91**, 16662g).

A. porrum Linn. syn. *A. ampeloprasum* Linn. var. *porrum* Regel

Eng.–*Egyptian garlic, leek.*

Alks. of Egyptian garlic and their toxicity (*Zentralbl Veterinaermed Reithe A*, 1966, **13**, 662; *CA*, 1967, **66**, 64219y).

Stems, essent. oil and several flavour compds. (*J Agric Food Chem*, 1976, **24**, 336). Leaves, kaempferol glycds. (*Z Lebensm Unters Forsch*, 1976, **161**, 25; *CA*, **85**, 59658d). β-Sitosterol in chloroplast (Wlth India, IA, 167).

A. sativum Linn.

Eng.–*Garlic.*

Garlic—effective drug for rheum. and catar. conditions (*Acta Phytother*, 1964, **11**, 147). Condiment and med., covering chem. constituents, antibact., antifung., antidiabetic, hypoten., antinflam., anticancer and pesticidal properties, rev., 68 refs. (*Indian Drugs*, 1977-78, **15**, 205); its usage; several preparations in various diseases (Med. Plants, 37; Herbal Med., 63; 67; 121; 124; 132-33; 136; 140; 147; 157; 181; 266). Raw garlic decreased glucose, total cholesterol, phospholipids, triglycerides, etc. in healthy individuals; activities regardless of age and sex, clin. trials (*Indian Med Gaz*, 1980, **114**, 157; *J Nat Integ Med Assoc*, 1978, **20**, 225). Garlic, useful in dyspep., clin. trials (*Antiseptic*, 1981, **78**, 197). Garlic, useful in cryptococcal meningitis in man (*Chin Med J*, 1980, **93**, 123). Antirickettsial activity (*Indian J Anim Res*, 1981, **15**, 93).

Garlic applied as resolvant to indolent tumours. Internally given with common salt in nervous diseases, headache, etc. Regular use kills harmful intestinal bacteria. Liniment beneficial in infantile convuls. and other spasmodic affections; in gout, sciatica, etc.

Juice—applied to bruises and sprains, used to relieve earache and to allay pain in otorrhoea [*Indian Fmrs' Dig*, 1978, **11**(6 & 7), 73]; of garlic and onion in hair-dressing compn. (Fr. Pat., 1967, 1481008; *CA*, **67**, 111344t); estrogenic in rats [*J Res Indian Med*, 1976, **11**(4), 7].

Fresh garlic inhibited mammary tumours in female C3H/He mice, allicin, active principle (*Acta Unio Int Contra Cancrum*, 1964, **20**, 855; *CA*, **61**, 16437c). Garlic enhanced phagocitic action of i.p. macrophages in mice; active principle, diallyl thiosulphonate (*in* Beal & Reinhard, 381). Effect of garlic pretreatment on isoprenaline-induced myocardial necrosis in albino rats (*Indian J Physiol Pharmacol*, 1980, **24**, 233).

Antibiot. content of garlic varies according to plant part (most in brood bulbs, less in true bulbs or garlic cloves and least in stems and leaves), strain, origin, etc.; activity 10-100 times greater in dermatophytes and yeasts, esp. *Candida* spp. than in bacteria. Garlic, superior than allicin as fungicide (*Pharmazie*, 1970, **25**, 266; *CA*, **73**, 117195r); aq. ext., antifung. against clin. isolates of *Candida albicans* (*Mycologia*, 1977, **69**, 793). Use of garlic ext. in cosmetic compn. preventing skin discoloration and wrinkling (Jpn Kokai, 1977, 77105224; *CA*, 1978, **88**, 41552s).

Antimicrob. and other related activities of preparation phytoncidin, from garlic (*Antibiotiki*, 1963, **8**, 832; *CA*, 1964, **61**, 16474c); of tablets containing lyophilized garlic (*Herba Pol*, 1969, **15**, 222; *CA*, 1970, **73**, 28968c); of garlic [*Indian Spices*, 1969, **6**(4), 19]; of crude juices of garlic and onion (*Qual Plant Mater Veg*, 1972, **22**, 29); bactericidal, insectic. and anthelm. properties and active compds., rev., 20 refs. (*Food Technol NZ*, 1973, **18**, 13; *CA*, **79**, 39169t); of aq. ext. against food-poisoning bacteria (*Lebensm Wiss Technol*, 1979, **12**, 330); of a preparation (*Varasarn Paesachasarthara*, 1979, **6**, 31; *CA*, 1980, **92**, 47166y); of young bulbs (*Acta Pharm Jugosl*, 1980, **30**, 205); of ext. stable beyond 48 hrs. (*J Food Sci Technol*, 1981, **18**, 44).

Pharmacol. and clin. studies, and literature survey (*Dtsch Apoth Ztg*, 1966, **106**, 1861; *CA*, 1967, **66**, 74823c). Nutritional and pharmacol. value, rev., 28 refs. (*Kagaku Kyoto*, 1966, **21**, 507; *CA*, 1968, **69**, 95110g). Chem. and med. aspects of *Allium*, rev., 67 refs. (*Pak J Sci Ind Res*, 1972, **15**, 81; *CA*, 1973, **78**, 47683a).

Exts. of garlic, by and large the same properties of garlic. Extensive pharmacol. investigations of garlic, its exts., etc. lend credence to their uses.

Antidiabetic activity of garlic ext. as reagent for urinary glucose detection (Jpn Kokai, 1974, 74120693; *CA*, 1975, **82**, 121267u); see *A. cepa* (onion) also. Powd. garlic, hypoglyc. in human after 4 weeks; elevated serum cholesterol and Mg (*J Shivaji Univ*, 1977, **17**, 125; *CA*, 1980, **93**, 147274w). Garlic powder of ISI-specifications [*Pharmatimes*, 1979, **11**(9), 25].

Allisatin, a conc. from bulb, slight antiarthritic (*Indian J Med Res*, 1966, **54**, 582). A preparation useful in rheum. (*Rheumatism*, 1976-77, **12**, 142; 1977-78, **13**, 24).

Anticholesteremic and other related properties of garlic, raw and boiled (*Indian J Nutr Diet*, 1976, **13**, 7); of aq. ext., on oral administration; activity due to allicin (*Indian J Exp Biol*, 1977, **15**, 489); garlic or aq. alc. ext., improved lipidogram patterns in hyperlipemic patients (*Acta Pharm Jugosl*, 1978, **28**, 137); of ext. in males with normal blood cholesterol level (*Indian J Physiol Pharmacol*, 1979, **23**, 211); aq. ext. of garlic (or onion), no significant effect on males' blood serum cholesterol level (*Mediscope*, 1979, **22**, 134); of ext. capsules; increased blood triglycerides and fibrinolylic activity and decreased blood cholesterol [*Int Congr Ser Excerpta Med*, 1980, 502 (Intern Med; Pt. 2), 1255; *CA*, **93**, 69484y]. Garlic, hypolipidemic agent (*Rajasthan Med J*, 1981, **20**, 73).

Onion and garlic in atherosclerotic heart disease; an appraisal [*Medikon*, 1977, **6**(5), 12; 17; *CA*, **87**, 116795p; *Atherosclerosis*, 1981, **40**, 175]; heavy consumption can produce nausea and bad breath; and raise cholesterol level in heart patients (*Drug Pharm Ind Highlights*, 1981, **4**, 7).

Essent. oil—from garlic. Used externally in paralytic pain [*Indian Fmrs' Dig*, 1978,**11**(6 & 7), 13]. It increased fibronolytic activity in patients with coronary artery disease (*Atherosclerosis*, 1977, **28**, 155; *CA*, 1978, **88**, 16128a); decreased serum cholesterol and blood sugar levels in adult human (*Bangladesh Med J*, 1981, **10**, 6); insectic. against housefly and *khapra* beetle (*J Food Sci Technol*, 1974, **11**, 153); antifung. effects of some components; antimicrob., stability of exts., yield (0.19 - 0.25%) (*Acta Pharm Jugosl*, 1978, **28**, 41; 1977, **27**, 35; *Indian Drugs*, 1977-78, **15**, 277); antibact. activity 10 times stronger than Hg chloride (*Dtsch Apoth*, 1968, **20**, 322; 324; *CA*, **69**, 109743v).

Leaves—ext., antifung. (*Indian Phytopath*, 1976, **29**, 448; *Sci Cult*, 1977, **43**, 487); fungitoxic activity of volat. fraction (*Indian Perfum*, 1979, **23**, 61).

From garlic, alloxol preparation (USSR Pat., 1968, 213030; *CA*, **69**, 46057b); sepn. of sulphur amino acids and peptides (*Acta Chem Scand*, 1968, **22**, 3333); 2 mercapto-L-cysteines; a biol. active thioglycd. (*Chem Pharm Bull*, 1964, **12**, 1114; 1969, **17**, 2193).

Anthocyanins (*J Food Sci*, 1975, **40**, 1101); glycds. of kaempferol and quercetin (*Z Lebensm Unters Forsch*, 1976, **161**, 25; *CA*, **85**, 59658d); saponin like substances (*Zesz Nauk Akad Ekon Poznaniu Ser 1*, 1975, **62**, 43; *CA*, 1976, **85**, 59614m); polysaccharides, str. (*Carbohydr Res*, 1978, **64**, 155; *CA*, **89**, 126115x); extn. and purification of alliinase (*Biokhimiya Moscow*, 1978, **43**, 1905). Sterols and hydrocarbons (*Riv Ital EPPOS*, 1980, **62**, 373; *CA*, 1981, **94**, 61791w).

Flavour components of garlic ext. (*J Agric Food Chem*, 1971, **19**, 273); antimicrob. and other biol. activities of S-containing aroma and flavour components of onion and garlic, rev., 6 refs. [*Indian Drugs Pharmac Ind*, 1978, **13**(2), 10].

Alliin—intact tissues contain non-volat. S-amino acid, alliin which on maceration rapidly attacked by allicin-lyase with release, within a few minutes, of pyruvic acid, ammonia and antimicrob. toxin allicin; role of these S-toxins in disease-resistance in *Allium* not yet clear (*in* Plant and Fungal Toxins, 750-52). Sepn. and purification of alliin homologues (Jpn Kokai, 1974, 7400221; *CA*, **80**, 108862y). Estn., yield 0.5-0.8%. In presence of allinase, alliin inhibited multiplication of T.B. bacilli, Gram +ve and Gram -ve bacteria and some fungi (*Jpn J Antibiot*, 1975, **28**, 638; *CA*, 1976, **84**, 111547n).

Allicin—diallyl disulphide oxide. Undergoes enzymic modification with loss of oxygen to give diallyl disulphide. Both allicin and diallyl disulphide, antifung.; most *Penicillium* spp. inhibited. Allicin, hypoglyc. comparable to tolbutamide in rabbits with mild alloxan diabetes (*Indian J Biochem Biophys*, 1973, **10**, 209). Detn. (*Elelmiszervizsgalati Kozl*, 1976, **22**, 23; *CA*, 1977, **86**, 41891k). Intratumoural injections of allicin or allithiamine (a product of allicin and thiamine) resulted in marked inhibition of sarcoma-180 tumour cells (*Taiwan I Hsueh Hui Tsa Chih*, 1981, **80**, 385; *CA*, **95**, 197366q). Diallyl disulphide & trisulphide, larvicidal principles (*Science*, 1971, **174**, 134); antifung. Stimulate certain soil fungi actually to grow sclerotia of *Sclerotium capivorum* to germinate, by release of diallyl disulphide from roots of onion and garlic (*in* Plant and Fungal Toxins, 752). Cholesterol-lowering effect of allitin (98% diallyl disulphide and 2% trisulphide) (*Indian J Exp Biol*, 1980, **18**, 858).

Other therapeutic compds. include sativin I & II; their extn. from garlic cloves (Ger Offen, 1976, 2528975; *CA*, **84**, 184882c). Scordinines A & B, extn. from fresh garlic; also scordinine A$_1$, A$_2$ and B (Jpn Pat., 1970, 7012876; 1972, 7215115; *CA*, **73**, 69836b; **77**, 45755f). Antimicrob. and antifung. agent, scordine extn.; from garlic and onion; sepn. from garlic (Jpn Pat., 1971, 7114918; 1972, 7229966; *CA*, **75**, 52793d; **77**, 130583t). Scormine, extn. and its conversion to antibact. compd. (Jpn Kokai, 1972, 7220159; *CA*, 1974, **78**, 30198y).

A. schoenoprasum Linn.

Eng.–*Chives*.

EtOH(50%) ext. of bulb, cardiac depress. (*Annu Rep CDRI Lucknow*, 1970-71, 24).

Gas chromatogr. of volat. oil of plant, several compds. (*Proc Am Soc Hort Sci*, 1964, **84**, 386; *CA*, 1965, **62**, 4529s; *Acta Chem Scand*, 1965, **19**, 1327; *Chem Ind Lond*, 1971, 556).

A. tuberosum Roxb.

Leaves, volat. oil constituents (*Nippon Nogei Kagaku Kaishi*, 1974, **48**, 385; *CA*, **81**, 152425c). Flavon. glycds. (*Agric Biol Chem*, 1980, **44**, 1405).

*A. victorialis Linn.

Plant used as carmin. in West Garhwal (*Khadi Gramodyog*, 1972-73, **19**, 269).

Himalayas from Kashmir eastwards to Sikkim between 2,100 and 3,900 m.

ALLOPHYLUS (*Sapindaceae*)

A monotypic genus of shrubs or trees, represented by polymorphic sp. *A. cobbe* and all other species considered synonyms (*Blumea*, 1967, **15**, 301; Wlth India, IA, 187).

A. cobbe (Linn.) Rausch.

Roots—used for treating piles and in nose-bleeding; roots and twigs utilized as chewsticks. In Nigeria, roots eaten for lactation. A hot infusion of rootbark used to check diar. and rheum. pains.

Leaves—eaten to induce lactation. Crushed ones inhaled as a sternutatory to relieve headache, colds and rheum. pains. Leaves and bark, a remedy for elephantiasis; pounded ones applied to dislocations; juice, vulnerary. A decoct. given in colic, or as a drink for babies and children with fever. To stupefy bees by keeping them at entrance of hives.

Fruits used against tapeworm (Wlth India, IA, 187). Plant, in fractures (*Sri Lanka For*, 1980, **14**, 145).

EtOH(50%) ext. of aerial parts, active against *Ranikhet* disease virus, and showed gross effects on CNS and hypothermia (*Indian J Exp Biol*, 1973, **11**, 43).

Leaves, Ph-acetamide and alks. (traces) (Wlth India, IA, 187).

Plant releases HCN (*Pharm Weekbl*, 1961, **96**, 577; *CA* 1962, **56**, 715g). Seeds, alks. (*Aust J Chem*, 1969, **22**, 1315). Stems, β-sitosterol (*Indian J Chem*, 1969, **7**, 308).

ALNUS (*Betulaceae*)

A. nepalensis D. Don

Eng.–*Indian alder, Nepalese alder.*

EtOH(50%) ext. of stem bark, hypoglyc. and spasmog. (*Indian J Exp Biol*, 1968, **6**, 232).

Bark contains tannin (7%) (Wlth India, IA, 188).

A. nitida Endl.

Eng.–*West Himalayan alder.*

EtOH(50%) ext. of bark, antivir. (*Indian J Exp Biol*, 1973, **11**, 43).

Bark, tannin (3%) (Wlth India, IA, 189).

ALOCASIA (*Araceae*)

*A. fornicata (Roxb.) Schott

Used medicinally (Wlth India, IA, 191). Cultivated in some parts of India.

A. macrorrhiza (Linn.) G. Don syn. *A. indica* (Lour.) Spach.; *A. odora* Koch; *Colocasia macrorrhiza* Schott

Eng.–*Giant taro.*

Application of Giant taro to stings of giant nettle (*Laportea gigas*) gives instant relief. In Java, chopped roots and leaves used as rubft. (Wlth India, IA, 190). Leaf used against tumour (*Lloydia*, 1967, **30**, 379); petioles contain HCN (up to 0.018%), used for toothache and their juice for coughs. In Fiji, stem juice, in earache; in Hawaii, corm, in stomach-ache (*Econ Bot*, 1969, **23**, 97; 1970, **24**, 279; 1971, **25**, 245).

Roots, skin irrit. (*Econ Bot*, 1974, **28**, 1). EtOH(50%) ext. of tubers, diur. (*Indian J Exp Biol*, 1977, **15**, 208).

Seed ext., antifung. (*Indian Drugs*, 1979-80, **17**, 210); antibact. [*Indian Drugs Pharmac Ind*, 1980, **15** (3), 41]; agglutinated trypsin treated red blood cells [*Ryuku Daigaku Nogakubu Gakujutsu Hokoku*, 1979, (26), 105; *CA*, 1980, **93**, 130339y].

Leaves, stalks, tubers and roots have high content of sol. oxalates and prolonged use of these in diet may cause Ca deficiency and oxaluria (Wlth India, IA, 190). Plant, a flavon. and a saponin (*Taiwan Yao Hsueh Tsa Chin, 1969, 21, 18; CA*, 1971, **75**, 126582h). All parts of plant except tubers contain cyanogenic principle; a mixt. of triglochinin & isotriglochinin (*Phytochemistry*, 1975, **14**, 1339); β-glucosidases, highly specific for hydrolysing triglochinin (*Hoppe-Seyler's Z Physiol Chem*, 1977, **358**, 859; *CA*, **87**, 147702k).

ALOE (*Liliaceae*)

Aloin content of leaves of some *Aloe* spp. grown in Indian gardens is as follows: *A. arborescens*, 11.5; *A. aristata*, 10.2; *A. ciliarias*, 8.6; *A. gracillis* 15.5; *A. jacksonii*, 16.1; and *A. lateritia*, 14.9 (*Biovigyanam*, 1978, **4**, 29).

A. barbadensis Mill. syn. *A. indica* Royle; *A. littoralis* Koening; *A. vera* Tourn. ex Linn.

Eng.–*Barbodos aloe, Curacao aloe, Indian aloe, Jafarabad aloe.*

Aloe varieties and their distribution (Wlth India, IA, 192; *Curr Sci*, 1979, **48**, 1001).

Betumi factory, Georgia produces three preparations of aloe, juice, emulsion and syrup with iron. Juice used for burns, suppurative wounds and trophic ulcers. Emulsion used in skin lesions. Syrup with iron used in anaemia [*East Pharm*, 1961, 4(46), 15].

Aloes are used in host of diseases, especially associated with digestive system. Aloe used in medicine, stands for its dried juice which flows from transversely cut bases of large leaves of various *Aloe* spp. Nature of aloe depends on spp. from which derived; it also depends on manner in which prepared. Slow drying in sun or on low fire gives amorphous opaque waxy ext. called 'hepatic' or 'livery' aloe; rapid concentration over a strong fire gives amorphous semitransparent mass called 'glassy' or 'vitreous' aloe (Wlth India, IA, 191).

Aloe, in menstrual diseases and stomach pain, tonic after pregnancy; not prescribed to expectant women. Contains glycd. barbaloin. Also details of aloe cultivation and med. properties: aloe produces pelvic congestion and used for uterine disorders, generally with Fe and carmin. Also as stomch. and in high fever. Root used in colic pain. Pulp used in menstrual suppressions. Mucilage used in painful inflam. Pulp keeps the nervous system under control if applied on head (*Indian Oil Soap J*, 1971-72, 37, 25; 63).

Aloe compd.(vet.), an ayurvedic non-hormonal compn. used successfully to treat irregularities of oestrous cycle in stud mares (*Indian Vet J*, 1980, 57, 762). Aloe compd., an indigeneous drug compn. useful in dysmen. without side effects, clin. trial (*Rajasthan Med J*, 1980, 19, 29). Aloe compn. useful in treatment of women sterility, clin. trial [*Med Surg*, 1981, 21(7), 22].

Aloe mixt. with other plant ext., a compn. for treating obstruction of lymphatic system (Ger Offen, 1969, 1963706; *CA*, 1971, 75, 91299 s).

A compn. of laxt.-hypnotic drug, which contains aloe ext. and other ingredients, allows for normal sleeping rhythm and useful in prophylaxis of drug abuse (Ger. Offen, 1972, 2128447; *CA*, 1973, 78, 62189n).

Various preparations from aloe ext., juice, polysaccharide, stabilized gel, etc. for topical use in burns, insect and fish bites, skin ailments, arthritis, myopathies, cosmetics, etc. [US Pat., 1963, 3103466; 1968, 3362951; 1975, 3898197; 3892853; *CA*, 1964, 60, 378g; 68, 89874n; 83, 48187g; 136932b; Neth Appl. 1965, 297511; *CA*, 1966, 64, 11032e; Aust. Pat., 1967, 273574; *CA*, 1968, 69, 61539d; *Acta Phytother*, 1972, 19, 83; *Farmatsiya Moscow*, 1978, 27(2), 40; Jpn Kokai Tokkyo Koho, 1979, 79119018; *CA*, 1980, 93, 99563v; *Seifen Oele Fette Wachse*, 1979, 105, 499; *CA*, 1980, 92, 220543u; *Cosmet Toiletries*, 1980, 95, 51; Fr. Demande, 1980, 2443835; *CA*, 1981, 94, 127150v].

Aloe meat eaten to alleviate colds; with salt keeps blood in good condition and relieves constip.; sap for same purpose. Aloes steeped with gomabush (*Stemodia maritima*) drunk to ease swellings and dropsy; leaves, as hot poultice to relieve swellings. In E. Africa, concoction to treat gonor. (*Econ Bot*, 1975, 29, 307; 1979, 33, 35).

Treatment of rats bearing guerin carcinoma with aloe alone, stimulated tumour growth, whereas treatment with aloe and benzotef markedly inhibited tumour; reoccurrence of tumour was also less common when mixt. was used for its inhibition (*Onkologiya Kiev*, 1971, No.2, 15; *CA*, 1972, 77, 70253y).

Antiinflam. compn. containing aloe ext. and steroids (Jpn Kokai, 1978, 7859019; *CA*, 89, 95018m); glycoprotein, alocutin A from aloe; may be used for cancer, inflam.; burns and skin diseases (*Eur. Pat. Appl.*, 1979, 2453; *CA*, 1980, 92, 11216a). Glycoprotein, alocutin A, its pharmacol.; had lymph-juvenating, haemagglutinating, cancer agglutinating and complement-activating; data on humans and animals given (*Jpn Kokai Tokkyo Koho*, 1979, 7973109; *CA*, 1980, **92**, 47211j); of alocutin B, a glycoprotein (containing 50% sugars) from aloe, haemagglutinating (*Jpn Kokai Tokkyo Koho*, 1979, 7973111; *CA*, 1980, **92**, 47212k). Glycoprotein from aloe, as anti-inflam. and anticancer (US Pat., 1980, 4225489; *Drug Pharm Patent Awareness Bull*, 1981, **4**, 136).

Alc. ext. of stem, antibact. against *E. coli, in vitro* [*J Res Indian Med*, 1974, **9**(2), 66]. Freeze-dried juice heated to 80° for 15 min. reported to inhibit growth of a number of bacteria (Wlth India, IA, 193).

Aloe ext. and vit., therapeutically favourable for glaucoma patients. (*Oftal'mol Zh*, 1967, **22**, 8; *CA*, **67**, 10311z).

A mixt. of aloe with cerebrolysin and vit. B$_{12}$ given to new-born rabbits enhanced density of the capillary network of cortex, stimulated nerve cell mitosis in cortex and cerebellum, and greatly reduced inhibitory effect of asphyxia on brain development (*Zh Nevropatol Psikhiatr im S S Korsakova*, 1970, 1815). Bradykininase activity of aloe leaves ext. (*Biochem Pharmacol*, 1976, **25**, 205). Aq. and alc. ext. of leaves showed antifert. activity in female rats (*Indian Drugs*, 1978-79, **16**, 124).

Aloin—cath. properties due to presence of a mixt. of glycds. called aloin; wide variation in aloin content of different varieties of aloes as also in different specimens of the same variety. This may be due to various methods of assaying used, and also due to the fact that aloin content varies with variety (Wlth India, IA, 192).

Aloin's principal constituent is w.-sol. crystalline glycoside, barbaloin [10(1)-deoxyglucosyl aloe-emodin anthrone]. Aloin also contains isobarbaloin and β-barbaloin.

Aloin detn., in dried juice by TLC (*Boll Chim Farm*, 1966, **105**, 767; *CA*, 1967, **66**, 79640c); comparison of methods (*Planta Med*, 1969, **18**, 36; *Herba Pol*, 1968, **14**,

243; *CA*, 1969, **71**, 42368x); colorim. (*Dtsch Apoth Ztg*, 1972, **112**, 1073; *CA*, **77**, 105664n); spectrophotom. (*Pharmazie*, 1973, **28**, 331).

Besides aloin, aloe contains aloe-emodin (hydrolytic product of barbaloin), isoemodin and resins. Resin fraction considered of equal importance as aloin, in cath. action of the drug (Wlth India, IA, 192). Assessment of purg. principles and aloe mixt. (*Planta Med*, 1970, **18**, 361).

Leaves of African aloe spp. contain aloesin (C-glycosyl-7-OH-chromone); glycosyl compds.; aloesone (aglycone of aloesin) (*Planta Med*, 1967, **15**, 342; 1969, **17**, 1; 1970-71, **19**, 322; 1972, **22**, 54; *J Chem Soc C*, 1970, 2581); from Japan, bitter glucd., aloenin (*Chem Lett*, 1972, 547; *CA*, **77**, 85571z).

Chem. compn. and biol. activity of aq. ext. of aloe (*Fiziol Akt Veschestva Respub Mezhvedom Sb*, 1971, 290; *CA*, 1972, **77**, 58742z). Phytochem. studies in Russian aloe grown at Ashkhabad (*Izv Akad Nauk Turkm SSR Ser Biol Nauk*, 1974, 83).

Colorim. detn. of 1,8-di-OH-anthracene (*Pharm Weekbl*, 1976, **111**, 1315; *CA*, 1977, **86**, 111220s). Leaves from plant grown in Egypt contain free and combined anthraquinones, carbohydrates and/or glycd. including barbaloin, chrysophanol glycd. and aloeemodin (*J Afr Med Pl*, 1977, No.1, 79). Juice, biogenic stimulator; it contains aloin, chrysophanic acid, aloeemodin and aloinoside A & B as major constituents. A liniment preparation from juice, clin. active in some skin ailments [*Farmatsiya Moscow*, 1978, **27**(2), 40].

Estn. of aloin in *A. barbadensis*, highest percentage of aloin (21.8%); and in *A. cilaris*, lowest (8.6%); sugars (4.5%), gums (8.2%), resin (5.7%), amino acid, etc. also determined; in addn. leaves contain sterols, triterps. (*Biovigyanam*, 1978, **4**, 29; *Lloydia*, 1978, **41**, 648); among others, substantial amts. of cholesterol, β-sitosterol, campesterol and lupeol (*Proc Okla Acad Sci*, 1978, **58**, 69; *CA*, 1979, **90**, 3177g). Str. of polysaccharide from leaves

(*Carbohydr Res*, 1979, **72**, 201; 1980, **86** 247; **87**, 249; *CA*, **91**, 35689n; 1981, **94**, 27388k, 2037g).

Aloe rev. of studies of aloes and other plants, 28 refs. (*Planta Med*, 1964, **12**, 260). Aloe detn. in commercial aloes and aloe exts. by TLC; identn. of aloes (*Arch Pharm Wien*, 1964, **297**, 681; *CA*, 1965, **62**, 7589f; *J Pharm Sci*, 1969, **58**, 197). Assay of aloe and its ext. (*Arch Pharm Wien*, 1965, **298**, 262; *CA*, **63**, 432h). Isolation of aloe prepn. (*Pharm Weekbl*, 1964, **99**, 1425; *CA*, 1965, **63**, 2051e). Aloes as arrow poison (*C R Acad Sci*, 1965, **260**, 4109). Chem. assay of aloes; and estn. of barbalovin in aloes (*Analyst Lond*, 1967, **92**, 593).

*A. christianii Reynolds

Indian studies of leaves gave aloin, 20.2%; aloin content almost equal to that from *A. barbadensis* (*Biovigyanam*, 1978, **4**, 29).

Grown in Indian gardens.

*A. ferox Mill.

Eng.–*African cape aloe.*

Important source of Cape aloes; uses similar to *A. barbadensis*. Sap (18 l) yields dried aloe (19.5 kg); inspissated juice as purg. for both man and beasts. Fresh leaf juice much valued by the African as a direct application to eye in opthalmia, also applied to sheep for treatment of scab. Leaf as a remedy for syphilis. Xhosa children fond of sucking sweet nectar from flower and if this is done to some extent it is said to produce a persistent weakness of joints; nectar is said to be narcotic. A preparation of leaf, for washing hair; leaf from Africa contains haemolytic sapogenin but not that grown in USA (Watt & Breyer-Brandwijk, 681-84).

A fraction of lyophilized aloe ext. *in vivo* inhibitory against sarcoma 180 and Ehrlich ascites carcinoma; pure active constituent alomicin more active (*Toho Igakkai Zasshi*, 1969, **16**, 365; *CA*, 1970, **73**, 75501e).

Leaves gave aloin, 12.4% (*Biovigyanam*, 1970, **4**, 28).

Cultivated in Indian gardens.

A. perryi Baker

Eng.–*Sucotrine or Zanzibar aloe.*

Plant aloin glycd., aloinoside B has same laxt. action as aloin (*Z Naturforsch*, 1964, **19B**, 222); aloe aloesin & its aglycone, aloesone (*Planta Med*, 1970-71, **19**, 322; 1972, **22**, 54).

A. succotrina Lamk syn. *A. perfoliata* var. *succotrina* Ait.; *A. vera* Mill., non Tourn. ex Linn.

Eng.–*Moka or Mocha aloes.*

Leaf juice—used in dysen., haemorrhoids. Remedy for haemor. congestion of stomach and spleen, valuable for uterine haemor. Useful in prolapsed uterus (*Bull Bot Soc Bengal*, 1972, **26**, 25). Mother tincture of plant, antimicrob. (*Indian J Exp Biol*, 1977, **15**, 338).

ALOYSIA(*Verbenaceae*)

*A. triphylla (L' Herit.) Britton syn. *A. citriodora* Ort. ex Pers.; *Lippia citriodera* H.B. & K.

Eng.–*Lemon verbena.*

Leaves—used for flavouring, seasoning food and in preparation of tisane. Also used in sachetts (Wlth India, IA, 195). A decoct. of leaves and flowers given as febge., sed. and antiflatulent. In Yemen, compresses of *Lavandula* sp. with *A. citriodora* used in mental agitation and dyspnoea (*Q J Crude Drug Res*, 1963, **3**, 395).

Essent. oil—leaves and flower tops yield essent. oil known as 'True oil of Verbena' or oil of verbena (0.1 - 0.7%), odour resembling lemon grass oil but more delicate (Wlth India, VI, 142). Spasmol. in isolated guinea-pig ileum and inhibited stim. effect of histamine (*Rev R Acad Farm Barcelona*, 1976, **14**, 39; *CA*, 1977, **86**, 65437t). Useful in conservative odontology; shows significant antimicrob. action against buccal cavity bacteria (*Plant Med Phytother*, 1980, **14**, 83).

Essent. oil contains citral (26-39%) as chief constituent (Wlth India, VI, 142); also sesquiterps. 15%, caryophyllane 2,6-oxide (*Helv Chim Acta*, 1976, **59**, 1803).

Leaves and flower tops contain, besides essent. oil, tannins, mucilage, acid phenols, flavons. and alks. (*Rev R Acad Farm Barcelona*, 1976, **14**, 39; *CA*, 1977, **86**, 65437t). Stems, stigmasterol, β-sitosterol and β-amyrin with their acetates; the last two, also as benzoates (*Curr Sci*, 1979, **48**, 534).

Indigenous to S. America, commonly grown in Indian gardens esp. in the hills.

ALPHONSEA (*Annonaceae*)

A. ventricosa Hook. f. & Thoms.

Leaves contain alks., galucine & nor-galucine (*Indian J Chem*, 1975, **13**, 306); roots, 16 poly-ynes (*Tetrahedron*, 1976, **32**, 737).

ALPINIA (*Zingiberaceae*)

A. calcarata Rosc.

Rhizome decoct., antiinflam. on carrageenin-induced hind paw oedema in rats (*Bull Med Ethno Bot Res*, 1980, **1**, 262).

A. galanga (Linn.) Willd. syn. *A. galanga* Sweet; *Amomum galanga* (Linn.) Lour.

Eng.–*Greater galangal.*

Rhizome (tuberous rootstocks) spray in ether, over a space showed high knockdown values against houseflies (*Bull RRL Jammu*, 1962-63, **1**, 169). Tuber, depress. to cardio-vascular system but stimulates respiration. Unani physicians consider it good for impotence (*Q J Crude Drug Res*, 1971, **11**, 1742). EtOH(50%) ext. of rhizome, anti-amphetaminic; diur. (*Indian J Exp Biol*, 1969, **7**, 250; 1977, **15**, 208).

EtOH ext. of plant antiinflam. [*Nagarjun*, 1977-78, **21**(11), 8]. Plant, antifung. (*Planta Med*, 1981, **42**, 140).

Essent. oil from rhizomes from Bangalore; 5.6% cineole, 2.6% Me-cinnamate and sesquiterps. (*Riechst Aromen*, 1963, **13**, 293, 375; *CA*, 1964, **60**, 1533g; 5271e);

from fresh rhizomes, 18 monoterps., of which α-pinene (22.5%), β-pinene(36.7%) and limonene (13.8%) were major and 17 oxygen containing monoterps. with cineol (69.0%), terpinen-4-ol, (8.7%) and α-terpineol (6.9%) as major compds. (*Sci Pharm*, 1981, **49**, 337).

Seeds contain antiulcer agents, 1′-OAc chavivol-OAc and 1′-OAc-eugenol-OAc (Jpn Kokai, 1974, 7436817; *CA*, **81**, 68544h); also caryophyllene oxide, caryophyllenol I & II, pentadecane, 7-heptadecane and fatty acid Me esters (*Chem Pharm Bull*, 1976, **24**, 2377).

A. nigra (Gaertn.) Burtt syn. *A. allughas*(Retz.) Rosc.; *Zingiber nigrum* Gaertn.

Rhizomes yield essent. oil, 0.05%; chief compds.: caryophyllene oxide, 23.0%; geraniol, 19.9%; eudesmol, 19.4%; and citronellyl OAc, 16.5% (*Riechst Aromen Koerperpflegem*, 1976, **26**, 139; 142; *CA*, 1977, **86**, 60387s).

A. officinarum Hance

Eng.–*Lesser galangal.*

Rhizomes, spicy in odour and pungent in taste resembling that of a mixt. of pepper and ginger (Wlth India, IA, 198). Rhizomes, constituent of Unani drug '*Jawarish Jalinoos*' used as diur., antimicrob. and for gastro-intestinal disorders [*J Res Indian Med*, 1979, **14**(3 & 4), 34].

A pharmaceutical compn. containing ZnCl, and dried rootstocks with those of *Sanguinaria canadensis* for treatment of skin cancer, caries and periodontal diseases, bilharziasis and *Pseudomonas aeruginosa* infections of skin (Eur Pat Appl, 1981, 25649; *CA*, **95**, 12795n).

Roots contain flavons.: galangin, kaempferide, kaempferol, quercetin and isorhamnetin (*Farm Aikak*, 1971, **80**, 95; *CA*, **75**, 59751x); and quercetin 3-Me ether, galangin 3-Me ether, kaempferol 7-Me ether and 7-OH-3, 5-di-OMe flavone (*Planta Med*, 1972, **22**, 145). Flavons. from rhizomes strongly antifung. against wide var. of pathogenic fungi including

Trichophyton rubrum, T. mentagrophytes, Epidermophyton floccosum, etc., responsible for major skin diseases in eastern India. Also active against a no. of Gram +ve & –ve bacteria, pathogenic and non-pathogenic yeasts; nontoxic to mice (*Indian J Exp Biol,* 1976, **14**, 712; 1975, **13**, 409).

Pungent principle in roots, 5-OH-7-(4-OH-3-OMe-Ph) - 1 - Ph - 3 - heptanone (*Yakugaku Zasshi,* 1978, **98**, 1255). 2 New and 3 known diarylheptanoids (*Chem Pharm Bull,* 1981, **29**, 2383).

Constituents of essent. oil (*Perfum Essent Oil Rec,* 1969, **60**, 88).

A. speciosa K. Schum.; see **Catimbium speciosum**

ALSOPHILA (*Cyatheaceae*)

*****A. australis** R. Br.

EtOH(50%) ext. of aerial parts, diur. (*Indian J Exp Biol,* 1974, **12**, 512).

Found in Tamil Nadu.

ALSTONIA (*Apocynaceae*)

Genus which is rich in indole alks. of multifarious skeletal patterns, can be divided into 3 well marked groups on the basis of major alk.; chief alk. of one group does not occur in other (Wlth India, IA, 199).

*****A. macrophylla** Wall. ex DC.

Eng.–*Match-stick tree.*

Bark, emmen., anticholeric and vulnerary. Administered as decoct., infusion or tincture. Leaves, greased with coconut oil, heated and applied hot to sprains, bruises and dislocated joints as a poultice (Wlth India, IA, 199-201).

Stembark yields monomeric indole alk., alstophylline; dimeric indole alk. villalstonine, macralstonine, macralstonidine; str. of villalstonine; monomeric quaternary alk. macrosalhine; dimeric macrocasalhine; macrocarpamine (*Helv Chim Acta,* 1965, **48**, 1349; 1966, **49**, 946; 1173; 1967, **50**, 1002; 1978, **61**, 337); some more alks.; total alk. content highest in stem bark and

lowest in leaves. Stembark of Indian plant yields villalstonine (0.8-1.0%) and macralstonine (0.06%). Macralstonine marked hypotens.; villalstonine, in a dose of 2mg/kg body wt of anaesthetised cat caused fall in B.P. which was unaffected by atropine. It is neuroleptic; 20mg/kg i.p. dose caused depletion of 5-OH- tryptamine on rat brain after 15 min. (*J Philipp Pharm Assoc,* 1967, **53**, 9; Wlth India, IA, 200).

Seeds, leaves, pods, stembark and roots, alk. pleiocarpamine (*Philipp J Sci,* 1968, **97**, 259).

Leaves yield indole alks. villalstonine, macralstonine and de-Me-alstophylline (*Nat Appl Sci Bull,* 1967, **20**, 225); from Indian plant, benzoylvincamajine (*Chem Ind Lond,* 1969, 1387); 3 monomeric affinisine, picrinine and picralstonine (*Phytochemistry,* 1972, **11**, 2605); an alk. quebrachidine and β-sitosterol (*Indian J Chem,* 1973, **11**, 706).

Roots also contain alks. (1.11% dry basis from Philippine sample) (Wlth India, IA, 201). Root alk. mixt., antihyperten. in animals and human with no side effect [*Sunday Times Magazine,* 1962, **18**(21), 44; *Philipp Abstr,* 1963, **4**, 5]. Total alks. given i.v. caused a fall in B.P. in dogs (*J Philipp Med Assoc,* 1964, **40**, 34; *Philipp Abstr,* 1964, **5**, 43). Roots, villalstonine, de-OMe-alstophylline; total alk. mixt. decreased 10-60% B.P. in dogs (*Nat Appl Sci Bull,* 1967, **20**, 225); macralstonine (*J Philipp Pharm Assoc,* 1967, **53**, 9).

Alks. of *A. macrophylla* (Wlth India, IA, 200).

Native to Malaysia, introduced and frequently planted in Indian gardens.

A. scholaris R. Br.

Eng.–*Devil's tree, dita bark tree.*

EtOH(50%) ext. of stem bark, hypoten. and anticancer (*Indian J Exp Biol,* 1968, **6**, 232).

Bark used in skin diseases (*J Sci Res Plants Med,* 1981, **2**, 101). Stem bark of *A. scholaris* and leaves of *Vitex negundo* used as poultice in bodyache and joint pains (*Ancient Sci Life,* 1981-82, **1**, 117).

Sap, gum and roots used in tumours and cancer (*Lloydia*, 1967, **30**, 407). In Assam, aq. ext. of bark latex used in tuberculosis; in New Guinea, milky, viscous white sap from stem used in ear sore. Sap mixed with water taken to cure cough and gonor. (*Q J Crude Drug Res*, 1979, **17**, 61; 1980, **18**, 33).

Aq. ext. of leaves significantly antimicrob. against *Mycobacterium tuberculosis (Philipp J Sci*, 1976, **105**, 205).

Various plant parts used in headache, pain in leg and loins, rheum., haemoplegia; cholera, broncht., phthisis and asthma, pleurisy, pneum., and lactation complaints (*Econ Bot*, 1970, **24**, 241). Plant used in treatment of skeletal fractures (*Sri Lanka For*, 1980, **14**, 145).

Trunk bark and fruit, rhazine (in both) (*J Indian Chem Soc*, 1969, **46**, 635). Stem bark, echitamine and a glycd. of venoterpine (*Indian J For*, 1978, **1**, 66).

Leaves, alk. picrinine (*Tetrahedron Lett*, 1965, 3633). Fresh leaves, alk. picralinal; crude ext. of the plant hypoten. and anticancer (*Experientia*, 1970, **26**, 1056); five alks. including picrinine (*Union Burma J Sci Technol*, 1970, **3**, 1; *CA*, 1972, **77**, 111466n). Leaves, alks. nareline, akuammidine, picralinal, picrinine and ψ-akuammigine (*Helv Chim Acta*, 1977, **60**, 1419). Leaves contain ψ-akuammigine, betulin, ursolic acid and β-sitosterol (*Indian J Chem*, 1977, **15B**, 390); flavon. and phenolic acids (*Indian J Exp Biol*, 1978, **16**, 512). Leaves, new indole alk., scholarine (*Phytochemistry*, 1981, **20**, 540).

Flowers, alks., picrinine (major), strictamine, tetrahydroalstonine and an unidentified indole alk.; picrinine, CNS depress. (*Planta Med*, 1976, **30**, 86); *n*-hexacosane, lupeol, β-amyrin, palmitic and ursolic acids (*ibid*, 1977, **31**, 33); strictamine, alk. from flowers, showed monoamine oxidase inhibitor activity *in vivo* and *in vitro*; and antidepress. in CNS (*Indian J Exp Biol*, 1979, **17**, 598).

Root and root-bark, echitamine chloride (*J Indian Chem Soc*, 1967, **44**, 639); α-amyrin, its -OAc, lupeol-OAc, stigmasterol, β-sitosterol and campesterol (*ibid*, 1968, **45**, 1183). Root bark of Thai plant yields indole alks., akamicine, its Nb-oxide & Nb-methiodide, ψ-akuammicine, Nb-di-Me-echitamine, tubotaiwine, echitamine (major) and some echitamidine isomers; stems, echitamine, its Me deriv., tubotaiwine, picrinine and echitamidine isomers (*Planta Med*, 1976, **29**, 380). Indian roots contain almost same alks. as those in Thai root (*Phytochemistry*, 1976, **15**, 821).

Chem. of *A. scholaris*, rev., 62 refs. (*Vishva Bharati J Res Sci*, 1979-80, **4**, 36). Alks. of *A. scholaris* (Wlth India, IA, 203).

A. venenata R. Br.

Stem bark contains 9 alks. including alstovenine & its C-3 epimer; their str. (*J Indian Chem Soc*, 1964, **41**, 638); pharmacol. of alstovenine (*Naturwissenschaften*, 1965, **52**, 187). Bark, indole alks., venenatine and isovenenatine (alstovenine) (*Tetrahedron*, 1965, **21**, 2951); reserpine, kopsinine, venalstonine, venalstonidine and echitovenine; str. of alk. venoxidine (*Tetrahedron Lett*, 1965, 2239; 159); alk., veneserpine (*Chem Ind Lond*, 1969, 1388); alks., 3-dehydroalstovenine and Δ^3-alstovenine (*Experientia*, 1973, **29**, 1337). Psychopharmacol. of 4-OMe- indole alks.; venenatine, sed. (*Planta Med*, 1975, **27**, 164). Stem bark, alk., tri-OMe-gallamide and anhydroalstonatine (*Indian J Chem*, 1977, **15B**, 183).

Fruit alks., echitovenidine and (+)-minovincinine; venoterpine (*Tetrahedron Lett*, 1966, 2483; 1968, 2763); ursolic acid and β-amyrin (*Curr Sci*, 1973, **42**, 606); also β-amyrin-OAc and lupeol ester of a β-hydroxy acid (*Indian J Pharm Sci*, 1979, **41**, 125); echitoserpine; new alks., (–)-echitoveniline, (–)-11-OMe-deriv., and (–)-11-OMe-echitovenedine (*Tetrahedron*, 1974, **30**, 2761; 1979, **35**, 1151).

Leaves, alk. echitovenaldine (*Chem Ind Lond*, 1973, 1032); echitoserpidine (*Phytochemistry*, 1974, **13**, 645); new alk., 19-*epi*-(+)-echitoveniline (*Tetrahedron*, 1981, **37**, 1243).

Root alks., alstovenine, venenatine, reserpine and 3- dehydroalstrovenine (*Indian J Chem*, 1975, **13**, 98).

Root bark, alk., 5, 22-dioxokopsane (*Indian J Chem*, 1979, **17B**, 651); new alks. 16-epivenenatine and 16-epialstovenine in addn. venenatine, alstovenine, etc. (*Phytochemistry*, 1981, **20**, 1981).

Alks. of *A. venenata*, rev., 50 refs. (*J Sci Ind Res*, 1978, **37**, 187; Wlth India, IA, 205).

ALTERNANTHERA (*Amaranthaceae*)

*A. pungens H.B. & K. syn. *A. repens* (Linn.)Link

Eng.–*Khaki-weed.*

In Argentina, plant used as diur. (*Lloydia*, 1972, **35**, 69); decoct. useful in gonor. (Wlth India, IA, 207).

Native to tropical America; introduced into India.

A. sessilis (Linn.) R. Br. ex DC.

Stems and leaves useful in eye trouble (*Bull Bot Soc Bengal*, 1968, **22**, 69). In Ghana, herb decoct. in gonor. Plant as enema for abdominal pains in pregnant women. With other ingredients herb used as abortif. Poultice of shoot used in swelling. Decoct. with little salt drunk to check vomiting of blood. Shoot with other ingredients used to restore virility. Poultice used for boils (*Ghana J Sci*, 1969, **9**, 119). Plant used for hazy vision, night blindness, malaria, post-natal complaints, *prolapsus ani, fistula ani,* diar., dysen., puerpeal fever, bite of rabid jackol or dog, and bone fracture (*Econ Bot*, 1970, **24**, 241); also in rheum. (*J Econ Tax Bot*, 1980, **1**, 137).

Pharmacol. (*Indian J Exp Biol*, 1971, **9**, 91). Herb ext., antiulcer in adrenalectomized rats (*Taiwan I Hsueh Hui Tsa Chih*, 1972, **71**, 256; *CA*, **77**, 96972g).

Herb contains hydrocarbons, ester and sterols (*Taiwan Yao Hsueh Tsa Chih*, 1975, **27**, 103; *CA*, 1976, **85**, 189263g); 24-Meenecycloartanol, cycloeucalenol, stigmasterol, campesterol, β-sitosterol, α-spinasterol, 5- α-stigmasta-7-enol and palmitates of sterols (*Hua Hsueh*, 1979, 22; *CA*, 1981, **94**, 117760e).

Roots, lupeol (*Pol J Chem*, 1978, **52**, 2495; *CA*, 1979, **91**, 207443w).

ALTHAEA (*Malvaceae*)

A. officinalis Linn.

Eng.–*Marsh mallow.*

Root—aq. ext. potentiated antiinflam. activity of dexamethasone (*Therapie*, 1966, **21**, 341; *CA*, **65**, 1267c). Syrup made from gummy matter of root, used in hoarseness, erosion of stomach and intestine for lubricating and relaxing the passage in nephritic and calculus complaints (*Indian J Hosp Pharm*, 1969, **6**, 102).

Polysaccharide compn. of plant mucilage (*Farmaco Ed Prat*, 1974, **29**, 83; *CA*, **81**, 47150m). Str. features of root mucilage (*Chem Pharm Bull*, 1980, **28**, 824).

Seed oil, malvalic acid (12.7%) [*J Oil Technol Assoc India*, 1974, **6**(1), 16].

A. rosea (Linn.) Cav.; see **Alcea rosea**

ALTINGIA (*Altingiaceae*)

A. excelsa Noronha

Et-OAc ext. of roots prevented gastric ulcers induced by different stressors in rats (*Bull Med Ethno Bot Res*, 1980, **1**, 250).

Resin from plant contains essent. oil, 4.4%; essent. oil from plant, 0.17% (*Perfum Essent Oil Rec*, 1967, **58**, 437).

ALYSICARPUS (*Fabaceae*)

*A. bupleurifolius DC.

G.–*Ad samerwo*; Mundari–*Nari jatanriba.*

In Bihar, herb crushed and fed to buffalo-calves as a vermicide (Wlth India, IA, 212).

Found all over India.

A. longifolius Wight & Arn.

Leaves, myricyl alc., β-sitosterol, its -OAc, pinitol, an aliphatic ester, rutin and a flavon. (*J Indian Chem Soc*, 1981, **58**, 819).

A. vaginalis DC.

Eng.–*Alyce clover*; G.–*Gaadar*; Mar.–*Dhakta dhampta*; Mundari–*Birbut*; Tam.–*Namappoondu.*

Leaf ext., anticancer (*Philipp J Sci*, 1967, **96**, 393). Plant used in treatment of skeletal fractures (*Sri Lanka For*, 1980, **14**, 145).

*A. vaginalis DC. var. **mummlarifolius** Baker

G.–*Bhoy samerwo*; Mundari–*Dudhi.*

Roots employed in Bihar for treating irregular menses (Wlth India, IA, 212).

Found in pastures of Rajasthan, and along the coasts.

AMARANTHUS (*Amaranthaceae*)

A. caudatus Linn. syn. *A. edulis* Speg.

Eng.–*Love-lies-bleeding, tassel flower.*

Used in dropsy and anasarca (*Econ Bot*, 1970, **24**, 241). Leaf, abortif.; as tea has been used for relieving pulmonary conditions (Wlth India, IA, 216).

Ferredoxine (*Biochim Biophys Acta*, 1970, **223**, 450). Fixed oil of seeds (*Indian Oil Soap J*, 1970-71, **36**, 273).

*A. graecizans Linn.

Eng.–*Prostrate amaranth, spreading pigweed.*

Herb is vulnerary, detergent and antiphl. Seeds used for pinole. Inflorescence, amarantin (Wlth India,IA, 222).

Native to Western USA, naturalized in India.

*A. hybridus Linn. ssp. **cruentus** Thell. syn. *A. cruentus* Linn. ; *A. paniculatus* Linn. Hook. f. (FBI) in part.

Eng.–*Red amaranth.*

Plant used in piles, to purify blood and in strangury as a diur. and antiscor. Leaves to relieve chest congestion and for local application in scrofulous sores (Wlth India, IA, 216).

Contains choline and betaine (*Poznan Tow Przyj Nauk Wyd Leb Pr Kom Farm*, 1966, **4**, 15; *CA*, 1967, **66**, 564n).

Grown as a leafy vegetable in Maharashtra, Nilgiri hills and Coorg.

*A. hybridus Linn. ssp. **hybridus** syn. *A. frumentaceus* Buch.-Ham.; *A. paniculatus* Hook. f. (FBI) in part non Linn.; *A. leucocarpus* Wats.

Eng.–*Green amaranth, pig weed.*

Fruits have distinct neck unlike the ssp. *cruentus*. Two vars. viz., *hybridus* syn. *A. chlorostachys* Willd. with green inflorescence and *erythrostachys* Moq. syn. *A. hypochondriacus* Linn. with red inflorescence.

Plant is detergent; used externally in ulcerated conditions of throat and mouth, as douche in leucor., as cooling wash for ulcers, sores, etc. Reported to be diur. (Wlth India, IA, 217).

Found in Himalayas, Madhya Pradesh, Gujarat, and in Nilgiris.

A. lividus Linn. syn. *A. blitum* Linn. var. *oleraceus* Linn.

Eng.–*Trailing amaranth, wild blite.*

EtOH(50%) ext. of aerial parts, diur. (*Indian J Exp Biol*, 1977, **15**, 208).

Leaves, alk., 0.63-0.70; stems, 0.40-0.45% [*Izuch i Ispol'z Lekarstv Rastit Resur SSSR* (Leningrad: Med) Sb, 164, 198; *CA*, 1965, **62**, 10821b].

*A. retroflexus Linn.

Eng.–*Red root amaranth, rough green pigweed.*

Plant—detergent, astrin.; relished by cattle but large quant. fatal. Nephrotoxic. Late summer cases of hay fever partly caused by this species (Wlth India, IA, 218; *Science*, 1977, **198**, 668).

Pollen ext. used as antigen in certain types of hay fever (Wlth India, IA, 218).

Roots, stems, leaves and flower contain choline, betaine and trigonalline (*Trav Soc Pharm Montpellier*, 1970, **30**, 203; *CA*, 1971, **74**, 72820t); roots also contain amaranthin, isoamaranthin, betanin and isobetanin (*Phytochemistry*, 1964, **3**, 547). Plant, KNO3, 6% (dry basis) (Wlth India, IA, 218).

Found in Khandala, Maharashtra.

A. spinosus Linn.

Eng.–*Spiny* or *thorny amaranth, spiny pigweed.*

EtOH(50%) ext. of plant, spasmog. (*Indian J Exp Biol*, 1969, **7**, 250). In Ghana, decoct. of herb used as mo uth-wash for tooth-ache; poultice mixed with native soap used as whitlow remedy; leaf infusion, diur. Plant, febge; suitable food for patients attacked by fever. Leaves used as enema, in stomach troubles, in curing piles and leprosy (*Ghana J Sci*, 1969-70, **9**, 119). Used in vomiting (*Econ Bot*, 1970, **24**, 241).

Pollen ext. useful in allergic asthma or allergic rhinitis in human patients (*Philipp J Sci*, 1972, **101**, 15).

Identn. of alkanes, sterols, acids, etc. by chromatogr. (*Curr Sci*, 1976, **45**, 481). Leaves and stems, hentriacontane and α-spinasterol. Root α-spinasterol and mixt. of saponins (*J Inst Chem India*, 1973, **45**, 205); also α-spinasterol octacosanoate and a saponin (*Indian J Chem*, 1979, **17B**, 180); 2 new saponins (*J Indian Chem Soc*, 1980, **57**, 417).

A. tricolor Linn. syn. *A. gangeticus* Linn.; *A. melancholicus* Linn; *A. polygamus* Linn., Hook.f. (FBI) in part; *A. tristis* Linn.

Plant astrin. Used as poultice in ulcerated throat and mouth. Also useful in toothache, sore throat and as a cooling agent (*J Agric Trop Bot Appl*, 1966, **13**, 251). Used in consumption, cough and bronch. (*Econ Bot*, 1970, **24**, 241).

A. viridis Linn. syn. *A. gracilis* Desf.

Eng.–*Green* or *wild amaranth, green pigweed.*

Shows vit. B12 like activity (*Indian J Biochem Biophys*, 1974, **11**, 71). Pet. ether ext. of plant possesses juvenomimetic activity (*Indian J Agric Sci*, 1978, **48**, 306).

In Ayurveda, root, as antifert. agent (*J Sci Res Plants Med*, 1981, **2**, 39).

Plant saponin (*Lloydia*, 1972, **35**, 288).

AMARYLLIS (*Amaryllidaceae*)

*A. belladonna Linn. syn. *Hippeastrum equestre* Herb.

Eng.–*Belladonna lily, cape belladonna.*

Bulbs—acrid and poisonous. In Java, they are used for poultice in swellings of the neck and contusions.

Bulbs contain an alk. bellamarin(e) identical with lycorine (Wlth India, V, 99). Indian bulbs, lycorine (0.02%) (*Indian J Chem*, 1967, **5**, 654); also ψ-lycorine and β-sitosterol (*Curr Sci*, 1969, **38**, 291); tazettine (*Planta Med*, 1972, **21**, 142).

Native of S. Africa; cultivated in India for its beautiful flowers.

AMBERBOA (*Asteraceae*)

*A moschata (Linn.) DC. syn. *Centaurea moschata* Linn.

Eng.–*Sweet sultan.*

EtOH(50%) ext. of seeds, toxic to *Alternaria alternata* and *Aspergillus niger* [*Environ India*, 1981, 4(I & II), 83]. Inflorescence, fragrant (Wlth India, IA, 222).

Herb, β-sitosterol (*Indian J Chem*, 1967, **5**, 523).

Native to E. Mediterranean region, cultivated in India for ornament.

*A. ramosa (Roxb.) Jafri

EtOH(50%) ext. of plant, anticancer (*Indian J Exp Biol*, 1980, **18**, 594).

Found in Kheri, U.P.

AMBROMA (*Sterculiaceae*)

A. augusta Linn. f. syn. *Abroma augusta* Linn.f.

Leaves used in homoeopathy; most effective uterine tonic, regulate irregular menses and pain (*Bull Bot Soc Bengal*, 1972, **26**, 25); paste used in Assam against ringworm (*Ethnomedicine*, 1980, **6**, 137).

Aq. ext. of roots, galact. in albino rats (*Indian J Pharm*, 1975, **37**, 153). Pet. ether ext. of roots showed antiimplantation and abortif. properties (*Indian J Med Res*, 1975, **63**, 378). Root powd., leaf juice estrogenic [*J Res Indian Med*, 1976, **11**(4), 7].

Leaves, taraxerol, its -OAc and β-sitosterol (*J Indian Chem Soc*, 1969, **46**, 849). Stem bark, friedelin and β-sitosterol (*ibid*, 1977, **54**, 647). Heartwood, β-sitosterol and glycol (*Curr Sci*, 1978, **47**, 301).

Roots, choline, betaine, β-sitosterol & stigmasterol (*Experientia*, 1970, **26**, 477). Root bark, β-sitosterol and polysaccharide (*Indian J Pharm*, 1975, **37**, 170).

Seeds, fixed oil (20.2%); fatty acid compn., linoleic (71.5%) having dietary role in the control of arteriosclerosis being anticholesteremic (*Planta Med*, 1971, **20**, 181).

AMBROSIA (*Asteraceae*)

*A. artemisiifolia Linn. syn. *A. elatior* Linn.

Eng.–*Dwarf* or *common ragweed, Roman wormwood.*

Plant—used in inflamn., and as detergent (Hocking, 11).

Pollen—causes pollinosis (Hocking, 11, 12). Preparation of therapeutic and diagnostic antigenic or allergenic exts. for use in hyposensitization therapy & diagnosis of allergies (US Pat., 1971, 3629397; *CA*, 1972, **76**, 90036n).

Plant, weakly active against KB cells; cytotoxic compds., psilostachyin and dihydroparthenolide (*Aust J Chem*, 1968, **21**, 1109); sesquiterp. lactones, ψ-guaianolides, cumanin, dihydrocumanin and peruvin (*Phytochemistry*, 1969, **8**, 793); germacranolides, artemisiifolin and isabelin (*ibid*, 1970, **9**, 199). Yugoslav plant, psilostachyin and psilostachyin C (*Glas Hem Drus Beograd*, 1972, **37**, 453; *CA*, 1974, **80**, 80080r); 2 new sesquiterp. lactones, their str. detn. (*Bull Acad Serbe Sci Arts Cl Sci Math Nat Sci Nat*, 1976, **54**, 43; *CA*, 1977, **87**, 35891q); sesquiterp. dilactone, psilostachyin B (*Planta Med*, 1977, **32**, 319); lactones from USSR plant

(*Khim Prir Soedin*, 1979, 578; *CA*, 1980, **92**, 143223k).

Pollen grains, hydrocarbons, sterols, triterp.; ambrosic acid, etc. (*Yakugaku Zasshi*, 1974, **94**, 362); ambrosic acid, a new irrit. peinciple (*Chem Pharm Bull*, 1974, **22**, 1435).

Found in Khasi and Jaintia hills in Meghalaya and also in Lucknow, U.P.

AMISCHOTOLYPE(*Commelinaceae*)

*A. hookeri (Hassk.) Hara syn. *Forrestia hookeri* (Hassk.) Hara

Mikir hills–*Chahalubor*; Nagaland–*Chagukadukhuan.*

Root paste applied to cuts (*Bull Bot Surv India*, 1976, **18**, 166).

Found in Assam and Nagaland.

AMMANNIA (*Lythraceae*)

A. auriculata Willd. syn. *A. senegalensis* DC.

Herb, hypoten. (*Indian J Exp Biol*, 1971, **9**, 91).

A. baccifera Linn.

Plant exts., antibact.; exts. of stem, leaf and inflorescence, more effective as compared to root and seed ext. (*Bull Bot Soc Univ Saugar*, 1978-79, **25-26**, 1).

Leaves contain lawsone (*Curr Sci*, 1972, **41**, 192).

AMMI (*Apiaceae*)

*A. majus Linn.

Eng.–*Greater ammi, bishop's weed.*

Fruit—also referred to as seed. Causes photosensitization in fowls and sheep (*Vet Rec*, 1975, **97**, 198; *Am J Vet Res*, 1978, **39**, 319). Dried fruit powd. or plant ext. used in vitiligo (leucoderma); clin. study [*J Sci Ind Res*, 1956, **15A**, Suppl., 1; *J Res Indian Med*, 1976, **11**(2), 75; 1978, **13**(1), 1]. Chief active principle, a furocoumarin, xanthotoxin (ammoidin).

Fruits contain ammoidin (xanthotoxin); ammidin (imperatorin) and majudin (bergapten); all the three compds. used in leucoderma; imperatorin, toxic to rabbits (*J*

Sci Ind Res, 1965, **15A**, Suppl., 1; 1962, **21C**, 132); the said 3 compds. and marmesin (*Acta Pol Pharm*, 1963, **20**, 321; *CA*, 1965, **62**, 399b); seed (fruit) furocoumarin detn.; their sepn. by paper chromatogr.; 4 furocoumarins, viz. marmesin, isopimpinellin, bergapten and xanthosin; imperatorin not found (*Med Promst SSSR*, 1963, **17**, 36; 44; 1965, **19**, 21; *CA*, 1964, **60**, 4449b; 850d; **62**, 14989f); isopimpinellin; also ammajin from Romanian fruits (*Naturwissenschaften*, 1966, **53**, 406; *Farmacia Buc*, 1966, **14**, 473; 1968, **16**, 213; *CA*, 1967, **66**, 118812g; **69**, 12987k). Highest amts. of furocoumarins present in fruits, while entire plantis green (*Sci Pharm*, 1966, **34**, 97; *CA*, **65**, 12562a). Preparation of ammifurin from seeds (USSR, 1970, 288229; *CA*, 1971, **74**, 130366n). Highest yield of xanthotoxin, 1.06; imperatorin; 0.8; and bergapten, 0.33% from air-dried mature unripe fruit from Cairo (Egypt); spectrophotom. estn. of furocoumarins (*Planta Med*, 1972, **22**, 122; 209; *Khim Pharm Zh*, 1967, **1**, 46; *CA*, **67**, 76348y). Fruit, minor furocoumarin majurin (*Tetrahedron Lett*, 1971, 1657). 5 Monohydroxylic coumarins: 7-isoPr-psoralene, dihydro-oroselone (both artefacts), ammirin, angenomalin (*Lloydia*, 1972, **35**, 469). Sepn. of ammajin and marmesin and their chem. estn. (*Planta Med*, 1973, **23**, 191). Antimicrob. activity of bergapten and nitrobergapten; gas chromatogr. estn. of fruit furocoumarins (*Egypt J Pharm Sci*, 1977, **18**, 167); also 12 psoralens including xanthotoxin, bergapten, isopimpinellin and isoimperatorin from Texas seeds (*J Agric Food Chem*, 1978, **26**, 1394). Chromatogr. method for furocoumarin detn. (*Khim Pharm Zh*, 1980, **14**, 78; *CA*, **93**, 21912j).

Essent. oil of seeds and its constituent; furocoumarin mixt., 60% (*Pak J Sci Ind Res*, 1979, **22**, 255).

Xanthotoxin—marketed under the trade name, 'oxsoralen'. Drug for leucoderma; effective orally in doses of 50mg t.d. or applied externally as 1% liniment followed by exposure of effected areas to sunlight or UV light for 2-hrs. Also used in 'suntan lotion' (*Indian J Pharm*, 1970, **32**, 165; Wlth India, IA, 225).

Detn. of xanthotoxin and isopimpinellin from leaves and/or fruits; also xanthotoxin and bergapten (*Farmacia Buc*, 1965, **13**, 331; 1967, **15**, 493; *CA*, 1966, **64**, 528e; **67**, 102702f). TLC-colorim. assay of xanthotoxin, imperatorin and bergapten in fruits (*Egypt J Pharm Sci*, 1975, **16**, 495; *CA*, 1978, **89**, 117614g); TLC-spectrophotom. det. of methoxsalen (xanthotoxin) in seeds (*Analyst Lond*, 1977, **102**, 779; *CA*,1978, **88**, 41715x). Extn. method (Indian Pat., 1976, 137495; *CA*, 1980, **92**, 116432u); CIMAP centre, Jammu method involves solvent extn. of powd. seeds followed by chilling and liq.-liq. extn., and chromatogr. sepn. after treatment with alc. HCl; bergapten, xanthotoxin and xanthotoxol separated, xanthotoxol methylated and total xanthotoxin (known as methoxsalen) purified. Max. xanthotoxin content, (1%) found in green fruits from Jammu (*Res Ind*, 1977, **22**, 12). Recovery from meladenine mixt., a byproduct of *A. majus* processing (*Egypt J Chem*, 1976, **19**, 533); meladinine, a drug containing both xanthotoxin and imperatorin, sold in various compns. increases pigmentation of normal skin and induces repigmentation in vitiligo (*J Ethnopharmacol*, 1980, **2**, 19). Xanthotoxin, imperatorin and umbelliferone, their sepn. and testing of antitumour activity (*Pharmazie*, 1981, **36**, 166).

Introduced into India; grown at Jammu and Delhi; plants naturalized under Jammu conditions.

A. visnaga (Linn.) Lamk syn. *Daucus visnaga* Linn.; *Visnaga daucoides* Gaertn.

Eng.–*Honeyplant, khella, tooth-pick ammi, tooth-pick fruit.*

Fruits—referred to as seeds, constitute the drug 'visnaga', 'khella' or 'khillia' consisting of mainly half fruits or pericarps mixed with a small quant. of unsplit fruits or cremocarps. Decoct. of fruit used by

Egyptians for expelling kidney stones and for renal colic (Wlth India, IA, 226). Used to bring relaxation of striated muscles in broncho-spasm (*Acta Phytother*, 1964, **11**, 111). Semi-purified exts. of plant tissue culture evoked pronounced vasodilation and bradycardia in rabbits ultimately resulting in death of animals (*J Pharm Pharmacol*, 1967, **19**, 760). 'Avisan', purified ext. of fruit, spasmol., diur., mild hypoten., in animals (*Farm Zh Kiev*, 1961, **16**, 51; *CA*, 1962, **56**, 13481e); extn. of 'Avisan' from fruits (USSR, 1969, 238098; 256461; *CA*, **71**, 42320 a; 1970, **73**, 7215 a). Chief active constituent in fruits (cremocarps) is a crystalline furocoumarin, bitter principle khellin (Wlth India, IA, 225).

Khellin—antisp., vasodilator, anthelm., antianaphylactic antiarteriosclerotic, antidiabetic, and antiulcerogenic (*J Ethnopharmacol*, 1980, **2**, 19). Used in treatment of angina pectoris and bronch. asthma. Commercially available as tablets and injections, but its use limited because of adverse side effects such as vomiting, dizziness, insomnia, vertigo, fatigue, etc. (Wlth India, IA, 226). But by manipulation of molecule, a compd. called 'Intal' (cromolyn sodium or di-Na-chromoglycate), largely removed toxic symptoms; prior inhalation of this compd. prevented immediate attacks against provocative inhalation of mixed pollen allergens (*Acta Allergol*, 1967, **22**, 487).

Fruits, active principles of *A. majus* are furocoumarins used in repigmentation in vitiligo while those of *A. visnaga* are chromones and furocoumarins showing spasmol. and coronary dilatory action (*Dtsch Apoth Ztg*, 1962, **102**, 733; *CA*, **57**, 16743 g). Highest % of total bitter principle as well as khellin in immature fruits, followed by flowers and mature unripe fruits; lowest in mature ripe fruits (*J Pharm Sci UAR*, 1968, **9**, 15; *Int Pharm Abstr*, 1970, **7**, 4830; *CA*, 1971, **74**, 1157 w). Chromone, khellin; furanochromone content of different Romanian plant parts;

inflorescence, 1.9-4.0; petals, 2.7-4.8; green fruits, 0.99-4.0%; mature fruits, 0.8-2.4%; extn. of khellin from green fruits recommended; also isolation of a ketol glucd. (*Farmacia Buc*, 1963, **11**, 375; 1968, **16**, 425; 1969, **17**, 617; *CA*, 1964, **60**, 6701d; **69**, 84071j; 1970, **72**, 70596j). Dihydroseselins assay in fruits and exts. (*J Pharm Sci*, 1969, **58**, 1545). Dental exts.: extn. of crude mixt. of furochromones, pyranocoumarins and flavon. (Fr Pat. 1970, 1588777; *CA*, 1971, **75**, 52794e). Quant. detn. of γ-pyrones (*Dtsch Apoth Ztg*, 1970, **110**, 44; *CA*, **72**, 118347h). Estn. of nonglycd. chromone and coumarin contents (*Planta Med*, 1970-71, **19**, 368). Spectrophotom. detn. of total furocoumarins (*J Natl Prod*, 1979, **42**, 366). Besides khellin, other imp. compds. are visnagin, khellinin, (khellol glucd.), etc.; visnagan, now resolved into 3 strongly vasodilating compds., visnadin, samidin and dihydrosamidin (Wlth India, IA, 226); rhamnazin (*Tetrahedron*, 1968, **24**, 2121); ketol glucd. from fruits of Romanian plant (*Farmacia Buc*, 1969, **17**, 617; *CA*, 1970, **72**, 70596j).

Khellin & visnagin, quant. detn. of khellin in wild plant (*Arch Ital Sci Farmacol*, 1965, **15**, 108; *CA*, 1967, **66**, 17033y). Biosynth. of visnagin from suspension culture (*Science*, 1965, **150**, 1731). Sepn. of khellin and visnagin and their assay in fruits, exts. and formulations (*Acta Pharm Jugosl*, 1966, **16**, 79; *CA*, 1967, **66**, 58868t; *J Pharm Sci UAR*, 1969, **10**, 189; 1970, **11**, 273; *CA*, 1970, **73**, 117046t; 1971, **75**, 137368u); by TLC (*J Pharm Sci*, 1970, **59**, 1025); micromethod (*J Drug Res*, 1971, **3**, 207; *CA*, 1972, **77**, 105656m).

Extn. of khellin from fruits by using 100-fold excess of 80° hot water, and 10% yield increase by ultrasonics (*Farmatsiya Sof*, 1971, **21**, 33; *CA*, 1972, **76**, 117455n). In RRL Jammu method, air-dried fruits, on extn. with solvent oil (bp 60- 80°) gave a fine powd. which on crystallization yielded a colourless crystalline khellin (0.98%) (*Res Ind*, 1977, **22**, 11). GLC detn. of khellin in fruits (*Pharm Acta Helv*, 1981, **56**, 223).

Leaves and flowers, several flavon. glucds. (*Planta Med*, 1964, **12**, 232).

AMOMUM (*Zingiberaceae*)

A. aromaticum Roxb.

Eng.–*Bengal or Jalpaiguri cardamom*.

EtOH(50%) ext. of rhizome and roots, hypoglyc. and anthelm. (*Indian J Exp Biol*, 1968, **6**, 232). Fruit paste applied to wounds and also against smallpox (*Bull Bot Surv India*, 1980, **22**, 161).

A. galanga (Linn.) Lour.; see **Alpinia galanga**

A. melegueta Rosc.; see **Aframomum melegueta**

A. subulatum Roxb.

Eng.–*Large* or *greater cardamom, Nepal cardamom*.

EtOH(50%) ext. of rhizome and roots, hypoglyc. (*Indian J Exp Biol*, 1968, **6**, 232). In Unani system, used as exhilarant for vital spirit; beneficial in fainting, insanity, nausea; dissolves gases [*East Pharm*, 1980, **23**,(272), 39].

Essent. oil from seeds, highly active against growth of keratinophilic fungi (*Nippon Kingakkai Kaiho*, 1978, **19**, 197; *CA*, 1979, **90**, 198238h).

Seeds, chalcone cardamonin and flavon., alpinetin (*Planta Med*, 1976, **29**, 391); petunidin-3,5-diglycd. and leucocyanidinglucd. (*J Indian Chem Soc*, 1976, **53**, 633); also a new aurone glycd., subulin (*Indian J Chem*, 1977, **15B**, 814).

Volat. oil from fruits contain a terp. (*Phytochemistry*, 1970, **9**, 665).

AMOORA (*Meliaceae*)

A. rohituka Wight & Arn.; see **Aphanamixis polystachya**

*A. wallichii King syn. *A. spectabilis* Hiern. non Miq.

H.–*Lalchini*; Ass.–*Amari*; B.–*Lalee, pitraj*; Trade–*Amari*.

EtOH(50%) ext. of stem, antivir., anthelm., and anticancer against human epidermoid carcinoma of nasopharynx in tissue culture and Friend's virus leukaemia (solid) in mouse (*Indian J Exp Biol*, 1968, **6**, 232).

Heartwood contains β-sitosterol (*Curr Sci*, 1976, **45**, 293).

Found scattered in evergreen forests of Sikkim, W. Bengal, Assam, Manipur and Andamans.

AMORPHOPHALLUS (*Araceae*)

A. campanulatus Blume ex Decne.

Eng.–*Elephant-root yam.*

In New Guinea fermented juice of petioles is drunk to treat diar. (*Econ Bot*, 1963, **17**, 16). Plant in earache, swelling of throat and difficulty in breathing, pimples, constip., cholera, haemor., septicemia, rinderpest, pain, kala-azar, enlarged spleen, intercostal neuralgia, pleur., pheum., puerperal fever, and diar. (*ibid*, 1970, **24**, 241).

Tubers used against abdominal tumours (*Lloydia*, 1967, **30**, 412).

Tubers contain protease inhibitors, trypsin and chymotrypsin (*Indian J Biochem Biophys*, 1975, **12**, 383). Corms, triacontane, lupeol, betulinic acid, stigmasterol, β-sitosterol & its palmitate, and glucose, galactose, rhamnose and xylose (*Indian J Pharm*, 1976, **38**, 109). Effect of purified starch on lipid metabolism in rats fed with atherogenic diet (*Indian J Biochem Biophys*, 1978, **15**, 423).

*A. dubius Blume

Eng.–*purple-stalked dragon*; Mal.–*Kattuchena, shena*; Sans.– *Kanana kanda*; Tam. – *Kattukarmei*.

Herb, in piles and apoplexy (Wlth India, IA, 234).

Found in Kerala.

A. sylvaticus (Roxb.) Kunth syn. *Synantherias sylvatica* Schott

Plant suspected to be poisonous to human beings and livestock (Chopra *et al*,

I, 35); used against tumours (*Lloydia*, 1967, **30**, 416).

AMPELOCISSUS (*Vitidaceae*)

*A. barbata (Wall.) Planch. syn. *Vitis barbata* Wall.

Lepcha–*Mikrum-rik.*

Crushed stems and tubers rubbed against swellings and body pains (*Bull Bot Surv India*, 1980, **22**, 161).

Found in hills of Assam and Meghalaya up to 1,200 m.

A. latifolia (Roxb.) Planch. syn. *Vitis latifolia* Roxb.

Used in muscular pain, sores, pneum., snakebite and bone fracture (*Econ Bot*, 1970, **24**, 266). Root decoct. taken in chr. dysen. (*Bull Bot Surv India*, 1973, **15**, 13). Roots applied in bone fractures and decoct. of stem bark given in stomach pain (*Bull Med Ethno Bot Res*, 1980, **1**, 8).

A. tomentosa (Heyne) Planch. syn. *Vitis tomentosa* Heyne

Used in swelling of head, leg and chest pain, spleen complaints, dropsy, anasarca, pimples, tubercular fistula, sores and carbuncle, dysen., neuralgia, pleur., pneum., rinderpest and bone fracture (*Econ Bot*, 1970, **24**, 266).

AMPELOPTERIS (*Thelypteridaceae*)

*A. prolifera Copeland syn. *Goniopteris prolifera* Presl; *Nephrodium proliferum* Keys.

Fronds used as alter. and aper. [*J Res Indian Med*, 1975, **10**(3), 68]; ext. inhibited formation of local lesions on *Chenopodium amaranticolor* by cucumber mosaic virus (*Indian J For*, 1980, **3**, 132).

Found throughout India on banks of rivers and ditches.

AMPHICOME (*Bignoniaceae*)

See **INCARVILLEA**

ANACARDIUM (*Anacardiaceae*)

A. occidentale Linn.

Eng.–*Cashewnut.*

Bark—ext., antihyperten. (Ger. Pat., 1971, 2034708; S. Afr. Pat., 1971, 7004836; *CA*, **74**, 91180a; **75**, 1154973e); antihyperten. principle from bark tannin (Rom. Pat., 1978, 63588; *CA*, 1980, **92**, 82416b). Bark ext. when given orally lowers blood sugar (Wlth India, IA, 245). Plants with hypoglyc. effects, rev. with med. properties of cashew and others, 32 refs. [*Leandra*, 1977, **6-7**, (7), 63; *For Abstr*, 1980, **41**, 256].

Bark exudes a pale yellow gum in stalictiform masses. Bark gum, partly w.-sol. and dextrorotatory. Gum, insectic. properties, used in pharmaceuticals and as a substitute for gum arabic (*Sci Cult*, 1966, **32**, 134; Wlth India, IA, 245); str. (*Indian J Biochem*, 1970, **7**, 68); Et-3,4,5-tri-MeO benzoate from gum (*J Indian Chem Soc*, 1971, **48**, 977). compn. of gum exudates (*Phytochemistry*, 1974, **13**, 2189). Bark, β-sitosterol (*Indian Oil Soap J*, 1969-70, **35**, 274).

Cashewnut shell—hexane ext., molluscicide for snails and toxic to fish (*Cienc Cult Sao Paulo*, 1974, **26**, 1054; *CA*, 1975, **82**, 134008k). Exts. caused high mortality against *Spodoptera litura* caterpillars (*Madras Agric J*, 1981, **68**, 270). Cashewnut shell yields gum; also cashewnut shell liquid and shell oil (yield, 25-30%) (Wlth India, IA, 244). Liquid-free nutshells, syringic and gallic acids and (+)-gallocatechin (*Curr Sci*, 1974, **43**, 341). Defatted nut shell yielded naringenin and prunin-6"-O-p-coumarate (*Phytochemistry*, 1978, **17**, 1064); new biflavon. glycd., occidentoside (*Indian J Chem*, 1981, **20B**, 150).

Cashewnut shell yields gum (9%), w.-sol. polysaccharide gum; hydrocolloid, acidic in nature which may find application in cosmetics, pharmaceutical industry, etc.; gum can be used for production of dulcitol, mucic acid and *D*-galactose having application in pharmacy (*Indian For*, 1972,

98, 710; *Res Ind*, 1975, **20**, 132; 1976, **21**, 243); str. of gum polysaccharide (*J Indian Chem Soc*, 1967, **44**, 1092; 1971, **48**, 567; 1972, **49**, 593; *Indian J Chem*, 1973, **11**, 996; 1974, **12**, 680; *Anal Chim Acta*, 1975, **79**, 185).

Cashewnut shell liquid (CNSL)—a vesicant juice (available commercially) a rich source of naturally occurring phenols, from which several new pesticides, drugs, etc. have been prepared (Wlth India, IA, 244; 245). Preparation of quaternary N-compds. from alkyl phenols, viz. cardanol, anacardic acid & their tetrahydro derivs.; also tetrahydrocardol (*Indian J Chem*, 1964, **2**, 265; 114; 337). Shell liquid, 90% anacardic acid and 10% cardol (*Trop Sci*, 1966, **8**, 79); isolation and detn. of anacardic acid (*Anal Chem*, 1968, **40**, 739); detn. of phenols in natural and tech. CNSL (*ibid*, 1976, **48**, 30). Variation of Compn. of CNSL obtained from different sources (*Lipids*, 1978, **13**, 525).

NMR of cardanol, cardol and other substances (*Indian J Chem*, 1972, **10**, 388). Recovery of cardanol (*Chem Age India*, 1976, **27**, 944). Simple liquid chromatogr. method for anal. and isolation of unsaturated components of anacardic acid (*J Liq Chromatogr*, 1980, **3**, 1497; *CA*, 1981, **94**, 71581s).

Cashewnut shell oil—(available commercially) dark brown viscous oil, sol. in org. solvents; a mosquito larvicide; addn. of 5% oil to kerosene or high speed diesel oil enhances antimosquito activity. Oil, mild purg. and used in treatment of hookworm (Wlth India, IA, 244). Also used for treatment of cracks on soles of feet, warts, corns and leprous sores; uses appear similar to tar obtained from bark (*Lloydia*, 1967, **30**, 394). Antibact. activity [*Indian Perfum*, 1971, **15**(2), 89].

Fruit or cashew apple—liquor made from apple valued as diur., having healthy effect on kidneys and advanced cases of cholera. It contains vit. C, 261.5 mg, and vit. E, 210 mg [*Indian Cashew J*, 1973, **10**(1), 9]. Also polyphenols of cashew apple juice (*Indian J Appl Chem*, 1962, **12**, 119; *Leath Sci*, 1978, **25**, 51).

Cashewnut—resinous juice useful in mental derangement, sexual debility, nervous prostration following seminal emission, morning sickness in pregnancy, palpitation of heart and rheum. percarditis, and loss of memory as a sequel to small pox (*Bull Bot Soc Bengal*, 1972, **26**, 25). Kernel good food for weak patients suffering from incessant and chr. vomiting; kernel oil good antid. for irrit. poisons [*Indian Cashew J*, 1973, **10**(1), 9]

Unsap. matter of lipids from cashewnuts contain squalene, cycloartenol, 24-methylene cycloartanol, β-amyrin, β-sitosterol and campesterol (*J Food Sci*, 1976, **41**, 190).

Husk (reddish brown testa) contains *D*-catechin, gallic, caffeic and quinic acids (*Leath Sci*, 1965, **12**, 396); polyphenols (*J Food Sci*, 1970, **35**, 140); (–)-epiafzelechin (*Indian J Chem*, 1975, **13**, 97); bioflavon., (–)- epicatechin, antiinflam. in rats; activity equivalent to Ph-butazone (*Indian J Pharm Sci*, 1981, **43**, 205). Flower polyphenols (*Phytochemistry*, 1969, **8**, 673); of leaves (*Plant Med Phytother*, 1977, **11**, 16; *CA*, **86**, 185967 m).

ANACYCLUS (*Asteraceae*)

A. pyrethrum DC. syn. *A. officinarum* Hayne

Eng.–*Spanish pellitory.*

Roots—used in rheum., toothache and in preparation of toothpaste (*Qual Plant Mater Veg*, 1962-63, **9**, 103). In Europe, tincture as local irrit. and rubft. Root as gargle in sore throat (*Acta Phytother*, 1971, **18**, 21). Constituent of indigenous drug, 'Amber Mezhugu' used in Tamil Nadu for treatment of many types of *Vatha* diseases (*Rheumatism*, 1976-77, **12**, 38). One of the constituents of an indigenus drug 'Fortege' used against sexual disorder in males (*Mediscope*, 1978, **21**, 140). Roots along with roots of *Withania somnifera* and *Vitis vinifera* used in epilepsy (*Q J Crude Drug*

Res, 1979, **17**, 61). Root ext., antibact. (*Fitoterapia*, 1980, **51**, 303).

Plant used as a drug in sexual disorders in male (*Nagarjun*, 1979-80, **23**, 170). Plant, polyacetylenic compds.

Roots, polyacetylenic compds.; 5 amides (*Chem Ber*, 1965, **98**, 1411; 1972, **105**, 1694); contain essent. oil, drug powerful stim. (*Q J Crude Drug Res*, 1971, **11**, 1742).

Roots contain pellitorine, anacyclin, enetriyne alc., hydrocarolin, inulin (*c*.50%), and (+)sesamin (Wlth India, IA, 248); N-(2′-*p*-OH-PhEt)deca-dodeca- & tetradeca-*trans*-2, *trans*-4-dienamides, a new series of tyramine amides corresponding to isobutylamides (*J Chem Soc C*, 1969, 2477).

Pellitorine, active principle of roots, intensely pungent; produces sialogogue effect. Physiologically analogous to piperine. A pharmacodynamic study of neuro-muscular toxic activity showed, it is more active on fish, crustacea, and cephalopod molluscs, while echinoderms are unaffected. Pellitorine is a mixt. of isoBu-amides (Chopra *et al*, I, 474).

Anacyclin has low insectic. effect towards grain insect, *Tenebrio molitor* (Wlth India, IA, 248). Anacyclin, isoBu-amide with acetylenic unsaturation pattern, takes on sialogogue and insectic. properties on semihydrogenation (*J Chem Soc C*, 1969, 2477).

ANAGALLIS (*Primulaceae*)

A. arvensis Linn.

Eng.–*Blue pimpernel, scarlet pimpernel.*

Herb used as piscic. (*Econ Bot*, 1970, **24**, 134). In Europe used as diur., diaphor., expect., in dropsy, rheum. and in hepatic and renal complaints, while in India used in gout and dropsy (*Acta Phytother*, 1971, **18**, 21). EtOH(50%) ext. of herb, hypoten., antivir., and diur. (*Indian J Exp Biol*, 1971, **9**, 91).

EtOH ext. of plant, potent uterine stim. on isolated guinea-pig uterus (*Indian J*

Pharm, 1962, **24**, 218). MeOH ext. of aerial parts, estrogenic in mice (*Farmacia Buc*, 1974, **22**, 499; *CA*, 1976, **84**, 65207b).

MeOH ext. inhibits herpes and poliomyelitis virus development; activity due to saponins (*Plant Med Phytother*, 1979, **13**, 122). Antifung. activity of herb ext. (*Geobios*, 1978, **5**, 49; *Acta Bot Indica*, 1979, **7**, 147). Antifung. activity of volat. fraction of leaf exts. (*Indian J Mycol Plant Pathol*, 1979, **9**, 250).

Antifung. agent from herb exts. (*Indian Phytopathol*, 1967, **20**, 64). Stems and leaves, heteroside (*C R Acad Sci Ser D*, 1969, **268**, 2279). Plant, triterp. anagalligenone B; also anagallin & its conversion into anagalligenin B (*Bull Soc Chim Fr*, 1971, 2320). Bitter cucurbitacin glycds., arvenin I & II and cucurbitacin E from whole plant (*Tetrahedron Lett*, 1977, 2099); also arvenin I, II, III & IV (*Chem Pharm Bull*, 1978, **26**, 3107). Cucurbitacin B, D & E, and probable presence of cucurbitacin I, L & R in herb (*Phytochemistry*, 1978, **17**, 1798).

Roots contain saponins of triterp. series (*Rastit Resur*, 1969, **5**, 380; *CA*, 1970, **72**, 63638w). Saponins had haemolytic index of 25000 (*Izv Akad Nauk Kirg SSR*, 1970, 54; *CA*, **73**, 106291t).

Aerial parts yield alk., 0.1% (*Pak J Sci Ind Res*, 1963, **6**, 53); *n*-hexacosane, rutin, β-sitosterol, stigmasterol, β-amyrin, lacceric acid, anagalligenin, glucose, arabinose and xylose [*Chem Era*, 1979, **15**(10), 10]. Flowers, stigmasterol, β-sitosterol, α-spinasterol 3-glucd., kaempferol, quercetin and rutin (*J Indian Chem Soc*, 1980, **57**, 761).

Chem. Compn. of seed oil; unsap. matter contain higher alkanols, stigmasterol & sitosterol [*Chem Era*, 1978, **14**(10), 455].

ANAMIRTA (*Menispermaceae*)

A. cocculus Wight & Arn.

Eng.–*Crow killer, levant/fish berry.*

Seeds and berries used as piscic. (*Econ Bot*, 1970, **24**, 134). EtOH(50%) ext. of aerial parts, anticancer and diur. (*Indian J*

Exp Biol, 1974, **12**, 512; 1977, **15**, 208).
Plant used in treatment of skeletal fractures
(*Sri Lanka For*, 1980, **14**, 145).

Alks., berberine, palmatine, magnoflorine and columbamine in stem and
roots; major tertiary alk. 1-8-
oxotetrahydropalmatine (*J Natl Prod*,
1981, **44**, 221).

ANANAS (*Bromeliaceae*)

A. comosus (Linn.) Merrill
Eng.–*Pineapple*.
Plant—fresh juice, excellent digest.; applied to horny excrescences on skin,
leprosy, elephantiasis; also found useful in
diphtheria (*Acta Phytother*, 1971, **18**, 21).
EtOH(50%) ext., spasmog. (*Indian J Exp
Biol*, 1973, **11**, 43). Alc. ext:, anthelm. *in
vivo* and *in vitro* against *Ascardia galli*
from infected pullet (*Indian Drugs*, 1978-
79, **16**, 234). Plant ext., nematicidal (*J Sci
Res Plants Med*, 1980, **1**, 18).

Fruits—blood purifier (*Econ Bot*, 1971,
25, 245). Juice of ripe fruit, diur., diaphor.,
and aper. (*Acta Phytother*, 1971, **18**, 21).
Juice, as also alc. and aq. exts. of unripe
fruits showed antifert. activity in female
albino rats (*Indian J Med Res*, 1970, **58**,
1285; *Indian J Exp Biol*, 1976, **14**, 623).

Rhizomes—pet. ether ext. and inorganic
fraction from alc. ext. of rhizomes showed
antifert. activity in exp. animals. (*Indian J
Exp Biol*, 1968, **6**, 252). Extn. procedure of
an antioedema substance from rhizome
juice (Ger Offen, 1969, 1913503; *CA*,
1970, **72**, 35777x); also with excellent activity from whole plant, fruits, and leaves
(Brit Pat, 1970, 1192773; *CA*, **73**, 59304b).

Addn. of 5% pineapple flower decoct.
and 2% ginseng root in cold creams can
control eczema and wrinkles (Fr Demands,
1971, 2073240; *CA*, 1972, **77**, 66111h).

Pineapple, volat. constituents: of juice
(*Aust J Chem*, 1964, **17**, 130); of canned
product (*J Sci Food Agric*, 1967, **18**, 106);
of essence detn. by gas chromatogr. (*J
Food Sci*, 1968, **33**, 284); of pineapple (*J
Agric Food Chem*, 1970, **18**, 306; *Helv
Chim Acta*, 1971, **54**, 1880); 3,4-ben-

zopyrene (very small amts.) (*Shokuhim
Eiseigaku Zasshi*, 1975, **16**, 187; *CA*, **83**,
162356m).

Leaves, ergosterol peroxides, 5-stigmas-
tene-3 β,7α-diol, β-sitosterol, campesterol,
stigmasterol and campestanol; first 2 compds. exhibit significant antifert. activity in
mice (*Indian J Chem*, 1975, **13**, 755).
Leaves of crown of fruit, 5-OH-tryptamine
(*Acta Bot Corat*, 1977, **36**, 83; *CA*, 1978,
88, 186093c); a novel steroid triterp. (*Diss
Abstr Int B*, 1976, **36**, 4497).

Stems contain enzyme bromelain and
starch, their method of extn. (*Taiwania*,
1972, **17**, 266; *CA*, 1973, **78**, 145173d); a
trihydroxy triterp. carboxylic acid called
ananasic acid (*Tetrahedron*, 1976, **32**,
1077); glyceryl esters of caffeic and *p*-
coumaric acids (*Lloydia*, 1976, **39**, 409).

Bromelain(s)—also called bromelin,
proteolytic enzyme and potent antiinflam.
agent (*Angiology*, 1962, **13**, 508). A mixt.
of proteases called bromolain A & B (*J
Biochem*, 1966, **59**, 463; Ger. East, 1967,
55405; *CA*, **67**, 84851x). Present in all
parts of the plants; commercially obtained
from stem. Useful in determining antibody
substances, dissolving necrogenic tissues,
treating digest. troubles; when applied as
an antiphl., it shows less after-effects (Wlth
India, IA, 260). Properties (*Z
Gastroenterol*, 1968, **6**, 185; *CA*, 1969, **70**,
54276h). Process developed by RRL, Jor-
hat for bromelain solutions from fruit flesh
[*Sem Rep*, 1974, **4**(4), 5]; isolation and
purification, rev., 15 refs. (*Methods Carbohydr Chem*, 1976, **7**, 175; *CA*, **85**,
88963e); industrial extn., rev., 26 refs (*Rev
Col Quim Ing Quin Coasta Rica*, 1976, **6**,
8; 11; *CA*, 1978, **89**, 55237a). Extn. and
activity (*MARDI Res Bull*, 1978, **6**, 172;
165; *CA*, 1979, **92**, 71733f; 104243b).

ANAPHALIS (*Asteraceae*)

*A. adnata DC.

Flower heads and plant hairs used to
stop bleeding (*Econ Bot*, 1971, **25**, 414).
Plant contains 4-OH-dehydrokawain and

campesterol (*Indian J Chem*, 1976, **14B**, 300).

Found in temperate Himalayas at 1,000 - 3,000 m, in Lushai hills, and in Andhra Pradesh.

*A. contorta Hook. f.

Flowers yield a kaempferol glucd., tiliroside & its acetate (*J Chin Chem Soc Taipai*, 1975, **22**, 383; 1976, **23**, 57). Whole plant, 5-OMe-7-OH-phthalide new phthalides, anaphatol and 5,7'-di-(OH)-phthalide and β-sitosterol (*Indian J Chem*, 1980, **19B**, 927).

Essent. oil from plant and its constituents; physical constants; cineol, 60; *d*-limonene, 24%, and others [*Indian Perfum*, 1974, **18**(Pt.2), 35; 1975, **19**(Pt.1), 33; 1977, **21**, 129; 1978, **22**, 16]. Essent. oil antibact., *in vitro*; also preliminary pharmacol. investigation (*Indian J Exp Biol*, 1977, **15**, 339; 1980, **18**, 594).

In temperate Himalayas; common in Sikkim.

*A. cuneifolia Hook.f.

EtOH(50%) ext. of plant, antibact. (*Indian J Exp Biol*, 1973, **11**, 43).

Found in Chamoli, U.P.

A. margaritacea Benth. & Hook. f. syn. *A. cinnamomea* C.B. Clarke

Kumaun–*Vernapata.*

Leaves applied to wounds and cuts (*Indian Drugs*, 1976-77, **14**, 47); contain steroid/terp. and flavan. (*Q J Crude Drug Res*, 1980, **18**, 17).

Found in temperate Himalayas at 1,200 - 2,700m and also in Aka and Khasi hills.

*A. triplinervis C.B. Clarke

EtOH(50%) ext. of plant, diur. (*Indian J Exp Biol*, 1974, **12**, 512).

Roots yield, biogenetically active triacetylene compds. (*Chem Ber*, 1966, **99**, 1648; *CA*, **65**, 3823a).

Found in temperate Himalayas, from Kashmir to Bhutan at 1,800 - 3,000 m.

ANCHUSA (*Boraginaceae*)

Source of heptatoxic pyrrolizidine alks. from *A. arvensis* Bieb. and *A. officinalis* Linn. (*J Natl Prod*, 1981, **44**, 129).

*A. capensis Thunb.

Eng.–*Bugloss, Cape forget-me not.*

Nutlets, fatty oil (29%); show +ve test for alks. (Wlth India, IA, 263).

Native to S. Africa, grown in Indian gardens for pot culture.

*A. italica Retz. syn. *A. azurea* Mill.

Nutlets yield fatty oil (21.4%) rich in cit. E (0.72%), content of which is more than wheat-germ oil (0.18%); gave +ve tests for alks. and tannins (Wlth India, IA, 263; *Chromatographia*, 1978, **11**, 193).

Flowers, anthocyanins; leafy stems, bornesitol (Wlth India, IA, 263).

Grown in Indian gardens.

*A. strigosa Labill.

Trade–*Gaozaban.*

Leaves and nutlets—stim., tonic, diur. and demulc., useful in cough, asthma, stones in bladder and kidney, and in bilious complaints. Drug administered as decoct. or syrup; pharmacognostic studies (Wlth India, IA, 263; *J Sci Ind Res*, 1962, **21C**, 317; *Indian J Pharm*, 1968, **30**, 167; *Q J Crude Drug Res*, 1970, **10**, 1581; 1971, **11**, 1818).

Pharmacol. (13th *Annu Confr Indian Pharmacol Soc RRL Jammu* 1980, Abstr. No.B8). Aq. ext. of flower, hypoten. (*Indian J Pharmacol*, 1981, **13**, 31).

Drug imported from W. Asia.

ANCISTROCLADUS (*Ancistrocladaceae*)

*A. heyneanus Wall. ex Grah.

Mar.–*Kardal, kardor.*

EtOH(50%) ext. of aerial parts, spasmol. (*Indian J Exp Biol*, 1974, **12**, 512; *Phytochemistry*, 1975, **14**, 578).

Roots contain alk. ancistrocladine; its str.; its -OMe deriv. (*Indian J Chem*, 1970, **8**, 567; 1971, **9**, 931; *Tetrahedron*, 1971, **27**, 1013); minor alks. ancistrocladinine; ancistrocladisine; ancistrocladidine (*Indian*

J Chem, 1971, **9**, 1421; 1972, **10**, 1117; 1973, **11**, 1190; 1976, **14B**, 473). Stereochem. of ancistrocladisine and ancistrocladinine; configuration of former and ancistrocladidine (*J Chem Soc Perkin Trans I*, 1974, 1413; 1975, 2134). Ancistrocladidine showed spasmol. activity on isolated guinea pig ileum at a concn. of 5 g/ml comparable with that of papaverine (*in* Wagner and Wolff, 213).

Roots also contain β-sitosterol; lupeol; a naphthaquinone, ancistroquinone; 1,8-di-MeO-3-Me-naphthalene; and a quinone, droserone (*Indian J Chem*, 1969, **7**, 308; 1971, **9**, 611; 1042; 1972, **10**, 1117; 1973, **11**, 840); leaves, octacosanol (*ibid*, 1970, **8**, 851).

Found in evergreen and semi-evergreen forests from Konkan to Kerala.

*A. tectorius (Lour.) Merrill syn. *A. extensus* Wall. ex Planch.

Leaves, arom. Boiled roots used in dysen. and malaria (Wlth India, IA, 264).

Plant, an alk. reported to be identical with ancistrocladine (*Phytochemistry*, 1975, **14**, 2699).

Stems and twigs, new alk. ancistrodine, ancistrocladine and hamatine; ancistrodine inhibited Walker 256 tumour in rats (*Acta Pharm Sin*, 1981, **16**, 519).

Found in dense forests on the sea coast of Andamans.

ANDIRA (*Fabaceae*)

A. araroba Aguiar

Chrysarobin, a mixt. of neutral principles obtained from Goa powd., a substance deposited in trunks, official as parasiticide in IP (IP, 1966, 130); effective as antipsoriatic (*Hautarzt*, 1969, **20**, 204; *CA*, **71**, 28935y). Main constituents of chrysarobin: chrysophanolanthrone, physcionanthrone, amodinanthrone, chrysophanol, physcion, emodin, chrysophanolidianthrone, physciondianthrone, and chryso- phanolphysciondianthrone (*Pharm Weekbl*, 1970, **105**, 61; *CA*, **72**, 59126k).

Imported in India.

*A. inermis H.B. & K.

Eng.–*Cabbage angelin tree.*

Wood, powerful anthelm., narcotic and purg. Seeds, same properties as wood; also used as febge. Bark, febge., anthelm. and purg.; poisonous in large doses and causes vomiting and delirium.

Wood, isoflavonoids biochanin A and inermin (de-Me-pterocarpin), and long chain fatty acids. Plant, alks. berberine and N-Me- tyrosine (angeline, andirine) (Wlth India, IA, 264).

Cultivated in Calcutta gardens and also; grown as a windbreak and for shade in coffee plantations.

ANDRACHNE (*Euphorbiaceae*)

A. cordifolia (Decne) Muell.-Arg. syn. *Leptopus cordifolius* Decne; *Arachne cordifolia* (Decne) Hurusawa

EtOH(50%) ext. of aerial parts, hypothermic (*Indian J Exp Biol*, 1973, **11**, 43); aq. ext. of branchlets, insectic. (Wlth India, IA, 264). Fruits, insectic. (*Nagarjun*, 1979-80, **23**, 177).

ANDROGRAPHIS (*Acanthaceae*)

A. echioides Nees

EtOH(50%) ext. of plant, diur. (*Indian J Exp Biol*, 1977, **15**, 208).

Plant, echioidin; echioidinin (*Tetrahedron*, 1965, **21**, 3715; 2633).

A. paniculata (Burm.f.) Wall. ex Nees
Eng.–*Creat.*

Kalmegh — official in IP; drug consists of dried leaves and tender shoots; yields not less than 1% of andrographolide on dry wt. basis (IP, 1966, 264).

Powd. plant mixed with *sarson* oil, applied in itching (*Econ Bot*, 1965, **19**, 244). Plant used in spleen complaints, colic, strangulation of intestine, constip., diar., cholera, phthisis, consumption and bite of rabid jackal (*ibid*, 1970, **24**, 244). Domestic medicine for flatulence and diar. of children. Used in tropidity of liver, neuralgia and convalescence after fever (*Bull Bot Soc Bengal*, 1972, **26**, 25).

Plant chief constituent of an Ayurvedic drug '*SG-I Switradilepa*' for dermatological diseases [*J Res Indian Med*, 1976, **11**(2), 66]. Constituent of drug 'Tefroli' used in viral hepatitis (*Antiseptic*, 1980, **77**, 643).

Leaf and stem exts. of *kalmegh*/andrographolide given s.c. or orally did not change blood sugar level of normal or diabetic rats (*Bangladesh Pharm J*, 1977, **6**, 21; *CA*, 1978, **88**, 315y). *Kalmegh* increased biliary flow and liver wt. in rats and decreased hexobarbital induced sleeping time; less potent than phenobarbital (*Indian J Exp Biol*, 1978, **16**, 830). Alc. ext. of plant prolonged the life of mice given cobra snake venom; ext. showed muscarinic activity in dog B.P., etc. (*Indian J Pharm Sci*, 1978, **40**, 132). Powd. stem showed antifert. activity in male mice (*Bangladesh Med Res Counc Bull*, 1979, **5**, 14). Leaf ext., hypoten. [*Acta Med Philipp*, 1980, **16**(2), 59].

Leaves, β-sitosterol glucd. and unknown compds. (*Pak J Sci Ind Res*, 1963, **6**, 152; *CA*, 1964, **60**, 13572 e). Alc. ext. of leaves andrographolide and panicolide (*Sci Res Dacca*, 1964, **1**, 65; *CA*, **61**, 16442h). Polyphenols, caffeic and chlorogenic acids, and a mixt. of dicaffeoylquinic acid from leaves (*Leath Sci*, 1978, **25**, 250).

Andrographolide — estn. of leaves; a better method than that given in I.P. (*Indian J Chem*, 1968, **6**, 359); faster method for estn. by TLC of liquid exts. of *kalmegh* leaves (*Indian J Appl Chem*, 1969, **32**, 25). Leaves, bitter substances (*Acta Pharm*, 1973, **4**, 36; *CA*, **79**, 118269d). Correction in str. of antimicrob. andrographolide Na bisulphite (included in Chinese Pharmacopoeia, 177) (*Yao Hsueh T'ung Pao*, 1980, **15**, 41; *CA*, 1981, **95**, 175611p).

Roots, flavones andrographin and panicolin, and α-sitosterol (*Sci Res Dacca*, 1964, **1**, 223; *CA*, 1965, **62**, 8119h); 5-OH-7,8,2',3'-tetra-MeO-flavone (*Indian J Chem*, 1969, **7**, 306); in addn., flavones,

apigenin 4,7-diMe ethers and mono-OMe-wightin (*Pak J Sci Ind Res*, 1972, **15**, 33; *CA*, 1973, **78**, 43200t).

Plant, diterp. glucd., neoandrographolide (*Tetrahedron Lett*, 1968, 4803); str. and stereochem. of neoandrographolide (*Tetrahedron*, 1971, **27**, 5081). Chem. examination of plant [*J Res Indian Med*, 1972, **7**(1), 93]. Ext. of plant gave 14-deoxy-11-oxoandrographolide and 14-deoxy-11, 14-didehydroandrographolide and 14-deoxyandrographolide (*J Chem Soc Perkin Trans I*, 1973, 1247). Rev. covering bot., chem. and biochem. details, 45 refs. (*Indian Drugs*, 1977-78, **15**, 187). 3 Flavones from cultures (*Phytochemistry*, 1979, **18**, 149). Apigenin 7,4'-di-OMe ether from plant exhibited antiulcer activity in Shay rats, histamine-induced ulcer in guinea pigs and aspirin ulcers in rats (*Indian J Pharm Sci*, 1981, **43**, 159).

*A. serpyllifolia Wight

Leaves, stems and roots, apigenin-7,4'-di-OMe ether; stems and roots, also tectochrysin and a new flavone, serpylin (*Tetrahedron*, 1968, **24**, 7027); apigenin-7,4'-di-OMe ether, antiulcer (*Indian J Pharm Sci*, 1981, **43**, 159).

Found in Tamil Nadu and Andhra Pradesh up to 900 m.

*A. wightiana Am. ex Nees

Stems and roots, flavone, wightin (5,3'-di-OH-7,8,2'-tri-MeO flavone); and leaves, echioidinin (*Tetrahedron*, 1965, **21**, 3237; *Indian J Chem*, 1967, **5**, 523). Plant, a bicyclic diterp. lactone, wightionolide (*J Chem Soc Perkin Trans I*, 1974, 2517).

Distributed in hills of Kerala, Tamil Nadu, and Karnataka up to 750 m.

ANDROPOGON (*Poaceae*)

A.citratus DC.; see **Cymbopogon citratus**

A.contortus Linn.; see **Heteropogon contortus**

A.halepensis Brot.; see **Sorghum halepense**

A. intermedius R. Br.; see **Dichanthium glabrum**

A. jwarancusa Jones; see **Cymbopogon jwarancusa**

A. muricatus Retz.; see **Vetiveria zizanioides**

A. nardus Linn.;see **Cymbopogon nardus**

A. nardus var. **flexuosus;** see **Cymbopogon flexuosus**

A. pertusus Willd.; see **Dichanthium pertusum**

A. sorghum Brot.; see **Sorghum bicolor**

A. squarrosus Hook.f.; see **Vetiveria zizanioides**

ANDROSACE (*Primulaceae*)

*A. sarmentosa Wall.
U.P.–*Gorabnurey*.
EtOH(50%) ext. of plant, spasmol. (*Indian J Exp Biol*, 1980, **18**, 594).
Chamoli, U.P.

ANEMONE (*Ranunculaceae*)

A.crinita Juz. syn. *A. narcissiflora* Linn.

Herb contains betulinic acid, oleanolic & its rhamnoside, β-amyrin and β-sitosterol (*J Indian Chem Soc*, 1979, **56**, 1041); 3 triterp. saponins, narcissiflorine, narcissiflorinine and narcissifloridine (*Phytochemistry*, 1981, **20**, 1675).

*A. japonica Sieb. & Zucc.
Eng.–*Japanese wind-flower*.

In China, roots used with other drugs for heart ailments. Fresh juice found to be effective against several pathogenic fungi; active principle of the juice is an unsaturated ester which is steam-volatile, greyish yellow liquid with irrit. odour. On exposure to air, it polymerises to form anemonin or higher w.-insol. polymers (Wlth India, IA, 268).

Introduced into Indian gardens for ornament.

A. obtusiloba D. Don

New triterp. saponin, obtusilobinin and obtusilobin; also new saponin, obtusilobicinin (*Phytochemistry*, 1979, **18**, 1539; 1980, **19**, 1244).

*A. rivularis Buch.- Ham. ex DC.
Khasi–*Bat-soh-plia*.
EtOH(50%) ext. of plant, anticancer (*Indian J Exp Biol*, 1980, **18**, 594).

Plant contains betulinic acid (*Proc Nat Acad Sci India*, 1975, **45A**, 300); and saponin, rivularinin (*Phytochemistry*, 1978, **17**, 1991).

Found in Eastern Himalayas, and hills of S. India.

*A. vitifolia Buch.-Ham. ex DC.
Eng.–*Vine-leaved anemone*.
EtOH(50%) ext. of plant, hypothermic(*Indian J Exp Biol*, 1973, **11**, 43). Plant ext., antifung. (*Geobios*, 1978, **5**, 49).

Found throughout the temperate Himalayas from Kashmir to Arunachal Pradesh, between 1,300 - 2,700 m.

ANETHUM (*Apiaceae*)

A. graveolens Linn.
Eng.–*Dill*.

Tea made from boiled seeds, given to loose bowels, to newborn children (*Econ Bot*, 1975, **29**, 321). Various dill preparations (Herbal Med., 86-87, 144, 171).

Seed essent. oil known as dill oil, used in preparation of gripe waters (Wlth India, IA, 269); antimicrob.(*Indian J Hosp Pharm*, 1978, **15**, 166); antifung.[*Indian Drugs Pharmac Ind*, 1978, **13**(1), 7; 1979, **14**(1), 3].

IP standards (IP 1966, 172-73). Characteristic data for seed oil from U.P. [*Indian Perfum*, 1967, **11**(Pt.II), 22; Wlth India, IA, 270]; from NBRI Lucknow (*Indian Perfum*, 1980, **24**, 124).

Cultivation investigations [*Perfum Essent Oil Rec*, 1969, **60**, 277; *Fert News*, 1971, **16**(2), 48]; agronomic studies[*Indian Oil Soap J*, 1970-71, **36**, 55; *Indian Perfum*, 1976, **20A** (Pt.I), 85].

Seeds of *A. graveolens* if cultivated in India, developed dillapiol (Wlth India, IA, 270); contradictory findings (*J Pharm Pharmacol*, 1969, **21**, 259). Chem. constituents of Kumaun seed essent. oil; of Indian seeds, carvone, 34.5% (*Flavour Ind*, 1970, **1**, 473; 1971, **2**, 241). Photom. detn. of dill oil (*Konserv Ovoshchesush Promst*, 1971, **26**, 30). Comparative study of essent. oils of seeds of *A. graveolens* and *A. sowa* (*Curr Sci*, 1972, **41**, 50). Essent. oil content max. at milk wax stage [*Rastenievud Nauki*, 1974, **11**(3), 69; *CA*, **81**, 111393 x].

Constituents of dill oil from different countries: from Egypt; contained dillapiol (*Acta Pharm Suec*, 1968, **5**, 155; *CA*, **69**, 45984q); from Hungary (*Acta Chim Acad Sci Hung*, 1974, **83**, 1; 1977, **94**, 1); from Alberta (*Can Inst Food Sci Technol J*, 1977, **10**, 208; *CA*, **87**, 182846g); from Romania (*Contrib Bot Univ Babes - Bolyai Cluj Gradina Bot*, 1980, 263; *CA*, 1981, **94**, 136149d).

Chem. studies of essent. oils from *A. graveolens* and *A. sowa* [*Indian Perfum*, 1971, **15**(Pt.I), 27]. Dill herb oil less important than dill seed oil (Arctander, 216). Constituent of weed oil from USA (*Taiwan K'o Hsueh*, 1978, **32**, 131; *CA*, 1979, **91**, 52719q). Variation of oil content with season (*Pharmazie*, 1977, **32**, 607; *CA*, 1978, **88**, 86130u).

Carvone—from dill oil (*J Inst Chem India*, 1967, **39**, 141). Spectrophotom. detn. in developing fruits (*J Pharm Pharmacol*, 1965, **17**, Suppl., 41). Gas chromatogr. estn. of carvone and dillapiol in fruits; dillapiol absent from European dill (even grown in India)(*ibid*, 1969, **21**, 259). Colorim. detn. in oil (*J Assoc Off Anal Chem*, 1979, **62**, 250). Insectic. and synergist compds.: *d*-carvone (only in aerial parts), apiol and dillapiol (in roots). Green dill exts. more active as insectic. and synergist than root ext.; high biol. activity of green parts due to *d*-carvone (*J Agric Food Chem*, 1974, **22**, 658). Carvone and limonene from dill oil [*Maslo-Zhir Promst*, 1980,(10), 28; *CA*, 1981, **94**, 71194t].

Fruit identn. by essent. oil constituents (*J Pharm Pharmacol*, 1964, **16**, 131). Fruits (so-called seeds) yield 14 coumarins and 3 phenolic acids; 6 flavons. including

vicenin (*Khim Prir Soedin*, 1969, **5**, 437; 1970, **6**, 268; *CA*, 1970, **72**, 75661m; **73**, 84627c); flavons. (*Phytochemistry*, 1972, **11**, 1741); a new xanthone glycd., dillanoside (*Chem Pharm Bull*, 1976, **24**, 220).

Aerial parts, scopoletin and a new coumarin; also from seeds (*J Chem Soc C*, 1967, 2593). Herb contains vit. C, 121.44 mg/100g (*Lucr Stiint Inst Agron Bucuresti Ser B*, 1973, **16**, 23; *CA*, 1976, **85**, 75175z). Leaves, flavon. glycds. (*Konservn Ovoshchesush Promst*, 1979, 31). Leaves and stems, carvone and *d*-α-phellandrene (*K'o Hsueh Nung Yeh Taipei*, 1979, **27**, 35; *CA*, 1980, **93**, 210148a).

Root lipid and essent. oil constituents (*Sci Pharm*, 1973, **41**, 102; *CA*, **79**, 75880b; *Planta Med*, 1975, **27**, 1; *Pharmazie*, 1979, **34**, 426).

A. sowa Roxb. ex Flem. syn. *A. graveolens* Linn. var. *sowa* Roxb.; *Peucedanum sowa* Roxb.

Eng.–*Indian dill, sowa*.

Intraspecific variability in Indian dill: *variyali sowa* or *fennel sowa* and *ghoda sowa* or *horse sowa* (*Curr Sci*, 1971, **40**, 328); chem. races in *variyali sowa* (*ibid*, 1975, **44**, 445). *Vizag sowa* (*Indian J Pharm*, 1972, **34**, 77).

EtOH(50%) ext. of fruits, hypoglyc. and spasmol. (*Indian J Exp Biol*, 1968, **6**, 232).

Essent. oil of seeds, antifung. (*Flavour Ind*, 1971, **2**, 484). Indian dill and its essent. oil made free from dillapiol, suitable as substitute for European dill and its essent. oil included in Indian Pharmacopoeia (*Indian J Pharm*, 1972, **34**, 69).

Chem. and utilization (*Indian Perfum*, 1965, **9**, 17). Fruits (so-called seeds) contain myristicin and apiol (*Phytochemistry*, 1969, **8**, 1729). Data on production and trade of dill seed and its oil in India (*Indian Oil Soap J*, 1969-70, **35**, 129). Seed fats, content of volat. octadecenoic acids, $\Delta^{5,6}$-octadecenoic acid (*Chem Ind Lond*, 1969, 1869; 1970, 831). Seed ext. contains 3,6-di-Me-tetrahydrocoumaran (*Taiwan K'o Hsueh*, 1978, **32**, 131; *CA*, 1979, **91**,

52719q). Metal content (*J Inst Chem India*, 1979, **51**, 236).

Essent. oil, characteristics, IS specifications (IS:3147 - 1965); from exotic plants raised in Kumaun; carvone as high as 69.8% (seed stored for 18 months which may have increased carvone appreciably) (Wlth India, IA, 274; *Perfum Essent Oil Rec*, 1968, **59**, 180); chem. of essent. oils from Indian seeds and herb, constituents and properties (*ibid*, 1967, **58**, 437). Burmese oil, carvone (39%), limonene (32%) and dillapiol (13%) (*Union Burma J Sci Technol*, 1968, **1**, 329); Jammu sample, (3%; at first stage, 3%), carvone, 19.1; *trans*-dihydrocarvone, 4.4; limonene, 19.7; and dillapiol (at final stages of distillation), 30% of total oil and other constituents (*Indian Perfum*, 1965, **9**, 17). Haldwani sample of fruit grown from improved strain had carvone, 20.7; dihydrocarvone, 14.3; *d*-limonene, 21.4; and undesirable ones: myristicin, 1; apiol(e), 5.7; and dillapiol(e), 8.6% (*Flavour Ind*, 1971, **2**, 363). Vizag fruit var. from Andhra Pradesh which in every respect resembles *variyali sowa* is dillapiol-free and with carvone content, 54-56%; having same flavon. pattern as *A. sowa* (*Indian J Pharm*, 1972, **34**, 77). Chem. races in *variyali sowa*: pale brown with yellowish broad wings and dark, carvone, 42, 23; dihydrocarvone, 5, 35; limonene, 39, 24; and dillapiol, 14, 18% (*Curr Sci*, 1975, **44**, 445). Constituents of Japanese oil (*Yakugaku*, 1974, **23**, 746; *CA*, 1975, **83**, 136696c). Quality standards of Indian dill (*J Inst Chem India*, 1980, **52**, 123). For carvone estn. see under *A. graveolens*.

Pharmacognosy of plant (*Curr Sci*, 1971, **40**, 328). Chem. studies of essent. oils from *A. graveolens* and *A. sowa* [*Indian Perfum*, 1971, **15**(Pt. I), 27].

Dillapiol(e)—carvone and dillapiol (1:2 by wt.) present in Indian dill from hexane extract (including that grown in Europe) (*J Pharm Pharmacol*, 1969, **21**, 259). Dillapiol considered undesirable. LD$_{50}$ in mice between 1 and 1.5 g/kg (*Indian J Pharm*, 1972, **34**, 69). Easy sepn. in fractionating column as it is heavier than water. Found to have a significant synergistic action with insecticides like pyrethrins and process patented for this formulation (Indian Pat., 1969, 128129; Wlth India, IA, 275).

ANGELICA (*Apiaceae*)

A. archangelica Linn. var. **himalaica** (C.B. Clarke) Krishna & Badhwar syn. *Archangelica officinalis* Hoffm. var. *himalaica* C.B. Clarke

Essent oil, antifung. and antimycotic (*Indian Drugs*, 1979- 80, **17**, 269; 1981-82, **19**, 34).

Roots from Kashmir contain 3 furocoumarins, angelican, prangolarin, and archangelin; 2 phenol compds.: angelicain and flavon. archangelicain; str. of archangelin (*Tetrahedron Lett*, 1964, 1961; 1972, 3811); in addn. ostruthol, and oxypeucedanin hydrate (*Indian J Chem*, 1968, **6**, 415); str. of ostruthol (*Sci Cult*, 1968, **34**, 460). Roots, flavon. archangelenone (*Chem Ind Lond*, 1971, 355); archangelenone, identical with 4'-prenyloxynaringenin (*Indian J Chem*, 1973, **11**, 407).

Volat. oil from roots, monoterp. hydrocarbon compn.; quant. detn. of pentadecanolide in roots (*Perfum Essent Oil Rec*, 1965, **56**, 224; 156).

Seeds contain umbelliprenin, isoimperatorin, bergapten, prangolarin, ostruthol oxypeucedanin hydrate and β-sitosterol (*J Indian Chem Soc*, 1967, **44**, 110); fruits isoimperatorin, imperatorin, bergapten, isopimpinellin, 8-OH-5- OMepsoralen, lupeol-OAc and α-amyrin-OAc (*Indian J Chem*, 1976, **14B**, 816).

Xanthotoxol from *A. archangelica* exhibited potent peripheral anti-5-OH-tryptamine activity in rat isolated fundal strip (*Indian J Physiol Pharmacol*, 1979, **23**, 142); also antihistaminic and antinicotinic activities on guinea-pig ileum (*Indian J Pharm Sci*, 1979, **41**, 247).

A. glauca Edgew.

Eng.–*Angelica.*

Herb—used in dyspep. and constip. (*Indian For*, 1964, **90**, 50); in ulcer of palate, infantile atrophy, dysen., menor. and rinderpest (*Econ Bot*, 1970, **24**, 244).

Root—powd., in stomach trouble of children and in vomiting. Used for flavouring curry or dal; the dal or curry gives strength and vitality to women after delivery [*Indian Perfum*, 1970, **14**(Pt.I), 41]. Cardiac stim., used in dyspep. and constip. (*Khadi Gramodyog*, 1976-77, **23**, 115).

Physical properties and constituent of fruit oil (*Indian Oil Soap J*, 1960, **26**, 6, 130). Pharmacognosy of root and rhizomes (*Indian J Pharm*, 1972, **34**, 171). Coumarins, isoimperatorin, prangolarin, and tert-OMe-oxypeucedanin hydrate (*Phytochemistry*, 1972, **11**, 475). Dimeric lingusticum lactone (*Planta Med*, 1980, **39**, 261).

ANGELONIA (*Scrophulariaceae*)

*A. grandiflora Hart.

EtOH(50%) ext. of plant, diur. (*Indian J Exp Biol*, 1977, **15**, 208).

Leaves contain a flavone glucd., angeflorin; salvigenin, balcalein and d-mannitol (*Indian J Chem*, 1976, **14B**, 463); also some rare methylated flavons. (*Phytochemistry*, 1978, **17**, 591).

Found in Coorg, Karnataka.

*A. sabicariaefolia Humb.

EtOH(50%) ext. of aerial parts, diur. (*Indian J Exp Biol*, 1977, **15**, 208).

Found in Calicut, Kerala.

ANISOCHILUS (*Lamiaceae*)

A. carnosus Wall.

Essent. oil, antitubercular (*Indian J Pharm*, 1967, **29**, 157). Alc. ext. of whole plant, antibact. (*Indian J For*, 1981, **4**, 115).

Leaves contain luteolin and apigenin (*Phytochemistry*, 1972, **11**, 452).

ANISOMELES (*Lamiaceae*)

A. indica (Linn.) Kuntze syn. *A. ovata* R.Br.

Plant decoct. used in animal dysen. (*Bull Med Ethno Bot Res*, 1980, **1**, 318). Crushed leaves applied to neck of bullock to cure inflam. caused by cart pulling (*J Econ Tax Bot*, 1981, **2**, 183).

EtOH(50%) ext. of herb, hypotheremic (*Indian J Exp Biol*, 1969, **7**, 250). Leaves, ext. antiinflam. and antiarthritic in albino rats (*Bangladesh Pharm J*, 1978, **7**, 5).

Leaves, diterps. ovatodiolide & its iso deriv. (*Bull Soc Chim Fr*, 1963, 1192; *Tetrahedron*, 1965, **21**, 2117; *J Org Chem*, 1977, **42**, 3824).

Roots contain stigmasterol and β-sitosterol; paraffins and fatty acids (*Taiwan Yao Hsueh Tsa Chih*, 1973, **25**, 57; 1975, **27**, 86; *CA*, 1976, **84**, 102343r; 1977, **86**, 2376b).

A. malabarica R. Br. ex Sims

Eng.–*Malabar catmint.*

Leaves infusion efficaceous in catarrh, intermittent fever and affections of bowels; essent. oil used for rheum.; and plant substitute of Unani drug *gaozaban* (*Q J Crude Drug Res*, 1970, **10**, 1581).

EtOH(50%) ext. of aerial parts, spasmog., diur. and anticancer; also spermic. against human and rat spermatozoa (*Indian J Exp Biol*, 1974, **12**, 512; 1977, **15**, 231).

Plant contains β-sitosterol (*Indian J Chem*, 1965, **3**, 237); 2 diterp. lactones, ovatodiolide and anisomelic acid (*ibid*, 1975, **13**, 1357); also monocyclic diterps., anisomelolide, malabaric acid, its 2-OAc deriv., anisomelyl-OAc and anisomelol (*ibid*, 1978, **16B**, 441). Aerial parts, an isoflavon., anisomelin identical with cirsillineol (*ibid*, 1979, **17B**, 84).

ANNONA (*Annonaceae*)

*A. cherimola Mill.

Eng.–*Cherimolia, cherimoyer*; Kan.–*Hanumaanaphala*; Tel.– *Hanumaana-phalamuchettu* (tree).

Fruit—pulp, subacidic, luscious with delicate arom. flavour, eaten raw or made into cooling-drinks; food value higher than mango, fig and grape. Sometimes fermented to prepare alc. beverage.

Seeds—emetic-cath. and insectic. Powd. seeds mixed with lard applied to body to destroy parasites. Seeds contain reddish fatty oil (7.8%); also caffeine and give on roasting, a smell like coffee, but cannot substitute coffee as they are emetic.

Flowers—dried flowers employed to flavour snuff in Jamaica (Wlth India, IA, 278-80).

Alc. ext. of fruit contains polyphenols which are astrin. and influence flavour of juice (*Z Lebensm Unters Forsch*, 1969, **140**, 129; *CA*, 1969, **71**, 79931b).

Twigs, alks. anonaine, liriodenine, norushinsunine (michelalbine) and reticuline (*Rev Latinoam Quim*, 1977, **8**, 133; *CA*, **87**, 180734v).

Leaves, condensed tannins and quercetin (*Qual Plant Mater Veg*, 1968-69, **17**, 384); an unnamed alk. (Wlth India, IA, 280).

Native to N. Andes in Peru, introduced and cultivated in S. India.

*A. glabra Linn. syn. *A. palustris* Linn.

Eng.–*Alligator-apple, monkey-apple, pond-apple.*

Ether exts. of wood and stem bark significantly inhibitory *in vitro* against cells derived from human carcinoma of nasopharynx; cytotoxic alk., liriodenine (*J Pharm Sci*, 1969, **58**, 637; *CA*, **71**, 69091p).

Stem bark and wood alks. [*Taiwan Yao Hsueh Tsa Chih*, 1973, **25**(1- 2), 1; *Proc Nat Sci Counc Taiwan*, Part 2, 1974, **7**, 177; *CA*, 1976, **84**, 102339u; 1977, **86**, 127149m].

Leaves, alks. (*Chin Chem Soc Taipei*, 1971, **18**, 133; *CA*, 1972, **77**, 16567r).

Native to C. America, introduced into Indian gardens.

*A. montana Macf.

Eng.–*Mountain soursop.*

Fruit, subacidic, with good flavour, juicy and refreshing, though inferior to that of *A. muricata.* Fruit, leaves and seeds, insectic. (Wlth India, IA, 295).

Native to W. Indies, introduced into IBG, Calcutta.

A. muricata Linn.

Eng.–*Soursop; prickly custard apple.*

In Philippines, ripe fruit, antiscor.; unripe fruit used in dysen. In Tonga, leaf infusion in stomach trouble (*Econ Bot*, 1971, **25**, 436).

Leaves—used as sed. and hypnotic; infusion given to crying babies to make them sleep (*J Pharm Pharmacol*, 1970, **22**, 116; *Chemtech*, 1972, **2**, 62). Flowers and leaves used in kidney ailments (*Econ Bot*, 1970, **24**, 354). In Exumas and Long Island, leaves with sugar grain made into tea given in nervousness or rapid heart beat. To reduce fever, leaves are crushed over a sickbed to induce sweating, or boiled with gale- of-wind (*Phyllanthus niruri*) and sub-abul (*Leucaena leucocephala*) for tea and given, or with those of tamarind to alleviate fever, chill and influenza, or with lime (*Citrus aurantifolia*), tamarind (*Tamarindus indica*) and pear (*Persea americana*) for colds (*ibid*, 1975, **29**, 316).

Venezuelan soursop, contains folic acid, 80.72 μg/100g (*Invest Clin Suppl*, 1979, **3**, 50; *CA*, 1980, **93**, 219570q). Physical properties of essent. oil from fruit pulp (*Flavour. Ind*, 1971, **2**, 305). Volat. constituents of fruits (*J Agric Food Chem*, 1981, **29**, 488).

Seeds, constitution of amyloid (*Phytochemistry*, 1967, **6**, 1665). Str. of galactomannans (*Carbohydr Res*, 1971, **20**, 329). Compn. of seed oil from Somaliland, oleic as major acid; sterols were β-sitosterol and stigmasterol; fatty oil (22.1%) can be used as food and in pharmaceutical preparation (*Qual Plant Foods Hum Nutr*, 1980, **30**, 163; *CA*, 1981, **94**, 190494a).

Bark, 3 alks. including reticuline, atherosperminine and an unidentified (*Philipp J Sci*, 1967, **96**, 399). Isoquinoline alks., from leaves, stem bark and roots: reticuline (main), coclaurine, coreximine, atherosperminine, stepharine, anomurine and anomuricine (*Planta Med*, 1981, **42**, 37).

*A. purpurea Moc. & Sesse

Eng.–*Negro-head, sonooya.*

EtOH ext. of leaves, active against *Mycobacterium* sp.(Wlth India, IA, 295). Leaves and stems contain alks.: isocorydine, O-de-Me-purpureine, glaziovine, norpurpureine, oxoglaucine, OMe-atheroline, oxopurpureine and stepharine; oxopurpureine active *in vitro* against 9KB tumour test system; glaziovine and oxoglaucine also active to a limited extent (Wlth India, IA, 295; *J Pharm Sci*, 1971, **60**, 1254).

Native to S. Mexico and C. America, introduced into IBG, Calcutta.

A. reticulata Linn.

Eng.–*Bullock's heart.*

Leaves used against inflam. tumours (*Lloydia*, 1967, **30**, 406). Exts. of leaves and stems, exhibited inotropic, +ve chronotropic and spasmol. activities; contain dopamine, salsolinol and coclaurine (*Plant Med Phytother*, 1981, **15**, 10).

Bark powerful astrin., used as antidysen. and vermifuge. Seed kernel, highly poisonous. Fruit pulp sweet and edible but its paste is used to kill lice on cattle (*J Econ Tax Bot*, 1981, **2**, 173).

EtOH(50%) ext. of aerial parts, spasmog. (*Indian J Exp Biol*, 1971, **9**, 91); insectic. against *Trinolium castereum* (*ibid*, 1978, **16**, 330).

Annona extractives, contact and stomach poisons, contact action equivalent to that of rotenone or nicotine; stomach poisoning, variable. Little or no ovicidal activity. Most effective applications against various aphide and human body pests such as lice (*in* Jacobson & Crosby, 218-19).

Biosynth. of coclaurine (*J Chem Soc Perkin Trans I*, 1979, 1515). Leaves,

polyprenols (*Acta Biochim Pol*, 1973, **20**, 343).

Fruit contains, I, 0.64; and F, 5.6 ppm (dry matter basis) (*Indian J Nutr Diet*, 1971, **8**, 66); and starch (19%) (*Starke*, 1976, **28**, 257; CA, **85**, 162276b).

Root bark contains alk., liriodenine (*Indian J Chem*, 1965, **3**, 237); and oxoushinsunine, anonaine, michelalbine, and reticuline; in addn. an unknown one [*Taiwan K'o Hsueh*, 1970, **24**(3-4), 99; *Pei I Hsueh Pao*, 1973, 130; *CA*, 1971, **75**, 45637c; 1974, **81**, 60846n].

Anonaine—insectic. principle. Aporphine (benzylisoquinoline) alk. isolated by initial extn. with alc., removal of resin followed by re-extn. with ether and precipitation as insol. HCl. Detailed toxicol. or pharmacol. not done (*in* Jacobson & Crosby, 216, 219).

Seed, a resinous mixt. highly toxic to aphids, toxic fraction nonnitrogenous, highly oxygenated and of c. 500 mol. wt (*in* Jacobson & Crosby, 218).

*A. senegalensis Pers.

In African folk med., plant used in V.D., dysen., dressing of sores and skin diseases; and as antipyr. and antid. Pet. ether ext. of root bark, marked inhibitory against sarcoma 180 ascites in mice. Ext., antibact. against *Staphylococcus aureus* and *Salmonella typhosa, in vitro* (*Planta Med*, 1975, **28**, 32).

In Nigeria, bark used for treatment of convuls. in children and against cancer; yields several kaurane-type diterps. (*Phytochemistry*, 1976, **15**, 1311; 1971, **10**, 3294). Leaf waxes. A sesquiterp. fraction from leaf, toxic to insect larvae (*J Sci Food Agric*, 1956, **7**, 203; *in* Jacobson & Crosby, 218).

Native to tropical Africa and introduced in IBG, Calcutta.

A. squamosa Linn.

Eng.–*Custard apple, sugar apple, sweetsop.*

Leaves—Leaves and fruits used against tumours (*Lloydia*, 1967, **30**, 406); ext. anticancer (*Philipp J Sci*, 1967, **96**, 393).

Leaf ext., insectic. (*Proc Nat Acad Sci India*, 1965, **35B**, 351); aq. and alc. exts. spasmog. and spasmol. and oxytocic; also cardiorespiratory in animals (*J Pharm Pharmacol*, 1970, **22**, 116); juice in treatment of animal wounds, as antisep.; in cows and other animals, paste applied to ulcers (*Bull Med Ethno Bot Res*, 1980, **1**, 318; 447). Leaves, seeds, immature dried fruits, as pesticidal against bed bugs and bird lice [*Macco Agric Digest*, 1981, **5**(9), 5].

Plant—used in cold, rheum., chancre and syphilis, carbuncle and puerperal fever; leaf tea to alleviate fever (*Econ Bot*, 1970, **24**, 241; 1975, **29**, 316). EtOH(50%) ext. of aerial parts, anticancer. Also insectic. against *Musca domestica* and *Tribolizen castereum* (*Indian J Exp Biol*, 1969, **7**, 250; 1978, **16**, 330).

Seeds—toxicological studies of ext.; toxicity varies with concentration of ext. (*Indian J Exp Biol*, 1971, **9**, 519); emet.; fruits, cooling and tonic [*J Res Indian med*, 1973, **8**(2), 74]; seeds, diur. in rats [*Indian Drugs Pharmac Ind*, 1981, **16**(1), 39]. Pharmacol. screening with ext.; antiimplantation activity in rats (*Planta Med*, 1975, **28**, 97; 1979, **35**, 283); ext. showed antifert. activity in albino mice (*Indian J Med Res*, 1979, **70**, 517). Powd. seeds alongwith leaves of *Plumbago zeylanica* used for abortion (*J Econ Tax Bot*, 1980, **1**, 137).

Leaves and tender stem of Indian plant, anonaine, roemerine, norcorydine, corydine, norlaureline, isocorydine, norisocorydine and glaucine (*Phytochemistry*, 1972, **11**, 1819). Also friedelin, alks., (–)-xylopine (+)-OMe-armepavine and lanuginosine; leaves and stems, nitroheteroside (*ibid*, 1980, **18**, 1584; 1251). Leaves tetrahydroisoquinoline alk., higenamine-HBr, which is cardiotonic in guinea pigs; stimulating -

adrenergic activity (*Planta Med*, 1980, **40**, 77; *J Natl Prod*, 1981, **44**, 53).

Essent. oil from leaves, constituents (*Perfum Essent Oil Rec*, 1967, **58**, 437); volat. constituents of Egyptian leaf oil; carvone (major) (*Egypt J Pharm Sci*, 1977, **18**, 1).

Fruit pulp polyphenols (*J Sci Food Technol*, 1970, **7**, 203). Fruits, folic acid, content (*Philipp J Sci*, 1966, **95**, 311); peel oil (0.1%), predominant terps., α- & β-pinenes and limonene (*ibid*, 1977, **106**, 37; *Lloydia*, 1975, **38**, 537).

Roots contain alks., anonaine, michelalbine, oxoushinsuine (liriodenine), L(+)-reticuline and analobine; also diazepine, squamolone (*J Chin Chem Soc Taipei*, 1970, **17**, 243; 1972, **19**, 149; *CA*, 1971, **74**, 121337b; 1973, **78**, 16151w). Also yield β-caryophyllene and five kaurane-related diterps. (*Chem Ber*, 1973, **106**, 841). Roots and bark, alks. corydine, isocorydine, anonaine, glaucine; β-sitosterol; camphor, borneol, and a new monoterp. which is laxt. in human, and volat. oil, antimicrob. (*Indian J Pharm Sci*, 1978, **40**, 170).

ANODENDRON (*Apocynaceae*)

A. paniculatum DC.

Plant ext., antifert. [*J Res Indian Med*, 1973, **8**(3), 73].

Leaves contain dambonitol (*Indian J Chem*, 1966, **4**, 457). TLC of wood gave 14 cardenolides including anodendrosides A, E_1, E_2, F, G, B_1 & B_2; str. of anodendroside A, E_1, E_2, F & G (*Helv Chim Acta*, 1970, **53**, 1253; 1972, **55**, 1696).

ANOGEISSUS (*Combretaceae*)

*A. acuminata (Roxb.) Wall. ex Guill. & Perr.

Eng.–*Button tree*; B.–*Chakwa*; Bihar, Kan. & Oriya–*Pansi(a)*; Tam.– *Nunnera*; Kondh–*Dehra, gora-hasel*; Rajasthan–*Dhauria*.

Seed ext., antibact. against human and plant pathogens [*Indian Drugs Pharmac Ind*, 1979, **14**(5), 17]; antifung. (*Bull Bot Soc Univ Saugar*, 1980, **27**, 24).

Powd. of dry bark with fruit of *Terminalia chebula* and common salt used as appetiser (*in* Jain, 24).

Found almost throughout India.

A. latifolia (Roxb.) Wall. ex. Bedd.

Eng.–*Button tree, dindiga tree, ghatti tree.*

Plant—in toothache, spleen enlargement, face cancer, dysuria, excessive perspiration, diar., cholera, cough and cold, and rinderpest (*Econ Bot*, 1970, **24**, 245). Pharmacol. (*Indian J Exp Biol*, 1971, **9**, 91). Plant as astrin., cooling: used in ulcers, diar., dysen., piles, and urinary disorders [*J Res Indian Med*, 1973, **8**(2), 74].

Gum — called 'Ghatti' or 'Indian gum' from plant used as tonic after delivery (*Bull Bot Surv India*, 1973, **15**, 13); gives stable oil-in-water emulsion and patented for incorporating oil-sol. vit. preparations (*J Indian Chem Soc*, 1976, **53**, 146).

Bark, heartwood and leaves, quinic and shikimic acids (*Leath Sci*, 1964, **11**, 178); leaves, gallotannin (*Aust J Chem*, 1964, **17**, 238). Polyphenols of bark, sapwood and heartwood (*Indian J Chem*, 1965, **3**, 308). Bark and heartwood steroids (*Econ Bot*, 1969, **23**, 274).

Bark, 3,3′,4-tri-OMe-flavellagic acid (*Curr Sci*, 1974, **43**, 544); and 2 glycds. (*Indian J Chem*, 1976, **14B**, 641). Heartwood contains gallic acid, ellagic acid, its derivs., quercetin and myricetin (*ibid*, 1981, **20B**, 1010).

Isolation method for pure aldobiouronic and aldotriouronic acids from plant mucilage (*ibid*, 1970, **8**, 48).

*A. pendula Edgew.

G.–*Dhau, dhaunkara*; H. & Rajasthan–*Dhaunkra*; Mar.–*Kardahi.*

Seed ext., haemagglutinating against human A, B and O red cells (*Indian J Med Res*, 1973, **61**, 1478). EtOH(50%) ext. of aerial parts, diur. and cardiovasular (*Indian J Exp Biol*, 1977, **15**, 208).

Tree yields 'Ghatti' or 'Indian gum' (Wlth India, IA, 302).

Found in N. and W. India.

ANREDERA (*Basellaceae*)

*A. baselloides (H. B. & K.) Baill. syn. *Boussingaultia baselloides* H.B. & K.

Eng.–*Lamb's tail, magnonette vine.*

In Philippines, roots used against corns (*Lloydia*, 1967, **30**, 436).

Native to S. America, grown in gardens all over India for its white fragrant flowers.

ANTHEMIS (*Asteraceae*)

A. cotula Linn.

Eng.–*Dog fennel, meyweed, wild chamomile.*

Leaves and seeds cause contact dermatitis. A good unguent for old sores (*Econ Bot*, 1974, **28**, 316).

Plant provides relief in inflam. of tissues. Dried powd. flowers effective against fleas, bed bugs and flies; leaves, insectic. Plant poisonous to cattle (Wlth India, IA, 303; Chopra *et al*, I, 475).

Sesquiterp. lactone (*Tetrahedron Lett*, 1969, 2417). Leaves, flavons. (*Naturwissenschaften*, 1969, **56**, 467); leaves and flowers, quercetin 5-glycd. (*Phytochemistry*, 1971, **10**, 1325). Dried flowerheads and flowering plant, volat. oil, mucilage and an antisp. substance (Med. Plants, 159). Plant and flowers contain alk. (*Planta Med*, 1976, **29**, 234).

A. nobilis Linn.

Eng.–*Roman chamomile, double chamomile.*

Chamomile in compn. used as liquid bactericide, deodorant and softener for skin hygiene (Fr Demande, 1974, 2224127; *CA*, 1975, **83**, 103280j). An ingredient of '*Majnoon-e-flasfa*', a Unani drug [*Nagarjun*, 1977-78, **21**(11), 23]. Japanese crude drug, screening for antitumour activity (*Shoyakugaku Zasshi*, 1979, **33**, 95). Flowers, as poultice in sprains, bruises and rheum. (Wlth India, IA, 303). Chamomile tea helps offset some reactions to alcohol drinking (Herbal Med., 119).

Essent. oil—improves appetite, but in large doses, violent poison. Prolonged use results in mental disturbance and madness (Med. Plants, 162).

Essent. oil content of different organs of plant (*Egypt J Pharm Sci*, 1975, **16**, 161). Progress in essent. oils; rev. on oil constituents of *A. nobilis* and others [*Perfum Flav*, 1981-82, **6**(2), 59]; 2 homologues of *p*-methene ketone, carvotanacetone (*Helv Chim Acta*,. 1981, **64**, 1488).

Hydroxyisonobilin, a cytostatically active sesquiterp. lactone from leaves (*Collect Czech Chem Commun*, 1977, **42**, 1065; *Pol J Pharmacol Pharm*, 1977, **29**, 419; *CA*, 1978, **88**, 94725g).

Essent. oil from flowers, 31 compds. (*Essenze Deriv Agrum*, 1973, **43**, 107; *CA*, 1974, **80**, 143045f). Sesquiterp. lactone, nobilin from flowers, partial str.; flowers yield sesquiterp. lactones, 3-epinobilin, 3-dehydronobilin and 1,10-epoxynobilin; str. revision of nobilin and eucannabinolide (*Collect Czech Chem Commun*, 1964, **29**, 3096; 1977, **42**, 1053; *CA*, 1965, **62**, 7805c).

Polyphenols, of capitula; of flowers, 7-glucds. of luteolin, apigenin and anthemoside; phenolic acids and coumarins; flavons. (of ligulated white, and yellow tubular flowers) (*Plant Med Phytother*, 1969, **3**, 167; 1971, **5**, 234; 1974, **8**, 306; 1973, **7**, 234; *CA*, 1970, **72**, 75687z; 1972, **76**, 56604m; 1975, **83**, 93831y; 1974, **81**, 1257y). Other constituents: *n*-nonacosane, *n*-heptacosane, lignoceryl alc., β-amyrin, and ψ-taraxasterol (*Acta Pol Pharm*, 1971, **28**, 621; *CA*, 1972, **77**, 2818m); of flowers from Egypt, scopoletin, β-sitosterol and hexacosanol besides apigenin, luteolin, their 7-glucds., apiin and kaempferol (*Qual Plant Mater Veg*, 1972- 73, **22**, 141); of plant, 2,3-di-OH-cinnamic acid & its glucose ester (*Plant Med Phytother*, 1970, **4**, 189; *CA*, 1971, **74**, 50555h).

ANTHOCEPHALUS (*Rubiaceae*)

A. chinensis (Lamk) A. Rich. ex Walp. syn. *A. cadamba* (Roxb.) Miq.; *A. indicus* A. Rich.

EtOH(50%) ext. of stem bark, anthelm. and hypoglyc. (*Indian J Exp Biol*, 1968, **6**, 232). Plant used in fever, anemia, pimples, sores, carbuncle, cholera, dysen. and rinderpest (*Econ Bot*, 1970, **24**, 245). Bark antidiur.; fruit, cooling, analg., decoct. in stomatistis [*J Res Indian Med*, 1973, **8**(2), 74]. Plant used to purify and improve semen quality (*Nagarjun*, 1979-80, **23**, 170). Flowers and roots used as abortif. (*Ancient Sci Life*, 1981-82, **1**, 67).

Leaves, str. of alks., cadambine & 3 α-dihydrocadambine; a glycd. alk., isodihydrocadambine (*Tetrahedron Lett*, 1974, 1957; 3335). Leaves yield hentriacontanol and β-sitosterol (*Labdev*, 1972, **10A**, 104); cadamine & its iso-deriv.; 3β- dihydrocadambine, cadambine, and 3 β- isodihydrocadambine (as acetates) (*Tetrahedron Lett*, 1976, 1629; 2723).

Root and bark, quinovic acid (*Indian J Chem*, 1969, **7**, 308). Stem bark, alk. (*Lloydia*, 1972, **35**, Suppl., 1); also a new pentacyclic triterp. acid, cadambagenic acid alongwith quinoric acid and β-sitosterol also saponins A; B; C & D, their str. detn. (*Indian J Chem*, 1974, **12**, 284; 1976, **14B**, 614; 1977, **15B**, 654; *J Indian Chem Soc*, 1978, **55**, 275).

Constituents of essent. oil from blossoms (*Parfuem Kosmet*, 1966, **47**, 198).

ANTHOXANTHUM (*Poaceae*)

A. odoratum Linn.

Eng.–*Sweet vernal grass.*

Flavone from leaves and nodes(stems) (*Agric Biol Chem*, 1973, **37**, 2663; *CA*, 1974, **80**, 45653h). Phytoestrogenic and toxic effects of grass on mouse (*Can J Zool*, 1980, **58**, 1575).

Grass yields essent. oil known as 'Flouve oil' with esters and coumarins as chief constituents, useful in perfume-compounding. Coumarin content varies with season and in different parts of plant; max. in leaves (up to 2.5% dry basis) followed by whole plant and stems (Wlth India, IA, 308).

ANTHRISCUS (Apiaceae)

*A. sylvestris Hoffm. syn. *A. nemorosa* Spreng.

Eng.–*Cow parsley.*

In Ladakh, smoke of plant powd. when inhaled, believed to cure rheum. and inflam. (*Bull Med Ethno Bot Res*, 1980, **1**, 301).

Roots contain furanocoumarin, apterin (*Phytochemistry*, 1976, **15**, 1079); a Ph-propanoid ester, anthriscusin (*Chem Pharm Bull*, 1978, **26**, 1337); lignans including anthricin & isoanthricin; Ph-propanoid esters, crocatone, and a new one, anthriscusin and an acycloxycarboxylic acid (*Yakugaku Zasshi*, 1978, **98**, 1486); and essent. oil, constituents (*ibid*, 1978, **98**, 1586).

Flowers and leaves contain essent. oil; constituents reported (*ibid*, 1979, **99**, 602).

Found in Himalayas from Kashmir to Garhwal, between 2,000-3,500 m.

ANTIARIS (Moraceae)

A. toxicaria Lesch. syn. *A. innoxia* Blume; *A. saccidora* Dalz.

Eng.–*Sacking tree, upas tree.*

Plant latex, used as arrow and dart poison (*Lloydia*, 1966, **29**, 172; *J Ethnopharmacol*, 1979, **1**, 367). Powd. wood boiled with *canjee* given in diar. (*Econ Bot*, 1973, **27**, 186). EtOH(50%) ext. of aerial parts, diur. (*Indian J Exp Biol*, 1974, **12**, 512).

Cardenolides from latex: antioside, α-antiarin, β-antiarin and 7 others including evomonoside; desglucocheirotoxin, convallatoxin and convallatoxol (*Helv Chim Acta*, 1962, **45**, 1183; 1206). Glycds. of latex from Java digitoxigenin-α-*L*-rhamnoside, convallatoxin and antioside and β-antiarin (*ibid*, 1963, **46**, 117). Seeds contain 34 cardenolides including cymarin,

cymarol, strophanthidin, periplogenin, peripalloside, strophalloside, etc. (*ibid*, 1964, **47**, 2164). Str. of 6 unknown compds. (*Ann Chem*, 1965, **685**, 253; *CA*, **63**, 13389a). Malayoside, antioside, α-antioside and bogoroside from latex; peripalloside, strophalloside, antiogoside and antialloside; glycds. from seeds produced typical digitalis like action in frog heart; mean LD_{50} in cats (0.107-0.160 mg/kg) demonstrated high potency of these compds. (*J Pharmacol Exp Ther*, 1965, **150**, 53). Latex yields convalloside (*Helv Chim Acta*, 1966, **49**, 2469).

Cardenolides of *A. toxicaria* latex and seeds with str.- sugar and activity correlation (Wlth India, IA, 310-11).

ANTICHARIS (Scrophulariaceae)

A. glandulosa Aschers.

Plant, a saponin, glanduloside, *d*-mannitol and hentriacontane (*J Chem Soc Pak*, 1981, **3**, 39).

*A. senegalensis (Walp.) Bhandari syn. *A. linearis* (Benth.) Hochst. ex Aschers.

Aq. ext. of semi-dried plant reported to exhibit marked variation in B.P. and stimulation of heart when injected into rats and dogs.

Plant said to be useful in treating diabetes.

Herb contains two OH-lactones, viz. linearin and linearoside, besides mannitol and triacontane (*Pak J Sci Ind Res*, 1970, **13**, 39).

Found in arid tract of Rajasthan, plains of Punjab and Haryana.

ANTIDESMA (Stilaginaceae)

A. bunius Spreng.

Eng.–*Chinese laurel, salamander tree.*

Leaves and stem contain friedelin; latter, also dammaro-20, 24- dien-3-ol (*Aust J Chem*, 1968, **21**, 2137).

*A. diandrum (Roxb.) Heyne ex Roth H.–*Matta-ara.*

EtOH(50%) ext. of aerial parts, spasmol. (*Indian J Exp Biol*, 1969, **7**, 250).

Used in whitlow, sores, dropsy and anasarca, carbuncle, muscular pain, adenitis axillaris, gravel, dysen., intercostal neuralgia, pleur., pneum. and bite of rabid jackal (*Econ Bot*, 1970, **24**, 241).

Trunk ext., sitosterol (*Phytochemistry*, 1973, **12**, 1819). Leaves, vit. B complex (*Bull Bot Surv India*, 1976, **18**, 247).

Found in Himalayas from Kumaun eastwards to W. Bengal and Sikkim; also common throughout peninsular India, up to 1,200 m.

A. ghesaembilla Gaertn.
Eng.–*Black currant tree*.
EtOH(50%) ext. of aerial parts, hypoten. and diur. (*Indian J Exp Biol*, 1974, **12**, 512).

*A. menasu Miq. ex Tul.
Kan.–*Kadivalasoppu*; Mal.–*Putharaval*.
Aerial parts yield a new pentacyclic triterp., antidesmanol, *n*- tritriacontane, friedelin, canophyllal and cyanophyllol; *n*-tritriacontane, antiinflam. (*Experientia*, 1980, **36**, 146); also 2 pentacyclic triterps, 16α-OH-3- & 3β-OH-16-ketoisomultiflorene; both exhibited 79% chlorothiazide diur. activity in rats (*Phytochemistry*, 1980, **19**, 2409).

Found in wet deciduous and semi-evergreen forests of Peninsular India, up to 1,800 m.

ANTIRRHINUM (*Scrophulariaceae*)

A. glaucum Stocks ex Wight; see **Schweinfurthia sphaerocarpa**

*A. majus Linn.
Eng.–*Snapdragon, dog flower*.
In Europe, leaves applied as poultices to tumours and ulcers (*Planta Med*, 1971, **20**, 108). Infusion of plant, cardiotonic, hypoten. and sed. (*Farmakol Toksikol Moscow*, 1971, **34**, 733; *BA*, 1973, **55**, 10072).

Aerial parts of flowering plant contain GABA (Swain, 271). Plant, choline; quant. detn.; 4 tertiary alks., 4-Me-2,6-napthyridine (major) (*Planta Med*, 1971, **20**, 108; 1972, **21**, 353; *Tetrahedron Lett*,

1970, 4773); iridoid glucds., antirrhinoside & its 5-O-β-D-glucd.(*Gazz Chim Ital*, 1969, **90**, 800).

Leaves yield a fat rich in linolenic acid and sterols with β-sitosterol as major (*Phytochemistry*, 1968, **7**, 1008); leaves and chloroplast alkanes (0.18%), both *n*-C_{16}-C_{35} & branched C_{25}-C_{35} - (*Phytochemistry*, 1968, **7**, 1008).

Flower pigments (*Phytochemistry*, 1971, **10**, 2848; 1973, **12**, 809; Wlth India, IA, 317).

Seed, a fixed oil, slightly inferior to olive oil (*Planta Med*, 1971, **20**, 108).

Cultivated in plains and in hills.

*A. oronitium Linn.
Herb similar properties as *A. majus*.; its use in med. recorded (Wlth India, IA, 317).

Aerial parts, choline chloride, 4-Me-2,6-naphthyridine, 2 unknown alks. (*Phytochemistry*, 1971, **10**, 2849); 7 tertiary alks. (*Planta Med*, 1972, **21**, 84; 1973, **23**, 182).

Found in plains of Punjab; N-E Himalayas and in Nilgiris.

APAMA (*Aristolochiaceae*)

A. siliquosa Lamk syn. *Bragantia wallichii* R. Br. ex Wight & Arn.
Root ext., antifung. (*Indian J Med Res*, 1961, **49**, 799).

Roots contain an alk., chakranine which is toxic on i.v. administration (LD_{50} in mice 2.2 mg/kg) but non-toxic orally (Chopra *et al*, 1958, 301); the alk. and alc. ext. of root, effective in cholera in young rabbits, although both failed to show any vibriocidal activity (*Indian J Med Res*, 1971, **59**, 1190). Root anal.; unsap. matter contains a thick brown resinous material and β-sitosterol (*Indian J Chem*, 1973, **11**, 840).

A. tomentosa (Blume) Engl. syn. *Bragantia tomentosa* Blume
Plant, extremely bitter, used as poultice for boils. Stems and leaves, diur.; juice (on pounding) given internally for cough (Chopra *et al*, II, 741).

APHANAMIXIS (*Meliaceae*)

A. polystachya (Wall.) Parker syn. *Amoora rohituka* Wight & Arn.

EtOH(50%) ext. of stem, anticancer (*Indian J Exp Biol*, 1968, **6**, 232). Bark ext., effective immunosuppressive drug in prevention of allergic orchitis in guinea pigs (*ibid*, 1977, **15**, 105; 1978, **16**, 758).

Plant used in eye diseases by tribals of Orissa (*Proc Indian Sci Congr*, 1981, III, 155).

Antibact. and antifung. activities of seed ext. (*Indian Drugs*, 1980-81, **18**, 79; 80).

Fruit shell, triterp., aphanamixin, str. (*Tetrahedron Lett*, 1967, 1471). Bark tetranortriterp. aphanamixinin (*Sci Cult*, 1968, **34**, 362); strs. of aphanamixin and aphanamixinin (*Tetrahedron*, 1970, **26**, 1859). Leaves contain diterp. alc., aphanamixol and β-sitosterol (*J Indian Chem Soc*, 1968, **45**, 208).

Seeds yield a limonoid, rohitukin; its str. (*J Chem Soc Chem Commun*, 1976, 909; *Tetrahedron Lett*, 1979, 721); str. detn. of several limonoids (*Phytochemistry*, 1978, **17**, 1995); limonoid polystachin (*J Chem Res Synop*, 1979, 294; *CA*, 1980, **92**, 129129c). Characterisation of a new alk. (*Proc Sci Program Joint Meet Soc Pharmacog Soc Econ Bot*, 1981, Abstr. 40). Seeds (Indian sample), a new saponin (*Phytochemistry*, 1981, **20**, 1749); a new glycd. (*Proc Indian Sci Congr*, 1981, III, 91).

APIUM (*Apiaceae*)

A. graveolens Linn.

Eng.–*Celery*.

Two varieties of celery known. *A. graveolens* var. *dulce* (Mill.) Pers. main variety under cultivation in India; and var. *rapaceum* (Mill.) Gaudich (called Celeriac), cultivated for root tubers, eaten after cooking (Wlth India, IA, 320).

Seeds—CNS depress.; alks. fraction (Dagandorff's test +ve) from seeds showed tranquilizing activity in animals (*Indian J Med Res*, 1970, **58**, 99). Decoct., popular household remedy for rheum. (Wlth India, IA, 323). Used for flavouring. India provides bulk of celery seed for world trade for distillation of essent. oil and preparation of oleoresinoids (*Curr Sci*, 1972, **41**, 856); essent. oil and oleoresins, for flavouring food products. Ext. showed antifert. activity in female rats (*Bull Med Ethno Bot Res*, 1980, **1**, 542).

Essent. oil from seeds—called celery seed oil, tranquilizing and anticonvuls. (*Indian J Med Res*, 1967, **55**, 1099); mild depress. in mice (*Indian J Physiol Pharmacol*, 1967, **12**, abstr. 37); significant antifung. activity against a no. of fungi [*Indian Spices*, 1969, **6**(2), 2; 7; *Indian Farming NS*, 1979, **14**(1), 26]; antifung., *in vitro* [*Indian Drugs Pharmac Ind*, 1979, **14**(1), 3]; antibact., *in vitro* (*Flavour Ind*, 1971, **2**, 111).

Herb—antioxidant (*J Food Sci*, 1964, **29**, 27); used as tonic, carmin., diur. and emmen. [*East Pharm*, 1980, **23**(272), 39]. Ingestion of celery suppressed testicular function w.r.t. sperm count in human (*J Med Assoc Thailand*, 1979, **62**, 164).

Antibact. properties of roots (*Indian Drugs*, 1977-78, **15**, 91).

Seed essent. oil, characteristics and compn. (*Perfum Essent Oil Rec*, 1967, **58**, 437; *Parfuem Kosmet*, 1968, **49**, 223; *Chem Ind Lond*, 1971, 1212); yield (3%), major constituent *d*-limonene (50%) (*Flavour Ind*, 1970, **1**, 783); sedanenolide (3-*n*-Bu-4,5- dihydrophthalide) & 3-*n*- Buphthalide, these two constituents show mild depress. activity on CNS (*J Org Chem*, 1977, **42**, 2333; *J Food Sci*, 1978, **43**, 143).

Fruits commonly called seeds yield a number of furocoumarins (Wlth India, IA, 323); rutaretin, apiumetin; bergapten and isopimpinellin; and isoimperatorin, also coumarins seselin, osthenol, and apigravin; new furanocoumarin glucd. apiumoside (*Phytochemistry*, 1978, **17**, 2135; 1979, **18**, 352; 1580; 1764); dehydroflurocoumarin glucd. celereoside; and a new coumarin, celerin; and 2 dihydrofurocoumarins including nodakenetin (*Planta Med*, 1980, **38**, 363; 186; 1981, **43**, 306).

Seed husk, graveobioside A & B (*Indian J Chem*, 1963, **1**, 410); seeds, fatty acids 7-octadecenoic acids; also compds. from seeds, rev. (*Chem Ind Lond*, 1969, 1869; 1971, 1212); stigmasterol (*Eiyo To Shokuryo*, 1973, **26**, 121; *CA*, **79**, 134358n); boar pheromone steroid (*Experientia*, 1979, **35**, 1674).

Essent. oil from celery (herb), constituents (*Proc Fl State Hortic Soc*, 1965, **78**, 249; *Pharmazie*, 1981, **36**, 374; 1974, **29**, 349; *CA*, **81**, 74928c). Essent. oil from leaves and stems inferior to that from seed (Wlth India, IA, 324).

Volat. flavon. compds. of herb juice; plant ext., antioxidant (*J Food Sci*, 1963, **28**, 484; 1964, **29**, 27). Celery contains rutin (*Prikl Biokhim Microbiol*, 1965, **1**, 594; *CA*, 1966, **65**, 4544a). Sucapigraveol from herb juice, diur. in dogs (*Herba Pol*, 1966, **11**, 8; *CA*, **65**, 15152c). Polyphenols of herb and leaves (*Z Lebensm Unters Forsch*, 1966, **132**, 193: 1979, **169**, 170; *CA*, 1967, **66**, 45594a; **91**, 171672d; *Phytochemistry*, 1972, **11**, 1741; *Konservn Ovoshchesuch Promst*, 1978, 28; 1979, 31).

Furocoumarins, detn. by paper chromatogr. (*Pharmazie*, 1964, **19**, 700; *CA*, 1965, **62**, 12137e); xanthotoxin and bergapten from celery infected with *Sclerotinia sclerotiorum* (*Appl Microbiol*, 1972, **23**, 852). Herb, xanthotoxin and isopimpinellin; quant. estn. of xanthotoxin may lead to its use for cure of vitiligo and for treatment of psoriasis (*Planta Med*, 1976, **29**, 164; Wlth India, IA, 324).

Root essent oil constituents, Buphthalide and neocnidilide (*Chem Pharm Bull*, 1963, **11**, 1317). Root polyacetylenes (*Chem Ber*, 1967, **100**, 3454).

*A. leptophyllum (Pers.) F. Muell. ex Benth.

Essent. oil used as carmin. and to scent hair-oil (Wlth India, IA, 325).

Plant essent. oil contains Me-ethers of thymol, carvacrol and thymoquinol (*Aust J Chem*, 1969, **22**, 495).

Fruits, bergapten and seselin (*Indian J Pharm*, 1973, **35**, 127); seeds (only), dihydrofurocoumarins, leptophyllidin, leptophyllin, its glucd. and umbelliferone, isopimpinellin and mannitol; leptophyllin & its glucd. identical with rutaretin and isorutarin resp.; anhydrorutaretin, marmesin and 9-OH-4-OMe-psoralen (*Indian J Chem*, 1978, **16B**, 563; 1979, **17B**, 647); they also contain *trans*-khellactone, marmesinin, sitosterol glucd. and skimmin (*Phytochemistry*, 1980, **19**, 1556).

Native to C. and S. America, common in waste places, roadsides and gardens.

A. petroselinum Linn.; see **Petroselinum crispum**

APODYTES (*Icacinaceae*)

*A. dinidiata Mey. ex Arn. syn. *A. benthamiana* Wight

Leaves, bitter and astrin; flowers, fragrant (Wlth India, IA, 326).

Bark, oleanolic acid and stigmasterol (*Indian J Chem*, 1967, **5**, 523).

Found in Assam; Khasi and Jaintia hills in Meghalaya and evergreen forests of Kerala, up to 1,500 m.

APORUSA (*Euphorbiaceae*)

*A. dioica (Roxb.) Muell.-Arg. syn. *A. roxburghii* Baill.; *A. villosula* Kurz

Ass.–*Bara heloch*; Cachar–*Khempasibaphang*; Garo–*Chhamolja*; Lushai–*Sontul*; Manipur–*Tamsir-arong*; Nepal–*Chipli*.

EtOH(50%) ext. of aerial parts showed respiratory and cardiovascular activities (*Indian J Exp Biol*, 1973, **11**, 43).

Occurs in tropical valleys of Eastern Himalayas.

A. lindleyana Baill.

EtOH(50%) ext. of plant, hypoglyc. (*Indian J Exp Biol*, 1980, **18**, 594)).

AQUILARIA (*Thymelaeaceae*)

A. malaccenisis Lamk syn. *A. agallocha* Roxb.

Eng.–*Agarwood, aloewood, malacca eaglewood.*

Used by traditional vaidyas as contracep. (*Nagarjun*, 1979- 80, **23**, 9). Leaves boiled in oil, taken for removing fish spines from throat (*Bull Bot Surv India*, 1980, **22**, 161). Wood, insect repellent [*Macco Agric Digest*, 1981, **5**(9), 5].

Str. of agarospirol, constituent of essent. oil (*Tetrahedron*, 1965, **21**, 115). Str. of agarotetrol, a chromone from wood (*Tetrahedron Lett*, 1978, 3921). Heartwood, 1,7-oxoaporphine, liriodenine (Indian Pat, 1979, 145857; *CA*, 1980, **93**, 80049f). Wood yields 2 sesquiterps., gmelofuran and agarol (*Phytochemistry*, 1980, **19**, 1869). Stem bark, 2 cytotoxic compds. (*J Natl Prod*, 1981, **44**, 569).

AQUILEGIA (*Ranunculaceae*)

A. vulgaris Linn. syn. *A. karelini* Baker

Eng.–*Common columbine.*

EtOH(50%) ext. of aerial parts, hypoten. (*Annu Rep RRL, Jammu*, 1970-71, 24).

Plant contains di-OH-di-MeO-aporphine (1.5%) (*Khim Prir Soedin*, 1967, **3**, 354; *CA*, 1968, **68**, 47002w). Seed oil, a trienoic acid, ranunculeic acid (*ibid*, 1970, **6**, 167; *CA*, **73**, 63191r).

ARABIDOPSIS (*Brassicaceae*)

A. thaliana (Linn.) Heynh. syn. *Sisymbrium thalianum* (Linn.) Gay & Monn.

Eng.–*Thalecress.*

Leaves and flowers, astrin., antiscor., stim.; used in asthma, throat and chest troubles (*Indian Drugs*, 1976-77, **14**, 47).

Seed oil (4.3%), fatty acid compn.; erucic acid 2% (*J Am Oil Chem Soc*, 1965, **42**, 817).

ARACHIS (*Fabaceae*)

A. hypogaea Linn.

Eng.–*Groundnut, monkeynut, peanut.*

Groundnut oil—depressed whole blood clotting time in human volunteers (*J Assoc Physicians India*, 1963, **11**, 213). Coronary atherosclerosis by hydrogenated oil; effect of peanut oil (*J Indian Med Assoc*, 1963, **41**, 477; *Atherosclerosis*, 1971, **14**, 53); intimal spindle cell lesions in rats, fed with 40% oil diet; effect of oil on atherosclerosis (*Exp Mol Pathol*, 1964, **3**, 421; 1976, **24**, 375); anticholesterimic studies in healthy young women (*Annu Rep Nat Inst Nutr Tokyo*, 1965, 1; *CA*, 1966, **65**, 20586g). Drug for haemophilia from oil [*Oil Oilseeds J*, 1966, **18**(10), 16]. Peroxidised oil, antineoplastic in inhibiting lymphomatosis (*Chim Ther*, 1968, **3**, 189; *CA*, **69**, 75425a). When present in diet of rats for 1 yr at 5.5% oil, it induced strong platelet aggregation, *in vitro* (*Rev Fr Corps Gras*, 1979, **26**, 171; *CA*, **91**, 69650h). Oil heated at temperatures higher than customarily used contains toxic factor, which caused liver hypertrophy and even death in rat (*in* Liener, 401). Oil, as a base for several drugs or medicine.

Peanuts—EtOH ext. of defatted peanuts shortened bleeding time; had excitatory effects on smooth muscles of exp. animals, but inhibitory effect on isolated frog heart (*Thromb Diath Haemorrh*, 1966, **16**, 265; 257). Peanuts contain protease inhibitors; antiplasmin activity is of particular interest in view of earlier reports that peanut fractions with antitryptic activity are effective haemostatic agent in patients with haemophilia (*in* Liener, 8, 27).

Peanut agglutinin(s)—contain a strong anti-P agglutinin for neuraminidase-treated cells (*Vox Sang*, 1964, **9**, 748); neuroleptic preparation; also nontoxic adjuvant to stimulate antibody reaction on all antigens and to keep antibody concentration for long period (Neth Appl, 1965, 294946; 6402687; *CA*, **63**, 6796c; 1966, **64**, 3290 g); lectin to study T-antigen (*in* Liener, 96); purification of anti-T lectin (*J Biol Chem*,

1975, **250**, 8518). Purification and properties of non-specific haemagglutinin (*Lloydia*, 1970, **33**, 270); aggregates blood platelets (*Biochem Biophys Res Commun*, 1977, **75**, 200).

Peanut meal—ext. in dogs, decreased clotting and recalcification time, higher heparin tolerance in plasma, increased thromboplastic and prothrombin activity and higher antihaemophilic globulin in blood; *in vitro* it did not accelerate clotting (*Farmakol Toksiol Moscow*, 1966, **29**, 568).

Peanut skin—haemostatic tincture; also haemostatic agent (Brit. Pat., 1965, 992753; *CA*, **63**, 5456h; Czech. Pat., 1967, 124782; *CA*, 1968, **69**, 38730a; Fr CAM, 1968, 233; *CA*, 1971, **74**, 103030s).

Oil, predominates in mono unsaturated fats; beneficial for cardiac patients, also preventive of heart attacks, yield, fatty acid compn., glycerides, carotenoids, tocopherols, triterps., sterols, phosphatides (a source of lecithin), etc. (Wlth India, IA, 361-65; *J Indian Leather Technol Assoc*, 1967, **15**, 338). Elaidic acid; sterols & Mc-sterols (*Oleagineux*, 1966, **21**, 225; 1974, **29**, 253); from Poland, erucic acid (*Rocz Panstw Zaki Hig*, 1979, **30**, 123; *CA*, **91**, 54838 b); α-tocopherol content, 9.7-14.1 mg/100g (*Int J Vitam Nutr Res*, 1980, **50**, 242).

Peanut cotyledons, arachins A & B, str. (*Biochem J*, 1965, **96**, 119); α-arachin, major globulin (*Anal Biochem*, 1969, **27**, 15). Milk substances (*Pak J Sci*, 1971, **23**, 172; *CA*, 1973, **78**, 70421x). Volat. components (*J Food Sci*, 1969, **34**, 635; *J Agric Food Chem*, 1971, **19**, 1020; 1025). I, 0.77 and F, 5.1 ppm & dry edible matter (*Indian J Nutr Diet*, 1970, **7**, 243; 1971, **8**, 66).

Peanut caused goitre in rabbits (*Postepy Hig Med Dosw*, 1965, **19**, 303; *CA*, **63**, 7554b). A phenolic glycd. named arachidoside isolated from red skins of groundnut kernels, goitrogenic in rats; counteracted by concommitant supplement of KI. Phenolic metabolites of glycd. get preferentially iodinated thereby depriving

the thyroid of available I (Wlth India, IA, 361; *Indian J Nutr Diet*, 1973, **10**, 303).

Shell, a folk med. for hyperten.; luleolin, β- sitosterol, daucosterol and an unidentified saponin present (*Yao Hsueh T'ung Pao*, 1980, **15**, 44; *CA*, 1981, **95**, 49262n); 5,7-di-OH-chromene, eriodictyol and luteolin (*Phytochemistry*, 1973, **12**, 2033).

Aerial parts and roots, pterocarpanoids (oxygen heterocyclics) having fungicidal properties; aerial parts, volat. compds. (*Phytochemistry*, 1973, **12**, 375; 950).

Aflatoxicosis—a particular case of mycotoxicosis; it is poisoning of man or animals by ingestion of foodstuffs contaminated with certain moulds of *Aspergillus flavus* and/or their metabolic products called aflatoxins. Mould-infected groundnut-kernels are toxic to most animals, in certain species of ducklings, rats and trouts. Moulds of *A. flavus* grow and produce aflatoxins in wide variety of crops, but appear to have special affinity for groundnuts (Wlth India, IA, 366; *in* Liener, 338); acute in calves fed peanut hay (*Aust Vet J*, 1980, **57**, 284).

Aflatoxins and other mycotoxins—aflatoxins and sterigmatocystins are a group of mould metabolites of polyketide type. Eight aflatoxins are known; chemically they are bifuranocoumarin metabolites. Aflatoxin B_1 is the most active and most toxic member; it is a hepatocarcinagen. Closely related sterigmatocystin has been isolated from *A. versicolor*. Toxins from fungus-infected groundnut damage animal liver [*Oil Oilseeds J*, 1969, **21**(12), 15]. There is strong circumstantial evidence for relationship between liver cancer incidence in human beings (*in* Wagner & Wolff, 86-87; *in* Liener, 331-47; 345). Anal. of groundnuts for aflatoxins, ochratoxins and sterigmatocystin (*Analyst Lond*, 1969, **94**, 136). Citrinin present in groundnuts occasionally infected with *Penicillium citrinum* (*Curr Sci*, 1974, **43**, 707); ochratoxins in market sample from Mysore (*J Food Sci Technol*, 1979, **16**, 113). Out of 150 isolates from

Indian peanuts, only 4 contained aflatoxin B₁ [*Mycotoxin Food Stuffs Proc Symp Mass Inst Technol*, 1964 (Pub. 1965), 251; *CA*, **63**, 17016c]. Chem. nature and biol. effects of aflatoxins, rev., 71 refs. (*Bacteriol Rev*, 1966, **30**, 460). Removal of aflatoxin from nut kernel (Indian Pat., 1971, 120257). Comparison of different methods of extn. of aflatoxin B in groundnut (*Indian Phytopathol*, 1972, **25**, 467); evolution of aflatoxin elimination methods, rev., 13 refs [*Cah Nutr Diet*, 1976, **11**(2 Suppl.), 105; *CA*, 1977, **87**, 37394d].

Using food-grade hexane for extn. and with right procedure, oil is nontoxic (*Indian J Med Res*, 1973, **61**, 422). Decontamination by adsorption-cum-filtration; removal, by activated kaolin [*Indian J Technol*, 1979, **17**, 440; *Huan Ching Pao Hu*, 1979, (4), 39; *CA*, 1980, **93**, 24712e].

Detn. of aflatoxin (*Nature Lond*, 1964, **203**, 862; *ISI Bull*, 1970, **22**, 199); TLC of aflatoxin B₁ (*Vet Rec*, 1964, **76**, 901; *CA*, 1965, **62**, 4531d); spectrophotom. (*Analyst Lond*, 1965, **90**, 155; 492); of aflatoxin B₁ in cake (*Boll Lab Chim Prov*, 1965, **16**, 619; *CA*, 1966, **65**, 1286c); in peanut products (*Pure Appl Chem*, 1973, **35**, 267); in peanuts (*J Sci Res Bhopal*, 1980, **2**, 119). HPLC (*Z Lebensm Unters Forsch*, 1976, **160**, 321; *CA*, **84**, 178319h); aflatoxin (*Prikl Biokhim Microbiol*, 1981, **17**, 759).

Aflatoxin and its heat stability in Indian cooking oils (*Trop Sci*, 1975, **17**, 229); oil, detoxification (*J Food Sci Technol*, 1975, **12**, 20); TLC removal of mycotoxins of oil (*J Assoc Off Anal Chem*, 1975, **58**, 620); oil contaminated with aflatoxin B₁, liver carcinogenic in rats (*Food Cosmet Toxicol*, 1981, **19**, 179).

Peanut food products, decontamination (Fr Demande, 1975, 2240695; *CA*, **83**, 112625c); aflatoxin-free food production (US Pat., 1977, 4035518; *CA*, **87**, 166367w). Codes of practice for control and prevention of aflatoxin contamination

in various operations, and groundnut products [IS: 9071 (Pt I-II) 1979].

Presence of substances around the embroys of freshly harvested nuts resistant to *A. flavus* reported, with possibilities of breeding *A. flavus*-resistant commercial varieties (Wlth India, IA, 367); 3 phytoalexins isolated from seeds including 2 novel isoprenylated stilbene derivs. (*Phytochemistry*, 1981, **20**, 1381).

ARACHNE (*Euphorbiaceae*)

See ANDRACHNE

ARALIA (*Araliaceae*)

*A. cachemirica Decne.

Kash.–*Khoree*; P.–*Banakhor*.

Plant, pimara-8(14), 15-dien-19-oic acid, exhibited antiinflam. activity; nonane, a hexacosane deriv., petroselinic acid, araloside A & B, stigmasterol & β-sitosterol [*Proc Indian Sci Congr*, 1980, part III, 163; *Indian J Chem*, 1976, **14B**, 475).

Temperate Himalayas from Kashmir to Sikkim at 2,100-4,000 m.

A. pseudo-ginseng Benth.; see **Panax pseudo-ginseng**

A. quinquefolia Decne.; see **Panax ginseng**

ARAUCARIA (*Araucariaceae*)

*A. araucana (Molina) Koch syn. *A. imbricata* Pav.

Eng.–*Chile pine, monkey puzzle*.

Bark, very resinous; resins from bark used med. by Araucanian Indians.

Resin, bicyclic diterps. (*J Chem Soc*, 1964, 3648; *Phytochemistry*, 1969, **8**, 633); terpenes of resin (*Naturwissenschaften*, 1965, **52**, 185; *Tetrahedron Lett*, 1965, 4623; 1966, 1901; *Gazz Chim Ital*, 1976, **106**, 1119).

Branches, essent. oil (0.06%); constituents (*Tetrahedron*, 1975, **31**, 1311). Heartwood, 2 substances both weak antifung. against *Poria vaporarius* (*An Fac*

Quim Farm Univ Chile, 1967, **19**, 12; *CA,* 1969, **70**, 69378s).

Native to S. America and introduced into India as an ornamental tree.

ARCHANGELICA *(Apiaceae)*

A. officinalis Hoffm. var. himalaica C.B. Clarke ; see Angelica archangelica var. himalaica

ARCTIUM *(Asteraceae)*

A. lappa Linn.

Plant—ext. caused a sharp long-lasting reduction of blood sugar with an increase in carbohydrate tolerance and less toxicity *(Farm Zh Kiev,* 1964, **19**, 52; *CA,* 1967, **66**, 1451e). Alc. ext., constituents of liquid compn. for treating psoriasis and seborrhoic eczemas (Czech. Pat., 1980, 185262; *CA,* 1981, **95**, 68027f). In Russia, for alopecia areata *(Farm Zh Kiev,* 1972, **27**, 78; *BA,* 1973, **56**, 56516).

Roots—tumour growth inhibitory mixt. *(Acta Univ Szeged Acta Phys Chem,* 1964, **10**, 91; *CA,* 1965, **62**, 6339e). EtOH(50%) ext., cardiac stim., diur. and spasmol. *(Annu Rep RRL Jammu,* 1970-71, 24). Pharmacognosy *(Indian J Pharm Sci,* 1979, **41**, 253).

Leaves, germakranolides *(Naturwissenschaften,* 1965, **52**, 209); bitter sesquiterp. lactone, arctiopicrin *(Diss Pharm Pharmacol,* 1968, **20**, 93; *Int Pharm Abstr,* **5**, 1397c); eremophilene, fukinone, petasitolone, fukinanolide, β-dudesmol, taraxasterol & its -OAc and palmitate esters, dehydrofukinone or 9(10)-fukinone and arcitol or 8α-hydroxyeudesmol *(Chem Lett,* 1972, 235; *CA,* **76**, 150982e).

Seeds yield sesquilignans, lappaol A & B *(Tetrahedron Lett,* 1976, 3961). Fruits, new sesquilignan derivs. Al-D and AL-F alongwith arctiin, arctigenin and mateiresinol *(Yakugaku Zasshi,* 1976, **96**, 1492); lappaol C, D & E *(Agric Biol Chem,* 1977, **41**, 1813).

Roots yield S-containing acetylenic acid, acetic acid and several volat. components *(Nippon Nogei Kagaku Kaishi,* 1970, **44**, 437; *CA,* 1971, **74**, 108136n). γ-Guanidino- n-butyric acid *(Phytochemistry,* 1975, **14**, 582). Root essent. oil *(Perfum Essent Oil Rec,* 1976, **58**, 437).

ARCTOSTAPHYLOS *(Ericaceae)*

A. uva-ursi (Linn.) Spreng.

Eng.–*Bearberry.*

Well known drug used for its diur. and antisep. properties in catar. of bladder (Chopra *et al,* I, 509). Dried leaves collected in autumn used as tonic. Also used as tea in some parts of Russia; known as *kutai* and *Caucasian* tea (Med. Plants, 112).

Leaf ext. (arbutin), efficient urinary disinfectant *(Planta Med,* 1969, **18**, 1). Preparation of liquid concentrate containing arbutin with diur. and antisep. activity *(Farmatsiya Moscow,* 1975, **24**, 40; *CA,* **83**, 32945s). One of the constituents of a compn. for improving form and appearance of feminine bust (Fr. Demande, 1976, 2296425; *CA,* 1977, **87**, 172722z).

Extensively investigated abroad w.r.t. constituents and arbutin content.

Arbutin—active principle, it is hydroquinone mono glucd. Also called arbutoside, from Bulgarian plant, 8.5% *(Acta Pharm Jugosl,* 1963, **13**, 117; *CA,* 1965, **63**, 9749e); in leaves, 5.9% *(Lek Sirovine,* 1968, **6**, 57; *CA,* 1971, **74**, 146291v); in leaves from wild plant growing in Yakutia (Russia), 18.1% (flowering period) *(Uch Zap Yakutsk Gos Univ,* 1971, No. 18, 41; *CA,* 1973, **79**, 2724 u). HPLC for sepn. and detn. of arbutin, Me-arbutin, hydroquinone & its mono Me ether *(Planta Med,* 1979, **35**, 253).

ARDISIA *(Myrsinaceae)*

A. colorata Roxb.

Garo–*Bol-simbal;* Lushai–*Rulthlu.*

Bark pigment used in Thailand as antileprous; bark contains rapanone (1%) and ilexol (*Shoyakugaku Zasshi*, 1967, **21**, 68; *CA*, 1968, **69**, 54264g).

*A. floribunda Wall. ex DC. non Kurz syn. *A. neriifolia* Wall.

EtOH(50%) ext. of aerial parts, diur., spermic., CNS depress. and anticancer (*Indian J Exp Biol*, 1977, **15**, 208; 231).

Bark contains friedelin, α-amyrin-OAc and isoarborinol-OAc (*Indian J Chem*, 1967, **5**, 523).

Sub-tropical Himalayas from Kumaun to Bhutan, and in Khasi Hills, up to 1,525 m.

*A. odontophylla Wall. ex DC.

Roots used in Malaysia and other eastern countries in diar., fever and rheum. (Wlth India, IA, 390).

Khasi and Jaintia hills of Meghalaya.

A. solanacea Roxb. syn. *A. humilis* C.B. Clarke non Vahl

EtOH(50%) ext. of aerial parts, antiacetylcholine (*Indian J Exp Biol*, 1969, **7**, 250).

Roots alongwith flowers of *Bauhinia purpurea* mixed in cow's *ghee*, given to asthma patient (*Nagarjun*, 1980-81, **24**, 1).

Roots and stem contain bauerenol, (*Indian J Chem*, 1967, **5**, 523); leaves, bauerenol, α- & β-amyrin (*Planta Med*, 1977, **32**, 162).

ARECA (*Aracaceae*)

A. catechu Linn.

Eng.–*Arecanut* or *betelnut palm, areca palm, Pinang palm.*

Plant—used in rhagades, smallpox, venereal sores, syphilis, cholera, and dysen. (*Econ Bot*, 1970, **24**, 241). Also used for fractured bones (*Sri Lanka For*, 1981, **14**, 145).

Nut—aq. ext. exhibits direct vasoconstriction and adrenaline potentiation in rats (*Curr Sci*, 1963, **32**, 455). Antimicrob. activity due to polyphenolic fraction (*Indian J Exp Biol*, 1965, **3**, 66). Ext. antifert. (*Indian J Med Res*, 1971, **59**,

302); a constituent of indigenous compn., 'Ayush-47' exhibiting antiimplantation activity in albino rats (*ibid*, 1979, **70**, 504), nut oil also showd antifert. activity in rats (*Planta Med*, 1974, **26**, 391). EtOH(50%) ext. of fruit and leaf, spasmog. (*Indian J Exp Biol*, 1973, **11**, 43; 1980, **18**, 594).

Seeds contain aflatoxins B_1 and G_1 (*Malay Agric J*, 1977- 78, **51**, 305). Carcinogenic effects of betel quid (*Experientia*, 1979, **35**, 384). Betel quid with tobacco-induced tumours in Swiss-strain mice (*Indian J Exp Biol*, 1980, **18**, 1159). *Aspergillus flavus*, a carcinogenic fungus contaminates betel nuts [*Hamdard*, 1981, **24**(1-2), 130].

Arecanut tannin potentiated the action of acetylcholine in ileum and uterus of rat, and noradrenaline on rat seminal vesicle at low concn. (*CNS Drugs Symp CSIR India*, 1966, 249). Mature nut (endosperm) contains, (+)-catechin, 2 monomeric and 6 polymeric leucocyanidins (*Phytochemistry*, 1964, **2**, 321); seeds, di-, tri- & tetrameric procyanidins (*J Chem Soc Chem Commun*, 1981, 781).

Seeds contain anti-P agglutinins (*Vox Sang*, 1964, **9**, 748); agglutinin, which resembles anti-T agglutinin of *Glycine max* (*Experientia*, 1965, **21**, 5).

Arecanut (chewing) good source of flouride (*Indian J Med Res*, 1971, **59**, 1966). Rev. on chem. and pharmacol. of betel nut, 214 refs. (*J Plant Crops*, 1979, **7**, 69; *CA*, 1980, **93**, 182759e).

Arecanut contains several alks. belonging to pyridine group. Most important being arecoline; also present are arecaidine, guvacine, isoguvacine, etc. (Wlth India, IA, 405-06); isoguvacine produces hypotension when given intracisternally in cumulative doses (*in* Beal & Reinhard, 275, 276).

Arecoline & arecaidine—both oily liquids; both contain a tetrahydropyridine nucleus; yield of arecoline (*c*. 1%) from dried ripe seed; that of arecaidine in smaller quant. Arecoline hydrolysed to arecaidine; esterification of arecaidine with MeOH yields arecoline.

Arecoline used as anthelm. for animals for treatment of tapeworm or roundworm infestation but not so for humans (Sim, 33-34). Pharmacol. (*Arzneim Forsch*, 1967, **17**, 1292; *CA*, **68**, 113138y). It has effect similar to pilocarpine; cholinergic, exerting sialogogue and diaphor. action in normal dosage, but in large doses CNS depress. and paralyses muscles. Sed. and CNS depress. (*Curr Sci*, 1967, **36**, 234). Mydriatic, but 1% sol. when dropped into the eye, constricted pupil like physostigmine. It may exert deleterious effect on dental enamel (Chopra *et al*, 1958, 282; *Taiwania*, 1973, **18**, 123). Possible carcinogenic action of alks., a rev. on betel nut alks. and their possible carcinogenic effects, 32 refs. [*Planta Med*, 1968, **16**, (Suppl.), 13].

Arecaidine has no parasympathomimetic effects but only stimulating properties; in higher doses, sed. (Chopra *et al*, 1958, 282). Nontoxic metabolic product of arecoline following liver degradation and perhaps chief pharmacol. agent in consumption of betel nuts (*Arzneim Forsch*, 1968, **18**, 222; *CA*, **68**, 113138y). Arecaidine and guvacine competitively inhibited uptake of GABA in rat brain slices (*Nature Lond*, 1975, **258**, 627). Arecaidine and arecoline gave +ve response to cell-transformation assay of styles; arecaidine, possible human carcinogen; may be more carcinogenic than arecoline (*Lancet*, 1979, 1, 112; *Excerpta Bot*, 1980, **34**, 135).

Arecoline & its metabolite arecaidine react with 3,4-olefinic bond with thiol groups, thus they are biol. alkylating agents and hence possibly carcinogenic (*Biochem J*, 1968, **113**, 123). According to Indian hypothesis, chewing of betel quid (excluding tobacco) enhances levels of nitrite in oral cavity, which may promote increased generation of carcinogenic nitrosamines (*Food Cosmet Toxicol*, 1980, **18**, 277).

ARECASTRUM (*Arecaceae*)

*A. romanzoffianum (Cham.) Becc. syn *Cocos romanzoffiana* Cham.; *C. plumosa* Hook.f.

Eng.–*Feathery coconut palm, queen palm.*

Unripe seeds reported to have caused scouring and death of calves in New S. Wales but in Florida, where palm is popular and fruits abundant, no such reports of toxicity available.

Kernel, fatty oil (52.2%) similar to coconut oil in odour and flavour; unsapon matter, 0.4%. Plant, scyllitol (Wlth India, IA, 413).

Native to Brazil, occasionally cultivated in Indian gardens.

ARENARIA (*Caryophyllaceae*)

A. serpyllifolia Linn. var. **serpyllifolia**

Plant contains an extremely active saponin with haemolytic activity remaining unaffected at different levels of pH; saponin present in root, stem and leaves in almost equal quantities (Wlth India, IA, 414).

ARGEMONE (*Papaveraceae*)

A. mexicana Linn.

Eng.–*Mexican poppy, prickly poppy.*

Root—ext., antifung. (*Geobios*, 1978, **5**, 49). Roots burnt to provide heat in treatment of piles; given in *pan* (*Piper betle*) for severe stomach-ache (*Bull Bot Surv India*, 1980, **22**, 201).

Seeds—pounded in '*Mahua* oil' and applied to eczema and itching (*Econ Bot*, 1965, **19**, 239). Ground seeds mixed with *Brassica* oil used for itch (*J Econ Tax Bot*, 1981, **2**, 191). Paper chromatogr. detection of argemone seeds in mustard seeds (*Curr Sci*, 1972, **41**, 465).

Plant—EtOH(50%) ext. antivir. (*Indian J Exp Biol*, 1968, **6**, 232). Plant used as anthelm., antileprotic, tonic, diur., antid; roots used for syphlitic infections and tapeworms; seeds in abdominal colic and dysen. [*J Res Indian Med*, 1973, **8**(2), 75].

Fruits of *Xeromphis spinosa* rubbed with juice of *A. mexicana* and applied to boils [*ibid*, 1978, **13**(4), 92]. Juice of stem and leaves alongwith *ghee* and *jira*, in skin diseases (*Bull Bot Surv India*, 1973, **15**, 13); ext. as a tea for difficult and burning urination (*Econ Bot*, 1975, **29**, 316). Tissue culture ext., antimicrob. (*Indian J Pharm Sci*, 1980, **42**, 113).

Latex—used in warts, tumours and cancer (*Lloydia*, 1970, **33**, 318); in eye diseases (*Bull Med Ethno Bot Res*, 1980, **1**, 318); yellow milky sap used to treat scabies. Leaf juice alongwith cow milk used to treat leprosy (*J Econ Tax Bot*, 1981, **2**, 173).

Seed oil—sanguinarine, toxic factor in seeds, cause of glaucoma with endemic dropsy (*Cesk Oftalmol*, 1966, **22**, 49; *CA*, **64**, 18108b). Oil obtained by screw pressing, toxic while that obtained by solvent extn., non-toxic (*Indian J Med Res*, 1971, **59**, 1676). Carcinogenicity of contaminates in indigenous edible oils (*Int J Cancer*, 1972, **10**, 652). Testing of carcinogenicity; toxicity in animals (*Indian J Med Res*, 1973, **61**, 428; 1975, **63**, 1353). Used to cure skin diseases (*Econ Bot*, 1978, **32**, 278).

Roots and stems contain protppine, berberine, resin and a toxic principle; pharmacol. studies with alks. (*J Pharm Sci*, 1963, **52**, 1172).

Argemone oil, detection in mustard oil; in edible oils [*Bull Calcutta Sch Trop Med*, 1965, **13**, 58; 1967, **15**(2), 65]; fatty acid compn. (*Fette Seifen Anstrichm*, 1972, **74**, 268; *CA*, **77**, 85578g; *Chem Phys Lipids*, 1977, **20**, 331); glyceride compn. (*J Am Oil Chem Soc*, 1965, **42**, 961); seed oil colorim. estn. and detection (*ibid*, 1972, **49**, 201; 1973, **50**, 543); detoxification (*ibid*, 1977, **54**, 322).

Sanguinarine—benzophenanthridine alk. tended to potentiate carcinogenic effects of a contaminated sample of mustard oil. Its postulated metabolite, 3,4-benzacridine, carcinogenic to rodents (*Indian J Cancer*, 1968, **5**, 183; *Nature Lond*, 1961,

189, 201). Procedure for removal of sanguinarine (*Indian J Med Res*, 1976, **64**, 1128). Sepn. of alks., sanguinarine and allocryptonine from seed oil (*Farmatsiya Moscow*, 1974, **23**, 36). Inhibition of human pregnancy plasma diamine oxidase with sanguinarine and berberine (*J Postgrad Med Bombay*, 1980, **26**, 28).

Alks. protopine and allocryptopine from aerial parts of flowering plant (*Khim Prir Soedin*, 1971, **7**, 208; *CA*, **75**, 31315j). Plant, several alks. norsanguinarine, norchelerythrine, cryptopine, berberine, coptisine, sanguinarine, chelerythrine, etc. (*Collect Czech Chem Commun*, 1975, **40**, 1576); benzophenanthridine alk. (*Z Chem*, 1976, **16**, 54; *CA*, **85**, 5917u).

Latex contains alk. berberine (0.74%), protopine (0.36%) and free amino acids (*Curr Sci*, 1971, **40**, 548).

Flowers, isorhamentin 3-glucd. & 3,7-diglucd. (*Indian J Chem*, 1965, **3**, 270); useful in whooping cough (*J Agric Trop Bot Appl*, 1966, **13**, 277).

*A. ochroleuca Sweet

Plant appears to have same properties as *A. mexicana*; seeds employed to adulterate those of mustard (Wlth India, IA, 417).

Alks. protopine, allocryptopine, berberine, coptisine, sanguinarine, etc. (*Collect Czech Chem Commun*, 1973, **38**, 2307).

Stems and flowers, berberine nitrate, 0.05; protopine nitrate, 0.05; isorhamnetin, 0.05 & its glycd., 0.07; K nitrate, 2.5; and Ca sulphate, 0.6%; ceryl alc., β-sitosterol, etc. (*Curr Sci*, 1966, **35**, 313).

Punjab, Haryana and Uttar Pradesh.

*A. subfusiformis Ownbey ssp. subfusiformis

Herb (without capsules), alks., allocryptopine, berberine, cheterythrine, protopine, sanguinarine and 3 unidentified bases (*Phytochemistry*, 1972, **11**, 3547).

Found in Rajasthan.

ARGYREIA (*Convolvulaceae*)

A. cuneata Ker-Gawl. syn. *Convolvulus cuneatus* Willd.; *Lettsomia cuneata* Roxb.; *Rivea cuneata* Wight

Eng.–*Purple convolvulus.*

Leaves effective in diabetes in animals; oral administration in man had little effect; contain mixt. of 3 polysterols which exhibit hypoglyc. and CNS depress. activity (Wlth India, IX, 48). Leaves, sitosterol (*Indian J Chem*, 1975, **13**, 97).

Seeds, ergoline alks. (*Phytochemistry*, 1973, **12**, 2435).

*A. hookeri C.B. Clarke

EtOH(50%) ext. of plant, hypoten. (*Indian J Exp Biol*, 1973, **11**, 43).

Found in Ratangiri, Maharashtra.

A. imbricata (Roth) Santapau & Patel syn. *A. aggregata* (Roxb.) Choisy; *Lettsomia aggregata* Roxb.; *L. mysorensis* C.B. Clarke

Kan.–*Uganballi*; Mar.–*Bondvel.*

Seeds contain hallucinogenic ergoline alks., chanoclavine, ergine, isoergine, ergometrine, etc. (*Lloydia*, 1967, **30**, 23).

*A. involucrata C.B. Clarke

EtOH(50%) ext. of aerial parts, diur. and anticancer (*Indian J Exp Biol*, 1977, **15**, 208).

Found in Bastar, M.P.

A. malabarica Choisy

Tam.–*Pay moostey.*

Leaves, antiphl.; used in same way as *A. nervosa.*

A. nervosa (Burm.f.) Bojer syn. *A. speciosa* Sweet

Eng.–*Elephant creeper, woolly morning-glory.*

EtOH(50%) ext. of seeds, hypoten. (*Indian J Exp Biol*, 1969, **7**, 250).

Plant—in stomach complaints, sores on foot, smallpox, syphilis, diar. and dysen. (*Econ Bot*, 1970, **24**, 241). One of the constituents of indigenous drug 'Fortege', used successfully against common sexual disorders in male, clin. trials [*Mediscope*, 1978, **21**(6), 140]; also of drug, 'Speman'

with anabolic-cum-androgen-like activity in mice (*Indian J Exp Biol*, 1976, **14**, 170).

Roots—bitter, diur., aphrodis. Pharmacognostic study, a paste of roots along with those of others used for chr. cough and cold, and in consequent fever (*Acta Phytother*, 1972, **19**, 46; Wlth India, IA, 419)

Fatty oil and its unsap. matter, antimicrob. [*Indian Drugs Pharmac Ind*, 1978, **13**(5), 29].

Seeds contain ergoline alks. (3 mg/g) (*Science*, 1965, **148**, 499); hallucinogens: isoergine, ergine and penniclavine (*Lloydia*, 1967, **30**, 31); lysergic acid amide & isolysergic acid amide (*J Assoc Off Anal Chem*, 1970, **53**, 123); also 19 ergoline alks.; ergine & isoergine main alks. (*J Pharm Sci*, 1973, **62**, 588). Seeds hypoten.; contain 3 alks. including ergometrine; caffeic acid and Et-caffeate (*Indian J Pharm*, 1974, **36**, 118).

Leaves contain 1-triacontanol, β-sitosterol, epifriedelinol & its -OAc (*Phytochemistry*, 1971, **10**, 1949).

*A. pomacea Choisy

EtOH(50%) ext. of aerial parts, hypoten. (*Indian J Exp Biol*, 1974, **12**, 512).

Found in Irruttapalyam, T.N.

ARISAEMA (*Araceae*)

*A. concinnum Schott

Tubers, irrit. due to Ca oxalate crystals; rendered edible by repeated boiling and discarding water (Wlth India, IA, 420).

Found in temperate Himalayas and in Meghalaya at 1,800 - 3,300 m.

*A. jacquemontii Blume

Garo–*Jinjok.*

Juice from tubers given to treat ringworms; also applied in various skin diseases (*Econ Bot*, 1981, **35**, 4).

Found in Khasi hills of Meghalaya.

*A. propinquum Schott syn. *A. wallichianum* Hook. f.; *A. costatum* Stapf non Mart.; *A. sikkimense* Stapf ex Chatterjee

Herb reported to possess anticancer activity (*Annu Rep CDRI Lucknow*, 1970, 76).

Tubers contain an alk. (0.25%) (*Pak J Sci Ind Res*, 1963, **6**, 53).

Temperate Himalayas from Kashmir to Bhutan at 2,000 - 4,000 m.

A. speciosum Mart.

Eng.–*Cobra-lily, snake-lily.*

Tubers poisonous to man and livestock; contain Ca oxalate crystals; liable to produce dermatitis (Chopra *et al*, II, 905).

Fruits reported to have deleterious effect on the mouth when eaten (Wlth India, IA, 421).

A. tortuosum (Wall.) Schott syn. *Arum curvatum* (Roxb.) Kunth

Eng.–*Cobra flower.*

Tubers—edible but highly irrit. due to Ca oxalate crystals (*Q J Crude Drug Res*, 1972, **12**, 1922); taken with black pepper in cold and cough. Credited with antifert., insectic. and insect-repellent properties (Wlth India, IA, 421; *Nagarjun*, 1979-80, **23**, 177).

Tubers contain a poisonous principle which is partially destroyed by fermenting tubers. Alc. ext. of fruit, alk. colchicine (0.21%) (*Nat Appl Sci Bull*, 1974, **26**, 25).

Pet. ether ext. of corms from Shimla contains *n*-alkanes, *n*-alkanols, stigmasterol, sitosterol, campesterol, cholesterol; EtOH ext., choline chloride and stachydrine-HCL (*Indian J Pharm*, 1978, **40**, 24).

ARISTOLOCHIA (*Aristolochiaceae*)

A. bracteolata Lamk syn. *A. bracteata* Retz.

Eng.–*Bracteated birthwort.*

Plant—every part, nauseous and persistently bitter (Chopra *et al*, II, 742); plant, insectic. or insect repellent due to presence of aristolochic acid (Wlth India, IA, 423); poisonous to man and livestock (Watt & Breyer-Brandwijk, 118). In Sudan, plant used against scorpion sting, and as purg. and anthelm. (*Fitoterapia*, 1981, **52**, 243).

Seeds—ground in water to form a lotion used for softening hair (*J Agric Trop Bot Appl*, 1966, **13**, 251); strong purg. (*J Econ Tax Bot*, 1980, **1**, 137); also antispasmol. and contain alk., sterol/triterp. (*Fitoterapia*, 1980, **51**, 143).

Leaf juice, vermifuge (*Econ Bot*, 1978, **32**, 278). Powd. root, in fertility control (*Ancient Sci Life*, 1981-82, **1**, 66).

Leaves and fruit contain ceryl alc. and β-sitosterol (*Indian J Pharm*, 1965, **27**, 264).

Seeds (Gujarat sample), non-drying oil (yield, 18.5%); unsap. matter (5.3%), with β-sitosterol. Defatted seeds, aristolochic acid (A.P. Sample, 0.011%; Sudanese sample, 0.19%) (Wlth India, IA, 423); 3 quaternery alks. including magnoflorine (*Planta Med*, 1970, **18**, 30).

*A. cathcartii Hook.f.

Garo–*Baro-nirkhut.*

Root juice mixed with root exts. of *Cyclea peltata* and *Coccinia grandis*, in small pox (*Bull Bot Surv India*, 1980, **22**, 161).

Found around Balphakram sanctuary in Meghalaya.

A. indica Linn.

Eng.–*Indian birthwort.*

Roots—decoct. used in impotency (*Q J Crude Drug Res*, 1971, **11**, 1742). Roots given in bowel complaints of children and in intermittent fever (*Bull Bot Soc Bengal*, 1975, **29**, 97). In large doses, acts as an irrit. provoking nausea and griping pains in the bowels and sometimes vomiting and tenesmus (Wlth India, IA, 426). $CHCl_3$ ext. of roots, antispermator. in mice (*Indian J Exp Biol*, 1977, **15**, 256); 100% interceptive (also pet. ether and alc. ext.) in mice and hamsters at 50 mg/kg dose level (*Indian J Med Res*, 1977, **66**, 991; *Indian J Exp Biol*, 1977, **15**, 428). One of the constituents of '*Majnoon-e-Flasfa*' a polypharmaceutical compn. of Unani system [*Nagarjun*, 1977-78, **21**(11), 23].

Roots, 100% antifert. activity in exp. animals (*Bull Med Ethno Bot Res*, 1981, **1**, 408); crushed and applied on the body against itching (*J Econ Tax Bot*, 1981, **2**, 183).

Plant—used as abortif. (*Q J Crude Drug Res*, 1972, **12**, 1922). EtOH(50%) ext., diur. (*Indian J Exp Biol*, 1977, **15**, 208); ext., antiinflam. [*J Res Indian Med*, 1977, **12**(2), 18]. Juice of fresh leaves useful in treating cough of children by inducing vomiting without depression (Wlth India, IA, 426).

Seeds, tasteless, useful in treating inflam., biliousness and dry cough (Wlth India, IA, 426).

Roots odour due to an essent. oil and bitter taste due to aristolochic acid. Latter, in varying amts. in samples of drug ranging from 0.06 to 0.7%(dry basis); variation in the yield, due to the varying amts. of stems in different drug samples. Besides aristolochic acid, roots also yield other phenanthrene derivs., alks., a no. of sesquiterps., stigmast-4-en-3-one, *p*-coumaric acid, etc. (Wlth India, IA, 423-25).

Phenanthrene derivs., aristolochic-acid-D & its Me ether lactam, aristololactam & its β-D-glucd.; aristolic acid & its Me ester, aristolamide, Me aristolachate & its 6-MeO deriv., besides aristolochic acid (*J Org Chem*, 1968, **33**, 3755; *Phytochemistry*, 1977, **16**, 1103; 1981, **20**, 1444).

Alk., aristolochine identified as *l*-curine; also unidentified ones, with mol. wts, 608, 622, 636 (*Indian J Chem*, 1967, **5**, 655).

Sesquiterps., ishwarone, str. (*Tetrahedron Lett*, 1969, 133); ishwarane; ishwarone & aristolochene (*Tetrahedron*, 1970, **26**, 615; 2371); ledol, str. (*Indian J Chem*, 1966, **4**, 457); 5 β H, 7 β,10 α-selina-4(14),11-diene (*ibid*, 1973, **11**, 971); ishwarol (*ibid*, 1971, **9**, 1310); (12*S*)-7-12-secoishwaran-12-ol along with (+)-ledol (*J Org Chem*, 1980, **45**, 4765).

Aristolochic acid—chief active principle of drug (roots); it is 8-OMe-3,4-methylenedioxy - 10-nitrophenanthrene-1-COOH; it is same as isoaristolochic, aristinic and aristolochic acids, aristolochia yellow but different from aristolochine; intensely bitter and optically inactive (Wlth India, IA, 424). The acid isolated by extracting roots with alc. (95%) or ammonium hydroxide (5%) and chromatographing ext. (*J Org Chem*, 1968, **33**, 3735). Extn. method and quant. detn. (from *A. maurorum*) by direct densitometric measuring of TLC plates described (*Fitoterapia*, 1981, **52**, 201).

Aristolochic acid, antitubercular (*Indian J Pharm*, 1967, **29**, 157). Antifeedant, male sterilant for some insects, toxic to houseflies (*Indian J Hort*, 1978, **35**, 406); feeding male houseflies with acid induced sterility (*Experientia*, 1980, **36**, 245). Study with 3 insects suggests mitotic death (*Indian J Exp Biol*, 1979, **17**, 354).

Exts. or isolates of *A. indica*, containing aristolochic acid, anticancer; compd. active against adenocarcinoma 755 ascites carcinoma in mice but inactive against a wide spectrum of exp. neoplasms (Wlth India, IA, 426).

It stimulates phagocytic function of reticuloendothelial system in rats (*Adv Exp Med Biol*, 1971, **15**, 87). Stimulates phagocytic activity in guinea pigs administered chloramphenicol, cyclophosphamide and to a small extent predinosone; clin. assessment terminated as a result of renal damages (*Progr Med Chem*, 1972, **9**, 26); tardolyt coated tablets which contain 0.3 mg of aristolochic acid increases phagocytosis in healthy male individuals (*Planta Med*, 1980, **39**, 234).

Aristolic acid & deriv.—roots also owe some of the pharmacol. properties to this compd. obtained from $CHCl_3$ ext., yield, 0.007% of market sample of root; effective antifert. agent in mature female albino rabbits; no adverse reaction in blood; antiestrogenic and prevents implantation in early stage of pregnancy in mice; its Me ester, strong abortif. but showed damage to liver and kidney; short term toxicity of Me ester (Wlth India, IA, 426; *Experientia*, 1978, **34**, 1377; 1192; *Indian J Exp Biol*, 1978, **16**, 1283; 1979, **17**, 437).

Roots, sesquiterp. exhibited interceptive (100%) and antiimplantation (91.7%) in mice and antiestrogenic (*Indian J Exp Biol*, 1977, **15**, 1197); *p*-coumaric acid, interceptive (100%) in mice (*ibid*, 1978, **16**, 1285).

*A. littoralis Parodi syn. *A. elegans* Mast.

Eng.–*Calico flower*.

Plant contains an alk. cryptopleurine, a substitute for colchicine in cytological work; alk. showed C-mitotic action on root tips of germinating onion seeds (Wlth India, IA, 427).

Roots and rhizomes, aristolochic acid and magnoflorine (*Eur J Biochem*, 1967, **1**, 70). Leaves from Sudanese plant, 5 unidentified alks. including 2 major, a phenolic compd. and β-sitosterol (*Planta Med*, 1974, **25**, 310).

Introduced into Indian gardens.

*A. macroura Gomez

Eng.–*Livid-flowered birthwort*.

Roots, emmen. Stems and leaves used as antirheum. and externally as antisep. (Wlth India, IA, 427).

Rhizomes, +ve test for steroids, triterp., traces of alks., saponins, etc. (*Lloydia*, 1972, **35**, 69).

Cultivated in Indian gardens.

A. tagala Cham. syn. *A. roxburghiana* Klotz.

Roots used for antifert. (*Lloydia*, 1975, **38**, 135); considered tonic and emmen.; they contain aristolochic acid and frequently used to adulterate *A. indica* for use in med. (Wlth India, IA, 427).

Aristolochic acid from plant, antineoplastic against *Ehrlich ascites* carcinoma in mice; activity more in female than male (*J Philipp Med Assoc*, 1970, **46**, 505); its toxicity study in mice (*Philipp Abstr*, 1971, **12**, 30).

ARMORACIA (*Brassicaceae*)

A. rusticana Gaertn. *et al.* syn. *A. lapathifolia* Gilib.; *Cochlearia armoracia* Linn.

Eng.–*Horseradish*.

Root—exts., B.P. depress. and spasmol. (*Eksp Med Morfol*, 1966, **5**, 47; *CA*, **65**, 4481b). Root, leaves and seeds used in various kinds of cancers (*Lloydia*, 1969, **32**, 79). Root ext. in treatment of athelet's foot (Jpn Kokai Tokyo Koho, 1979, 79143514; *CA*, 1980, **92**, 135407h).

Essent. oil—known as horseradish oil, broad-spectrum antibiot. due to allyl isothiocyanates and allied compds. (Miller, III, 62); internally given as stim., sudorific and diur. Cytotoxic and carcinostatic and inhibits germination and growth of higher plants. Antifung. (Wlth India, IA, 428-29).

Plant—used for treatment of gout, increases excretion of uric acid; contains alkyl isothiocyanate, its glucd., sinigrin, etc. (*Riv Ital Essenze-Profumi Piante Off*, 1964, **46**, 159; *CA*, **61**, 11225d). Juice inhibited tobacco mosaic virus (*Tocz Nauk Roln Ser A*, 1969, **95**, 417; *CA*, 1970, **72**, 65753d).

Leaf—boiled in wine with olive oil used as poultice for hard swellings of liver and spleen (Wlth India, IA, 428).

Volat. constituents of roots (*J Sci Food Agric*, 1972, **23**, 527). Volat. components; main component allyl isothiocyanate (*Nippon Shoukuin Kogyo Gakkai-Shi*, 1970, **17**, 361; 1981, **28**, 365; *CA*, 1971, **75**, 150407a; **95**, 167284x).

Leaves, polyphenols (*Khim Prir Soedin*, 1969, **5**, 320; 1970, **6**, 636; *CA*, 1970, **72**, 39764p; 1971, **74**, 39170h; *Konservn Ovoshchesuch Promst*, 1979, 31).

ARNEBIA (*Boraginaceae*)

A. benthamii Johnston syn. *Macrotomia benthamii* DC.

Plant—expect. and used for cardiac disorders. Aq. ext., *sherbet* and jam of flowering shoots useful in fever; dry plant yields essent. oil (Wlth India, VI, 207).

Root—used as antisep. and antibiot. in healing of cuts and wounds when applied as a poultice; also for subsiding swelling of organs [*J Res Indian Med*, 1973, **8**(1), 76].

A. euchroma Johnston syn. *Macrotomia perennis* Boiss.

Plant used in Afghanistan in toothache and earache. Root alongwith that of *Onosma hispidum* and other roots constitute *ratanjot* of Punjab and N.W. Himalayas (Wlth India, VI, 207).

Plant contains Ac-shikonin ad 4 related compds. Ac-shikonin inhibited histamine-induced capillary permeability, rat paw oedema and cotton pellet granuloma and also antinflam. effects in rats (*Peiching I Hsueh Yuan Hsueh Pao*, 1980, **12**, 101; *CA*, **93**, 143008q). Alkannin-β, β-di-Me-acrylate, antipyr. and antimicrob; its estn. (*Yao Hsueh T'ung Pao*, 1981, **16**, 14;1980, **15**, 3; *CA*, **95**, 156425q; **94**, 71295b).

*A. gutta Bunge syn. *A. tibetana* Kurz

Roots yield a dye, in Ladakh as cough medicine (Wlth India, IA, 430); *d*-alkanin known as shikonin (4.16%) (*Sb Nauch Rab Vses Nauch Issled Insr Lek Rast*, 1970, No.1, 175; *CA*, 1972, **76**, 70042h).

Found in northern parts of Kashmir.

*A. hispidissima DC.

Vitexin from flowers, potent hypoten., antiinflam. and antisp. in rats (*Planta Med*, 1981, **43**, 396).

A roots sample from Hastinapur (U.P.), *dl*-alkanin (shikalkin, 0.04% air-dry basis) (*Bull Nat Inst Sci India*, No.28, 1965, 52; Thomson, 248).

Found in plains of N-W India.

*A. nobilis Rachinger

Trade–*Ratanjot*.

Roots—used as anthelm., in diseases of eye, broncht., abdominal pain, itch, fever, wounds, and eruptions; also valued in vet. med. for its wound healing action; antimicrob. (*Indian J Pharm*, 1966, **28**, 302); EtOH(50%) ext., antimicrob. (*Indian J Exp Biol*, 1969, 7, 250). Aq. ext. inhibited aflatoxin production in liquorice flour medium (*ibid*, 1979, **17**, 1151).

EtOH ext. of roots, antibiot.; contains naphthaquinones, arnebin-1 (alkannin β, β-di-Me-acrylate), arnebin-3 (alkannin mono-OAc), and tiglic acid ester of dihydro-OH-alkannin (*Experientia*, 1969, **25**, 357). 3 Naphthaquinones; their strs.(*Phytochemistry*, 1971, **10**, 1909); other than naphthaquinones, hexacosanol, heptacosanoic acid and sitosterol (*ibid*, 1972, **11**, 2621). Alc.(50%) ext. of roots or naphthaquinones arnebin I & III effective against rat Walker carcinosarcoma 256 *in vivo*, and each naphthaquinones inhibited tumour cells *in vitro* (*Indian J Cancer*, 1972, **9**, 50). A naphthaquinone, arnebin-7 from roots (*Indian J Chem*, 1973, **11**, 528).

Roots imported into India from Afghanistan.

ARNICA (*Asteraceae*)

A. montana Linn.

Eng.–*Arnica, mountain tobacco*.

Plant—homeopathic mother tincture, antimicrob. (*Indian J Exp Biol*, 1977, **15**, 338); wound healing and antiinflam. (*Aptech Delo*, 1963, **12**, 38; *CA*, 1964, **61**, 11000le). Alc. ext. with other ingredients as smoking preventive (Belg. Pat., 1965, 668319; *CA*, **65**, 3678h). Plant ext. active in blood coagulation (Fr. Demande, 1974, 2201082; *CA*, 1975, **82**, 64483k); in pharmaceutical compn. for treating various skin diseases (Ger. East, 1974, 109, 511; *CA*, 1975, **83**, 120859x; Czech Pat., 1980, 185262; *CA*, 1981, **95**, 68027f); plant produces contact allergy (*Contact Dermatitis*, 1978, **4**, 3; *CA*, **89**, 48296r).

Flower—ext., protected mice from fatal infections with *Listeria monocytogenes* (*Fortschr Veterinaermed*, 1974, **20**, 98; *CA*, **81**, 130910e); inflorescence ext., antimicrob. and useful in cosmetics (*Herba Hung*, 1980, **19**, 165; Fr Demande, 1976, 2296425; *CA*, 1977, **87**, 172722z).

Roots—evaluation of tinctures (*Acta Pharm Jugosl*, 1981, **31**, 177).

Essent. oil—present in all plant parts; extensive investigations (Wlth India, IA, 430).

Reviews (*Pharm Weekbl*, 1968, **103**, 769; 1971, **106**, 190; *CA*, **69**, 33500r; **74**, 136330t); new results of Arnica researches, 37 refs. (*Herba Pol*, 1981, **27**, 75).

ARRHENATHERUM (*Poaceae*)

*A. elatius (Linn.) Presl syn. *Avena elatior* Linn.

Eng.–*Tall* or *false oat-grass*.

Seed ext. haemolyzes red blood cells [*Univ Wyoming Agr Exp Sta Laramie Sci Monograph*, 1971, **24**, II, 1; *CA*, 1972, **76**, 70197n].

Fruits yield a fatty oil similar to that from *Avena sativa*; unsap. matter, 4.3-6.9% (Wlth India, IA, 431); acid phosphatase F1 (*Acta Soc Bot Pol*, 1977, **46**, 481; *CA*, 1978, **88**, 165895a).

Introduced into Assam.

ARTABOTRYS (*Annonaceae*)

A. hexapetalus (Linn.f.) Bhandari syn. *A. odoratissimus* R. Br. ex Ker-Gawl. non Blume

EtOH ext. of fruits, cardiac depress. followed by cardiac stim., hypoten. and spasmog. (*Indian J Med Res*, 1971, **59**, 635). EtOH(50%) ext. of aerial parts, fruit and root, spasmog. (*Indian J Exp Biol*, 1974, **12**, 512; 1980, **18**, 594).

Leaves, EtOH exts., weak estrogenic (at 75 mg/kg) and antiestrogenic (at 150 mg/kg); benzene ext., strong antiestrogenic in rats (*Curr Sci*, 1978, **47**, 659; *Indian J Exp Biol*, 1978, **16**, 1214). Volat. fraction of ext., antifung. (*Indian J Mycol Plant Pathol*, 1979, **9**, 250; *Acta Bot Indica*, 1979, **7**, 147). Flower ext., strong antifung. (*Indian Biol J*, 1980, **2**, 109).

Roots, yingzhaosu A & B (*Hua Hsueh Hsueh Pao*, 1979, **37**, 315; 231; *CA*, 1980, **92**, 146954k; 164104n).

ARTEMISIA (*Asteraceae*)

Artemisias, popularly known as *Sage Brush* or *Wormwood* are bitter aromatics; some of them a source of volat. anthelm. drug, santonin (Wlth India, IA, 434); al-most all spp. elaborate sesquiterp. lactones which might be involved in toxicity in live-stocks (*in* Plant and Fungal Toxins, 572).

A. absinthium Linn.

Eng.–*Absinthe, madarwood, worm-wood*.

Plant—historical survey on uses in gynaecology, 90 refs. (*Sven Farm Tidskr*, 1965, **69**, 669; *CA*, **63**, 14633h). EtOH(50%) ext. of herb, diur. (*Annu Rep RRL Jammu*, 1970 - 71, 25). In Europe, tincture used as stomch., febge., anthelm. and in debility (*Acta Phytother*, 1971, **18**, 21); also used for brain concussions (*Farm Zh Kiev*, 1972, **27**, 78; *BA*, 1973, **56**, 56516). In Unani system, leaves, stem, and flowering tops, in chr. fevers, swellings and inflam. of viscera (*Indian J Pharm*, 1973, **35**, 208). Drug available in Indian market, greyish white material having broken stem, leaves and flowerheads (Wlth India, IA, 434).

Essent. oil—ointment based on chamazulene from herb effective in treatment of human periodontal infections (*Farmacia Buc*, 1965, **13**, 471; *CA*, 1966, **64**, 4141d). Herb fragrance when inhaled for a long time exercises a powerful influence over the nervous system; shows a tendency to produce headache and other nervous disorders (Wlth India, IA, 434); leaf oil, antibact. and antifung. in 1:1000 dilution (*Indian J Pharm*, 1976, **38**, 21).

Herb flavons. artemitin and rutin (*Diss Pharm*, 1965, **17**, 53; *CA*, 1966, **64**, 18028h).

Aerial parts, sesquiterp. lactone, artabsin; also artabin & its str.; lactone arabsin & its str. (*Khim Prir Soedin*, 1969, 57; 1970, 622; 691; 1972, 245; 1976, 548; *CA*, **71**, 10280w; 1971, **74**, 50523w; 12239u; **77**, 85567c; 1977, **86**, 16805c). Lignans, ketopelenolide and a sesquiterp. lactone from Yugoslav plant (*Glas Hem Drus Beograd*, 1976, **41**, 287; *CA*, 1977, **87**, 98796h). New diguaianolide, anabsin & its str.; crystal str.; new guaianolide, artemoline from leaves and flowers (*Symp IUPAC Int Symp Chem Natl Prod*, 11th,

1978, **2**, 421; *Khim Prir Soedin*, 1979, 495; 731; 658; *CA*, 1980, **92**, 59025q; 129115v; 1981, **94**, 175299x; 80214b); isoabsinthin (*Tetrahedron Lett*, 1981, **22**, 2269).

Essent. oil known as 'Absinth or Wormwood oil' (yield, 0.12-0.51% fresh basis) (Wlth India, IA, 434); 3,6- & 5,6-dihydrochamazulene (*Tetrahedron*, 1968, **24**, 2079); leaf oil monoterpenes (*Planta Med*, 1971, **20**, 147); oil constituents, chief compd. thujyl alc. (20.23%) (*Indian Perfum*, 1979, **23**, 1); rev. [*Perfum Flav*, 1978-79, **3**(6), 21; 1981-82, **6**(2), 59]. Components (*Z Naturforsch*, 1981, **36C**, 369).

Absinthin—a bitter taste of herb due to this guaianolide lactone, important in pharmacy (*in* Wagner & Wolff, 159); oil and bitter principle stimulate gastric secretion and improve appetite (Med. Plants, 162); TLC sepn. from bitter substance, anabsinthin (*Pharm Ztg*, 1975, **120**, 1262; *CA*, **83**, 197867f); estn. of absinthin and artemetin; pharmacol. (*J Afr Med Pl*, 1977, 137; 121); from leaves, along with artabsin and matricin (*Dtsch Apoth Ztg*, 1979, **119**, 977; *CA*, **91**, 71726f); str. (*Tetrahedron Lett*, 1980, **21**, 3191).

Seeds, a fatty oil (yield 33.4%) with usual fatty acids and OH- dienic acids (Wlth India, IA, 435; *Khim Prir Soedin*, 1974, 701; *CA*, 1975, **82**, 144814j). Sterols of unsap. matter (*Egypt J Pharm Sci*, 1978, **19**, 323).

Roots, new acetylenic esters and thiophene deriv. (*Phytochemistry*, 1978, **17**, 806).

A. annua Linn.

Plant—antipyr.(*Yao Hsueh T'ung Pao*, 1980, **15**, 39; *CA*, **95**, 121030e).

Plant contains artemisinin, benzyl isovalerate, β-farnesene, a new compd. artemisininic acid, etc.; artemisinin, antimal. [*Chung Yao T'ung Pao*, 1981, **6**(2), 31; *CA*, **95**, 175616u]. Artemisinin, TLC detn. from leaves (*Yao Hsueh T'ung Pao*, 1980, **15**, 8; *CA*, 1981, **95**, 68092y).

Essent. oil from aerial parts, compn. (*Clujal Med*, 1980, **53**, 331); constituents

(*Acta Pharm Sin*, 1981, **16**, 366). Plant, sesquiterp. lactone, arteannuin B (*Tetrahedron Lett*, 1973, 3038); its str. (*Glass Hem Drus Beograd*, 1977, **42**, 227; *CA*, **87**, 168213a); a new sesquiterp. lactone (*K'o Hsueh T'ung Pao*, 1977, **22**, 142; *CA*, **87**, 98788g); arteannuin and arteannuin B (*Hua Hsueh Hsueh Pao*, 1979, **37**, 129; *CA*, 1980, **92**, 94594w; *Acta Pharm Sin*, 1981, **16**, 65).

Aerial parts also contain coumarins and flavons. (*Khim Prir Soedin*, 1970, **6**, 758; *CA*, 1971, **74**, 35433h; *Phytochemistry*, 1975, **14**, 1873; *Glass Hem Drus Beograd*, 1979, **44**, 615; *CA*, 1980, **92**, 211806e; *Yao Hsueh T'ung Pao*, 1980, **15**, 39; *CA*, 1981, **95**, 121030e; *Acta Pharm Sin*, 1981, **16**, 65).

Introduced into India; reported to be recently cultivated in J. & K.

*A. brevifolia Wall. ex DC.

Contains santonin (0.5-1.0%) (*Indian Drugs*, 1979-80, **17**, 318); Santonin is an anthelm. drug (Wlth India, IA, 434).

Grown in abundance in Kashmir and Kumaun.

A. dracunculus Linn.

Eng.–*Dragon mugwort, estragon, tarragon.*

Essent. oil called 'Oil of Tarragon' used for flavouring vinegar sauces, salad dressings, etc. (Wlth India, IA, 435).

Properties and constituents of essent. oil (*Perfum Essent Oil Rec*, 1967, **58**, 437). Monoterps. of leaf oil (*Planta Med*, 1971, **20**, 147). Extn. of eugenol from herb [*Maslo- Zhir Promst*, 1973, (3), 33; *CA*, **78**, 163932e]. Volat. constituents (*Chem Mikrobiol Technol Lebensm*, 1973, **2**, 184; *CA*, 1974, **80**, 144505t; *Z Naturforsch*, 1981, **36C**, 724). Estragole(1-allyl-4-MeO-benzene), major component of oil, weak hepatocarcinogen to young mice by s.c. injection (*J Nat Cancer Inst*, 1976, **54**, 1323).

Herb flavons. including rutin, artemitin, hyperoside, etc. (*Diss Pharm*, 1965, **17**, 503; *CA*, 1966, **64**, 18028h; *Khim Prir*

Soedin, 1969, 323; 1970, 629; *CA*, 1970, **72**, 63619r; 1971, **74**, 50530w).

Leaf constituents including scopoletin, herniarin, etc. (*Z Lebensm Unters Forsch*, 1968, **138**, 146; *CA*, 1969, **70**, 26407h); isocoumarin artemidin from aerial parts; also artemidinal; artemidiol from roots; artemedinol; 8-OH-capillarin from herb; acetylenes and dehydrofalcarinone derivs. from roots (*Khim Prir Soedin*, 1970, 467; 531; 1971, 120871; 1974, 720; 811; *CA*, 1971, **74**, 10344g; 76270m; **75**, 115871a; 1975, **82**, 121665x; 1977, **86**, 136302h; *Phytochemistry*, 1977, **16**, 795; 1979, **18**, 1244; 1319).

A. gmelinii Weber ex Stechm. syn. *A. sacrorum* Ledeb.

Leaves, internally in abdominal pains (*Khadi Gramodyog*, 1972-73, **19**, 275).

Aerial parts, umbelliferone and genkwanin (*Curr Sci*, 1965, **34**, 609). Shoots, scopoletin (*Khim Prir Soedin*, 1972, 643; *CA*, 1973, **78**, 108211u).

*A. macrocephala Jacq. ex Bess.

Ladakh–*Khanpa*.

In Ladakh, herb applied as a paste on joints to cure rheum. and other pains (*in* Atal & Kapur, Med. Plants, 519).

Kashmir and Himachal Pradesh.

*A. maritima Linn. var. **fragrans** (Willd.) Ledeb.

This variety is non-santonin yielding earlier described as var. *thomsoniana*; it has greyish stems in early stages of growth (Wlth India, IA, 436).

Essent. oil from leaves and flowering tops of the santonin-free type (var. *fragrans*) from Bashahr (H.P.), physicochem. properties; cineol (14-22%) (*Perfum Essent Oil Rec*, 1966, **57**, 14).

Found in Himachal Pradesh.

*A. maritima Linn. var. **thomsoniana** C.B. Clarke

Eng.–*Wormseed*.

This santonin-yielding variety resembles in every respect to var. *fragrans*, except that stems of this var. are reddish in early stages of its growth. It occurs in Kashmir, earlier referred to by Badhwar as forma *rubricaule*. It is tetraploid (2n = 36) (Wlth India, IA, 436; Chopra *et al*, I, 477-78).

Plant — powerfully arom. producing severe headache in persons unaccustomed to its influence in field as well as in godown; symptoms lasting for a few days (Chopra *et al*, I, 479). It is stomch. and acts as cardiac and respiratory stim. against *Ascaris* in combination with *Chenopodium* (*Nagarjun*, 1978-79, **22**, 136). Flowers a good source of santonin (*Pak J Sci*, 1979, **31**, 64).

Flowering tops or buds—anthelm, useful in ascites and in hiccough; and paste with water, externally applied to inflam. swellings by Mohammedan physicians.

Herb, santonin (0.5-1.0%) (*Indian Drugs*, 1979-80, **17**, 318); santonin is an anthelm. drug (Wlth India, IA, 434).

Santonin—a sesquiterp. lactone, is classical remedy for treatment of *Ascaris* and *Oxyuris* infections. In man, large doses (more than 0.3g) cause poisoning; in children small doses of 1 grain (0.06g) produced serious and in some cases fatal poisoning. Regarded inferior to hexyl resorcinol and chenopodium (Chopra *et al*, I, 481-82), however combination of santonin and chenopodium, more effective than either of these drugs on *Ascaris*. Santonin usually administered in very small doses; it causes xanthopsy (yellow vision) and sometimes also violet vision. Antifert. activity; but contradictory findings also reported (Wlth India, IA, 438).

Unlike Kurrum *Artemisia* of Pakistan where immature flowerheads are important source of santonin, in Kashmir *Artemisia*, leaves are important, though both contain santonin. Roots, stems and twigs are devoid of santonin (Chopra *et al*, I, 478). Method and time of collection of material important, as there is variation in santonin content; max. yield being in spring and summer in leaves, and in buds in preflowering period; flowering period varies from place to place.

Santonin extn. from steam-distilled essent. oil (Wlth India, IA, 437; *Kogyo Kagaku Zasshi*, 1965, **68**, 1224; *CA*, **63**, 14629h). Extn. from buds and leaves (*Farmatsiya Sof*, 1968, **18**, 6; *CA*, 1969, **71**, 19514h).

Leaves and buds also contain β-santonin (a stereoisomer at C_{11} position), less anthelm.; herb ψ-santonin and another bitter principle artemisin (7-OH-santonin) (Wlth India, IA, 437-38)

Essent. oil contains besides santonin, cineol (9.3%) and others (*Kogyo Kagaku Zasshi*, 1965, **68**, 1224; *CA*, **63**, 14629h).

A. maritima varieties contain essent. oil varying in quant. and compn. Essent. oil, valuable ingredient in flavour of liqueurs and pharmaceutical compn. Commercial oil, a byproduct of santonin factories and rich in cineol (*Parfuem Kosmet*, 1967, **48**,64); monoterps. (*Planta Med*, 1971, **20**, 147); sesquiterp. lactone, artemin (*Phytochemistry*, 1977, **16**, 1836); plant contains a new germacranolide, gallicin (*J Chem Soc Perkin Trans 1*, 1978, 1243); a new sesquiterp. ketone, devanone (*Arch Pharm Wein*, 1979, **312**, 435; *CA*, **91**, 74732r).

Found wild in Kashmir.

A. nilagirica (C.B. Clarke) Pamp. syn. *A. vulgaris* Linn. var. *nilagirica* C.B. Clarke

Eng.–*Indian wormwood.*

Herb—antilithic and alexipharmic properties and assists parturition; also used as febge. and as an inferior substitute for cinchona in fevers; a weak decoct. given to children suffering from measles. Externally used as fomentation in skin diseases and ulcers; leaves applied as haemostatic and to allay burning sensation in conjunctivitis (Wlth India, IA, 439). Compost, useful in controlling grubs of beetles; plant employed to keep away fleas and other insects [*J Res Indian Med*, 1974, **9**(3), 101].

Essent. oil—good larvicide like kerosene and a feeble insectic.; freshly distilled oil from air-dried leaves, antibact.

and antifung. in 1:1000 dilution (*Indian J Pharm*, 1976, **38**, 21).

Essent. oil from plant, physico-chem. properties of oil from W.Bengal (*Parfuem Kosmet*, 1964, **45**, 63). Another sample (0.34%) containing *p*-cymene, *l*-linalool, β-thujone azulene, thujyl alc. and an unidentified hydrocarbon; yield of the oil in and around Nainital at different altitudes varied from 0.07 to 0.2%; from Garampani area (U.P.), plants at lower altitude had more % of cineol, thujone, thujyl alc. and citral whereas from higher altitude, terpenes in higher % (*Perfum Essent Oil Rec*, 1968, **59**, 866).

*A. pallens Wall. ex DC.

Kan., Mar. & Tam.–*Davana*; Tel.–*Davanamu.*

Two distinct types: (i) with short stature having basal leaves entire and early-flowering, and (ii) tall (*c.*60 cm.) with leaves highly dissected and late flowering (*Curr Sci*, 1964, **33**, 346).

Davana marketed as sachet powd. for preserving delicate fabrics against moths [*Perfum Flav*, 1980, **5**(2), 23]. Seeds, slightly sweet-smelling devoured by ants (*Farm Bull CIMAP*, 1978, No.12, 1).

Leaves and flowers yield essent oil known as 'Oil of Davana' having delicate aroma and used in high-grade perfumes.

Essent. oil, yield, 0.22 - 0.58% (Wlth India, IA, 440). Its commercial production and marketing by CIMAP centre at Haldwani (U.P.) and Bangalore. Physicochem. properties of oil from exp. cultivated plants at Haldwani and constituents, including artemone and davanone [*Perfum Essent Oil Rec*, 1967, **58**, 523; *Flavour Ind*, 1971, **2**, 370; *Tetrahedron Lett*, 1970, 502; *Recl Trav Chim Pays-Bas*, 1968, **87**, 715; *Indian Perfum*, 1980, **24**, 101; *Perfum Flav*, 1980, **5**(2), 23]. Antimicrob. action (*Indian Perfum*, 1981, **25**, 110; 112).

Found in Karnataka, Tamil Nadu, Andhra Pradesh, and also near Pune.

*A. parviflora Roxb.

H.–*Pati.*

EtOH(50%) ext. of herb, diur. (*Annu Rep RRL Jammu*, 1970- 71, 25); also antivir. (*Indian J Exp Biol*, 1973, **11**, 43).

Plant coumarins, 6,7-di-Me-aesculetin, aesculentin and scopoletin (*Curr Sci*, 1976, **45**, 640).

Found throughout greater part of India up to 3,000 m.

A. persica Boiss.

Leaves and stem, scopoletin (*Khim Prir Soedin*, 1969, **5**, 319; *CA*, **72**, 63625q).

A. roxburghiana Wall. ex Bess. syn. *A. grata* Wall.

Aerial parts, hentriacontane, hentriacontanol, α- & β-amyrin and β-sitosterol (*Indian J Pharm Sci*, 1978, **40**, 102).

A. scoparia Waldst. & Kit.

Flower heads, coumarin lactone, scoparone (*Farmatsiya Sof*, 1964, **14**, 18; *CA*, **61**, 11959a); also capillarin besides scoparone; roots, β-sitosterol, oxalic acid and a lactone (*Khim Prir Soedin*, 1971, 376; *CA*, **75**, 115850t); leaves and flowers, capillin, 1-Ph-2,4-hexàdiyne-1-ol, vanillin and scoparone (*Phytochemistry*, 1973, **12**, 2996); flavon. [*Fenol' nye Soedin Ikh Fiziol Svoistva Mater Vses Simp Fenol' nym Soedin*, 2nd, 1971 (Pub'73), 76; *CA*, 1975, **82**, 54138r]; detn. (*Rastit Resur*, 1980, **16**, 187; *CA*, **93**, 41537u); flavons. of inflorescence (*Planta Med*, 1981, **43**, 310).

Air-dried flowering tops from Jammu, essent. oil (0.5%) with characteristic odour of eugenol (30% of oil); and various constituents: dillapiol, carvone, etc. (*Perfum Essent Oil Rec*, 1969, **60**, 301; 1967, **58**, 437; *Indian J Pharm*, 1968, **30**, 283; *Curr Sci*, 1970, **30**, 182).

Scoparone—it is 6,7-di-MeO-coumarin, has marked hypoten. action with tranquillizing and sleep-inducing effects on exp. animals through various routes; also antihyperten.; action partly central and partly peripheral. No tolerence to hypoten. activity after repeated administration; therapeutic ratio, LD_{50}/ED_{50}, 20. Hypoten.

activity compares well with that of α-Me-DOPA (ALDOMET). At higher dose levels, marked analg. and hypothermic. Also anticonvuls. (*Annu Rep RRL Jammu*, 1975, 71; *Indian J Med Res*, 1972, **60**, 763); because of uncertainty of availability of plant material, method of synth. for promising hypoten. drug scoparone developed by methylation of aesculetin (obtained by condensation of 1,2,4-tri-OAc-benzene with malic acid) (*Res Ind*, 1975, **20**, 129).

Active constituent of plant, *p*-OH-acetophenone promotes secretion of bile and bile salts (*Chin Med J*, 1981, **94**, 237).

A drug preparation, artemisol, used against urolithiasis (*Urol Nefrol*, 1966, **31**, 37).

A. siversiana Ehrh. ex Willd.

Aerial parts, guaienolide, sieversin (*Zh Prikl Khim*, 1965, **38**, 2372; *CA*, 1966,**64**, 3608g); green parts or essent. oil, sesquiterps., sesquiterp. α-lactone, sieversinin, a stearic isomer of arborescin (*Khim Prir Soedin*, 1966, 399; *CA*, 1967, **67**, 32803p); α-lactone, antimicrob.(*Rastit Resur*, 1966, **2**, 216; *CA*, **65**, 14140f). Absinthin, artabsin and a compd. (mp 156°), rutin, isoquercetin, etc. (*Tr Nauch Konf Tomsk Otd Vses Khim Obshchest*, 1968, 271; *CA*, 1970, **73**, 91191j).

*A. vestita Wall. ex DC.

Garhwal–*Chamaria, kundja.*

Plant—EtOH ext. of herb, anticancer (*Annu Rep CDRI*, Lucknow, 1970, 76; *Cancer Res*, 1971, **31**, 1649). In Europe, plant used as emmen., diur. and diaphor.; in India, as antisep., expect. and anthelm. (*Acta Phytother*, 1971, **18**, 21); arom.; leaves applied externally as haemostatic (Wlth India, IA, 442; *Khadi Gramodyog*, 1972-73, **19**, 276); plant used in stomachache (*Nagarjun*, 1979-80, **23**, 242).

Essent. oil—antibact. and antifung. in 1:1000 dilution (*Indian J Pharm*, 1976, **38**, 21); active against dermatophytes; also antimycotic (*Indian Drugs*, 1979-80, **17**, 269; 1981-82, **19**, 34).

Essent. oil from air-dried leaves and flowering tops, from Jammu & Kashmir (yield, 0.9%) characteristics and constituents which include among others artemisol, 4.4% (*Soap Perfum Cosm*, 1964, **37**, 889).

Essent. oil from leaves from Kumaun (yield 0.08-0.2%) with physicochem. characteristics (*Perfum Essent Oil Rec*, 1967, **58**, 437; 1968, **59**, 866; *Flavour Ind*, 1971, **2**, 539; *Indian Perfum*, 1978, **22**, 11; 16).

Flowering tops, essent. oil (0.09-0.2%), properties and constituents (*Indian Oil Soap J*, 1969-70, **35**, 229); compn. of oil (*Planta Med*, 1976, **30**, 211; *Chim Ind Milan*, 1977, **59**, 23; *CA*, **87**, 135977r).

Besides essent. oil, Indian plant contains fernenol (*Aust J Chem*, 1968, **21**, 1931); α-amyrin & its -OAc, (−)thujone, β-sitosterol, stigmasterol α- & β-pinenes and 3 hydrocarbons (*J Indian Chem Soc*, 1969, **46**, 584); sesquiterp. lactone, vulgarin, antitumour (*Phytochemistry*, 1976, **15**, 1573).

Found in Western Himalayas from 2,100 to 3,000 m.

ARTHROCNEMUM (*Chenopodiaceae*)

*A.fruticosum Moq. syn. *A. glaucum* Ung.-Stemb. non Woodr.

Plant used in Greece in garlic porridge. Contains same sterols as those in *A. indicum* (Wlth India, IA, 444).

Found in marshy coast of Tamil Nadu.

A. indicum Moq. syn. *A. glaucum* Woodr. non Ung.- Stemb.

Stigmastane type 3 C_{29} sterols including fucosterol (*Egypt J Chem*, 1974, **17**, 869).

ARTOCARPUS (*Moraceae*)

*A. communis J.R. & G. Forst. syn. *A. altilis* (Park.) Fosberg

Eng.–*Breadfruit.*

In Hawaii, sap from tree used for cuts, scratches, scaly or cracked skin and ulcers. In Fiji Islands, infusion of root bark used in treatment of internal fractures. In Tonga, bark infusion used in relapsed illness. Gum from stem used against boils (*Econ Bot*, 1971, **25**, 245; 442).

In Samoa, root used in diar. and dysen.; also for swollen testicles. Petiole used for eye wounds, sores, irrit. and itch. Leaf and twig for eye splinters. Twig smoke, for baby with fever and running stool. Root bark, an ingredient of drug for backache; leaves externally for headache, stomachache also for fever with high temp. (*Econ Bot*, 1974, **28**, 21; 1975, **29**, 314).

EtOH(50%) ext. of aerial parts, diur. (*Indian J Exp Biol*, 1974, **12**, 512). Aq. ext. of branchlets and leaves, very toxic to American cockroaches; pet. ether and chloroform exts., toxic to black carpet beetle larvae (Jacobson, 178).

Heartwood phenolics, morin, norartocarpetin, artocarpin and cycloartocarpin; distribution of cycloartocarpenol & related compds. (*Phytochemistry*, 1972, **11**, 1571; 1973, **12**, 2725); fresh fruits, α-amyrin, cycloartenol, cycloart-23-ene-3β, 25-diol & -3β-24-diol (*ibid*, 1976, **15**, 829).

Indigenous to Malaysia, commonly cultivated in S. India.

A. heterophyllus Lamk syn. *A. integrifolia* Hook.f. non Linn.; *A. heterophylla* Pers.; *A. integra* auct. non Merrill

Eng.–*Jackfruit, jack tree.*

Fruit—unripe fruit acrid, carmin. and tonic. Ripe fruit, cooling, fattening and useful in biliousness.

Seeds—diur. (Wlth India, IA, 452). Ext., pharmacol. active; may possess Accholine activity (*Arch Intern Pharmacodyn*, 1964, **148**, 397; *CA*, **61**, 1121h); preliminary pharmacol. (*Indian J Exp Biol*, 1969, **7**, 250).

Leaves—ash useful in healing ulcers (Wlth India, IA, 452). Leaves, estrogenic (*Indian J Physiol Allied Sci*, 1967, **20**, 6). Young leaves and shoots with *gur* as lactag. in women (*Nagarjun*, 1980-81, **24**, 1).

Latex—from tree, bacteriolytic; from young branches, less active. Mixed with vinegar, promotes healing of abscesses.

Root—useful in skin diseases, asthma and diar. (Wlth India, IA, 451-52).

Various plant parts, used in toothache, caries, stomach complaints, sores, smallpox, carbuncle, sterility in women, and postnatal complaints (*Econ Bot*, 1970, **24**, 241).

Seed, lectin extn. potent and selective stimulation of distinct human T and B cell functions (*J Immunol*, 1981, **127**, 427); 2 isolectins, their purification (*Biol Plant*, 1981, **23**, 186); dipeptide, aurantiamide-OAc (*J Indian Chem Soc*, 1981, **58**, 103).

Leaves contain cycloartenone, cycloartenol and β- sitosterol (*Bull Calcutta Sch Trop Med*, 1967, **15**, 100).

Heartwood of Indian plant, flavons., artocarpesin and norartocarpetin; their strs. (*Tetrahedron Lett*, 1965, 663; *Indian J Chem*, 1966, **4**, 406); also di-Me ethers of artocarpin & iscartocarpin, and dihydrocycloartocarpin (*Beitr Biochem Physiol Naturstotten Festschr*, 1965, 317; *CA*, 1966, **64**, 17563a); cycloartocarpesin & oxydihydroartocarpesin (*Indian J Chem*, 1969, **7**, 101); and some phenolics (*Phytochemistry*, 1972, **11**, 1571). Heartwood of Indonesian sp. *A. integra*; flavon. integrin, cyclointegrin & oxyisocyclointegrin (*Indian J Chem*, 1976, **14B**, 69).

Bark, flavons., including cycloheterophyllin & its iso-deriv. (*ibid*, 1971, **9**, 7; 1973, **11**, 298); distribution of cycloartenol & related compds. (*Phytochemistry*, 1973, **12**, 2725).

A. hirsutus Lamk

Eng.–*Wild jack*.

EtOH(50%) ext. of aerial parts, diur. (*Indian J Exp Biol*, 1974, **12**, 512).

A. lakoocha Roxb.

Eng.–*Monkey jack*.

Plant used in spleen complaints and bone fracture in cattle (*Econ Bot*, 1970, **24**, 241). Preliminary pharmacol. (*Indian J Exp Biol*, 1971, **9**, 91). Seeds, haemagglutinating (*Indian J Med Res*, 1973, **61**, 1478).

Stems, 2,4,3',5'-tetra-OH-stilbene(11-13%), a vermifuge for tapeworm (*J Natl Res Counc Thailand*, 1962, **3**, 245). Stem bark, lupeol-OAc and α-amyrin-OAc (*Bull Calcutta Sch Trop Med*, 1966, **14**, 16). Distribution of cycloartenol & related compds. in bark (*Phytochemistry*, 1973, **12**, 2725).

Root bark, a new glycoflavonol; lupeol and β-sitosterol (*Planta Med*, 1979, **37**, 86; *Indian J Chem*, 1979, **18B**, 473).

*A. rigidus Blume ssp. **rigidus**

Latex, as vet. med. (Wlth India, IA, 455).

Cultivated for its edible fruit.

ARUM (*Araceae*)

A. curvatum (Roxb.) Kunth; see **Arisaema tortuosum**

ARUNCUS (*Rosaceae*)

A. dioicus (Walt.) Fernald var. **triternatus** (Maxim.) Hara; syn. *A. sylvester* Kostel; *Spiraea aruncus* Linn.

Eng.–*Goat's beard*.

Flowers, leaves and roots used in gall diseases (Hocking, 20).

Roots and leaves contain prunasin (*Planta Med*, 1981, **41**, 313).

ARUNDO (*Poaceae*)

A. donax Linn.

Eng.–*Spanish-bamboo-reed, giant-bamboo-reed*.

EtOH ext. of rhizome produced hypoten. and antisp. effects.

Rhizome, indole-3-alkylamine bases, including bufotenidine & dehydro- bufontenine (*J Med Chem*, 1969, **12**, 480). Plant, indole-3-alkylamines including a polymer of gramine N-oxide and bufotenine (*Chem Ind Lond*, 1967, 2046). Leaves, sterols and triterps. Leaves, seeds, fruits and roots, w.-sol. bases (*Phytochemistry*, 1970, **9**, 1895; 2137; 429).

Flowers, alks. gramine, its methohydroxide, eleagnine, N, N-di-Me-tryptamine methohydroxide, and 3,3'-bis(indolyl-Me)-di-Me-ammonium hydroxide (*ibid*, 1971, **10**, 2852); indole bases/alks. produced hypoten. and respiratory depress. effect; gramine, tryptamine derivs., etc. from different plant parts (*Planta Med*, 1972, **21**, 22; 200).

*A. donax Linn. var. **versicolor** Stokes
Eng.–*Ribbon grass.*

The variety may possess same properties as *A. donax* (Wlth India, IA, 457).

Frequently cultivated in gardens for ornament.

ASARUM (*Aristolochiaceae*)

*A. himalaicum Hook.f. & Thoms. ex Duch. syn. *A. canadense* Linn.

Rhizome essent. oil constituents (*J Pharm Sci*, 1967, **56**, 336). HPLC detn. of Ph-propane deriv. in plant tincture; *trans*-Me-eugenol detected (*Dtsch Apoth Ztg*, 1980, **120**, 1859; *CA*, 1981, **94**, 20478f); *in vitro*, studies on expect. effect of Ph-propane derivs. (*Planta Med*, 1981, **42**, 155).

Reported from Eastern Himalayas.

ASCLEPIAS (*Asclepiadaceae*)

Cardenolides (*in* Plant and Fungal Toxins, 43-83).

A. curassavica Linn.
Eng.–*Blood flower; West Indian ipecacuanha.*

Various plant parts, as also plant latex used against warts and cancers (*Lloydia*, 1967, **30**, 430); plant latex, bactericidal (Wlth India, IA, 467). Leaf juice, in abdominal pain and externally in piles. Root powd. mixed with *Acorus* root cures chr. ulcers [*J Res Indian Med*, 1973, **8**(1), 76].

Stem and leaves exts., anticancer (*Philipp J Sci*, 1964, **93**, 57). Exts. of roots, leaves, flowers and stems; as also alc. ext. of plant can destroy human cancer cells in culture; activity due to calotropin (*J Inst Chem India*, 1965, **37**, 261; *Science*, 1964, **146**, 1685).

Cardiotonic effects of Chinese native, in rats due to cardiac glucd., curassavicin (*Yao Hsueh Hsueh Pao*, 1964, **11**, 80; *CA*,

61, 3574h). Mech. of cardiovascular response to root ext.; increased B.P. and heart rate in dogs [*J Res Indian Med*, 1977, **12**(3), 30].

Alc. ext. of plant from Dehra Dun (U.P.), strong cardiotonic and contains 22 Kedde +ve substances in defatted ext., including calotropin, uzarin & their free genins, calactin, coroglaucigenin, a new genin (substance B) and its 4 glucds. (glucorhamnosides H_1 & H_2 and glucds., I & J); the remaining 11 compds. could not be isolated pure; oleanolic acid, β-sitosterol & its glucd. in lipid ext.; cardenolides differ from those of Brazilian plant (*Indian J Chem*, 1969, **7**, 1105); a rev., 10 refs. (*Q J Crude Drug Res*, 1976, **14**, 61). High speed chromatogr. for resolution of glycds./labriformin, labriformidin and eriocarpin (*J Chromatogr*, 1978, **140**, 521). Cardiac glycds./aglycones, viz. uzarin, uzarigenin and frugoside (*Egypt J pharm Sci*, 1980, **21**, 77).

Asclepin—chief active principle, excellent cardiotonic, having longer duration of action than digoxin (a single oral dose of asceplin persisted for 96 h in cat, as against that of digoxin for 72 h) and cumulative toxicity lower than that of digoxin; also produced emesis in pigeons and showed spasmog. activity (*Annu Rep CDRI Lucknow*, 1970, 64; 73; *Indian J Pharmacol*, 1973, **3**, 8). Str. of asclepin (substance B of 1969 work); a genin, but itself a glycd.; it is 3′-OAc-calotropin, yield, 0.011% (*Phytochemistry*, 1972, **11**, 757). LD$_{50}$, 0.236 mg/kg (*Arzneim Forsch*, 1978, **28**, 1365); see also *Asclepia* cardenolides (*in* Plant and Fungal Toxins, 43-83).

*A. physocarpa Schlecht.

Severe gastrointestinal irrit., poisonous and causes death (Chopra *et al*, I, 573).

Leaf and stem reported to contain an alk. (Wlth India, IA, 467).

Found in Tamil Nadu.

ASPARAGUS (*Asparagaceae*)

A. adscendens Roxb.

Root bark taken with milk for vitality and strength. Stem, aphrodis. (*Econ Bot*, 1971, **25**, 420). An ingredient of indigenous drug 'Geriforte' used in senile pruritus and against fatigue (*Rajasthan Med J*, 1980, **19**, 23; *Indian Drugs*, 1980-81, **18**, 346).

Root, asparagine (*Indian For*, 1964, **90**, 50). Root saponin (steroidal), *in vitro*, antimicrob.(*Indian Drugs*, 1976-77, **14**, 103).

Fruits, β-sitosterol, sarsasapogenin and diosgenin (*Pharmazie*, 1980, **35**, 711).

A. filicinus Buch.- Ham. ex D. Don

EtOH(50%) ext. of plant, antiprot. and spasmog. (*Indian J Exp Biol*, 1968, **6**, 232). Plant ext., antifung. (*Labdev*, 1971, **9B**, 136).

A. gonocladus Baker

Leaves alongwith other ingredients, strong sterilizer (*Econ Bot*, 1970, **34**, 273).

Flowers contain malvin and asparagine (*J Indian Chem Soc*, 1978, **55**, 520).

Aerial parts, apigenin, kaempferol, rutin, 4,6,4'- tri-OH-aurone and a new chalcone glycd. (*Indian J Chem*, 1981, **20B**, 1008); saponin(*Phytochemistry*, 1981, **20**, 1687).

A. officinalis Linn.

Eng.–*Asparagus*.

Berries decoct., contracep. (*Planta Med*, 1973, **23**, 167). Antimicrob. substance from tissue culture (*Lloydia*, 1968, **31**, 180).

Flavons., extn. from various parts (*Farm Zh Kiev*, 1966, **21**, 44; *CA*, 1967, **66**, 44249e). Flowers contain flavons. rutin (2.5%), quercetin and hyperoside & their glycds.; same glycd. from fruits but no free quercetin. Leaves yield rutin; roots, a steroidal glycd.(*Curr Sci*, 1968, **37**, 287). Plant, main glucd. rutin; quercetin, 1.4% and kaempferol, 0.05% dry basis (*Z Lebensm Unters Forsch*, 1974, **155**, 151; *CA*, **81**, 118771c).

Seeds polysaccharides, str. (*Phytochemistry*, 1969, **8**, 1783); α-mannosidase activity (*C R Acad Sci Ser D*, 1969, **269**, 1419; *CA*, 1970, **72**, 39748m).

Asparagusic acid, 35 ppm from roots; nematicidal (*Chem Lett*, 1975, 43). Roots contain β-sitosterol, sarsasapogenin and 9 steroidal glycds., asparagosides A-I (*Khim Prir Soedin*, 1976, 400823; *Dokl Akad Nauk SSSR*, 1976, **231**, 1479; *CA*, **85**, 90178w; 1977, **86**, 68399t; 103064d); hexasaccharides (*Phytochemistry*, 1981, **20**, 2581).

Volat. components, rev. (*Chem Ind Lond*, 1971, 556).

Etiolated shoots, diosgenin and yamogenin (*Phytochemistry*, 1981, **20**, 2209; 1969, **8**, 493); plant growth regulators asparagusic acid & its derivs. (*Tetrahedron Lett*, 1972, 2549; 1973, 1073; *Plant Cell Physiol*, 1972, **13**, 923). Shoots, furostanol saponins, asparasaponins I & II (*Agric Biol Chem*, 1977, **41**, 1); also 2 cysteine derivs. (*Phytochemistry*, 1981, **20**, 2209).

*A. plumosus Baker

Eng.–*Asparagus fern.*

Rhizomes, and its var. contain hecogenin and diosgenin (*An R Soc Esp Fis Quim Ser B*, 1967, **63**, 951; *CA*, 1968, **68**, 33148m).

Native to S. Africa; grown in Indian gardens.

A. racemosus Willd.

Tubers—used in fever (*Econ Bot*, 1965, **19**, 246). Aq. ext. of roots, nematicidal; EtOH(50%) ext. of aerial parts, anticancer (*Indian J Exp Biol*, 1967, **5**, 59; 1968, **6**, 232). Roots used as sexual tonics [*J Res Indian Med*, 1973, **8**(2), 75]; decoct. for fever (*Bull Bot Surv India*, 1973, **15**, 13); ext., antifung. (*Geobios*, 1978, **5**, 49). Various med. preparations in various ailments (Herbal Med., 78, 155, 161, 163). Powerful tonic; constituents of an indigenous drug 'Geriforte' used against senile pruritus and fatigue (*Indian Drugs*, 1977-78, **15**, 145; 1980-81, **18**, 346; *Rajasthan Med J*, 1980, **19**, 23). Root used in rheum. (*Khadi Gramodyog*, 1981, **27**, 401).

Plant—an ingredient in compn. for curing impotency; used against ulcerated tongue, pain in limbs or bones, ardor of body, gravel, pleur. and rinderpest (*Econ Bot*, 1965, **19**, 246; 1970, **24**, 241). In Ayurveda, used in diabetes, jaundice and other urinary disorders (*Acta Phytother*, 1972, **19**, 141). Clin. trials of preparation '*Shatavari*' promising antidiar. and potent gastric sed. [*J Res Indian Med*, 1974, **9**(3), 23]; drug effective in hyperacidity (*Sachitra Ayurveda*, 1980- 81, **33**, 40). In skelatal fractures (*Sri Lanka For*, 1980, **14**, 145).

Bark, antibact. and antifung. (WIth India, IA, 471).

Str. of disaccharide from roots (*Indian J Chem*, 1970, **8**, 588).

Fresh leaves yield diosgenin (*Curr Sci*, 1969, **38**, 414). Plant, 4 saponins, viz. shatavarin I to IV; shatavarin IV is a glycd. of sarsasapogenin with 2 mols. of rhamnose and 1 mol. of glucose; shatavarin I has an additional glucose mol.; shatavarin IV, antioxytoxic (*in* Wagner & Wolff, 221; *Arch Int Pharmacodyn Ther*, 1969, **179**, 121; *CA*, 1970, **72**, 20334b).

Flowers and fruits, glycds. of quercetin (also free in former), rutin, and hyperoside; ripe fruit, cyanidin 3-glycds. (*Curr Sci*, 1968, **37**, 287). Indian fruits, sitosterol, stigmasterol, their glucds. and sarsasapogenin; 2 spirostanolic and 2 furostanolic saponins (*Pharmazie*, 1981, **36**, 709).

*A. sprengeri Regel

Roots and other parts contain diosgenin (*Phytochemistry*, 1969, **8**, 493).

Native of S. Africa, cultivated in Indian gardens.

ASPERUGO (*Boraginaceae*)

*A. procumbens Linn.

Ladakh–*Til.*

Seeds used in rheum.

Plant contains delphinidin and other compds. (*Plant Med Phytother*, 1977, **11**, 5; *CA*, **86**, 185965k).

Found from Punjab to Kashmir.

ASPHODELUS (*Liliaceae*)

A. tenuifolius Cav. syn. *A. fistulosus* Linn. var. *tenuifolius* Baker

Plant, insectic. (*Nagarjun*, 1979-80, **23**, 177).

Seed oil contains β-amyrin, β- sitosterol (both, major), campesterol and stigmasterol (*J Pharm Pharmacol*, 1968, **20**, 646; *Curr Sci*, 1975, **44**, 723). Str. of ester, 1-0-17-Mc-stearylmyoinositol from seeds (*Indian J Chem*, 1974, **12**, 1325).

Anthraquinones (*Z Naturforsch*, 1974, **29**, 351); their identn. in leaves, seeds and tubers (*Pharmazie*, 1974, **29**, 609).

Plant yields lupeol (*J Inst Chem India*, 1976, **48**, 296); also quercetin [*J Res Indian Med*, 1976, **11**(4), 13]

ASPIDIUM (*Aspidiaceae*)

A. filix-mas Linn.; see **Dryopteris filix-mas**

ASPIDOPTERYS (*Malpighiaceae*)

*A. indica (Roxb.) Hochr. syn. *A. roxburghiana* A. Juss(FBI) in part.

EtOH(50%) ext. of aerial parts, hypoten. (*Indian J Exp Biol*, 1980, **18**, 594).

Found in Eastern Himalayas, Orissa, Deccan and Western Ghats extending up to Kerala.

ASPLENIUM (*Aspleniaceae*)

A. adiantum-nigrum Linn.

Eng.–*Black spleen/wort.*

Plant used against knots, swellings and induration of lever (*Lloydia*, 1970, **33**, 385); in enlargement of spleen, calculus, jaundice, malaria and as diur., rhizome used as anthelm. [*J Res Indian Med*, 1975, **10**(3), 68; 1974, **9**(4), 39]; also as contracep. (*Planta Med*, 1973, **23**, 167); and in treatment of hiccough (*Indian Drugs*, 1976-77, **14**, 136).

Fronds, aliphatic and triterp. hydrocarbons (*Phytochemistry*, 1972, **11**, 2519). OH-cinnamic acid-sugar deriv.; fresh fronds, a xanthone-O-glucd. (*Chem Ind Lond*, 1979, 553; 1980, 465); fern, 3,7,8-tri - OH - xanthone - 1 - O-β - laminaribioside (*Phytochemistry*, 1980, **19**, 2030).

A. ceterach Linn.; see **Ceterach officinarum**

*A. laciniatum D. Don

Alc. ext. has burning effect on skin.

Plant, octatriacontane, vit. K3, β-sitosterol & its glucd., phthiocol and stearic acid (*Curr Sci*, 1976, **45**, 44); also 3,3'-bi-(2-Me-1,4-naphthoquinone (*Indian J Chem*, 1977, **15B**, 394).

Found in Eastern Himalayas, hills of S. India and also in Maharashtra.

*A. macrophyllum Sweet

Fronds decoct., powerful diur. for defective urinary secretion, esp. when induced by beri-beri (Wlth India, IA, 474).

Found in Anaimalai hills, T.N.

*A. nidus Linn. syn. *Thamnopteris nidus* (Linn.) Presl

Eng.–*Bird's nest fern.*

Plant, depuritive and sed.(Wlth India, IA, 475).

Found in Eastern Himalayas, Tamil Nadu and Karnataka.

A. ruta-muraria Linn.

Eng.–*Wall-rue, white maiden hair.*

Herb used in induration of liver, knots and swellings (*Lloydia*, 1970, **33**, 385).

A. trichomanes Linn.

Plant used in abscess of uterus (*Lloydia*, 1970, **33**, 385); as anthelm. and for hypochondriac affections (*Indian Drugs*, 1976-77, **14**, 136).

Fern, aliphatic and triterp. hydrocarbons (*Phytochemistry*, 1972, **11**, 2519); 2 kaempferol diglycds. and kaempferitrin (*Experientia*, 1979, **35**, 1134). Fronds, catechol, pyrogallol and gallic acid, main phenolic compds. (*Sci Cult*, 1979, **45**, 452).

ASTER (*Asteraceae*)

*A. albescens DC.

EtOH(50%) ext. of plant, spasmog. (*Indian J Exp Biol*, 1973, **11**, 43).

Found in Chamoli, U.P.

A. indamellus Grierson syn. *A. amellus* auct. non Linn.

Aq. alc. ext., diur. as strong as norphylline; weak hypoten. and good spasmol. (*Farmatsiya Sof*, 1965, **15**, 301; *CA*, 1966, **64**, 16492f).

*A. molliusculus Wall. ex C.B. Clarke

Essent. oil from herb antibact. and antifung; also ester fraction, antifung. [*Indian Perfum*, 1969, **13**(1), 17; *Indian Phytopathol*, 1979, **32**, 104]. Antifung. activity of essent. oil and hydrocarbon, ester and alc. fractions [*Indian Drugs Pharmac Ind*, 1979, **14**(5), 19].

Found in Western Himalayas from Kashmir to Kumaun between 1,500 – 2,400 m and also in Sikkim.

*A. peduncularis Wall.

Essent. oil from leaves, moderate antifung. and antibact. [*J Res Indian Med*, 1978, **13**(3), 122].

Found in Kumaun.

*A. thomsonii C.B. Clarke

Eng.–*Thomson's aster.*

Essent. oil from leaves, compds; moderate antibact. and antifung. [*J Res Indian Med*, 1978, **13**(3), 122; 71].

Found in Shimla and Kashmir up to 3,000 m.

ASTERACANTHA (*Acanthaceae*)

See **HYGROPHILA**

ASTILBE (*Saxifragaceae*)

*A. rivularis Buch.-Ham. ex D. Don
Khasi–*Padh.*

Leaves eaten raw in toothache; for blood purification (*Econ Bot*, 1981, **35**, 4).

Rhizomes contain bergenin,β-peltoboykinolic, astilbic & OAc-β-peltoboykinolic acids (*Indian J Chem*, 1977, **15B**, 494).

Temperate Himalayas from Kashmir to Bhutan up to 2,700 m.

ASTRAGALUS (*Fabaceae*)

*A. candolleanus Royle

H.–*Rudanti, rudrawanti.*

Root powd. and decoct. used in T.B., in skin diseases, cough and as blood purifier (*Khadi Gramodyog*, 1972-73, **19**, 277).

Found in Western Himalayas.

*A. chlorostachys Lindl.

EtOH(50%) ext. of plant, antiinflam. (*Indian J Exp Biol*, 1980, **18**, 594).

Found in Chamoli, U.P.

*A. graveolens Buch.-Ham.

Plant reported to possess cardiac depress. and diur. properties (*Annu Rep RRL Jammu*, 1970-71, 24).

Found in temperate regions of Western Himalayas at 1,200-1,750 m.

*A. oplites Benth. ex Parker syn. *A. cicerifolius* Royle ex Bunge non Royle ex Fischer

Plant, cardiac depress. (*Annu Rep RRL Jammu*, 1970-71, 24).

Western Himalayas from 3,000 to 5,100 m.

ASYSTASIA (*Acanthaceae*)

*A. dalzelliana Santapau

Heated leaves are used as a bandage on boils and swellings (*J Econ Tax Bot*, 1981, **2**, 188).

Western peninsular India.

*A. gangetica T. Anders. syn. *A. coromandeliana* Wight ex Nees; *A. violacea* Dals. non C.B. Clarke

EtOH(50%) ext. of plant, antiacetylcholine (*Indian J Exp Biol*, 1969, **7**, 250).

Petals contain luteolin 7-glucd., isosalipurposide & its glycd. (*Phytochemistry*, 1966, **5**, 111).

ATALANTIA (*Rutaceae*)

A. monophylla (Roxb.) DC.

Essent. oil from leaves, antitubercular (*Indian J Pharm*, 1967, **29**, 157); antifung. (*Flavour Ind*, 1972, **3**, 368).

Root bark contains a tetranortriterp., atalantin; stigmasterol (*Indian J Chem*, 1969, **7**, 870; 1970, **8**, 851); also xanthyletin, marmesin and γ-sitosterol (*J Indian Chem Soc*, 1970, **47**, 600); 2 tetranortriterp. and a C-12 lactone alongwith capaene, α-*trans*- bergamotene, β-bisabolene, etc. (*Indian J Chem*, 1975, **13**, 24); limonoids, atalantin, dehydroatalantin & cycloepiatalantin (*Tetrahedron*, 1976, **32**, 2367); revised str. of atalantolide and atalantin (*J Chem Soc Perkin Trans I*, 1977, 1875).

Root bark also contain acridone alks., atalaphylline & its N-Me deriv. (*Tetrahedron*, 1970, **26**, 2905); minor alk. N-Me- bicycloatalaphylline (*J Org Chem*, 1972, **37**, 3035); acridone base atalaphylline; atalaphyllidine, atalaphylline-3,5-di-Me-ether (*Phytochemistry*, 1975, **14**, 835; 1976, **15**, 2367; 1981, **20**, 867); str. of atalaphyllidine (*Experientia*, 1975, **31**, 1387).

Leaves, essent. oil, properties and constituents (*Perfum Essent Oil Rec*, 1967, **58**, 437). They yield friedelin and epifriedelanol and a mixt. of stigmasterol & γ- sitosterol; also *n*-Bu-palmitate (*J Indian Chem Soc*, 1970, **47**, 600; 1981, **58**, 1123).

Heartwood yields β-sitostenone, β-sitosterol, 10-nonacosanone, angelicin and psoralen (*Indian J Chem*, 1980, **19B**, 424); palmitic, stearic and arachidic acids (*J Indian Chem Soc*, 1981, **58**, 1123).

Fruits, alk. severine (*Tetrahedron*, 1980, **36**, 827).

*A. racemosa Wight & Arn.

EtOH(50%) ext. of aerial parts, antivir. (*Indian J Exp Biol*, 1971, **9**, 91).

Plant, racemosin (a pyranocoumarin), xanthyletin and xanthotoxin (*Proc Indian Acad Sci*, 1978, **87A**, 173).

Found in Western Peninsula.

ATHYRIUM (*Athyriaceae*)

*A. dialatatum (Blume) Mulde

EtOH(50%) ext. of plant, diur. (*Indian J Exp Biol*, 1977, **15**, 208).

Found in Chamoli, U.P

A. filix-femina (Linn.) Roth

Fronds contain Ca (large amt.) (*Flora Jena*, 1981, **171**, 1; *CA*, **95**, 765603y).

ATRIPLEX (*Chenopodiaceae*)

A. hortensis Linn.

Eng.–*Mountain spinach, orache.*

Estn. of ascorbic & dehydroascorbic acids and total vit. C in plant (*Ernaehr Umsch*, 1981, **28**, 187; *CA*, **95**, 148869x).

ATROPA (*Solanaceae*)

A. acuminata Royle ex Lindl. syn. *A. belladonna* C.B. Clarke (FBI) in part non Linn.

Eng.–*Belladonna, deadly nightshade, Indian belladonna.*

Belladonna in brain fever or encephalitis (*Hahnemannian Gleanings*, 1980, **47**, 259).

EtOH(50%) ext. of leaves, antiprot., antivir. and hypoglyc. (*Indian J Exp Biol*, 1968, **6**, 232). Homoeopathic mother tincture, antimicrob. (*ibid*, 1977, **15**, 338); plant ext., antifung (*Geobios*, 1978, **5**, 49).

Plant, extremely poisonous and contain alks.; hyoscyamine, and to a lesser extent atropine'and hyoscine (sopolamine), most important alks., although other minor alks. also contribute to activity (Med. Plants, 137; Wlth India, IA, 484); considerable variations in alk. content among different plants of same species and also variations in alk. content between younger and older plants (Sim, 37); cultivated herb, alk. content, 0.324% (dry basis) (*CIMPO Lucknow*, 1975, 5).

Leaves, alk. content of commercial samples of (0.42-0.55% dry basis) as also of roots (0.03-0.67% dry basis; may contain stem bases) (*Indian J Chem*, 1969, **7**, 414). Concentration of tropane alks. in leaves decreases with maturity (*Rev Med Targu-Mures*, 1968, **14**, 451; *CA*, 1969, **71**, 10380d). Alk. content of leaves increases after flower abscission (*Farmacia Buc*, 1971, **19**, 431; *CA*, 1972, **76**, 23166s).

Total belladonna alks.—called tropane (tropine) or solanaceous alks. Prophylaxis of carbontetrachloride hepatotoxicity (*J Egypt Med Assoc*, 1966, **49**, 59); parasympatholytic or cholinergic-blocking and consequently relax bronch. and intestinal smooth muscles (antisp.); inhibit contraction of iris muscles of eyes to produce mydriasis, and decrease salivary and sweat gland secretions. These alks. and plant drugs, sometimes used in combination with sed. to inhibit secretions, for mydriasis, and for diar. (Sim, 45). Plant ext. of alk. mixt. in compn. for drug of anti-stress, antifatigue, etc.; also for treatment of neurovegetative dystonia (Rom. Pat., 1972, 56379; 60376; 1973, 55773; 1978, 64161; *CA*, 1974, **81**, 68550g; 1975, **82**, 7652r; 1978, **89**, 30776n; 1980, **92**, 64773m); alks. as additive to tranquilizers enhancing activity and reducing side-effects (Brit. Pat., 1976, 1425969; *CA*, **85**, 25387z). Formulations containing plant ext. and antacids (*Farmatsiya Moscow*, 1974, **23**, 20). Proprietary pharmaceutical compn. to treat diseases like gastro-intestinal hypermotility, hyper-secretion, peptic ulcer, spastic constip., spastic dysmenor., nocturnal enuresis, bronch. asthma and whooping cough (Wlth India, IA, 487).

Ultrasonic extn. of total alks., from leaves (*Farmatsiya Sof*, 1963, **13**, 36; *CA*, 1964, **61**, 6858e); extn. from roots and leaves (*Bull Tech Gattefosse SFPA*, 1970, No.65, 25; *CA*, 1971, **74**, 57222f); electrochem. extn. (*Khim Prir Soedin*, 1972, 334; *CA*, **77**, 161675d); by percolation (*Rev Cubana Farm*, 1976, **10**, 249; *CA*, 1978, **88**, 11789g); large scale extn. procedure from leaves (*Res Ind*, 1970, **15**, 257; Indian Pat., 1975, 130818; *CA*, 1980, **92**, 55355z).

TLC sepn. of alks., hyoscyamine, atropine and hyoscine (*Formatsiya Sof*, 1964, **14**, 57; *CA*, 1965, **62**, 14988g). Atropine, hyoscyamine, scopolamine, etc. in belladona exts., chromatogr. (*Trav Soc Pharm Montpellier*, 1968, **28**, 211; *CA*, 1969, **70**, 99577y). Several other methods for detn. (*Farm Vestn Ljubljana*, 1967, **18**, 161; *Arch Pharm Ber Dtsch Pharm Ges*, 1972, **305**, 273; *Dtsch Apoth Ztg*, 1974, **114**, 1171; *Bull Soc Pharm Bordeaux*, 1973, **112**, 135; *CA*, 1968, **68**, 62725c; 1972, **77**, 39316x; 1974, **81**, 101500r; 1975, **83**, 136966r). Sepn. of alks. from leaves, in acidic medium [*Mitt Dtsch Pharm Ges*, 1970, **40**, 176; *Rev Farm Buenos Aires*, 1975, **117**(7-9), 66; *CA*, **73**, 84469e; 1976, **85**, 2154g]. Detn. of hyoscine, hyoscyamine and atropine in total alks. [*J Inst Chem India*, 1971, **43** (Pt I), 5]. Gas chromatogr. detn. of tropane alks. in different organs (*Planta Med*, 1977, **31**, 249); method for assay of alks. (*Indian J Pharm Sci*, 1981, **43**, 228).

Hyoscyamine (75-99% of the total alk. naturally present), occurs in laevo form and racemized to atropine (*dl*-hyoscyamine) with age of plant. In other countries, both alks. manufactured from *A. belladonna* or *Hyoscyamus* spp., but in India, both manufactured from *Physochlaina praealta*. Atropine and its sulphate official in IP as anticholinergic and sed. (Wlth India, IA, 455).

Pharmacol. of propionylatropine Me nitrate, 15 times as potent as papavarine (*Acta Pharmacol Toxicol*, 1963, **20**, 357). Effect of atropine and hyoscine on cardiovascular system in man (*Anesthesiology*, 1964, **25**, 123; 1965, **26**, 299); prior administration of atropine reduced early bradycardial effects of digitalis glycds. (*Boll Soc Med Chir Catania*, 1963, **31**, 308; *CA*, 1965, **63**, 3520f). Atropine useful for treatment of dimethoate poisoning in humans (*Arzneim Forsch*, 1966, **16**, 492; *CA*, **65**, 2882h). Atropine Me nitrate or bromide, as med. agent (Sim, 41).

A no. of minor alks. apoatropine (atropanine) (an anhydride of atropine) and belladonnine, thought to be dimeride related to apoatropine or its isomer, also present. Heating the plant or plant parts for 30 min. at 120° or direct dehydration of hyoscyamine or atropine yields these alks. Hyoscyamine, when heated at 120-30° changes successively into atropine, apoatropine and belladonnine. Apoatropine, beneficial effect on encephalitis; belladonnine, weak parasympatholytic in action; anticonvuls. and serves as a cure for Parkinson's disease (Wlth India, IA, 486; Sim, 41).

Roots of Indian and Greek belladonna plants also contain cuscohygrine (Wlth India, IA, 486).

Hyoscyamine-N-oxide and hyoscine-N-oxide present in roots, leaves and seeds (*Phytochemistry*, 1975, **14**, 999). A tropane alk. precursor, 8-N-Me-ornithine (*ibid*, 1981, **20**, 2064); role of hormones on tropine production (*Indian J Pharm Sci*, 1981, **43**, 175).

Leaves and flowers, flavons. (*Dtsch Apoth Ztg*, 1965, **105**, 1685; *Pharm Acta Helv*, 1966, **41**, 670; *CA*, 1967, **66**, 95361t, 95362u); leaves as well as flower flavons.; roots and seeds devoid of flavons. (*C R Acad Sci Ser D*, 1976, **282**, 53). Decomposition products of flavons. in commercial belladonna drugs (*Arch Pharm*, 1965, **298**, 107; *CA*, **62**, 12978h).

Seeds contain almost same alks. as leaves; highly poisonous, prescribed as specific antid. to opium and muscarine poisoning (Wlth India, IA, 487; Chopra *et al*, II, 640). Although only leaves and roots used commercially, seeds can also prove a promising source of alks. (*Bul Univ Shteteror Tiranes Ser Shkencat Mjekesore*, 1974, 199; CA, 1975, **82**, 144874d). Seeds, fatty oil (25%) and also an arom. oil (Wlth India, IA, 486).

ATYLOSIA (*Fabaceae*)

*A. lineata Wight & Arn.

EtOH(50%) ext. of plant, spasmog. and diur. (*Indian J Exp Biol*, 1977, **15**, 208).

Found in Tirupati, A.P.

*A. mollis Benth.

Plant used in dropsy, anasarca, pain in leg, pain and swelling during pregnancy and rinderpest (*Econ Bot*, 1970, **24**, 245).

Sub-Himalayan region from Himachal Pradesh to Sikkim, up to *c.* 2,000 m and also in Maharashtra.

A. scarabaeoides Benth.

Plant used for pain in leg, night fever, dropsy, anasarca, anaemia, hemiplegia, burns, wounds, smallpox, venereal sores, syphilis, gonor., spermator., gravel, cholera, dysen., snakebite and rinderpest (*Econ Bot*, 1970, **24**, 245).

*A. trinervia Gamble syn. *A. candollei* Wight & Arn.

Kan.–*Kaaduthogari*; Tam.–*Kattuthuvarei.*

EtOH(50%) ext. of aerial parts, CNS depress. (*Indian J Exp Biol*, 1974, **12**, 512).

Plant yields lupenone, lupeol, β-sitosterol and an antibact. substance, atylosol (*Indian J Pharm*, 1977, **39**, 165; *Phytochemistry*, 1978, **17**, 2001).

Nilgiris and Kerala at 1,500 - 2,400 m.

*A. volubilis Gamble syn. *A. mollis* Baker (FBI) in Part non Benth.; *A. crassa* Prain

Mundari–*Bir-rambara*; Santal–*Birmanthan.*

Root eaten in Bihar in bite of mad dog (Wlth India, IA, 490).

Punjab and Dehra Dun to Assam and in Bihar, Orissa, Andhra Pradesh, Madhya Pradesh and Maharashtra up to 900 m.

AUCUBA (*Aucubaceae*)

*A. japonica Thunb.

Plant, antifung. Aq. ext. of leaves inhibits growth of *E. coli*, *Micrococcus pyogenes* var. *aureus*, and *Mycobacterium tuberculosis* (Wlth India, IA, 490).

Aucubigenol glucd. (aucuboside) content of leaves decreases when dried with IR light as compared to air-drying (*Ann Pharm Fr*, 1965, **23**, 297; *CA*, **63**, 9752e). Fruit contains glycds. of pelargonidin and cyanidin (*Experientia*, 1971, **27**, 1006). All parts of plant contain iridoid glucd., aucubin (*Tetrahedron Lett*, 1976, 4279).

Aucubin—antibiot. activity under influence of β-glucosidase (e.g. emulsin); against a culture of *Staphylococcus aureus*, 1 ml of 2% aq. solution of aucubin had in presence of β-glucosidase, the same effect as 600 I.U. penicillin; aucubin yields an aglucone, aucubigenin in presence of β-glucosidase or on acid hydrolysis, whether the activity is due to aglucone or its products is not known (in Wagner & Wolff, 148-49; *Pharm Acta Helv*, 1969, **44**, 453; *CA*, **71**, 73968x); purg. activity, 50% cath. dose ED_{50}, 0.39 g/kg, and onset of diar., 6h; delayed action due to OH-group at 6 position (*Planta Med*, 1974, **25**, 285).

Grown in Indian gardens.

AVENA (*Poaceae*)

A. elatior Linn.; see Arrhenatherum elatius

A. fatua Linn.

Eng.–*Wild oat.*

Preliminary pharmacol. (*Indian J Exp Biol*, 1977, **15**, 208). Grass, toxic (*J Sci Res*, 1980, **2**, 171).

Triterp. & related compds. (*Yakugaku Zasshi*, 1980, **90**, 390). Leaves and roots contain saponins avenacoside A & B; both membranolytic (*Agnew Bot*, 1976, **50**, 49). Plant aflatoxin B_1; see also *Arachis (Nord Veterinaermed*, 1978, **30**, 482; *CA*, 1980, **92**, 145106y).

Grains, 4-OH-phthalide; sterols (*Nature Lond*, 1966, **210**, 1261; *Phytochemistry*, 1968, **7**, 2067). Seed endogenous hormones (*Can J Bot*, 1980, **58**, 1016).

Wild oat grits contain pangamic acid, 106mg/100g (*Z Lebensm Unters Forsch*, 1970, **143**, 411; *CA*, 1971, **74**, 75359k).

A. sativa Linn.

Eng.–*Oats*.

Oats—ext. enhanced the carcinogenic activity of Me- cholanthrene in male mice (*Nature Lond*, 1965, **208**, 598). Fresh seed used in spermator., impotency and sexual weakness; also in heart palpitation, in sleeplessness, and in haggard looks (*Bull Bot Soc Bengal*, 1972, **26**, 25). Standardization of. homoeopathic tincture used as nervine tonic (*Hahnemannian Gleanings*, 1979, **46**, 75). Large amts. of rainfall tended to increase estrogenic activity of oats [*Dokl Vses Akad S-kh Nauk im V I Lenina*, 1980, (9), 23]. Oats, common cause of photosensitization in pigs; may be unjustly labelled as hepatotoxic causing secondary photosensitization; when detecting hepatotoxic compd., any possible fungi the plant product harbouring should be studied (*in* Plant and Fungal Toxins, 352).

Oat hulls—inhibited exp. caries in rats; cariostatic (*Arch Oral Biol*, 1964, **9**, 219; *J Dent Res*, 1974, **53**, 1398). Alc. ext., ulcer preventing in swine and potent inhibitor of gastric acid secretion in pig (*J Anim Sci*, 1971, **32**, 1160).

Plant—hay ext., antiestrogenic in rats (*Acta Endochrinol*, 1965, **49**, 90). Ext. of fresh plant cut before harvest, reduced habit of cigarette smoking, clin. trials (*Nature Lond*, 1971, **233**, 496).

Seeds and aerial parts, two saponins, avenacoside & its degluco deriv. (*Z Naturforsch*, 1966, **21B**, 896); steroid saponin, avenacoside B (*Chem Ber*, 1971, **104**, 3549).

Persons exposed to grain dust for long time developed respiratory complaints (*J Occup Med*, 1964, **6**, 319; *CA*, 1965, **62**, 3312d). Grains, two allergenic compds. (*Int Arch Allergy Appl Immunol*, 1967, **31**, 546; *CA*, **67**, 51036g). Seeds possess α-mannosidase and α- & β-glucosidase activities (*C R Acad Sci Ser D*, 1967, **264**, 1036).

Seed sterols, cholesterol, brassicasterol, β- sitosterol, campesterol, stigmasterol, Δ^7-stigmasterol, and stigmastdienols

(*Phytochemistry*, 1965, **4**, 857; 1967, **6**, 407; 1968, **7**, 2067); β-sitosterol *D*-glucd. and others (*Herba Pol*, 1979, **25**, 57).

Oats, 3 phenolic antioxidants; diferulates of long chain diols (*Chem Ind Lond*, 1965, 1763); gluceryl esters of caffeic and ferulic acids; oat flour antioxidant uneffected by heat (*J Sci Food Agric*, 1968, **19**, 710; *Inf Grasas Aceites*, 1977, **17**, 27; *CA*, **87**, 182888x). Oat polyphenol compn. prevented the increase of cholesterol and β- lipoprotein of blood serum of fasting rabbits (*Ukr Biokhim Zh*, 1972, **44**, 376; *CA*, **77**, 122090q). Flavons. from different organs of plant (*Z Pflanzenphysiol*, 1977, **85**, 103). Effect of ascorbic acid and polyphenols from oats on respiration and oxidative phosphorylation in liver mitochondria of rats with alloxan diabetes (*Ukr Biokhim Zh*, 1978, **50**, 50; *CA*, **88**, 88015j). HPLC of flavone derivs. (*J Chromatogr*, 1979, **176**, 270).

Colororim. detn. of aconitic acid (*J Agric Food Chem*, 1970, **18**, 546). OH-hentriacontanediones (*Phytochemistry*, 1972, **11**, 2654).

Oat mycotoxins, low levels of aflatoxin (*Cereal Chem*, 1969, **46**, 446); patulin; sterigmatocystin, TLC sepn. (*J Assoc Off Anal Chem*, 1970, **53**, 686; 1977, **60**, 104); estn. of ochratoxin A in Swedish oat products (*Var Foeda*, 1976, **28**, 206; *CA*, 1977, **86**, 138091n). Penicillic acid from oat meal (*Z Lebensm Unters Forsch*, 1981, **172**, 110; *CA*, **94**, 101463z).

Avenacine, antifung. compd. from oats [*Chem Can*, 1967, **19**(8), 20]. Oat, antibiot. glycd. avenacine A & B (*Tetrahedron*, 1973, **29**, 629). Bitter tasting monoglycerides of stored oat flour (*ibid*, 1979, **169**, 22; *CA*, **91**, 139088g).

Leaves, stems and inflorescences, C-glycosylflavones, including vitexin, isovitexin, isoswertisin 2"-rhamnosides and · isoorientin 2"-arabinosides (*Phytochemistry*, 1977, **16**, 1112; 2041); leaves, 4 saponins, avenacosides A, B, C & D (*Z Naturforsch*, 1981, **36C**, 1072). Estn. of prussic acid of leaves and caryopses in oat vars. (*Z Lebensm Unters Forsch*, 1981, **173**, 176; *CA*, **95**, 147204q). Leaves, N-containing phytoalexins avenalumin I, II & III; str. detn. of I (*Tetrahedron Lett*, 1981, **22**, 2103).

Roots contain chelidonic acid (*Aust J Biol Sci*, 1965, **18**, 437). New amino acid, avenic acid (*Tetrahedron Lett*, 1980, **21**, 3071); saponins avenacosides A .& B (*Angew Bot*, 1976, **50**, 49).

Production of furfural; acetic acid from oat husks (*Chem Age India*, 1976, **27**, 521; Jpn Tokkyo Koho, 1979, 7912539; *CA*, **91**, 73158w).

AVERRHOA (*Averrhoaceae*)

A. bilimbi Linn.

Eng.–*Cucumber tree, bilimbi.*

Fruit, in whitlows (*Loydia*, 1970, **33**, 313).

A. carambola Linn.

Fruit—juice effect on rat (*Asian Symp Med Plants and Spices*, 1980, 159). Ext. caused dose-related increase in hypnosis in mice (*Med J Malays*, 1980, **34**, 279); eaten in Assam for jaundice (*Q J Crude Drug Res*, 1979, **17**, 61).

Plant—EtOH(50%) ext. of aerial parts, preliminary pharmacol. (*Indian J Exp Biol*, 1977, **15**, 208); used in fractured bones (*Sri Lanka For*, 1981, **14**, 145).

Fruit, protein and amino acid compn. (*J Agric Food Chem*, 1980, **28**, 1217); vit. C (*J Food Technol*, 1980, **15**, 459); oxalic acid, Ca and P, estn. (*Qual Plant Mater Veg*, 1972- 73, **22**, 335).

Plant, phytochemical anal. [*An Fac Farm Univ Fed Pernambuco*, 1976, (Pub. 1977), **15**, 39; *CA*, 1979, **91**, 16729j].

Flowers, rutin and quercetin 3-glucd. (*J Indian Chem Soc*, 1979, **56**, 944).

AVICENNIA (*Avicenniaceae*)

*A. alba Blume syn. A. officinalis Linn. var. alba

B.–*Baen.*

Bark contains tannins (6% in a Malaysian sample); leaves and bark, same constituents as *A. officinalis* (*J Indian Chem Soc*, 1979, **56**, 111).

Found in tidal forests of eastern coast.

*A. marina Vierh.

Tam.–*Venkandan*; Tel.–*Mada.*

Plant juice used as abortif. (*Econ Bot*, 1973, **27**, 189).

Bark, tannins (12.5% in Nigerian sample) and triterps. including betulinic acid (0.3% dry wt basis) (Wlth India, IA, 503).

Found along the coast in tidal waters and salt-swamps.

A. officinalis Linn.

EtOH(50%) ext. of aerial parts, antiprot. (*Indian J Exp Biol*, 1980, **18**, 594).

Kernels contain a naphthaquinone deriv., lapachol (1%) which possesses antitumour properties (*Cancer Res*, 1968, **28**, 1952).

Aerial parts yield β-sitosterol, friedelin, lupenone, lupeol, betulinic and ursolic acids (*Indian J Pharm*, 1974, **36**, 105). Distribution of triterps. in bark and leaves (*J Indian Chem Soc*, 1979, **56**, 111). Leaves yield betulin (*Indian J Chem*, 1981, **20B**, 632).

AZADIRACHTA (*Meliaceae*)

A. indica A. Juss. syn. *Melia azadirachta* Linn.

Eng.–*Indian lilac, margosa tree, neem tree.*

Bark—EtOH(50%) ext., anticancer, antivir. & spasmog. (*Indian J Exp Biol*, 1969, **7**, 250; 1971, **9**, 91). Ext., antibact. against *E. coli* [*J Res Indian Med*, 1974, **9**(2), 66]. Aq. ext., contracep. for male [*ibid*, 1978, **13**(2), 104]. Used in syphilis (*Nagarjun*, 1979-80, **23**, 9).

Gum—proteolytic activity (Wlth India, IA, 506). Compn. (*Indian J Biochem*, 1967, **4**, 181).

Leaves—antivir. (*Indian J Med Res*, 1969, **57**, 495). Antineoplastic [*Proc Nat Acad Sci India*, 1976, **46B**(Pt IV), 527]. Fungitoxicity (*Geobios*, 1978, **5**, 49); ext., antifung. [*Indian Phytopathol*, 1981, **34**, 385; *Labdev*, 1970, **8B**, 58; *Proc Nat Acad*

Sci India, 1972, **42B** (Pt III), 300]; see seed oil also. Leaves cause dermatitis (*Indian J Med Res,* 1978, **68,** 650). Alc. ext., useful in eczema, ringworm and scabies (*Antiseptic,* 1979, **76,** 677). Ext., very effective anthelm. in ascariasis, clin. trials (*Antiseptic,* 1980, **77,** 274). Fresh leaves' ext., antifert. in male mice (*J Postgrad Med Bombay,* 1980, **26,** 167). Ext., 100% mosquito larvicidal at 1% concentration (*Indian J Pharmacol,* 1981, **13,** 96).

Ext., decreased heart rate in rabbit, also weak antiarrhythmic (*J Pharm Sci,* 1978, **67,** 1476); also hypoglyc. and antihyperglyc. (*Indian J Pharmacol,* 1978, **10,** 247); leaves form one of the constituents of a compn. for diabetic patients (*Maharashtra Med J,* 1981, **28,** 165). Aq. ext. of leaves along with those of *Ziziphus jujuba* used against falling hair (*Q J Crude Drug Res,* 1979, **17,** 61).

Seeds—powd. kernel, protectant against stored grain pests (*Indian J Entomol,* 1965, **27,** 160; 1967, **29,** 21). Repellent against various insects (*Andhra Agric J,* 1969, **16,** 107). Seeds, feeding-inhibitors against pest of sesame, *Antigastra catalaunalis (East Afr Agric For J,* 1977, **42,** 257). Suspension of kernel in w., antifeedant against tobacco caterpillar (*Indian J Agric Sci,* 1978, **48,** 19). Kernel ext., larvicidal; also ovipostitional repellent for moths of tobacco caterpillar (*Phytoparasitica,* 1978, **6,** 85; 1979, **7,** 199); neem ext., pesticide [*Pestology,* 1980, **4**(3), 16]; neem seeds with oleoresin from *Chrysanthemum cinerariaefolium* flowers, toxic against housefly, pulse beetle and lesser grain borer [*Pesticides,* 1980, **14**(3), 11]. Kernels, one of the constituents in hair compn. useful in preventing hair loss and treatment of dandruff (Brit. U.K. Pat. Appl. 1979, 2000971; *CA,* **92,** 11100h).

Kernel oil—official in IP for local application (IP, 1966, 324); greenish yellow to brown, acrid, bitter fixed oil (40-49%) called oil of margosa or neem oil, having a strong disagreeable odour resembling garlic (Ketkar, 1976, 5). Use of oil and ext. in

Indian pharmacy, a report on chem. and therapeutic properties (*Seifen Oele Fette Wasche,* 1963, **59,** 894; *CA,* 1965, **63,** 5449b); oil or leaves' smoke inhibited growth of *Aspergillus flavus* [*J Res Indian Med,* 1978, **13**(1), 127]. Neem oil boiled with nuxvomica seeds useful in eczema [*ibid,* 1979, **14**(3-4), 74]; ext., mosquito larvicidal and toxic to insectivorous fish and tadpoles. Neem oil and leaves' exts., strong antifeedant against desert locust (*Indian J Entomol,* 1980, **42,** 371; 469). Infants ingesting neem oil developed toxic symptoms (*Lancet,* 1981, 1, 487). Oil useful in diabetes (*Drug Pharm Ind Highlights,* 1979, **2,** 214); see also nimbidin.

Seed cake—used as insectic. and nematicide, possesses vermicidal properties. Gives protection from grain moth, lesser grain borer and red flour beetle; reduces gall formation (Wlth India, IA, 510); alc. ext., repellent against migratory as well as desert locusts (*Bull RRL Jammu,* 1963, **1,** 176). Addn. of aq. ext. of de-oiled seed to pyrethrum formulations increased insectic. strength (*Pyrethrum Post,* 1976, **13,** 119).

Flowers—flowers and fruits, purg. (*Indian For,* 1964, **90,** 50). Cure rheum. pains [*J Res Indian Med,* 1977, **12**(4), 53]; one of the constituents of indigenous drug, '*Amber Mezhugu*' useful against rheum., clin. trials (*Rheumatism,* 1976-77, **12,** 38); an indigenous preparation with *Piper nigrum* used as anthelm., clin. trials (*Sachitra Ayurveda,* 1977-78, **30,** 327).

Essent. oil—anti-T.B. (*Indian J Pharm,* 1967, **29,** 157); from flowers, antibact. (*Bull Bot Soc Univ Saugar,* 1976-77, **23-24,** 74); from seeds, antimicrob. (*Indian J Hosp Pharm,* 1978, **15,** 166); essent. oil from seeds and from leaves, antifung.; former, against keratinophilic fungi [*Indian Drugs,* 1977-78, **15,** 41; 1981-82, **19,** 245; *East Pharm,* 1977, **20**(232), 147].

Various plant parts—used in inflam. of gums, sores, fever, spleen complaint, tumours, strangulation of intestine, head scald, measles, smallpox, diar., cholera, nausea, failure of lactation, fever in labour and anthrax (*Econ Bot*, 1970, **24**, 258). Dental compn. containing exts. of wood, bark or leaves, useful for preventing and curing gingivitis and periodontitis (Brit. Pat., 1973, 1314136; *CA*, **79**, 45789m). Cosmetics containing exts. of bark, leaf, flower, stem and root skin(bark), beneficial for skin (Jpn Pat., 1977, 7728853; *CA*, 1978, **88**, 11747s). Tree powd. useful in white leprosy [*J Res Indian Med*, 1977, **12**(4), 53]. Plant used in skeletal fractures (*Sri Lanka For*, 1980, **14**, 145). Plant, antilithic (*Proc Indian Sci Congr*, 1981, pt III, 156). Wood, as contracep. (*Ancient Sci Life*, 1981-82, **1**, 72; *J Sci Res Plants Med*, 1981, **2**, 39).

Reviews—marvellous margosa, rev. with production, med uses, etc., 12 refs. (*Indian Oil Scap J*, 1967-68, **23**, 298). Neem-insectic. of the future, covering uses of *neem* products against stored grain pests, 37 refs. [*Pesticides*, 1981, **15**(10), 19]. Components of *neem* in pest control, many refs. (*Meded Fac Landbouwwet Rijksuniv Gent*, 1981, **46**, 39; *CA*, **95**, 198837f). Vegetative fallows and potential value of *neem* tree, 64 refs. (*Econ Bot*, 1981, **35**, 398).

Bark, bitter principles, penta-nortriterp., nimbin & 6-de-Ac- nimbin (*Indian J Chem*, 1967, **5**, 460; *Tetrahedron*, 1968, **24**, 154; *Chem Ber*, 1981, **114**, 2375). Trunkwood, nimbolin A & B (*J Chem Soc D*, 1969, 1166). Heartwood sterols (*Fitoterapia*, 1977, **48**, 166).

Nigerian leaves, a meliacin, nimbolide (*J Chem Soc Chem Commun*, 1967, 808); leaves, quercetin and β- sitosterol glucd. (*J Indian Chem Soc*, 1968,45, 466); *n*-hexacosanol, glucds. of quercetin and kaempferol (*Phytochemistry*, 1971, **10**, 2842). Ca, P and oxalate contents of Indian leaves (*Qual Plant Mater Veg*, 1972, **12**, 335). Leaf ext., antifeedant, active principles, meliantriol and azadirachtin (*Indian J Entomol*, 1980, **42**, 469). Isolation of petanortriterp., nimbinene, 6-de-Ac-nim-

binene and nimbandiol its-6-de-OAc-deriv. (*Chem Ber*, 1981, **114**, 2375).

Berries, str. detn. of azadirone, azadiradione, epoxyazadiradione, and gedunin (*Tetrahedron*, 1971, **27**, 3927). Fruits(berries) contain hexacyclic tetranortriterp. vilasinin (*Chem Lett*, 1974, 357). Insect antifeedant, azadirachtin and salanin (*Recent Adv Phytochem*, 1975, **9**, 283). Str. of triterp. isolated from fruit pulp (*Z Naturforsch*, 1975, **30B**, 961); also of steroidal compd., 17-OH-azadiradione & 17β-OH-azadizaradione (*Tetrahedron Lett*, 1978, 611; 2395).

Seeds, 6 new tetranortriterps. (*Phytochemistry*, 1981, **20**, 117); azadirachtin (Wlth India, IA, 508).

Seed oil contains an active antifeeding principle, meliantriol (*J Chem Soc Chem Commun*, 1967, 910); and nimbin, str. (*Tetrahedron*, 1968, **24**, 1517); a compd. vepinin; tiglic acid (*Indian J Chem*, 1969, 7, 187; 1979, **17B**, 169). Components of neem oil, known to raise oxidation potential of erythrocytes and thus prevent propagation of malaria parasites within them; may act in the same way in gingival sulcus, so that microorganisms responsible do not proliferate (*Med Anthropol*, 1979, **3**, 401; 431). Str. of 3-de-Ac-salanin & 1,3-di-Ac-vilasinin (*Justus Liebigs Ann Chem*, 1981, 181). Pentanortriterp., nimbinene, its 6-de-Ac deriv., nimbandiol & its 6-OAc-deriv.(*Chem Ber*, 1981, **114**, 2375).

Azadirachtin—active compd. from seeds; feeding inhibitor for desert locust; completely inhibited in 40 μg/l dose (*J Insect Physiol*, 1971, **17**, 969). A potent rejectant for desert locust (*Nature Lond*, 1971, **232**, 402). Antifeedant, very active insect phagorepellent and systemic growth disruptor (*Recent Adv Phytochem*, 1975, **9**, 283; *Phytoparasitica*, 1981, **9**, 27); its effect on moulting process of last instar nynphs of *Periplanata americana* (*Indian J Exp Biol*, 1978, **16**, 1141).

Partial str. of azadirachtin (*J Chem Soc Perkin Trans I*, 1972, 2445); str. (*Recent*

Adv Phytochem, 1975, **9**, 283; *J Am Chem Soc*, 1975, **97**, 1975).

Reversed-phase liq. chromatogr. for isolation of azadirachtin from seed kernels (*J Liq Chromatogr*, 1979, **2**, 875; *CA*, **91**, 137185n).

Nimbidin—tetranortriterp., nimbidin a bitter fraction from seed oil (*Tetrahedron Lett*, 1970, 2761; *Phytochemistry*, 1971, **10**, 857); from neem oil, effective drug in acute and chr. inflam. (*Planta Med*, 1981, **43**, 59); effective in psoriasis, clin. trials (*Indian Med J*, 1978, **72**, 180; *J Res Ayur Siddha*, 1980, **1**, 52); analg. & antipyr. in rats (*Bull Med Ethno Bot Res*, 1980, **1**, 393). Oil and nimbidin, hypoglyc. in rabbits (*Indian J Med Res*, 1980, **74**, 931; *Indian J Pharmacol*, 1981, **13**, 91). Nimbidin, as also nimbin inhibited potato virus X growth (*Acta Microbiol Pol Ser B*, 1974, **6**, 9). Oil and nimbidin, antibact., latter more potent (*Indian J Pharmacol*, 1981, **13**, 102).

Na-nimbidinate—obtained from nimbidin, diur. and antiinflam. When administered i.m. in congestive cardiac failure with anasarca, good response observed. Produces uterine contraction. Reduced B.P. in animals. Nimbidin and Na-nimbidinate kill *Paramaecium caudatum* in 1/500 dilution; the latter w.-sol., more active. Na-nimbidinate and Na-nimbinate, spermic. (Wlth India, IA, 509).

Nimbidol — one of the by-products of extn. of main constituents of the oil; it is a mixture of nimbidin, odourous S- containing constituents and fatty impurities, both oil and nimbidol, antiarthritic (Wlth India, IA, 510).

Flowers, essent. oil, constituent (*Agra Univ J Res*, 1963, **12**, 299); quercetin-3-galatoside, kaempferol-3-glucd. and myricentin-pentoside (*Indian J Chem*, 1972, **10**, 452).

AZANZA (*Malvaceae*)

A. lampas (Cav.) Alef. syn. *Hibiscus lampas* Cav.; *Thespesia lampas* (Cav.) Dalz. & Gibs.; *T. macrophylla* Blume

Preliminary pharmacol. (*Indian J Exp Biol*, 1973, **11**, 43). Seeds, anthelm. (*Econ Bot*, 1965, **19**, 239). Plant used by Santals, in nosebleed, limb or bone pain, fever, sores, stab wound, ulcer, carbuncle, *prolapsus ani, fistula ani*, dysen., consumption, cough and broncht. (*ibid*, 1970, **24**, 265). Leaf decoct., antiinflam. (*ibid*, 1978, **32**, 278). Pounded root given to stop bleeding in haemor. (*Nagarjun*, 1980-81, **24**, 1).

Seeds yield a fatty oil (16.9%); all parts of plant contain gossypol, toxic principle of cottonseed (*Gossypium* spp.; for properties see *Gossypium*); roots, 2.75; stems, 0.16; leaves, 0.98; flower buds, 1.95; and seeds, 1.74%; these values than those in *Thespesia populnea* but than those in *Gossypium hirsutum* (*Econ Bot*, 1967, **21**, 128; *IDMA Bull*, 1980, **11**, 229).

AZIMA (*Salvadoraceae*)

A. tetracantha Lamk

EtOH(50%) ext. of aerial parts, spasmog. (*Indian J Exp Biol*, 1968, **6**, 232).

Leaves contain alks. azimine, azcarpine and carpine (*Tetrahedron Lett*, 1967, 3465). Str. of azimine and azcarpine (*Tetrahedron*, 1968, **24**, 6417).

Leaves and roots yield friedelin, lupeol, glutinol and β-sitosterol; no alk. detected (*Curr Sci*, 1978, **47**, 857).

AZOLLA (*Azollaceae*)

*A. pinnata R. Br. syn. *Salvinia imbricata* Roxb.

Plant pharmacol. (*Indian J Exp Biol*, 1969, **7**, 250); ext. antifung. [*Indian Drugs Pharmac Ind*, 1978, **13**(3), 21]; antibiot. (*Econ Bot*, 1980, **34**, 288).

Throughout India, in shallow freshwater lakes, ponds, ditches, etc.

BACCAUREA (*Euphorbiaceae*)

*B. ramiflora Lour. syn. *B. sapida* Muell.-Arg.; *B. wrayi* King ex Hook.f.

Ass.–*Leteku;*B.–*Letka*; H.–*Kataphal*; Garo–*Dojuka*; Manipur–*Moktok*; Mikir–*Damiyu-arong*; Tripura–*Bhubi*.

EtOH(50%) ext. of aerial parts, pharmacol. (*Indian J Exp Biol*, 1973, **11**, 43). Bark useful in constip.; adults chew it; children take its sap (*Bull Bot Surv India*, 1976, **18**, 66).

Bark contains friedelin, epifriedelanol, Me-betulinate, β-sitosterol and an unknown ester (*J Indian Chem Soc*, 1967, **44**, 728).

Wild or cultivated in sub-Himalayan regions, Assam and Andamans, chiefly in moist tropical forests.

BACOPA (*Scrophulariaceae*)

B. monnieri (Linn.) Wettst. syn. *Gratiola monniera* Linn.; *Herpestis monnieria* (Linn.) H.B. & K.; *Moniera cuneifolia* Michx.

Plant—Alc. ext., tranquillizer in rats and dogs; smooth musculature relaxant and antisp. (*Indian J Pharm*, 1961, **23**, 2; *Indian J Med Res*, 1967, **55**, 473). Effect of EtOH(50%) ext. of plant on cerebral amino acid levels in mice; Ac-cholinesterase activity of mice cerebral tissues and mouse brain; ext., also anticancer (*Indian J Exp Biol*, 1966, **4**, 216; 1967, **5**, 36; 1969, **7**, 250). Treatment with plant produced improvement in maze-learning of albino rats (*Indian J Physiol Allied Sci*, 1976, **30**, 88).

In Ayurveda, plant used for dermatosis, anaemia and diabetes (*Acta Phytother*, 1972, **19**, 141). Plant, in boils and as blood purifier [*J Res Indian Med*, 1973, **8**(1), 82]. Brain tonic, sharpens dull memory; used in catar. complaints; also a safe cardiac tonic (*Bull Bot Soc Bengal*, 1972, **26**, 25; 1975, **29**, 97);gives relief to patients from anxiety neurosis [*J Res Indian Med*, 1979, **14**(3-4), 1,8; *J Res Ayur Siddha*, 1980, **1**, 133; *Probe*, 1980- 81, **20**, 201]; juice alongwith ginger juice, sugar and bark ext. of *Moringa oleifera*, given to children in stomach disorders (*J Econ Tax Bot*, 1981, **2**, 181).

Leaves—decoct. in cough (*Bull Bot Surv India*, 1973, **15**, 19). Used in rheum. (*Indian Drugs*, 1977-78, **15**, 145).

Plant, 2 saponins, bacoside A & B; betulic acid, *d*-mannitol, stigmasterol, β-sitosterol and stigmastanol; another sample, a saponin, monnierin, betulinic acid and *d*-mannitol and an alk.; constitution of bacoside A; becoside B, like bacoside A, gave on hydrolysis, bacogenins A_1, A_2, A_3 & A_4; also str. of A_1, A_2; str. of tetrasaccharide of monnierin (*Indian J Chem*, 1963, **1**, 212; 408; 1965, **3**, 24; 1967, **5**, 84; 1975, **13**, 309; 1968, **6**, 471). Neuropharmacol. effects of hersaponin (*Indian J Physiol Pharmacol*, 1967, **11**, 33). Plant contains nicotine, 3-formyl-4-OH-2H-pyran, luteolin & its glucd. (*Phytochemistry*, 1972, **11**, 2649). Constitution of bacogenin A_1 & A_4; isolation of bacogenin A_3; A_1 & A_3 epimers. Smith-de Mayo degradation of bacoside A gave jujubogenin & ψ-jujubogenin (*ibid*, 1973, **12**, 887, 2074; 1977, **16**, 141; 1978, **17**, 287).

BAECKEA (*Myrtaceae*)

*B. virgata Andr.

Leaves and twigs of Queensland plant yield an essent. oil (*c.* 1%) with α-*d*-pinene, 50-60; cineol, 30%; and others (Wlth India, IIB, 3).

Introduced into Nilgiris.

BALANITES (*Balanitaceae*)

B. roxburghii Planch. syn. *B. aegyptiaca* Delile; *B. aegyptiaca* var. *roxburghii* Duthie

Eng.–*Desert date.*

Chemotaxon.—seed hydrocarbons; of *B. aegyptiaca* and *B. roxburghiana* (*Phytochemistry*, 1970, **9**, 1087); w.r.t alks. and flavons. of *B. aegyptiaca* and *B. roxburghiana* (*Biochem Syst Ecol*, 1977, **5**, 121; *CA*, **87**, 180727v). Systematic position (*Curr Sci*, 1978, **47**, 968).

Plant—used as arrow poison by Fali Tinguelin of N. Cameroun (*C R Acad Sci*, 1965, **260**, 4109); in Sudan, for bilharziasis and as purg. (*Fitoterapia*, 1981, **52**, 243).

Fruit—edible. Used as soap substitute (Wlth India, IIB, 3). Administration of EtOH(50%) ext. of ripe fruit pulp in dogs resulted in mass atrophy of spermatogenic elements (*Indian J Exp Biol*, 1981, **19**, 918). Fruit useful in boils, leucoderma and other skin diseases; pulp, in whooping cough.

Seed kernel oil—in Uganda, for sleeping sickness, and in Spain, as purg. (*J Agric Trop Bot Appl*, 1966, **13**, 281); oil applied in burns, ulcers, etc. [*J Res Indian Med*, 1973, **8**(2), 75]; oil and unsap. matter, antimicrob. [*Indian Drugs Pharmac Ind*, 1978, **13**(1), 15].

Bark—fish poison, bactericide (Wlth India, IIB, 3). EtOH(50%) ext. of bark, spasmol. (*Indian J Exp Biol*, 1973, **11**, 43).

Fruit, as standby source of diosgenin; fruit from Egypt contains 4.08%; diosgenin/yamogenin (44:56) (Asolkar & Chadha, 53).

Kernels and also leaves, 6 diosgenin glucds.; fruit wall, steroidal sapogenins, 1.2% (dry basis); yamogenin, major (*Phytochemistry*, 1969, **8**, 261; 1970, **9**, 645). Extn. of saponins & their genins (Brit. Pat., 1971, 1239555; *CA*, **75**, 109011d); see *Dioscorea* also. Estn. of sapogenin in fruit epicarp and mesocarp; yamogenin, major. Fruit pulp richer in sapogenins than seeds (*Econ Bot*, 1972, **26**, 169); pulp, 5 diosgenin glycds., balanitisins A, B, C, D & E (*Indian J Pharm*, 1977, **39**, 125; 1979, **41**, 122). Fruits from Jodhpur, yielded diosgenin (3.65% dry basis) (*J Bombay Natl Hist Soc*, 1981, **78**, 194).

Extn. of sapogenins from nuts (US Pat., 1969, 3449328; *CA*, **71**, 64086f). Seed kernel, a saponin of diosgenin (also in leaves) (*Indian J Pharm*, 1975, **37**, 103); also incubation with water and ultrasonic insonation increase diosgenin yield; diosgenin content of pericarp (0.1%) and that of defatted seeds (0.4%); incubation with

water, treatment with 2,4-D also increase yield; non-edible fatty oil (44%) from seed kernel [*East Pharm*, 1978, **21**(244), 191; *Indian J Pharm Sci*, 1978, **40**, 228]. Spermic. activity of saponins (*Indian Drugs*, 1979-80, **17**, 6).

Stem bark, steroidal sapogenin, 0.7% (dry basis); nitrogenin glucd. (*Phytochemistry*, 1970, **9**, 645; 1971, **10**, 2829); sesquiterp., balanitol (*J Indian Chem Soc*, 1978, **55**, 1148); bergapten and d-marmesin (*Planta Med*, 1981, **43**, 92).

Roots, steroid sapogenin, 1%; IR. spectrophotom. estn. of diosgenin & yamogenin (*Phytochemistry*, 1970, **9**, 645; *Planta Med*, 1972, **22**, 78; 1974, **25**, 22).

Plant, diosgenin & yamogenin levels in different plant parts (*Planta Med*, 1976, **30**, 118). Growth regulators for diosgenin production in callus culture (*Indian J Exp Biol*, 1980, **18**, 1207; 1981, **19**, 611). Cytotoxic and antitumour principle, isolation and identn. (Univ. Microfilms Int., No. 7908323; *CA*, 1979, **91**, 35691g).

BALANOPHORA (*Balanophoraceae*)

*B. polyandra Griff.

In Thailand, plant used as antiasthmatic.

Plant, coniferin (*Phytochemistry*, 1969, **8**, 913); coniferin effective in cough syrups (*Chem Pharm Bull*, 1971, **19**, 207).

Found in Nagaland and Manipur, W. Bengal, Orissa, Bihar and Andhra Pradesh up to 2,000 m.

BALDINGERA (*Poaceae*)

See **PHALARIS**

BALIOSPERMUM (*Euphorbiaceae*)

B. montanum Muell.-Arg. syn. *B. axillare* Blume; *Croton polyandrus* Roxb.

A preparation from leaves given in abdominal tumours (*Lloydia* 1969, **32**, 157). Preliminary pharmacol. (*Indian J Exp Biol*, 1971, **9**, 91). Latex used in rheum. (*Ancient Sci Life*, 1981-82, **1**, 177).

EtOH ext. of roots showed *in vivo* activity in p-388 lymphocytic leukaemia (*Lloydia*, 1966, **40**, 609).

Roots yield 5 new phorbol esters belonging to diterp. hydrocarbon, tigliane skeleton viz., montanin, baliospermin, 12-deoxyphorbol and 12-deoxy-16-OH-phorbol as 13-palmitates, 12-deoxy-5 β-OH-phorbol-13-myristate; esters, *in vitro* anticancer (*Planta Med*, 1978, **33**, 128); biol. activities of tiglianes along with other diterps. (*Lloydia*, 1978, **41**, 193).

BALLOTA (*Lamiaceae*)

See **OTOSTEGIA**

BALSAMODENDRON (*Burseraceae*)

See **COMMIPHORA**

BAMBUSA (*Poaceae*)

B. arundinacea Roxb. syn. *B. bambos* Druce

Eng.–*Spiny bamboo.*

Culms soot mixed with lime and applied to cuts and wounds (*Econ Bot*,1965, **19**, 246). Used as expect., tonic, stim., aphrodis., and in blood T.B., broncht., and asthma (*Q J Crude Drug Res*, 1970, **10**, 1555).

Hollow internodes accumulate a substance called *tabashir* (liq. accumulation) or *banslochan* (a solid) given in T.B., asthma and leprosy (Wlth India, IIB, 34; *Bull Bot Soc Bengal*, 1975, **29**, 97).

EtOH(50%) ext. of aerial parts, preliminary pharmacol. (*Indian J Exp Biol*, 1973, **11**, 43). Aerial parts (stem and leaves) used by Ayurvedic physicians as blood purifier and in leucoderma and inflam. conditions. Fresh young shoots, insectic.; lethal to mosquito larvae (*Nagarjun*, 1979-80, **23**, 177; *Bull Bot Soc Bengal*, 1975, **29**, 97). Antibact. activity of plant (*Indian J Pharm*, 1975, **37**, 176). Decoct. of stem joints used for fertility control (*Ancient Sci Life*, 1981-82, **1**, 67).

Shoots—young and tender ones, considerably acrid, although relished like asparagus, they may be poisonous to both humans and cattle, as they contain benzoic acid (0.23%) and a cyanogenic glucd. yielding HCN (0.03%) on endogenic enzymic hydrolysis. Cooking destroys enzyme (Chopra *et al*, II, 928).

Contains cynogenic glucd., taxiphyllin (*Proc K Ned Akad Wet Ser C*, 1978,**81**, 347; *CA*, **89**, 211962r). If plant proves teratogenic by feeding trials, cyanide could be responsible in view of teratogenic propensity of hypoxia and the ability of cyanide to induce hypoxic state (*in* Plant and Fungal Toxins, 187, 198).

*B. nutans Wall. ex Munro

H.–*Mala bans*; Ass.–*Bidhuli*; B.–*Makla*; Mikir–*Chak*.

EtOH(50%) ext. of aerial parts, anticancer and hypoglyc. (*Indian J Exp Biol*, 1980, **18**, 594).

From Himachal Pradesh to Arunachal Pradesh and Meghalaya up to 1,500 m.

*B. tulda Roxb.

Eng.–*Calcutta cane, common bamboo of Bengal*; H.–*Deobans*; Ass.– *Bejli*; B.–*Jowa*; Mal.–*Makor*; Garo–*Wati*; Lepcha–*Bleeng*; Tripura– *Jowa*.

Plant, in tetanus (*Econ Bot*, 1970, **24**, 241).

Wild in E. India, hills of Andhra Pradesh and Orissa, up to 600 m. Cultivated in plains of N. India.

B. vulgaris Schrad. ex Wendl. non Nees

Leaves used in burns and wound (*Econ Bot*, 1974, **28**, 5).

Shoots, cyanogenic compd., taxiphyllin. Lipid ext., β-sitosterol, campesterol and stigmasterol (*Chem Ber*, 1976, **109**, 3379).

BAPHICANTHUS (*Acanthaceae*)

B. cusia Bremek. syn. *Strobilanthes cusia* Imlay; *S. flaccidifolius* Nees

Eng.–*Assam indigo, Assam rum*; Ass.–*Rampat, rum*; Lushai–*Tiny*; Manipur–*Khum*; Mikir–*Bukangda*.

Leaves—astrin., diur. and lithotriptic (Wlth India, IIB, 38). Fresh juice contains an antifung. substance, tryptanthrin, and employed in Japan to kill dermatophytes causing 'athlete's foot' (*Planta Med*, 1979, **36**, 85).

BARBAREA (*Brassicaceae*)

*B. verna (Mill.) Aschers. syn. *B. praecox* R.Br.

Eng.–*Beele-Isie cress, early winter cress, scurvy cress.*

Leaves—pectoral and detergent. Antiscor., rich in vit. C (130mg/100g); herb contains a glucd., an enzyme and Ph-Et-mustard oil (*Econ Bot*, 1977, **31**, 76; Wlth India, IIB, 39).

Native to Europe, introduced into Nilgiris.

B. vulgaris R. Br. syn. *B. vulgaris* var. *taurica* Hook. f. & T. Anders.

Eng.–*Bitter winter cress, hedge mustard, yellow rocket.*

Herb—diur., anthelm. and stomch. (Wlth India, IIB, 39); preparation method of agent for stimulating spermatogenesis from pulverised herb (USSR Pat., 1979, 663401; *CA*, 1980, **92**, 220686t). Ingestion of plant in large quantities causes gastroenteritis in horses (Kingsbury, 158). Estrogen and toxic effect of herb ext. on exp. animals (*Can J Zool*, 1980, **58**, 1575).

Leaves, rich in vit. C (130mg/100g) (*Econ Bot*, 1977, **31**, 76). Ascorbic acid content of plant parts (*Ernaehr· Umsch*, 1981, **28**, 187; *CA*, **95**, 148869x). Roots contain sinigrin (Wlth India, IIB, 39).

BARLERIA (*Acanthaceae*)

B. buxifolia Linn.

EtOH(50%) ext. of plant, spasmog. (*Indian J Exp Biol*, 1974, **12**, 512).

B. cristata Linn. syn. *B. ciliata* Roxb.

Root decoct. given in anaemia (*in* Jain, 24). EtOH(50%) ext. of plant, spasmog. and hypoglyc. (*Indian J Exp Biol*, 1968, **6**, 232).

Violet flowers contain apigenin, its glucuronide, naringenin and malvindin 3,5-diglucd. (*J Indian Chem Soc*, 1972, **49**, 825). Roots contain 2 anthraquinones, bar-

lacristone and cristabarlone (*Indo-Soviet Symp on Chem of Natl Prod*, 1981, 84).

*B. cuspidata Heyne ex Nees

EtOH(50%) ext. of plant, CNS depress. (*Indian J Exp Biol*, 1974, **12**, 512).

Found in Western Peninsula.

B. dichotoma Roxb. syn. *B. cristata* var. *dichotoma* Prain

Flowers contain apigenin 7-glucuronide (*J Indian Chem Soc*, 1972, **49**, 825).

B. prionitis Linn.

Leaves—tribals apply infusion to soles of their feet to harden them to tolerate extreme heat, cold and rough soil (*Econ Bot*, 1978, **32**, 283). Crushed fresh leaves applied to wounds; juice with coconut oil applied on pimples [*J Sci Res Plants Med*, 1979-80, **1**(2), 37]. Leaves, as also flowering tops, diur.; leaf juice given in urinary and paralytic affections, and stomach disorders; applied to lacerated sole.

Bark—fresh juice, diaphor. and expect.

Roots—febge; as decoct. used as mouthwash in toothache (Wlth India, IIB, 47); for poisoning rat.

Plant—in whooping cough [*J Res Indian Med* , 1973, **8**(2), 75]; as decoct. in cough T.B. and toothache (*J Econ Tax Bot*, 1980, **1**, 143). Plant, antisep.(Wlth India, IIB, 47).

Plant contains β-sitosterol (*Bull Calcutta Sch Trop Med*, 1970, **18**, 7). Flowers, scutellarein-7-rhamnosylglucd. (*Phytochemistry*, 1971, **10**, 2822). Leaves and stems, iridoids, barlerin & Ac-barlerin (*Tetrahedron Lett*, 1975, 1995).

B. strigosa Willd.

Root decoct. in cough and broncht. (*Indian J For*, 1981, **4**, 115).

Plant mild antisep. (Wlth India, IIB, 48); contains β- & γ-sitosterol (*Bull Calcutta Sch Trop Med*, 1969, **17**, 120).

BARRINGTONIA (*Barringtoniaceae*)

B. acutangula Gaertn.

Eng.–*Indian oak.*

EtOH(50%) ext. of root, hypoglyc. and that of stem bark, antiprot. (*Indian J Exp Biol*, 1968, **6**, 232). Plant used against cholera (*Econ Bot*, 1970, **24**, 246).

Heartwood, triterp. dicarboxylic acid, barringtonic acid (*Indian J Chem*, 1964, **2**, 463). Triterp. barrigenic acid (*Phytochemistry*, 1976, **15**, 1780). Wood, hexa-OH-triterp., tanginol (*Tetrahedron*, 1967, **23**, 3837). Branch wood, barringtogenol E and triterp. acid, barrinic acid (*J Indian Chem Soc*, 1967, **44**, 991; 1972, **49**, 519).

Leaves, acutangulic and barringtogenic acids, and stigmasterol glucd. (*Curr Sci*, 1976, **45**, 518); also tangulic and oleanolic acids, β-amyrin, β-sitosterol & stigmasterol (*J Indian Chem Soc*, 1978, **55**, 1169).

Fruits, barringtogenol D, C & B; their constitutions (*Tetrahedron*, 1963, **19**, 1727; 1965, **21**, 381; 1968, **24**, 1113); triterp., barrigenic acid (*Phytochemistry*, 1976, **15**, 1780).

B. asiatica Kurz syn. *B. speciosa* J.R. & G. Forst.

Eng.–*Queen of the shores*; Andaman–*Dod-da.*

Fruit and root used against wounds. Fruit, as vermifuge. Fruit or bark for yaws; bark to treat T.B. Seeds against ringworm (*Econ Bot*, 1974, **28**,16).

Fruits, bartogenic acid (*Phytochemistry*, 1981, **20**, 333).

B. racemosa (Linn.) Spreng.

Toxic principle of bark concentrated mainly in resinous fraction (Watt & Breyer-Brandwijk, 534). Bark contains ellagic acid & its mono-, di-, & tri-OMe derivs.; flowers, cyanidin- and delphenidin-3-sambubiosides (*Phytochemistry*, 1968, **7**, 1803; 1976, **15**, 513).

BASELLA (*Basellaceae*)

B. alba Linn.

Eng.–*Indian spinach*, *Malabar nightshade.*

Used against syphilitic ulcer in nose (*Econ Bot*, 1970, **24**, 246). Root, poisonous (*Q J Crude Drug Res*, 1972, **12**, 1922).

B. alba. Linn. var. **rubra** Stewart syn. *B. rubra* Linn.

In Java, fruit juice of red var. applied to eyes in conjunctivitis.

Roots, rubft. and used as poultice to reduce local swellings; sap in acne. A decoct. of root given to stop bilious vomiting and in intestinal complaints (Wlth India, IIB, 52).

Leaves, extn. of w.-sol. polysaccharides (*Sci Res Dhaka*, 1969, **6**, 63; *CA*, 1970, **72**, 28398w). Loss of ascorbic acid content of leaves on heating (*Ecol Food Nutr*, 1973, **2**, 35; *CA*, 1974, **80**, 58545z). Herb, antivir. substance (*Shokubutsu Boeki*, 1977, **31**, 219; *CA*, 1978, **88**, 32465p); fats and sterols (*Bangladesh J Biol Sci*, 1979, **8**, 17; *CA*, 1980, **93**, 237544p).

BASILICUM (*Lamiaceae*)

*B. polystachyon (Linn.) Moench syn. *Moschosma polystachyon* Benth.

Crushed leaves applied to sprains; decoct. as sed. for epilepsy, palpitation of heart, neuralgia and convuls.; cause sores in mouth. In W. Africa, plant juice used in curing headache in children (Wlth India, IIB, 52).

From W. Bengal, Bihar southwards to Peninsular India.

BASSIA (*Sapotaceae*)

See **AISANDRA** and **MADHUCA**

BAUHINIA (*Caesalpiniaceae*)

*B. acuminata Linn.

Eng.–*Dwarf white bauhinia*; Mal.–*Velutthamandarom*; S.–*Sivamalli*; Tam.–*Vellaimandarai.*

Plant, juvenomimetic (*Entomon*, 1977, **2**, 259).

Decoct. of bark or leaves used in biliousness, in bladder stone, leprosy and asthma. It improves digestion; decoct. of root boiled with oil and applied to burns (Wlth India, IIB, 58).

Found almost throughout India.

B. foveolata Dalz.; see **Piliostigma foveolatum**

B. malabaricum Benth.; see **Piliostigma malabaricum**

*B. phoenicea Heyne

Roots used in preparation of ointment against itches and abscesses (Wlth India, IIB, 58).

Moist areas of Western Ghats of Karnataka and Kerala.

B. purpurea Linn.

Eng.–*Butterfly tree, geranium tree, orchid tree.*

Used in dropsy, anasarca, pain, rheum., thigh swelling, deer-epilepsy, convuls., delirium febris, datura intoxication, blackness of lip or tongue, animal bite (tiger, crocodile, snake, lizard, etc.), haemor., septicaemia, rinderpest, stupefication (*Econ Bot*, 1970, **24**, 241). Plant, antithyroid-like in exp. animals [*J Res Indian Med*, 1979, **14**(3-4), 67]. Ext. of stems and branches rubbed on fractured parts and also given for drinking to set right bones (*Bull Bot Surv India*, 1980, **22**, 161).

Flowers contain astragalin, isoquercitrin and quercetin (*Curr Sci*, 1967, **36**, 574); also pelargonidin 3-glucd. & 3-triglucd. (*Vijnana Parishad Anusandhan Patrika*, 1978, **21**, 177); butein galactoside (*Phytochemistry*, 1979, **18**, 689). Plant releases volat. Hg (*Org Geochem*, 1980, **2**, 99; *CA*, **92**, 194777b).

Seeds, alks.[*Lloydia*, 1970, **33**(3A), Suppl., 104]; trypsin and chymotrypsin inhibitors (*Phytochemistry*, 1974, **13**, 779); also two chalcone glycds. (*ibid*, 1979, **18**, 689; 1981, **20**, 2051).

B. racemosa Lamk

Bark, in glandular inflam., ulcers, skin diseases; efficacious remedy for goitre. Flowers, in haemor., piles, cough and as laxt.; leaves in worms [*J Res Indian Med*, 1973, **8**(2), 70].

EtOH(50%) ext. of seeds, anticancer (*Indian J Exp Biol*, 1968, **6**, 232). An ext. of seed agglutinated *Pseudomonas aeruginosa* isolates (*Jpn J Exp Med*, 1980, **50**, 263).

Stem bark, octacosane, β-amyrin and β-sitosterol (*Curr Sci*, 1976, **45**, 705).

*B. rufescens Lamk

Bark, used as an astrin. for treating diar. and dysen. Bark, tannins (18-20%). Decoct. of root or bark, for leprosy. Leaves, in eye troubles (Wlth India, IIB, 58).

Madhya Pradesh and Tamil Nadu.

B. semla Wunderlin syn. *B. retusa* Roxb.

Used in cholera, snake-bite and rinderpest (*Econ Bot*, 1970, **24**, 241). Preliminary pharmacol. (*Indian J Exp Biol*, 1971, **9**, 91).

Str. of gum (*Indian J Chem*, 1976, **14B**, 113). Protein isolate from seeds, hypocholesteremic and hypoglyc. in young normal as well as alloxan-induced diabetic albino rats (*J Indian Med Assoc*, 1977, **68**, 201). Bark, quercetin glucd. and rutin (*Proc Nat Acad Sci India*, 1978, **48A**, 183).

B. tomentosa Linn.

Eng.–*Bell/yellow bauhinia, St. Thomas tree.*

Leaves, an ingredient of a plaster applied to abscesses; seeds, tonic.

Seeds yield a fatty oil called 'Ebony oil', a w.-sol. mucilage, 7.4% and saponins (Wlth India, IIB, 55).

Flowers, isoquercitrin (6%), rutin (4.6%) and quercetin (small amts.); can be exploited commercially for rutin (*Indian J Chem*, 1963, **1**, 450; Wlth India, IIB, 55).

B. vahlii Wight & Arn.; see **Phanera vahlii**

B. variegata Linn.

Eng.–*Buddhist bauhinia, mountain ebony, orchid tree.*

Preliminary pharmacol. (*Indian J Exp Biol*, 1969, **7**, 250). Decoct. of root bark for lessening fatness and against tumours. Flower buds against tumours (*Econ Bot* 1971, **25**, 420); as laxt. (*Bull Bot Surv*

India, 1973, **15**, 13). W.-sol. portion of alc. ext. of plant, preventive against goitre in rats [*J Res India Med*, 1975, **10**(3), 12; 19]. Exts. of buds, flowers and bark, antibact. (*Indian Drugs*, 1978-79, **16**, 295). Leaves, as condiments. Seed ext. agglutinates human blood (*Econ Bot*, 1960 **14**, 232; Wlth India, IIB, 57).

BEAUMONTIA (*Apocynaceae*)

*B. grandiflora (Roxb.) Wall.

Eng.–*Easter-lily vine, Herald's trumpet, Nepal trumpet flower*; Lepcha–*Chomrik*.

Seeds yield 4 cardenolide glycds., oleandrin, wallinchoside, beauwalloside and beaumontoside; detn. of cardiotonic activity of beaumontoside (*Helv Chim Acta*, 1963, **46**, 505; *J Med Chem*, 1970, **13**, 1029); fermented seeds of Indian plant contain 8 additional cardenolides including digitoxigenin and oleandrigenin (*Pharm Acta Helv*, 1964, **39**, 168; *CA*, **61**, 7361h).

Leaves contain quercetin and tamarixetin (*Indian J Exp Biol*, 1978, **16**, 512); also *n*-hentriacontane, *n*- triacontane, palmitic, linoleic, and ursolic acids, β-sitosterol & its glucd. (*J Indian Chem'Soc*, 1981, **58**, 927). Stems or twigs, an alk. (Wlth India, IIB, 74).

Indigenous to Eastern Himalayas, grown in gardens throughout India for its beautiful foliage and fragrant flowers.

*B. jerdoniana Wight

Flowers, fragrant. Plant contains cardiotonic glycds. (Wlth India, IIB, 75).

Occurs throughout Western Ghats from Konkan to Kerala; also cultivated elsewhere as an ornamental.

*B. khasiana Hook.f.

Plant contains cardiotonic glycds. (Wlth India, IIB, 75).

Found in Meghalaya.

BEGONIA (*Begoniaceae*)

*B. cucullata Willd. var. **hookeri** Smith & Schubert

Aq. ext. of leaves and flowers active against Gram +ve and –ve bacteria (*Econ Bot*, 1959, **13**, 286).

Leaves contain oxalic, fumaric, malic, succinic and 3 other unidentified acids (*Ann Sci Univ Besancon Bot*, 1965, No.2, 24; *CA*, 1966, **65**, 7622h).

Native of S. America, introduced into India for ornament.

*B. heracleifolia Cham. & Schlecht. syn. *B. longipila* Lamk

Aq. ext. of leaves and flowers active against Gram +ve and –ve bacteria (*Econ Bot*, 1959, **13**, 286).

Native to Mexico, introduced into India.

*B. josephi DC.

Khasi–*Jajew*.

Bulbs eaten raw in stomach pain and indign. (*Econ Bot*, 1981, **35**,4).

Moist places and on roadsides near Elephant Falls in Shillong, Meghalaya.

*B. luxurians Scheidw.

Plant eaten as potherb. Decoct. of leaves used in fevers in Brazil (Uphof, 72).

Native to Brazil, introduced into Indian gardens.

*B. palmata D. Don var. **gamblei** Hara

B.–*Hooirjo*; Nagaland–*Teisu*.

Decoct. against fever and liver complaints; fresh shoots for tooth troubles (Wlth India, IIB, 102).

Found in N-E regions of India.

*B. picta Smith

Mundari–*Luncliara*; Oraon–*Pakkan chatta*.

Leaves—acidic in taste; used as a remedy for colic and dysen. (Hedrick, 85).

Almost throughout India up to 2,000 m.

B. rex Putz.

Leaves contain cyanidin 3-xylosylglucd. and rutin (*Phytochemistry*, 1964, **3**, 453).

*B. roxburghii DC.

Ass.& Meghalaya–*Kamchal.*

Tubers together with the fruits of *Solnea heterophylla* are boiled and decoct. taken in fever; rootstock, in fecal discharge in bile dysen. (*in* jain, 127, 140).

Khasi and Jaintia hills in Meghalaya.

*B. rubro-venia Hook.f.

Juice of roots taken as a cure for dysen. Plant used in diar., dysen. and other diseases (*in* Jain, 127).

Assam and Meghalaya.

BELAMCANDA (*Iridaceae*)

B. chinensis DC.

Eng.–*Blackberry lily, leopard lily.*

Rhizome—acrid, antipyr., expect., deobstruent, carmin., alexipharmic and diur. Used in gonor., pulmonary complaints and as blood purifier (Wlth India, IIB, 103). In China, used in laryngeal tumour and tumours of faces; also against breast cancer (*Lloydia*, 1969, **32**, 251).

Herb ext. useful in skin and cosmetic preparations (Jpn. Kokai, 1977, 7779032-33; *CA*, **87**, 157011y-12z). Stem chewed in food poisoning (*Ethnomedicine*, 1980, **6**, 143). Leaves and flowers contain glycoflavone (Wlth India, IIB, 103-104).

Chem. anal., confusing; drug (rhizomes) of Chinese and Indian origin, isoflavone glucd., shekanin (1.5% dry wt basis) identical with tectoridin, inactive both in pure and crude form (alc. ext.). Japanese plant known as *Hsieh-yu*, glucds., belamcamdin (should be belamcandin, Ed.) and iridin but no tectoridin. Plant, known in China as *Shehkan*, gave glucd. belamacamdin (*sic*) which on hydrolysis gave a penta-OH-mono-MeO isoflavone, belmacamgenin (should be belamcangenin, Ed.), *shehkan*, botanically referred to as *Belmacamda sinensis* is obviously a misnomer for *Balamcanda chinensis* (Wlth India, IIB, 103-04).

BENINCASA (*Cucurbitaceae*)

B. hispida (Thunb.) Cogn. syn. *B. cerifera* Savi

Eng.–*Ashgourd.*

Fruit—fruit as also seeds used in tumours (*Lloydia*, 1969, **32**, 92). In China, flesh, as demulc., thirst-quenching; and cooling in fever; raw flesh, remedy for facial eruptions. Juice, antid. for Hg and alc. poisoning. In Philippines, syrup, in respiratory afflictions (*Proc Fla State Hort Soc*, 1971, **84**, 104). Fruits made into '*Kushmanda lehyam*' can be stored for several years; recommended for epilepsy, constip., piles, dyspep., syphilis and diabetes (Wlth India, IIB, 108).

Seeds—in China, seed-kernel used as one of the ingredients in drug preparation for appendicitis (*Q J Crude Drug Res*, 1963, **3**, 437); EtOH and aq. exts., anthelm. (*Indian J Pharmacol*, 1981, **13**, 89); habitual consumption of seeds prevents hunger and prolongs life; kernel used against skin eruption, and seed ash, as remedy for gonor.

Leaves—purg.; juice or poultice used in bruises (*Proc Fla State Hort Soc*, 1971, **84**, 104).

Pollen, allergenic (*Indian J Med Res*, 1962, **50**, 881).

Ext. antivir. against Columbia S.K. virus in mice; activity due to non-dialyzable material in aq. ext. (*Med Pharmacol Exp*, 1967, **16**, 407).

Fruit, *n*-triacontanol, mannitol, several amino acids, glucose, rhamnose, lupeol and β-sitosterol (*Q J Crude Drug Res*, 1976, **14**, 163).

BENTHAMIDIA (*Cornaceae*)

*B. capitata Hara syn. *Cornus capitata* Wall. var. *khasiana* C.B. Clarke

H.–*Bamora, tharbal*; Ass.–*Dieng-sóh-japhon.*

Leaves and twigs contain an iridoid glucd., verbenalin (cornin, 0.07%) and phlorin (Phloroglucinol- β-glucd., 0.38%) (*Phytochemistry*, 1973, **12**, 2301; Wlth India, IIB, 108).

Distributed from Kashmir to Bhutan and in Meghalaya.

BERBERIS (*Berberidaceae*)

Genus commonly known in Eng., as *Barberry* or in vern. as *Kashmal* or *kinjosa*.

Roots—alongwith stem bark a reputed drug in Ayurvedic med. Contain several alks. including berberine.

Rasaut—locally prepared drug from root bark, root chips and lower stemwood by boiling with w., straining and evaporating till a dark brown sticky mass like opium, is obtained. It is bitter, tonic, cholag., stomch., laxt., diaphor., antipyr. and antisep. Administered in indolent ulcers and haemor. (Wlth India, IIB, 115). In Unani system, used in leprosy (*J Nat Integ Med Assoc*, 1981, **23**, 43).

Berberine—chief active alk. from roots and stembark. Manufactured in India mostly from roots of *B. aristata* and *B. asiatica.*

B. aristata DC.

Roots—EtOH(50%) ext. of root, hypoglyc. and anticancer (*Indian J Exp Biol*, 1968, **6**, 232). *Raswat*, a crude dried preparation inhibited cholera toxin-induced diar. in rats (*Indian J Med Res*, 1977, **65**, 133; 305). In Tibet, decoct. used in piles, gastric disorders and other allied complaints (*Nagarjun*, 1978-79, **22**, 190; *Bull Med Ethno Bot Res*, 1980, **1**, 455). Root and root bark, gastro-irrit. (*Am Pharm NS*, 1981, **21**, 42). Berberis ext., one of the minor ingredients of drug 'Geriforte', useful in senile pruritus (*Rajasthan Med J*, 1980, **19**, 23); antifatigue in rats (*Indian Drugs*, 1980-81, **18**, 346); with exts. of *Iris germanica* and *Terminalia chebula* used as contracep. (*Ancient Sci Life*, 1981-82, **1**, 72).

Plant—used as fish poison (*Nagarjun*, 1979-80, **23**, 177). In Unani system, in enlargement of spleen and as emmen. [*East Pharm*, 1980, **23**(272), 39]. In '*Charak Samhita*', plant preparation, for regulating fat metabolism (*Q J Crude Drug Res*, 1972, **12**, 1988). Ingredient of indigenous drug 'Vitafix', useful in premature ejaculation (*Indian Pract*, 1980, **33**, 81); an indigenous preparation '*Madhudarvyadhi*',

useful in conjunctivitis, clin. trial (*J Nat Integ Med Assoc*, 1980, **22**, 135); in jaundice, clin. trials (*Indian J Pharmacol*, 1981, **13**, 61).

Fresh berries—laxt. and antiscor.; useful in piles, sores and eye diseases. Mixed with bark of *Cinnamomum tamala* given in leucor. Decoct. as mouth-wash for treating, swollen gums and toothache (Wlth India, IIB, 115). Fruit useful in stomach disorders (*Khadi Gramodyog*, 1972-73, **19**, 273).

Bark in liver complaints (*Acta Phytother*, 1964, **11**, 141).

Berberine—produces long lasting, dose ·related fall in B.P. of anaesthetised rabbits. Also useful in oriental sores. As HCl and sulphate used in drugs for cholera, diar., dysen., and eye complaints. They help in diagnosis of latent malaria (Wlth India, IIB, 114). Anti-T.B. (*Indian J Pharm*, 1960, **22**, 34; *ibid*, 1967, **29**, 157); useful in acute cholera [*East Pharm*, 1967, **10**(110), 42]; sulphate antibact. against *Staphylococcus aureus* (*Arch Immunol Ther Exp*, 1972, **20**, 353; *CA*, **77**, 135606n). Thiophosphamide derivs., antitumour (*Farm Zh Kiev*, 1975, **30**, 40; *in* Wagner & Wolff, 650). Infusion of berberine given i.v. to rats, B.P. lowering (*Gen Pharmacol*, 1979, **10**, 177). As HCl useful in lesions and sores, a clin. study (*Indian J Dermatol Vernereol Leprol*, 1980, **46**, 163).

Berberine, extn. from *B. vulgaris* (*Yakugaku Zasshi*, 1969, **89**, 1286); quant. detn. (*Farmatsiya Moscow*, 1971, **20**, 28); TLC- fluorim. detn. (*Shoyakugaku Zasshi*, 1976, **30**, 127; *CA*, 1977, **87**, 29066h). TLC and UV spectrophotom. in different spp. [*Indian Drugs Pharmac Ind*, 1979, **14**(2), 17]. Quant. detn. in drugs by HSLC (*Herba Pol*, 1978, **24**, 199). Extn. of berbamine, oxyacanthine and berberine from bark (Rom. Pat., 1978, 63426; *CA*, 1979, **90**, 76555p). Spectrofluorim. detn. (*Acta Pharm Jugosl*, 1980, **30**, 31).

B. asiatica Roxb. ex DC. non Griff.

EtOH(50%) ext. of roots, spasmol. and anticancer (*Indian J Exp Biol*, 1968, **6**, 232).

Ayurvedic drug for conception (*J Sci Res Plants Med*, 1981, **2**, 39). Stems used in rheum. Berries mildly laxt. and given to children (Wlth India, IIB, 117).

Roots contain berberine, palmitine, jatrorrhizine, columbamine, tetrahydropalmitine, berbamine, oxyberberine and oxyacanthine (*Indian J Chem*, 1968, **6**, 123). Optimum conditions for production of berberine from roots [*J Res Indian Med*, 1976, **11**(4), 34].

Berbamine (obtained from *B.poiretii* root from China) increased leucocytes (*Acta Bot Sin*, 1978, **20**, 255; *Chin Pharm Bull*, 1979, **14**, 381).

*B. chitria Lindl. syn *B. aristata* auct. Hook.f. & Thoms. (FBI) in part, non DC.

Roots and stem bark richest source of alks. (5% and 4.2% resp. as berberine) (Wlth India, IIB, 117).

In Himalayas, from Kashmir to Nepal at 1,500 - 2,400 m.

B. insignis Hook. f. & Thoms. var. **shergaonensis** Ahredt.

EtOH(50%) ext. of aerial parts, diur. (*Indian J Exp Biol*, 1974, **12**, 512).

B. lycium Royle

EtOH(50%) ext. of roots, antiprot., antivir., spasmol. and anticancer (*Indian J Exp Biol*, 1968, **6**, 232).

Roots, alks., berbenine, berbericine and berbericinine (*Pak J Sci Ind Res*, 1966, **9**, 343). Pharmacol. of berbenine; shows depress. action on isolated rabbit heart; B.P. falls with cardiac depress. [*ibid*, 1967, **10**, 34; *Life Sci*, 1969, 8(Pt. 1), 933]. Berbericine identical with berberine-acetone complex (*Indian J Chem*, 1971, **9**, 503). Anal. for alk. (*Pak J For*, 1972, **22**, 43; *CA*, **77**, 149688c). Artefact alks., berberinechloroform and palmatinechloroform, and oxyberberine (*Phytochemistry*, 1973, **12**, 1822).

Pharmacognosy of roots; chief alks., umbellatine and berberine; also contains berbamine (*Pak J For*, 1978, **28**, 25).

B. pachyacantha Koehne syn. *B. thunbergii* DC.; *B. vulgaris* auct. non Linn.

Antibiotic activity of plant ext. and its alk. (*Clujul Med*, 1973, **46**, 627). Plant ext., antiinflam. (*Yakugaku Zasshi*, 1974, **94**, 796).

Alks.—ext. with other alk. mixt. used for treating obstruction of lymphatic system (Ger. Offen, 1971, 1963706; *CA*, **75**, 91299s). Anal. (*Pak J For* 1972, **22**, 43; *CA*, **77**, 149688c). TLC- spectrophotom. detn. (*Farmatsiya Moscow*, 1974, **23**, 27); sprectrophotom. detn. of protoberberine alks. of different plant parts (*Acta Pol Pharm*, 1974, **31**, 683; *CA*, 1975, **82**, 121750w); gravimetric detn. (*Planta Med*, 1975, **27**, 213). Extn. of alks. from bark (Rom. Pat., 1978, 63426; *CA*, 1979, **90**, 76555p).

Roots, magnoflorine and columbamine (*Acta Pol Pharm*, 1971, **28**, 81; *CA*, **75**, 1320q). Chem. compn. of fruits (*Rastit Resur*, 1974, **10**, 237; *CA*, **81**, 60875w). Seeds, alks. (*Chem Zvesti*, 1980, **34**, 259; *CA*, **93**, 91881x). Berbamine-HCl hypoten. in animals (*Acta Pharm Sin*, 1980, **15**, 248).

Berberine extn. and detn., see *B. aristata*. Leaf pigments [*Bull Torrey Bot Club*, 1969, **96**, 594; *Ekologiya*, 1971, (2), 45]; carbohydrates (*Carbohydr Res*, 1972, **23**, 379; *CA*, **77**, 84753y).

B. petiolaris Wall. ex G. Don

Roots used as diur.; yielded berberine 0.43%, berbericine, 0.78%; berbericinine, 0.67% and polar alk., 0.4% (*Sci Res Dacca*, 1968, **5**, 75; *CA*, **69**, 61516u); also berbamine, berberine chloride and palmitine (*Pak J Sci Ind Res*, 1970, **13**, 49).

B. umbellata Wall.

Root contains 2,5-bis-(2′-OMe-5′-MePh)furan (*Phytochemistry*, 1981, **20**, 295).

BERCHEMIA (*Rhamnaceae*)

B. edgeworthii M.A. Laws. syn. *B. lineata* M.A. Laws. non DC.

Leaves and needles, as source of catechols (*Prikl Biokhim Microbiol*, 1972, **8**, 207).

BERGENIA (*Saxifragaceae*)

B. ciliata(Haw.) Stemb. syn. *B. ligulata* Engl.; *Saxifraga ligulata* Wall.

S.–*Pashanabheda*; H.–*Pakharbhed*; Dharchula–*Silpano*.

Rhizomes—dried rhizomes, astrin., tonic, antiscor., and laxt.; given in ulcers, cough and spleen enlargement (Wlth India, IIB, 120). Powd. taken with water in dysurea and menor. Also used sometimes in urinary diseases (*Khadi Gramodyog*, 1980-81, **27**, 401).

EtOH(50%) ext. of rhizome, spasmog., antiprot. and anticancer (*Indian J Exp Biol*, 1968, **6**, 232).

Powd. root mixed with water applied on burns and cuts; mixed with soybean (*Glycine max* seeds), given to cattle in diar. (*Econ Bot*, 1971, **25**, 421). Pharmacognosy of Pashanbhed (*Q J Crude Drug Res*, 1971, **11**, 1683). Alc. ext. of roots, antilithic. Acetone ext. of root bark, cardiotoxic, CNS depress. and antiinflam.; in mild doses diur. but antidiur. in higher doses [*J Res Indian Med*, 1974, **9**(2), 1; 1975, **10**(4), 7]. One of the main constituents of indigenous drug 'Cystone' used successfully for urinary tract infections (*Probe*, 1979-80, **19**, 270).

Leaves—juice used in earache (Wlth India, IIB, 120). In Himalayan region, plant used in vertigo, headache, dizziness; leaves for dissolving kidney stones (*Nagarjun*, 1979-80, **23**, 242).

Roots contain (+)-afzelachin (*Ann Ist Super Sanita*, 1969, **5**, 555; *CA*, 1970, **73**, 117127v); bergenin (0.6%), a C-glycd. and β-sitosterol (*Indian J Chem*, 1974, **12**, 1038). Bergenin prevented stress-induced erosions in rats and lowered gastric outputs (*Gen Pharmacol*, 1980, **11**, 361).

*B. **purpurascens** Engl. syn. *Saxifraga purpurascens* Hook. f. & Thoms.

Rhizomes—used as a tonic and as a styptic (Uphof, 74).

Found from Nepal to Arunachal Pradesh between 3,000-5,000 m.

*B. **stracheyi** Engl. syn. *Saxifraga stracheyi* Hook.f. & Thoms.; *S. ciliata* Lindl. non Royle

Rhizome used in menor. and in urinary diseases (*Khadi Gramodyog*, 1972-73, **19**, 277); contains bergenin (0.75%), β-sitosterol and (+)-catechin 3-gallate (Wlth India, IIB, 120; *Indian J Chem*, 1974, **12**, 1038).

Commonly found from Kashmir to Uttar Pradesh between 2,400-4,800 m.

BERGIA (*Elatinaceae*)

B. suffruticosa Fenzl syn. *B. odorata* Edgew.

Poultice of leaves applied to sores (Wlth India, IIB, 120). Plant paste as antid. against scorpion sting (*Econ Bot*, 1978, **32**,278).

BERRYA (*Tiliaceae*)

*B. **cordifolia**(Willd.) Burret syn. *B.ammonilla* Roxb.

Eng.–*Trinocomalee wood*; Tam–*Charandalai*; Tel.–*Sarala-devadaaru.*

EtOH ext. of seeds, insectic. against European corn bores (*J Econ Entomol*, 1979, **72**, 541).

Native to Sri Lanka, frequently found in Andamans and S. India.

BETA (*Chenopodiaceae*)

B. vulgaris Linn. var. **alba** DC. & var. **saccarifera** Alef.; ssp. **esculenta** (Salisb.) Gurke var. **altissima** Rossig. Eng.–*Sugarbeet.*

Pectic substances from bulb; pulp useful as blood plasma substitute (*Org Khim Puti Razvit Khim Proizvod Kirg*, 1976, 89; *CA*, 1978, **88**, 158334p). Root ext., +ve test for antifert. activity (*Indian J Med Res*, 1979, **70**, 517). Plant causes oxalate poisoning in

cattle [*Indian Farming*, 1966, **16**(9), 43].
Antimicrob. substance from plant tissues
(*Lloydia*, 1967, **30**, 177).

Root uronic acid, 7.16% dry basis (*Zh
Prikl Khim*, 1964, **37**, 462). Gas
chromatogr. of saponins (*Period Polytech
Chem Eng*, 1969, **12**, 347; *CA*, **71**,
111636x). Saponins of raw sugarbeet (*Glas
Hem Drus Beograd*, 1970, **35**, 313; *CA*,
1971, **75**, 7705r). Str. of beet sapogenin
(*Cukoripar*, 1970, **23**, 71; *CA*, **73**, 73088b).
Extn. of saponins and sapogenins; saponin
detn. (*Tehnika*, 1970, **25**, 534; 1971, **26**,
16; *CA*, **73**, 16578n; **75**, 78400y). Tuber,
triterp. glucds. (*Khim Prir Soedin*, 1970, **6**,
272; *CA*, **73**, 63200t).

Biochem. and use of beet constituent,
betaine, rev., 138 refs. (*Zucker*, 1972, **25**,
48; *CA*, **76**, 122991p).

Leaves, ferulic, caffeic and chlorogenic
acids, paper chromatogr. detn. (*Z Lebensm
Unters Forsch*, 1966, **132**, 193; *CA*, 1967,
66, 45594a); 3 polyphenols
(*Phytochemistry*, 1976, **6**, 417); growth
stimulator with panthothenic activity
[*Nauch Dokl Vyssh Shk, Biol Nauki*, 1967,
(12), 103; *CA*, 1968, **68**, 57606k]; isolation
and identn. of active principle responsible
for estrogenicity (*Planta Med*, 1971, **19**,
208). Leaves contain oxalic acid (*Z
Labensm Unters Forsch*, 1978, **166**, 153;
CA, **89**, 2614q); volat. compds.
(*Phytochemistry*, 1981, **20**, 2292).

Plant, source of vit.A (*ISI Bull*, 1967,
19, 393). Seeds, α-glucosidase (*Agric Biol
Chem*, 1978, **42**, 241).

B. vulgaris Linn. var. **atrorubura** syn. *B.
vulgaris* Linn. ssp. *esculenta* (Salisb.)
Gurke var. *rubra* (Linn.) Moq.

Eng.–*Beet root*.

Fat-sol. beetroot ext., useful in humans
to treat vascular and metabolic disorders
(Fr Demande, 1974, 2187325; *CA*, **81**,
58449s).

Basic proteins and a new "blue" pas-
tocyanin-like protein from red beets.
Proteins, having isoelectric points 9.1 and
9.7, had a tumour growth-retarding effect
(*Proc Hung Annu Meet Biochem*, 1975, 83;
CA, 1976, **85**, 119628f).

Beet root pigment (betanin) and uric
acid crystals, and relation of findings to
nephrolithiasis discussed (*Isr J Med Sci*,
1976, **12**, 73). Cardiovascular and hypoten.
effect of beetroot (betanin) in rats (*Food
Cosmet Toxicol*, 1980, **18**, 363).

BETULA (*Betulaceae*)

B. alnoides Buch.-Ham. ex D. Don syn. *B.
acuminata* Wall.

Eng.–*Indian birch, naga birch*.

Preliminary pharmacol. (*Indian J Exp
Biol*, 1980, **18**, 594).

B. utilis D. Don syn. *B. bhojpatra* Wall.

Eng.–*Birch tree*.

Resin mixed with water, administered
with butter after menstrual cycle, works as
oral contracep. Used on cuts and burns
(*Econ Bot*, 1971, **25**, 414).

Used for alimentary disorder of animals.
Bark, arom.; possess antifert. activity
(Wlth India, IIB, 148). As fumigant to
produce postpartum contraction (*Khadi
Gramodyog*, 1972-73, **19**, 276).

Preliminary pharmacol. (*Indian J Exp
Biol*, 1980, **18**, 594).

Stem bark, irrit. poison; contains alk.,
volat. oil and betuline (*Q J Crude Drug
Res*, 1972, **12**, 1922). Outer bark contains
leucocyanidin, betulin, lupeol, oleanolic &
Ac-oleanolic acids (*Indian J Chem*, 1968,
6, 231). Bark, betulin and karachic acid
(*Phytochemistry*, 1973, **12**, 214; 1975, **14**,
789; *Pak J Sci Ind Res*, 1975, **17**, 195).

Chem. of birch tree, rev., 54 refs. [*East
Pharm*, 1970, **13**(149), 127].

BIDENS (*Asteraceae*)

*****B. bipinnata** Linn. syn. *B. pilosa* Linn.
var. *bipinnata* Hook. f. (FBI) in part.

Eng.–*Beggar lice, Spanish needles*.

Plant—warmed juice of fresh plant used
in earache and conjunctivitis, and as styptic
on wounds. Aq. ext. of stem, leaves and
flowers., antibiot. against *Micrococcus
pyogenes* var. *aureus*, and yeast. Young

plant relished by cattle, but rich in a volat. oil with objectionable odour which may taint milk.

Seed—emmen., expect., stim., antisp. and used in asthma; also act as local irrit. Root used for same purpose as seeds (Wlth India, IIB, 149).

Found almost throughout India.

*B. biternata (Lour.) Merrill & Sherff ex Sherff syn. *B. chinensis* Willd.; *B. pilosa* auct., non Linn.

H. & P.–*Chirchitta*; G.–*Samara kokadi*; Oriya–*Magha latenga*; H.P.– *Chor pushi*; Mundari – *Huring sargujia ba*.

Plant given in leprosy and skin diseases. Also useful in fistulae, pustules, tumours, phthisis, coughs, bites, stabs and other wounds. Infusion of leaf and root, a remedy for colic. Juice of leaves applied to heal ulcers and to cure eye and ear complaints. Dried flower buds used in toothache. Flowers, in diar. Achenes cause dermatosis. Seeds, anthelm. to animals (Wlth India, IIB, 150).

Bruised leaves applied to forehead in headache (*Bull Bot Surv India*, 1976, **18**, 166). Roots reduced toothache; plant juice, for eyesores (*J Econ Tax Bot*, 1980, **1**, 137).

Throughout India as weed up to 2,000 m.

*B. cernua Linn.

Eng.–*Burr marigold*.

Essent. oil, diur. and laxt.; applied for healing wounds (Wlth India, IIB, 150).

Essent. oil, antimicrob.; activity due to arom. hydrocarbons and 1-Ph-hepta-1,3,5-triyne. Triyne inhibits Gram +ve bacteria, dermophytes, certain yeast and mould fungi in dil. from 1:100,000 to 1:200,000 (*Antibiotiki*, 1968, **13**, 167; *CA*, **68**, 85073c).

Herb contains tannin, 4.5-5.8; ascorbic acid, 121.7-139.3; carotene, 0.4-1.5 mg/100g; five flavons., 0.5-2.9% [*Issled Lek Prep Prir Sint Proiskhozhd Mater Mezhvuz Nauchn Konf*, 1974 (Pub. 1975), 4; *CA*, 1977, **86**, 167869c].

Western Himalayas from Kashmir to Chamba at 1,500-1,800 m.

*B. pilosa Linn. var. **minor** (Blume) Sherff syn. *B. pilosa* Linn. var. *bipinnata* Hook. f. (FBI) in part.

Plant used as cure for leprosy and various skin diseases. Seeds administered as anthelm. to animals [*J Res Indian Med*, 1973, **8**(1), 76].

Plant from Taiwan contains β-sitosterol, stigmasterol, phytosterin-B and hentricontanol [Wlth India, IIB, 150; *Hua Hsueh*, 1975, (2), 38; *CA*, 1976, **84**, 176691z].

Phytosterin B, hypoglyc. like insulin in normal and diabetic rats (*Taiwan I Hsueh Hui Tsa Chih*, 1967, **66**, 58; *CA*, 1968, **68**. 20822b).

Plant contains several polyacetylenes, phototoxic to bacteria, fungi and human fibroblast cells; toxic principle, Ph-heptatriyne (*J Natl Prod*, 1979, **42**, 103).

Uttar Pradesh, Sikkim and Meghalaya.

B. tripartita Linn.

Eng.–*Burr marigold*; *three-lobed butterburr*.

Herb—antiscor., diaphor., emmen., diur., antisep., aper., febge., sed., and mild narcotic. Particularly useful in dropsy, gout, haemat. Very effective as respiratory and uterine haemor.; addn. of ginger enhances its usefulness (Wlth India, IIB, 150).

Seeds—emmen., expect., diur. and also for kidney and gall stones.

Root—aper. (Hocking, 28).

Herb contains tannins, 2% and essent. oil, 0.11% (Wlth India, IIB, 150). Several flavons. (*Acta Pol Pharm*, 1963, **20**, 357; *CA*, 1965, **62**, 1510c); luteolin & its 7-glucd.; butin glucds. and buteine glucd.; also coumarins umbelliferon, scopoletin and dihydroxycoumarin; and identn. of flavon., as isookanin glucd. (*Khim Prir Soedin*, 1972, **8**, 121; 440; 668; 1975, **11**, 144; *CA*, **77**, 58828g; 1973, **78**, 1987z; 94851p; **83**, 93862j). Flavon., isocoreopsin (*Farm Zh Kiev*, 1975, **30**, 88; *CA*, **83**, 128660w).

Catechol tannins (6.5-12.0%), flavons. (0.5%) and volat. oil (0.05-0.11%) of herb and fruits (*Acta Pharm Jugosl*, 1976, **26**, 253; *CA*, 1977, **86**, 27646c).

Leaves, ascorbic acid (134.4 mg/100g). Fruits, fixed oil (19.5%) similar to sunflower oil (Wlth India, IIB, 150).

BIEBERSTEINIA (*Biebersteiniaceae*)

*B. odora Steph. ex Fisch. syn *B. emodi* Jaub. & Spach

Ladakh–*Drakspose.*

Plant used in healing of wounds, ulcers, cuts and in peptic ulcer (*in* Atal & Kapur, Med. Plants, 521).

Western Himalayas up to 5,000 m.

BIGNONIA (*Bignoniaceae*)

*B. capreolata Linn. syn. *B. alliacea* Lamk; *Adenocalymna alliaceum* Miers.

Eng.–*Cross-vine; quarter vine.*

Root—substitute for sarsaparilla; decoct. as detergent, aper. and diur. (Wlth India, IIB, 151).

Essent. oil from flowers and leaves contain allyl sulphides; leaves, alliin (*Phytochemistry*, 1978, **17**, 1660; 1980, **20**, 822). Flower flavons. (*Indian J Pharm Sci*, 1978, **40**, 226; *Curr Sci*, 1980, **49**, 468).

Native to N. America, grown as an ornamental.

BIOPHYTUM (*Oxalidaceae*)

*B. reinwardtii Klotzsch

Mundari–*Durumbihir;* Oraon–*Lajauri.*

Herb decoct. used in fevers. In Bihar, leaves and roots given in insomnia (Wlth India, IIB, 151).

Distributed from Kumaun to Arunachal Pradesh up to 1,800 m and extending up to peninsular India.

B. sensitivum DC. syn. *Oxalis sensitiva* Linn.

Plant—tonic and stim.; used in chest complaints, convuls., cramps, burning pain and burns (Wlth India, IIB, 151; *Econ Bot*, 1970, **24**, 246); also in inflam. tumours (*Lloydia*, 1970, **33**, 313). Dried and powd.

plant given to cattle to stop excess salivation [*J Sci Res Plants Med*, 1979-80, **1**(2),37]. Pounded plant given in insomnia (*Nagarjun*, 1980-81, **24**, 1).

Leaves—astrin. and antisep.; pounded or bruised or their juice used in dressing burns and contusions. Decoct. given in asthma and phthisis. Aq. ext. inhibited *Mycobacterium tuberculosis* 607 (Wlth India, IIB, 151); saline ext. hypoglyc. in rabbit (*Planta Med*, 1972, **21**, 364). In Gujarat, tribals believe that dried leaves smoked with tobacco render man infertile while excessive use makes him impotent (*Econ Bot*, 1978, **32**, 378). Paste applied to wounds and cuts to stop bleeding. Also as a tonic.

Root decoct. in fever (*J Econ Tax Bot*, 1981, **2**, 173).

*B.umbraculum Welw. syn. *B. petersianum* Klotzsch

Mundari–*Durumbihir;* Oraon–*Lajauri.*

Plant used as remedy for snake-bite; also given to women to increase fertility. Leaves and roots, purg. In Bihar, they are given in insomnia (Wlth India, IIB, 152).

Found in Meghalaya, Bihar, Orissa, Andhra Pradesh, Tamil Nadu, Karnataka, and Kerala.

BISCHOFIA (*Bischofiaceae*)

B. javanica Blume

Eng.–*Bishop wood.*

Bark—in Samoa, taken for cough. Inner bark for throat ailments, high fever, diar. in children, burns and cracks on the soles of feet.

Plant, in gastro-diar.; leaves, to treat sores, eye diseases and toothache (*Econ Bot*, 1974, **28**, 12). Seed ext., haemagglutinating (*Aust J Exp Biol Med Sci*, 1981, **59**, 195).

Bark contains epifriedelanol-OAc, friedelin, betulinic acid and β-sitosterol (*J Indian Chem Soc*, 1969, **46**, 757). Root, β-amyrin, ursolic acid and β-sitosterol (*Curr Sci*, 1971, **40**, 11).

Leaves contain tartaric acid, 8-10%; and vit.C, 136 mg/100g (Wlth India, IIB, 152). Yield ellagic acid, β-sitosterol, friedelin, friedelan-3β-ol, friedelan-3α-ol & its -Ac deriv.(*Aust J Chem*, 1968, **21**, 1675).

BISTORTA (*Polygonaceae*)

*B. affinis Greene syn. *Polygonum affine* D. Don

Leaves, 7 flavon., including flavone, isoaffinetin (*Z Pflanzenphysiol*, 1976, **79**, 372; 465).

Himalayas from Kashmir to Nepal at 2,400-4,800 m.

*B. amplexicaulis Greene syn. *Polygonum amplexicaule* D. Don

Eng.–*Mountain fleece*; Garhwal–*Amli*; Kash.–*Ajbar*; U.P.–*Durpa tandar.*

Root-stock sold as the drug '*Anjubar*', roots used medicinally in cough and dysen. (*Khadi Gramodyog*, 1972-73, **19**, 276). In Tibetan system of medicine, powd. roots used as a diur., blood purifier, and in post-natal diseases, and also to reduce billiousness (*Nagarjun*, 1978-79, **22**, 19); used as a substitute for sarsaparilla, reported to be useful in oesophageal cancer (Wlth India, IIB, 157).

Sub-alpine and alpine Himalayas from Jammu & Kashmir to Bhutan, between 1,800 and 4,200 m.

*B. macrophylla Sojak syn. *Polygonum macrophyllum* D. Don

Herb good astrin(Wlth India, IIB, 157).

Distributed in Himalayas from Garhwal to Bhutan at 3,300–4,600 m.

BIXA (*Bixaceae*)

B. orellana Linn.

Eng.–*Annatto, arnato, Chinese dye tree, lipstick tree, monkey turmeric, roucou, safron tree.*

Root—roots when used as a meat flavouring, impart a saffron-like taste and colour. Pulverised, antisecretary; aq. ext. antisp. and hypoten. (Wlth India, IIB, 159). EtOH ext. of defatted root bark, an-timicrob., weak CNS-depress. and spasmog. (*Llyodia*, 1972, **35**, 35).

Seed—pulp, haemostatic, antidysen., diur., laxt., febge., digest. Prescribed in epilepsy and skin diseases. Fresh pulp applied to burns to prevent blisters and scars. Antid. to cassava and physic nut poisoning. Seed fatty oil used in leprosy (Wlth India, IIB, 159). Pulp, useful in kidney diseases (*Perfum Essent Oil Rec*, 1969, **60**, 247).

Leaves—decoct. used as a gargle for sore throat; infusion in dysen. Popular febge. Pounded leaves on maceration in w. yield a gummy substance used in gonor., and as diur. Twigs, in liver diseases and as emol. (Wlth India, IIB, 159). HCl ext., anticancer (*Philipp J Sci*, 1967, **96**, 393); poultice applied to cuts and gashes as scar-preventive; in Columbia, bixa paste considered aphrodis. (*Econ Bot*, 1971, **25**, 240; 1970, **24**, 355).

Seeds, a carotenoid, bixin (70-80% of total pigments (Merck Index, 158).

Bixin—oil-sol. and occurs in unstable *cis*-form and changes to *trans*-form also called isobixin; on saponification gives w.-sol. product, norbixin. Annatto dye, nontoxic and non-carcinogenic. Used in colouring food, cosmetics, pharmaceutical ointments and as mosquito repellent (Wlth India, IIB, 159).

In Hawaii, dry wood used against fainting, mouth sores, and impure blood (*Econ Bot*, 1971, **25**, 245). Preliminary pharmacol. of plant (*India J Exp Biol*, 1977, **15**, 208).

Roots, triterp. tomentosic acid and another unidentified one (*J Org Chem*, 1965, **30**, 2856).

Leaves, essent. oil (0.4%), which contains sesquiterp., bixaghanene (ishwarane) (*Perfum Essent Oil Rec*, 1969, **60**, 247; *Phytochemistry*, 1973, **12**, 2995). Leaves, flavons., 7-bisulphates of apigenin, luteolin and hypolaetin (*ibid*, 1975, **14**, 1331).

BLACHIA (*Euphorbiaceae*)

*B. denudata Benth.

Preliminary pharmacol. (*Indian J Exp Biol*, 1974, **12**, 512).

Reported from Jogfall, Karnataka.

*B. umbellata Baill.

EtOH(50%) ext. of aerial parts, diur. (*Indian J Exp Biol*, 1977, **15**, 208).

From Western Ghats to Coorg southwards.

BLECHNUM (*Blechnaceae*)

*B. occidentale Linn.

EtOH(50%) ext. of plant, hypoten. and diur. (*Indian J Exp Biol*, 1977, **15**, 208).

Vaythri, Kerala.

B. orientale Linn.

H.–*Hathethazori*; Lushai–*Vomban*.

EtOH(50%) ext. of plant, spasmol. (*Indian J Exp Biol*, 1969, **7**, 250).

Rhizome used for urinary disorders (Wlth India, IIB, 162); and as a cure of *sanipat* (delirium) (*J Sci Res BHU*, 1969-70, **20**, 227).

Chlorogenic acid (*Phytochemistry*, 1968, **7**, 1825).

BLEPHARIS (*Acanthaceae*)

B. linariefolia Pers. syn. *B. sindica* Stocks ex T. Anders.

Plant boiled with milk taken as tonic (*J Agric Trop Bot Appl*, 1966, **13**, 249).EtOH(50%) ext. of flower, anticancer (*Indian J Exp Biol*, 1980, **18**, 594).

B. persica (Burm.f.) Kuntze syn. *B. edulis* Pers.

Leaves useful in wounds, ulcers, nasal haemor., asthma, throat inflam., ascites, liver and spleen complaints and as purg. Roots, diur.; beneficial in urinary discharges and dysmenor. (Wlth India, IIB, 162).

Seeds, deobstruent and useful in strangury and conjunctivitis (Wlth India, IIB, 162).

Plant used in rheum. and impotency (*Sachitra Ayurveda*, 1980-81, **33**, 670).

Seeds contain isocoumarin glucd., blepharin (*Chem Ind Lond*, 1969, 328); a saponin, which on hydrolysis gave lupeol (*Indian J Appl Chem*, 1969, **32**, 72); also β-sitosterol glucd. and blepharigenin [*J Res Indian Med*, 1973, **8**(4), 27].

*B. repens (Vahl) Roth

Leaf paste applied to forehead for curing headache [*J Econ Tax Bot*, 1981, **2**, 188].

Common in Palamalai, T. N.

BLEPHARISPERMUM (*Asteraceae*)

*B. sub-sessile DC.

Decoct. of herb, tonic (*Econ Bot*, 1965, **19**, 242).

Bastar, M.P.

BLIGHIA (*Sapindaceae*).

B. sapida Koenig & Sims syn. *Sapindus obovatus* Wight & Arn.

Eng.–*Akee apple*.

Fruits and seeds—poisonous; ingestion causes vomiting sickness due to toxic principles, hypoglycin(e) A & B. Unripe fruit more toxic than ripe. Parboiled aril, consumed on frying; pleasant, slightly nutty in flavour; this preparation considered a delicacy. Belief that ripe, cooked aril is non-toxic has been supported in some exp., but contradicted by other findings (*Curr Sci*, 1964, **33**, 323; Kingsbury, 22, 217); improperly prepared fruit retains hypoglyc. compd. (*J Agric Food Chem*, 1969, **17**, 492).

Bark—used as liniment for oedemas and intercostal pains; seasoned with Guinea grains and ginger, eaten to allay orchitis pain. Alongwith chillies, ground bark used in Ghana, for rubbing on body as stim.

Leaves—pulp of leaf-tips applied on forehead in migraine. Leaf juice used as eye drops (Wlth India, IIB, 164).

Vomiting sickness due to 2 toxic principles, hypoglycine A & B. Unripe fruit contains higher amts. (0.11%) of hypoglycin A than ripe fruit (0.008%) [Wlth India, IIB, 164; *J Pharm Pharmacol*, 1968, **20**, 974; *Life Sci*, 1979, **19**(Pt. II),

1305]. Ripe husk of fresh fruit yields a saponin, hederagenin (1.5-2%), a naphthaquinone deriv., blighinone, etc. (*Planta Med*, 1967, **15**, 74); blighinone, str. (*Tetrahedron Lett*, 1968, 1549); fruit pulp, hypoglycin(e) A (*West Indian Med J*, 1969, **18**, 147); also hypoglycin(e)s A & B (*J Pharm Pharmacol*, 1974, **26**, 639). Saponin from fruit, spermic. in human; spasmol. (*Indian Drugs*, 1979-80, **17**, 6; 1981-82, **20**, 51).

Seeds, cyclopropane amino acids, hypoglycin(e) A & B; peptides (*Phytochemistry*, 1969, **8**, 437; 1043).

Hypoglycin(e)s — cyclo-Pr amino acids. Hypoglycin A[2-(methylene-cyclo-Pr)alanine] twice as toxic as hypoglycin B, (N- γ-glutamyl-3) deriv. as 9 Cl; *L*-form teratogen (Dictionary Org. Compds., III, 3271). Both compds. strong hypoglyc.; A has antisarcoma properties (*J Pharm Pharmacol*, 1968, **20**, 974); also teratogenic in rats and rabbits (*Nature Lond*, 1968, **217**, 471; *West Indian Med J*, 1968, **71**, 52); mech. of teratogenic action; hypoglycin-A-induced deformities can be prevented by riboflavin phosphate (*Experimentia*, 1971, **27**, 414). Toxic substances of *Akee* (name of fruit in Jamaica), rev. (*West Indian Med J*, 1969, **18**, 238; *J Sci Res Counc Jam*, 1971, **2**, 4); spectrophotom. estn. of hypoglycin A (*ibid*, 1980, **5**, 1); detn. of hypoglycin A in *Akee* (*J Food Sci*, 1974, **39**, 1057); hypoglycin A (from mature aril) and its relation to Jamaican vomiting sickness; 24 refs; estn. using amino acid analyzer (*Pan-Am Assoc Biochem Soc Symp*, 1975, **3**, 1; 11; 21; *CA*, 1976, **85**, 117425p; 117426q; 1977, **86**, 713k). Biosynth. (*Phytochemistry*, 1981, **20**, 2161).

Leaves and twigs, vomifoliol (*Phytochemistry*, 1976, **15**, 332); and gave +ve test for alk. (*Lloydia*, 1972, **35**, 1).

BLUMEA (*Asteraceae*)

*B. aurita DC. syn. *Laggera aurita* Sch.-Bip. ex C.B. Clarke
Mundari–*Soan pura*.

In Angola, strongly arom. and sticky infusion used in rheum. pains (Watt & Breyer-Brandwijk, 207).

Essent. oil, inhibitory against *E. coli* and *Klebsiella aerogenes* (*Indian J Pharm*, 1975, **37**, 129).

Essent. oil from plant (0.04%), constituents identn. (*Curr Sci*, 1975, **44**, 571). Plant, new secondary alc., laggerol, triterps., alkanes and alcs. (*Indian J Chem*, 1976, **14B**, 64); ether, 2,3-diMeO-*p*-cymene (*ibid*, 1976, **14B**, 711).

Found in waste places almost throughout India.

B. balsamifera DC. syn. *B. densiflora* Hook. f.(FBI) in part.

Leaves—in treatment of body-swelling. Hypothermic; stomch., given in intestinal diseases such as diar., cholera and colic. Ext. in chest trouble, headache, dropsy, hyperten. and as tranquillizer. Fresh leaf juice, used as eye drops in chr. eye diseases (Wlth India, IIB, 165); sap of young leaves in bowel disorder in infants (*Bull Bot Surv India*, 1976, **18**, 166).

Alc. ext. of plant, antibact. against *E. coli* [*J Res Indian Med*, 1974, 9(2), 66]. Roots, in beri-beri and colds (Wlth India, IIB, 165).

Leaves, contain 2 quercetin derives. (*J Natl Prod*, 1981, **44**, 541). Leaves alongwith those of *Vitex negundo* and *Careya arborea* used for fomentation (Wlth India, IIB, 166).

B. densiflora DC.

Juice of fresh leaves, insect-repellent; protects skin from mosquito-bites for some times (Wlth India, IIB, 167).

B. eriantha DC.

Leaves alongwith those of *Vitex negundo* and *Careya arborea* used for fomentation (Wlth India, IIB, 166).

Essent. oil—*in vitro*, antibact.; antifung. (*Planta Med*, 1971, **20**, 118; 1972, **22**, 136); from leaves, insectic. against *Culex pipiens* and *C. fatigans* larvae (*J Commun Dis*, 1980, **12**, 39).

Flowers, a flavonol, erianthin, str.; identical with artemetin (*J Indian Chem Soc*, 1968, **45**, 851). Seeds, essent. oil (Wlth India, IIB, 168).

*B. fastulosa Kurz syn. *B. glomerata* DC.

EtOH(50%) ext. of plant, diur. (*Indian J Exp Biol*, 1974, **12**, 512). Essent. oil, CNS depress. (Wlth India, IIB, 168).

Steam non-volat. fraction of plant ext. yields a mixt. of *n*-alkanes from C_{27} to C_{35} (*Indian J Pharm Sci*, 1978, **40**, 227).

Found throughout India.

B. flava DC.; see **Blumeopsis flava**

B. lacera DC. Hook.f. (FBI) in part.

Preliminary pharmacol. (*Indian J Exp Biol*, 1969, **7**. 250). Leaf juice mixed with black pepper given in piles [*J Res Indian Med*, 1973, **8**(2), 76]. Leaves used to prepare astrin. eyewash. Alc. ext. of herb exhibited marked antiinflam. activity against carrageenin- and bradykinin-induced inflam. in rats (*Indian J Pharmacol*, 1981, **13**, 73).

Essent. oil from leaves, antimicrob. (*Indian J Pharm*, 1975, **37**, 175). Antifung. and insect repellent.

Root, astrin. and febge. (Wlth India, IIB, 167).

Leaves contain coniferyl alc. deriv. (*Tetrahedron Lett*, 1969, 69); campesterol (*Phytochemistry*, 1972, **11**, 1855); flavons. (*Planta Med*, 1977, **31**, 235). Leaves essent.oil (0.5%), cineol, 66 & *d*-fenchone, 10% (Wlth India, IIB, 167)

Non-sapon. fraction of EtOH ext. of aerial parts, hentriacontane, hentriacontanol, α-amyrin, lupeol & its -OAc and β-sitosterol; root and rootbark, triterp. and sterols (*Proc Indian Sci Congr*, 1980, Pt. III, **90**; 93).

*B. lacera var. **blumei** DC. syn. *B. laciniata* DC.

Plant used against mouth diseases of cattle (Wlth India, IIB, 167). Contains essent. oil; antibact. and antifung. (*Planta Med*, 1974, **26**, 196; *Indian J Pharm*, 1975, **37**, 175).

Punjab to Arunachal Pradesh, Mizoram and peninsular India up to 1,350 m.

B. lanceolaria(Roxb.) Druce syn. *B. myriocephala* DC.; *B. longifolia* DC.

Leaves decoct. with leaves of *B. sessiliflora*, *B. balsamifera* and *Mikania cordata* used for bathing to cure body pain (*Bull Bot Surv India*, 1976, **18**, 166). Leaves as poultice in rheum.

Herb, antiberiberi agent. In China, plant used as carmin., obstipation and antibact. (Wlth India, IIB, 168).

Saponin from plant, haemolytic on human blood. Stem and root contain α-spinasterol (*Kuo Li Taiwan Ta Hsueh I Hsueh Yuan Yen Chiu Pao Kao*, 1972, **17**, 42; *CA*; 1973, **78**, 69220z).

Herb contains essent. oil. (Wlth India, IIB, 168).

*B. malcolmii Hook.f.

Volat. oil from aerial parts, constituents and antibact. activity; also insectic. against stored grain insects and insect- attractant for housefly (*Indian Drugs*, 1978-79, **16**, 204; Wlth India, IIB, 168).

Maharashtra, Karnataka and Kerala.

*B. membranacea (DC.) Hook.f.

Leaves yield an essent. oil with antibact. properties (*Sci Cult*, 1979, **45**, 327; *Indian Drugs*, 1979-80, **17**, 14). Essent. oil from plant, antibact. (*Indian J Med Res*, 1976, **64**, 854); *in vitro*, antifung. activity [*Indian Drugs Pharmac Ind*, 1979, **14**(2), 21]; wide range in antifung.(*Indian Drugs*, 1978-79, **16**, 21).

Herb contains sitosterol (*Indian J Chem*, 1976, **14B**, 473).

From Himachal Pradesh and Punjab to Sikkim.; in Assam and Peninsular India.

*B. mollis (D.Don) Merrill syn. *B.wightiana* DC. Hook.f. (FBI) in part.

Kan.–*Gobbusoppu*; Mundri–*Ote jetang*.

Boiled herb used by Mundas to treat diar. (Wlth India, IIB, 168). Preliminary pharmacol. (*Indian J Exp Biol*, 1974, **12**, 512).

Essent. oil from herb, antibact. and antifung. against several human pathogenic bacteria and phytopathogenic fungi (*Indian Drugs* 1977-78, **15**, 253).

Plant contains stigmasterol (*Indian J Chem*, 1975, **13**, 97).

Essent. oil, 2,3-di-MeO-p-cymene (*Parfuem Kosmet*, 1981,**62**, 392); from USSR plant (*Khim Prir Soedin*, 1981, 50; *CA*, **95**, 3373w).

Found from Kashmir to Assam and also in Peninsular India.

*B. obliqua Druce

EtOH(50%) ext. of plant, diur. (*Indian J Exp Biol*, 1974, **12**, 512).

Parasnath, Bihar.

*B. oxyodonta DC.

Mundari–*Huring kuru*.

Herb used as fish poison by Mundas (Wlth India, IIB, 169). EtOH(50%) ext. of plant, diur. (*Indian J Exp Biol*, 1974, **12**, 512). Essent. oil from leaves, insectic. (*J Commun Dis*, 1980, **12**, 39).

Garhwal and Kumaun, Rajasthan and in Peninsular India up to 1,500 m.

*B. riparia DC. syn. *B. chinensis* DC. Hook.f. (FBI) in part; *B. pubigera* Merrill

Decoct. of leaves given in colic and beri-beri (Uphof, 79).

Eastern Himalayas up to 1,300 m and in Andaman and Nicobar Islands.

BLUMEOPSIS (*Asteraceae*)

*B. flava Gagnep. syn. *Blumea flava* DC.; *Laggera flava* Benth.

Mundari–*Bocho tupuri*.

Plant used with mustard oil in dropsy (Wlth India, IIB, 169).

Almost throughout India.

BOEHMERIA (*Urticaceae*)

*B. macrophylla Hornem. non D. Don syn. *B. platyphylla* D. Don

H.–*Gargela*; Garhwal–*Khaksha*; H.P.–*Samrali*.

Leaves ground with black pepper excellent drug for all types of eczema [*J Res Indian Med*, 1973, **8**(1), 76]. Preliminary pharmacol. (*Indian J Exp Biol*, 1973, **11**, 43).

Plant contains alk., 3,4-di-OMe-w-(2'-piperidyl)acetophenone; cryptopleurine and secophenanthroquinolizidine, minor alks.; cryptopleurine, cytotoxic against Eagle's 9KB carcinoma of nasopharynx in cell culture (*Aust J Chem*, 1968, **21**, 1397; 2579; 1969, **22**, 1805). Leaves and twigs, pomolic and oleanolic acids, lupeol, 5α-stigmastane-3,6-dione, and β- sitosterol (*J Indian Chem Soc*, 1981, **58**, 815).

Found throughout India up to 1,500 m.

B. nivea Gaud.

Roots contain palmitic, stearic, behenic, ursolic & 19α-OH-ursolic acids, β-sitosterol, its glucd., etc. (*Yakugaku Zasshi*, 1974, **94**, 150; *CA*, **80**, 105909h).

*B. rotundifolia D. Don

EtOH(50%) ext. of aerial parts, diur. (*Indian J Exp Biol*, 1980, **18**, 594).

Rhenock, Sikkim.

BOENNINGHAUSENIA (*Rutaceae*)

*B. albiflora Reichb. ex Meissn. syn. *Ruta albiflora* Hook.

H.P.–*Pissu mar*; Kumaun–*Upaniya jhar*.

Plant—mild insectic. and insect repellent (*Bull RRL Jammu*, 1962-63, **1**, 156). EtOH(50%) ext., hypoglyc. and spasmog. (*Indian J Exp Biol*, 1968, **6**, 232).

Essent. oil—from leaves and from plant, dog-flea repellent (*Indian For*, 1966, **92**, 295; *Nagarjun*, 1979-80, **23**, 177); antibact. and antifung. [*Indian Perfum*, 1976, **20**(1A), 45].

Root—powd. root paste applied to worm infested wounds (*Econ Bot*, 1979, **33**, 52). In China, roots as also leaves used as antiper. (Wlth India, IIB, 173).

Essent. oil from plant (0.14-0.2%), components (*Indian Oil Soap J*, 1969-70, **35**, 207); constituents (*Parfuem Kosmet*, 1972, **53**, 125). Essent. oil from leaves and stems, β-myrcene, α-phellandrene, β-caryophyllene, cadiene, cadalene, caryophyllene oxide, sapthulenol, 7-OMe-2,2-di-Mechromene and ageratochromene (*Phytochemistry*, 1975, **14**, 308).

Plant contains rutin (c. 0.004%) (*Kyoto Yakka Daigaku Gakuho*, 1962, **10**, 17; *CA*, 1964, **60**, 3264b). Aerial parts, coumarin, 3-(1,1-di-Me-allyl)xanthyletin; leaves and stems, 6 coumarins, xanthyletin, bergapten, xanthotoxin, etc.; 2- isoprenyl coumarins, angenomalin and micropubscin from plant (*Phytochemistry*, 1973, **12**, 2073; 2312; 3010); also minor coumarins (*ibid*, 1975, **14**, 836). Leaves, 2 isomeric coumarins and chalepensin, isolation and str. detn. (*ibid*, 1977, **16**, 291). Plant, 3-(1,1-di-Me-allyl)xanthyletin, bergapten, chalepin-OAc, octacosanoic acid and β-sitosterol; coumarins, spasmol. on guinea pig ileum (*Indian J Pharm Sci*, 1977, **41**, 205); see also distribution of furocoumarins (psorelens) in plants; photosensitization (*J Invest Dermatol*, 1962, **39**, 225; *Biochem Biophys Acta*, 1969, **195**, 197).

Aerial parts contain 6 alks.: rutacridone, noracronycine, 1-OH- acridone, 1-OH-N-Me-acridone, 1-OH-7-OMe-acridone & 1-OH-3-OMe-N- Me-acridone and lignane justicidin B (*Fitoterapia*, 1981, **52**, 37).

Root, 3 acridone alks. including 1-OH-N-Me-acridone and rutamarine; also rutacridone, noracronycine, 1-OH-acridone & 1,7- di-OH-N-Ne-acridone (*Pharmazie*, 1975, **30**, 753; *CA*, **84**, 56523z; *Phytochemistry*, 1978, **17**, 169).

From Kashmir to Arunachal Pradesh, Meghalaya and Mizoram, between 660 and 2,600 m.

BOERHAVIA (*Nyctaginaceae*)

*B. chinensis Aschers. & Schweinf. syn. B. rependa Willd.

Mundari–*Piri kecho ara.*

Roots—pharmacognosy; contain alks., 0.1-0.15% [*J Res Indian Med*, 1972, **7**(1), 1]. Roots, antileucor. in human beings (*Proc Nat Acad Sci Biol Sci*, 1978, 91; *Indian J For*, 1979, **2**, 370). Antispermator. and anthelm., clin. trials [*J Sci Res Plants Med*, 1980, **1**(1 & 2), 29].

Found throughout India as a common weed.

B. diffusa Linn. syn. *B. repens* Linn.

Roots—leaf ash and roots taken to cure nightblindness (*J Agric Trop Biol Appl*, 1966, **13**, 276). EtOH(50%) ext. of roots and plant, spasmol. (*Indian J Exp Biol*, 1968, **6**, 232). Root, for restoration of virility in man ; its poultice mixed with palm kernel oil applied to boils (*Ghana J Sci*, 1969, **9**, 119). Roots and leaves more diur. and antiinflam. than stems and whole plant [*J Res Indian Med*, 1974, 9(2), 57]; activity max. in rainy season (*Planta Med*, 1975, **32**, 283); ext., antivir. (*Can J Bot*, 1979, **57**, 926); anticonvuls. in albino rats (*Q J Crude Drug Res*, 1979, **17**, 84). Vermifuge (*Nagarjun*, 1979-80, **23**, 9).

Leaves—used in opthalmia and in eye wounds, in muscular pain; in dropsy (see also roots) and also in gonor.; to purify blood and hasten delivery (*Indian Drugs*, 1977-78, **15**, 145). Diur. and antiinflam. activity of leaves from plants with or without flowers [*J Res Indian Med*, 1974, 9(2), 57; 1977, 12(4), 108]. Paste taken orally to check bleeding after delivery (*J Econ Tax Bot*, 1980, **1**, 144). Dry and powd. leaves mixed with *Brassica* oil used for external application on itch and eczema (*ibid*, 1981, **2**, 191). Boiled with rice, garlic and water rubbed on body to cure rheum. (*Econ Bot*, 1981, **35**, 4).

Plant—drug for oedema and ascites resulting from early cirrhosis of liver and chr. peritonitis (Wlth India, IIB,174). In Ghana, decoct. cooked with shea butter drunk to relieve asthma (*Ghana J Sci*, 1969, **9**, 119). Powd. used against abdominal tumour and cancer (*Lloydia*, 1970, **33**, 297). Significant antiinflam. activity similar to hydrocortisone (*Q J Crude Drug Res*, 1970, **10**, 1555). Used in epilepsy, pain in abdomen due to congestion of blood, *prolapsus ani* and *fistula ani*, dysen., poison of scolopendrids and otitis media suppurativa (*Econ Bot*, 1970, **24**. 246). Useful drug in inflam. renal diseases and nephrotic syndrome. EtOH ext., cardiotonic, raises B.P. and relaxant; its non-w.-sol. ext., antiinflam.; ext., antibact. [*J Res Indian Med*, 1972, **7**(3), 13; 17; 28; 1974, **9**(2), 66]. In Samoa, used in dropsy (*Econ Bot*, 1974, **28**, 22). Plant ext. for increasing memory (*Bull Bot Surv India*, 1976, **18**, 161). One of the ingredients of following indigenous drugs: of a drug useful in polycythaemia, clin. study [*J Res Indian Med*, 1976, **11**(1), 117]; 'Biliarin' used in liver disorders, clin. trials (*Indian Pract*, 1978, **31**, 683); and also minor constituent of 'Styplon' used in the prevention of excessive bleeding in tonsillectomy (*Probe*, 1979-80, **19**, 281). Haematinic and growth promoter in children (*J Res Ayur Siddha*, 1980, **1**, 370).

Plant ext., protective against potato virus (*Biol Plant*, 1980, **23**, 205). Decoct. used in treatment of nodules, in the body (*Bull Med Ethno Bot Res*, 1980, **1**, 1). Aspirin- and prostaglandin-induced *in vitro* enhancement of fibrinolytic activity of menstrual fluid inhibited by ext. of *B. diffusa* [*Indian J Biochem Biophys*, 1981, **18**(4 Suppl.), 47]; punarnovoside, present in plant exhibits significant antifibrinolytic activity (*Annu Rep CDRI Lucknow*, 1981-82, 9).

Flowers and seeds as contracep. in Ayurveda [*Nagarjun*, 1976-77, **20**(2), 17; *Ancient Sci Life*, 1981-82, 1, 72].

Chem. difference between *B. diffusa* and *B. punarnava* (*Indian J Pharm*, 1965, **27**, 41). Plant, β-sitosterol [*J Res Indian Med*, 1972, **7**(3), 34]. 2 Alks, punarnavine-1 & -2 (*Indian J Exp Biol*, 1974, **12**, 509). Myricyl alc., myristic acid, oxalic acid and alk. (*Bangladesh Counc Sci Ind Res*, 1974, **9**, 47; *CA*, 1975, **82**, 13974p).

Hypoxanthine-9-*L*-arabinofuranoside—isolation from root, str., synth.; compd. lowered serum uric acid levels in adult male rats, chicks and human volunteers (*Pak J Biol Agric Sci*, 1968, **11**, 41; *CA*, 1971, **74**, 61602x); its isolation, identn. and cardiovascular action (*Abstr Paper Int Symp Med Plants*, 1981, 43).

Roots, also hentriacontane, ursolic acid and β- sitosterol (*Phytochemistry*, 1971, **10**, 3318). Amino acid compn. of roots and herb; aspartic and glutamic acids possible agent for dissolving calculi of Ca-oxalate (*J Inst Chem India*, 1979, **51**, 214). Virus inhibitor from roots, its properties; and also isolation; occurrence of highly antivir. agent in plants, treated with *B. diffusa* inhibitor (*Can J Bot*, 1979, **57**, 926; 1214; 1980, **58**, 2141).

*B. rubicunda Steud. syn. *B. elegans* Choisy

Leaves used as diur. (Wlth India, IIB, 176).

Some parts of Rajasthan and Punjab.

BOLBOSCHOENUS (*Cyperaceae*)

B. martimus Rolla Rao syn. *Scirpus martimus* Linn.

Decoct. of plant given in fever (*J Econ Tax Bot*, 1980, **1**, 137).

Pet. ether ext. of rhizomes, on steam distillation yields essent. oil, 2.7% and phellonic acid (*Pak J Sci Res*, 1966, **18**, 57).

BOLUSANTHUS (*Fabaceae*)

*B. specious Harms syn. *Lonchocarpus specious* Bolus

Eng.–*Wild wistaria*; H.–*Gul- inilam*.

Decoct. of bark used as aphrodis. (Wlth India, IIB, 176). Leaves and pods contain alks., cytisine & its N-Me deriv. (*Tydskr Naturwet*, 1970, **10**, 213; *CA*, 1971, **74**, 95432g).

Endemic to S. Africa, introduced into India for ornament.

BOMBAX (*Bombacaceae*)

B. ceiba Linn. syn. *B. malabaricum* DC.; *Salmalia malabarica* Schott & Endl.

Eng.–*Silk cotton tree*.

Various plant parts used in smallpox, bleeding gums, toothache and carries, sores in mouth, pain in leg, fever, enlarged spleen, atrophy, emaciation, rheum., spermator., haemat., cholera, pneum., pleur., intercosal neuralgia, leprosy and rinderpest (*Econ Bot*, 1970, **24**, 241). In Taiwan and Kwangton, plant used in enteritis, dysen., menor., lymphoadenoma, hepatitis, etc. [*Taiwan K'o Hsueh*, 1970, 24(1-2), 15; *CA*, 1971, **74**, 121328z].

Flowers—astrin. and cooling. Paste of flowers as also of leaves applied in cutaneous troubles.

Young tap roots, astrin., and used in dysen. (Wlth India, IIB, 184).

Bark—infusion used as demulc., and tonic. Externally used as styptic and for fomenting wounds. Paste of bark applied in skin eruptions (Wlth India, IIB, 184); applied on boils, acne and pimples (*J Econ Tax Bot*, 1981, **2**, 193). Aq. ext. with curd given in blood dysen. (*Bull Bot Surv India*, 1973, **15**, 14). Used in gonor. and syphilis (*Q J Crude Drug Res*, 1979, 17, 61).

Young fruits—expect., stim. and diur.; beneficial in calculous affections, chr. inflam. and ulceration of bladder and kidneys (Wlth India, IIB, 185).

Seeds—used in gonor., chr. cystitis and other catar. affections (Wlth India, IIB, 185). Hot aq. exts., moderate oxytocic (*Indian J Pharm*, 1968, **30**, 165). Seeds contain hexacosanol, tocopherol, terps., etc. (*Planta Med*, 1976, 29,148). Bark contains mucilage which is used for haemoptysis in pulmonary T.B., and in influenza (Wlth India, IIB, 185).

Lupeol and β-sitosterol in stembark (*J Indian Chem Soc*, 1971, **48**, 769); also present in rootbark besides a naphthoquinone compd. (*Curr Sci*, 1971, **40**, 630); phenolics of rootbark, str.; and a lactone (*Indian J Chem*, 1973, **11**, 825; 1976, **14B**, 616); 4 sesquiterps. (*Phytochemistry*, 1981, **20**, 1877). Root yields triacontanol, β-sitosterol and a new glycd. (*Can J Chem*, 1980, **58**, 328).

Fresh petals, essent. oil, hentriacontane, hentriacontanol, quercetin, kaempferol, β-sitosterol & its glucd. (*J Pharm Sci*, 1972, **61**, 807); also glucds. of pelargonidin and cyanidin (*Planta Med*, 1973, **24**, 196); 3

biosides, flavons., etc. (*Arzneim Forsch*, 1974, **24**, 285; *CA*, **81**, 1286g).

BORAGO (*Boraginaceae*)

*B. officinalis Linn.

Eng.–*Beebread, borage.*

Herb, febge., nervine, laxt., demulc., emol., diur. and diaphor. Tender leaves and flowers relished as pot herb; they impart pleasant flavour and cooling effect to beverages.

Seeds, protein, 20.9 and fatty oil, 38.3% (Wlth India, IIB, 187); contain an octadecatetraenic acid (*Naturwissenschaften*, 1964, **51**, 164). Leaves and flowers, choline (*Planta Med*, 1968, **16**, 411).

Chromatogr. investigation of flavons. (*Acta Pol Pharm*, 1969, **26**, 559; *CA*, 1970, **72**, 107779z). Study of polyphenols and alks. (*Plant Med Phytother*, 1977, **11**,5). Plant contains cyanophoric principles, dhurrin (*Proc K Ned Acad Wet Ser C*, 1979, **82**, 171). Chemotaxonomy of some Boraginaceae: pyrrolizidine alks. and phenolic compds. (*Plant Syst Evol*, 1981, 137, 127).

Introduced into India and cultivated in gardens for ornament.

BORASSUS (*Arecaceae*)

B. flabellifer Linn.; Becc. & Hook.f. (FBI) in part.

Eng.–*Palmyra palm, brab tree.*

Plant in heat stroke, headache, earache, pain, epilepsy, convuls., adenitis scrofulosa colli, sores, scabies, burns, syphilis, ulcer of palate, nausea and vomiting, spiderlick, menor., and haemor. septicaemia (*Econ Bot*, 1970, **24**, 241).

Root, diur. and anthelm., used as a cure for gonor. Decoct. of young root and juice from young terminal buds and leaf-stalks used in gastritis and hiccups.

Powd. of burnt bark or decoct. in dentifrice. In Kampuchea, flower and root as sinapism in tumours of uterus. Gum, emol. in indurations. An ext. of central axis of male inflorescence, with mustard oil, used in rheum.

Toxic effects of plant in rats (*Br J Exp Pathol*, 1971, **52**, 524).

Ash of spathe alongwith other demulc. applied for enlarged liver and spleen.

Useful as antacid in heart burn and as antiper. A substance obtained from the base of leaves applied on wounds (Wlth India, IIB, 187). Aq. MeOH ext. of young shoots contains heat-stable toxin; edible part of young shoot, neurotoxic to rats (*Food Cosmet Toxicol*, 1980, **18**, 483).

Fruit juice—tonic for asthmatic, anaemic and leprosy patients, improves general health, suppl. for Fe and vit. deficiency. Sap prescribed in digest. troubles and chr. gonor. and in Hansen's disease; slightly fermented juice given in diabetes. Excellent source of biologically available riboflavin (Wlth India, IIB, 187). EtOH(50%) ext. of fruit, diur. (*Indian J Exp Biol*, 1974, **12**, 512).

Fruit jaggery (*gur*)—energy providing food for convalescents, laxt. and useful in anaemia, *gur* sol. excellent food for typhoid patients; laxt. Nutr. properties of *gur*, palm and *neera*, rev. 30 refs. (*Indian J Nutr Diet*, 1970, **7**, 44). Jaggery sol. may be used in hyperten. and oedema due to heart and liver diseases. Sugar, antibil. and alter., used in hepatic disorders and gleet. Palm candy used in coughs and pulmonary affections and a laxt. for children (Wlth India, IIB, 187).

BORRERIA (*Rubiaceae*)

B. articularis Williams syn. *B. hispida* K. Schum.; *Spermacoce hispida* Linn.

Plant—used in ophthalmia, inflam. of eye and gums, blindness, earache, otitis media suppurativa, fever, spleen complaints, pimples, sores, dysen. and stings (*Econ Bot*, 1970, **24**, 264). EtOH(50%) ext. of plant, diur. (*Indian J Exp Biol*, 1974, **12**, 512). Crushed leaves used in stomach pain (*Bull Bot Surv India*, 1979, **22**, 161).

Plant contains β-sitosterol and ursolic acid (*Indian J Appl Chem*, 1969, **32**, 402);

and *d*-mannitol (*Phytochemistry*, 1971, **10**, 2125). Seeds, isorhamnetin [*J Res Indian Med*, 1979, **14**(1), 131].

Decoct. of herb in headache and, of roots as mouthwash to cure toothache. Leaf juice used in conjunctivitis. Leaf ext., astrin. in haemor. and gall stones. Seeds, demulc., given in diar. and dysen. (Wlth India, IIB, 202).

*B. verticillata (Linn.) Mey.

In Nigeria, plant used as anti-eczematic; a volat. oil from aerial parts inhibited growth of Gram +ve and Gram -ve bacteria; oil constituents (*Q J Crude Drug Res*, 1979, **17**, 135). Stems and leaves, emetic and antisep. (Wlth India, IIB, 202).

Aerial parts, alk., borrerine & its dimer borreverine (*Phytochemistry*, 1973, **12**, 2308); alk., borreline (*Tetrahedron Lett*, 1977, 1219). Leaves, alks., borrerine & its 2 dimers (*Lloydia*, 1978, **41**, 655). Borreverine (*J Chem Soc Chem Commun*, 1977, 261); alk., antibact. (*C R Seances Soc Biol*, 1980, **174**, 925; *CA*, 1981, **94**, 25644s).

Leaves contain rutin, quercetin, ursolic acid, β- sitosterol, its glucd., etc. (*J Indian Chem Soc*, 1981, **58**, 202).

Rootbark, 7 iridoids, daphylloside, asperuloside, its de-Ac deriv., feretoside, Me-de-Ac-asperulosidate, asperulosidic & de- Ac-asperulosidic acids (*Planta Med*, 1981, **42**, 260).

Introduced from tropical America, common on wastelands in Western Ghats of Karnataka.

BOSWELLIA (*Burseraceae*)

B. serrata Roxb. ex Colebr. syn. *B. glabra* Roxb.

Eng.–*Indian olibanum tree.*

Gum—stim., antisep.; useful in diar., dysen. and piles. Used in ointment for syphilis. Non phenolic fraction, antitumour (Wlth India, IIB, 208).

Nonsap. fraction of bark ext., β- sitosterol (*Indian J Pharm*, 1970, **32**, 48).

Plant—cardiotonic, purifies vital spirit, dissolves wind, increases intellect and remedies forgetfulness [*East Pharm*, 1980, **23**(272), 39]. In epilepsy, snakebite and rinderpest (*Econ Bot*, 1970, **24**, 247); ext., antibact. (*Bull Bot Soc Univ Saugar*, 1980, **27**, 57).

Bark—in diar., piles, skin diseases, ulcers and cough [*J Res Indian Med*, 1973 **8**(2),67]. EtOH ext., active against potato virus x (*Technology, Sindri*, 1971, **9**, 415).

Gum-resin—as an ointment for sores (*Bull Bot Surv India*, 1973, **15**, 13); properties (*Indian Drugs*, 1979-80, **17**, 225); antiinflam., antiatherosclerotic and antiarthritic in animals (*Indian J Pharmacol*, 1981, **13**, 63, 67). Nonphenolic fraction of gum-resin, marked sed. and analg. in rats (*Planta Med*, 1970-71, **19**, 333); it produced a marked and long-lasting hypoten. in anaesthetised dogs [*Indian Drugs Pharmac Ind*, 1977, **12**(4), 17].

Essent. oil—from gum-resin, antifung. (*Indian J Pharm*, 1974, **36**, 46; *Indian Drugs*, 1978-79, **16**, 24); antibact. (*Curr Sci*, 1978, **47**, 453).

Grain used in plaster form for indurated as also ulcerated breast, condylomata, cancer and scirrhous and uterine tumours (*Lloydia*, 1967, **30**, 394). EtOH(50%) ext. of fruit and stem, hypoglyc. and of root, anticancer (*Indian J Exp Biol*, 1968, **6**, 232).

Bark contains β-sitosterol (*Agric Res Delhi*, 1963, **3**, 110).

Gum resin, a diterp. alc., serratol; 8 tetracyclic triterp. acids, viz. β-boswellic, Ac-β- boswellic, 11-keto-boswellic, Ac-11-keto-boswellic acids, etc. (*Indian Drugs*, 1978-79, **16**, 80).

BOTHRIOCHLOA (*Poaceae*)

B. intermedia(R.Br.) A. Camus; see **Dichanthium glabrum**

B. pertusa A. Camus; see **Dichanthium pertusum**

BOTRYCHIUM (*Ophioglossaceae*)

B. lunaria Swartz
Eng.–*Moonworf.*

Juice of roots and fronds reported to be used for treatment of breast cancer (Wlth India, IIB, 209).

B. termatum Swartz
Fleshy roots applied to cuts and bruises (Wlth India, IIB, 209).

B. virginianum Swartz
Eng.– *Rattlesnake fern.*

Fern used in dysen. (Wlth India, IIB, 209). EtOH(70%) ext. of vegetative pinna active against *Bacillus subtilis* (*Econ Bot*, 1980, **34**, 284).

BOUSSINGAUI.TIA (*Basellaceae*)

See **ANREDERA**

BRACHIARIA (*Poaceae*)

*B. mutica Stapf syn. *Panicum muticum* Forsk.

B.–*Nardul*; Kan.–*Mauritius hullu*; Mal.–*lombopullu*; Tam.– *Niradipul.*

Grass, slightly estrogenic (*Indian Vet J*, 1974, **51**, 610); and cynogenic (Wlth India, IIB, 213).

Cultivated all over India.

*B. reptans Gardner & Hubbard syn. *Urochloa panicoides* Beauv.

Tam.–*Shanipillu.*

Grain contains cyanidin 3-monoside. In Tanzania; dried whole plant burnt and ashes applied over scarification in snakebite (Wlth India, IIB, 214).

Found throughout the plains.

BRACHYACTIS (*Asteraceae*)

*B. roylei Wend. syn. *B. umbrosa* Benth. Ladakh–*Sathi.*

Plant used for treatment of rheum. (*in* Atal & Kapur, Med. Plants, 521).

Himalayas from Kashmir to Karakoram up to 3,500 m.

BRAGANTIA (*Aristolochiaceae*)

See APAMA

BRASENIA (*Cabombaceae*)

B. schreberi J.F. Gmel. syn. *B. peltata* Pursh

Eng.–*Frogleaf, waterleaf.*

Leaf ext., antimicrob. against Gram +ve bacteria and yeast. Poultice of stems and leaves applied to boils and abscesses. Seeds, cooling, digest. and antidysen.; their decoct. allay thirst, and strengthen gums (Wlth India, IIB, 215).

Plant contains low amts. of vit. B_{12} (*Shokuhin Eiseigaku Zasshi*, 1964, **5**, 39; *CA*, **61**, 6279d). Extn. of neoplasm inhibitors from whole plant; inhibitors, esp. effective against gastric ulcer and skin tumour (Jpn Kokai, 1978, 7818714; *CA*, **88**, 197638k). Str. of polysaccharide of mucilage (*Agric Biol Chem*, 1979, **43**, 1269).

BRASSAIOPSIS (*Araliaceae*)

*B. hainla Seem.

EtOH(50%) ext. of aerial parts, diur. (*Indian J Exp Biol*, 1974, **12**, 512).

Bomdila, Arunachal Pradesh.

BRASSICA (*Brassicaceae*)

B. alba (Linn.) Boiss. syn. *Sinapis alba* Linn.

Bitter principle, sinapin thiocyanate (*Nippon Nogei Kagaku Kaishi*, 1966, **40**, 236; *CA*, **65**, 6199h). Seeds, *p*-OH-benzyl isothiocyanate (*Chem Ind Lond*, 1965, 308); method of detn. (*Agric Biol Chem*, 1971, **35**, 959; *J Sci Food Agric*, 1971, **22**, 523). Bound phenolic acids (*J Food Sci*, 1975, **40**, 820); sinapine and sinalbin (*Egypt J Pharm Sci*, 1975, **16**, 113); sinapine content (*Angew Bot*, 1980, **54**, 47).

B. campestris Linn. ssp. **chinensis** (Rupr.) Olsson

Eng.–*Celery* or *Chinese mustard, pakchoi*; Mundari–*Risakuhi.*

Turnip aper., diur. and oil, rubft. [*Bull Med Ethno Bot Res*, 1981, **2**(4), 17].

Folic acid content (*Philipp J Sci*, 1966, **95**, 311). From Japanese leaves carcinogenic 3,4-benzopyrene (*Shokuhin Eiseigaku Zasshi*, 1974, **15**, 18; *CA*, **81**, 36653b); cystine synthase (*J Biochem Tokyo*, 1975, **77**, 1107; *CA*, **83**, 39312s).

*B. campestris Linn. ssp. **pekinensis** (Lour.) Olsson syn. *B. pekinensis* Linn.

Eng.–*Celery* or *Chinese cabbage, petsai.*

Chinese cabbage, antiscor., resolv.; seeds, stim. and laxt. Seed oil stimulates hair growth (Wlth India, IIB, 270).

Indole deriv. in infected clubroots (*Agric Biol Chem*, 1970, **34**, 1590). Edible parts and seed glucosinolates (*J Agric Food Chem*, 1979, **27**, 34); and seed, sinapine (*Angew Bot*, 1980, **54**, 47).

Grown as a vegetable in some parts of India.

B. juncea (Linn.) Czern. & Coss.

Eng.–*Brown* or *Indian mustard.*

Histpathology of thyroids and livers of rats and mice fed with seed glucosinolates (*Can J Anim Sci*, 1972, **52**, 395); sinigrin, gluconapin and sinalbin (*Egypt J Pharm Sci*, 1975, **16**, 113).

Volat. compds. of plant (*Yakugaku Zasshi*, 1973, **93**, 453; *Phytochemistry*, 1976, **15**, 763); constituents of essent. oil from various parts; isothiocyanates in raw and salted (*Nippon Nogei Kagaku Kaishi*, 1980, **54**, 99; 1979, **53**, 261; *CA*, **92**, 194443q; 74550a).

Seeds, 2 antithiamine compds., one of them Me-sinapate (*Biochem Biophys Acta*, 1974, **343**, 211). Flavonol glycds. of *Brassica* spp. (*Phytochemistry*, 1973, **12**, 1091); *p*-OH benzoic acid (*Z Lebensm Unters Forsch*, 1981, **172**, 253; *CA*, **95**, 78676f).

B. napus Linn.

Eng.–*Rape, colza.*

Rapeseed oil—nutritive value, rev. (*J Am Oil Chem Soc*, 1971, **48**, 728); myocardial effects, rev., 53 refs. [*Cah Nutr Diet*, 1971 **6**(3), 85; *CA*, 1972, **76**, 81585p]; effect on cardiac tissue, rev., 76 refs. (*Modif Lipid Metab Symp*, 1974, 43; *CA*, 1976, **85**, 4095n; *Vet Ital*, 1974, **25**, 195; *CA*, 1975, **82**, 123791; *Can J Comp Med*, 1975, **39**, 261; 1976, **40**, 360; *Acta Med Scand*, Suppl, 1975, **585**, 51; *Lipids*, 1977, **12**, 951; *J Nutr*, 1978, **108**, 273; *Ann Nutr Aliment*, 1977, **31**, 291; *CA*, 1978, **88**, 61387v). Rapeseed oil, ingredient of compn. for treating osteoarticular rheum. inflam. and collagenic patients (Fr.M., 1968, 6043; *CA*, 1970, **72**, 24623t); meta-·bolic effect in man [*Cah Nutr Diet*, 1972, 7(1), 67; *CA*, **77**, 112835x]; effect on hepatic hexobarbital metabolism in rats (*Nutr Metab*, 1975, **18**, 272); heated compd. fraction, fatal for rats (*Ann Biol Anim Biochem Biophys*, 1974, **14**, 855; *CA*, 1975, **82**, 165650t); biochem. and nutritional aspects (*Rev Fr Corps Gras*, 1978, **25**, 175; *CA*, **89**, 41148k); toxic effects in animals (*J Am Oil Chem Soc*, 1978, **55**, 711); substance from unsap. fraction causes focal cardiac degeneration (*Ann Med Nancy*, 1978, **17**, 335; *CA*, **89**, 145180f); unsap. matter, analg. effects[*Indian Drugs Pharmac Ind*, 1977, **12**(5), 33].

Seed meal—effect on thyroid, glucosinalate level and iodine content of milk in cattle (*J Nutr*, 1979, **109**, 1129). Toxic effects, rev., 54 refs.; other similar studies (*Br Vet J*, 1979, **135**, 3; *Ernaehrungsforschung*, 1972, **16**, 541; *CA*, 1973, **78**, 70573y; *Can J Anim Sci*, 1979, **59**, 133; *Br Poult Sci*, 1979, **20**, 231; 239; *CA*, **91**, 139507t; 139508u; *Rev Vet Sci*, 1980, **28**, 330; *CA*, **93**, 93955y; *Lipids*, 1979, **14**, 773); see also seed meal (*in* Liener, 1050).

Bran ext., anticoagulant; also essent. oil (*An Fac Quim Farm Univ Chile*, 1964, **16**, 92; *CA*, 1966, **64**, 13084d).

Erucic acid—(Z)-form of 13-decosenoic acid, important fatty acid of seed fats of *Cruciferae* (Dictionary Org. Compds, II, 2385); content in various seed fats; in rapeseed, 0 to 60% with proper attention to genetic factors (*in* Swern, I, 29-30; 415-18). A rapeseed sample from Hissar yielded fatty oil (39%) with erucic acid, c.

32.7% of oil; from Indore sample, 37.6% (*Indian J Nutr Diet*, 1975, **12**, 85; Wlth India, IIB, 255); its content and myocardial changes in male rats (*Lipids*, 1976, **11**, 9); biochem. and functional damage in rats fed with erucic acid-rich oil (*Boll Soc Ital Biol Sper*, 1972, **48**, 1201; *CA*, 1974, **81**, 34249a); erucic acid-poor oil, pathophysiol. effects on adrenal glands of rats; effects on platelet aggregation; effect in human (*Ann Nutr Aliment*, 1977, **31**, 69; *Rev Fr Corps Gras*, 1979, **26**, 171; *CA*, **87**, 195106r; **91**, 696650h; *J Med NY*, 1978, **9**, 471).

High content of erucic acid (40-55%) in fatty oil from black mustard affects metabolism; poor digestibility due to slow rate of absorption of oil in rats (*Indian J Genet Plant Breeding*, 1975, **35**, 417); in compn. of appetite depress. (Ger. Offen, 1976, 2511643; *CA*, **85**, 182423a); increase in adrenal cholesterol in rats; marked localization of the acid resulting in myocardial lesions in heart muscle (*Int Symp Rapeseed and Mustard Mysore*, 1976, 5; 16; 1979, 84). See erucic acid (*in* Swern, I, 413- 22).

Rapeseed oil, triterp., and sterols (*J Am Oil Chem Soc*, 1973, **50**, 122; 300); brassicasterol (*Lipids*, 1973, **8**, 453); tocopherol and sterols (*Prikl Biokhim Mikorobiol*, 1975, **11**, 805). Brassidic acid and thioglucds. (*Quad Merceol*, 1976, **15**, 189; *CA*, 1977, **86**, 154210f). Dihydrosterols (*Kyushu Daigaku Nogakubu Gakugei Zasshi*, 1977, **32**, 21; *CA*, 1978, **89**, 22487d); 7- oxosterols (*Glas Hem Drus Beograd*, 1978, **43**, 567; *CA*, 1979, **90**, 134249e). Tocopherol detn.; sterols (*Fette Seifen Anstrichm*, 1967, **69**, 559; 1981, **83**, 123; *CA*, **67**, 101260y; **94**, 188647j).

Rapeseed alk., sinapine; its content (*Bull Soc Pharm Bordeaux*, 1961, **100**, 238; 1964, **60**, 13093g; *Angew Bot*, 1980, **54**, 47); extn. of toxic substance (US Pat, 1971, 3615648; *CA*, 1972, **76**, 33045r). Polyphenols (*Can Inst Food Sci Technol J*, 1975, **8**, 160; *CA*, **83**, 176913c; *Z Naturforsch*, 1976, **31C**, 622); triterp. alc. and sterols (*Phytochemistry*, 1976, **15**, 1781; 1977, **16**, 1448; *Fette Seifen Anstrichm*, 1978, **80**, 383; *CA*, 1979, **90**, 164703r).

Flowers, glycd. brassicoside (*Chem Ber*, 1967, **100**, 2301). Leaf and stem, goitrin, barbarin and napoleiferin (5-allyl-2-thioxo- oxazolidone) (*Phytochemistry*, 1967, **6**, 749). Brassinolide, a plant growth-promoting steroid from pollen (*Nature Lond*, 1979, **281**, 216).

Glucosinolates—thioglucds.;sinigrin, sinalbin and progoitrin, responsible for pungent flavour. Some of them associated with endemic goitre-hypothyroidism with enlargement of thyroid gland. Various aspects including their toxic products such as oxazolidinethiones, thiocyanates & isothiocyanates, nitriles, rev. (*in* Liener, 103-42). Glucosinolates in seeds of Swedish *Brassica* spp. and var. (*Acta Agric Scand*, 1968, **18**, 97); effect of var. and environment; seed, detoxification (*J Sci Food Agric*, 1968, **19**, 564; 1970, **21**, 143). Toxicity in seed (*Can J Anim Sci*, 1971, **51**, 187). Extn. methods; diffusion extn. (*Med Welt*, 1972, **28**, 502; *Can Inst Food Sci Technol J*, 1972, **5**, 149; 101; *CA*, 1973, **78**, 2848s; 41760b; **77**, 73850b); glucds. of Indian *Brassicae* (*Plant Biochem J*, 1974, **1**, 26); anal. (*Z Pflanzenzuecht*, 1977, **79**, 331); variation, in rapeseed and mustard (*Indian J Agric Sci*, 1981, **51**, 23).

Goitrogens—goitre-producing compds. including 5-vinyl-2- oxazolidinethione (vinyl thiooxazolidone, 5-vinyl-OZT); its *S*- form, goitrin E, etc., from rapeseed (*Tluszcze Srodki Piorace*, 1962, **6**, 273; *CA*, 1964, **60**, 14829e). Vinyl-OZT detn.; in seed and cake; of isothiocyanates and OZTs in seeds (*Can J Biochem* 1969, **47**, 817; *Rev Fr Corps Gras*, 1970, **17**, 677; *CA*, 1971, **74**, 43757u; *J Sci Food Agric*, 1967, **18**, 510); extn. from seeds of var. *oleifera* (*Nippon Shokuhin Kogyo Gakkaishi*, 1968, **15**, 129; *CA*, **69**, 74478h). S-containing compds. in seeds, rev., 31 refs (*Riv Ital Sostanze Grasse*, 1973, **50**, 277; *CA*, 1974, **80**, 44434a); also isothicyanate and vinyl thiooxazolidone contents of rapeseed and oil (*Nahrung*, 1975, **19**, 583; *CA*, **83**, 95146c). OZTs inhibit incorporation of iodine into precursors of thyroxine; in contrast to activity of thiocyanate ion, antithyroid effect of -OZTs is not overcome by larger amts. of I in diet (*in* Liener, 122-23). Isothiocyanates, irritating and vesic. at higher concentration and therefore it would be surprising if amts. large enough to cause malfunction of thyroid could be eaten. However if intact glucosinolates consumed and later isothiocyanates released in intestinal tract, they might act as goitrogens, esp. in cases of iodine-deficient diet (*in* Liener, 124). Other goitrogens, 5-allyl-OZT occur in turnip greens and Chinese cabbage.

B. nigra (Linn.) Koch

Eng.–*Black* or *true mustard*.

Glucosinoles, chem. and goitrogenic property, rev. (*Planta Med*, 1972, **21**, 35).

Plant, a common weed ingested by livestock may produce severe gastroenteritis, pain, salivation, diar. and irritation of mouth (*Lloydia*, 1975, **38**, 63).

Insect control capacity of volat. oil, rev. (*Indian Perfum*, 1978, **22**,139).

*B. oleracea Linn. var. **acephala** DC.

Eng.–*Cury kale*.

Plant feeding causes severe anaemia in sheep (*Br Vet J*, 1969, **125**, 472); toxicity to ruminants (*ARC Res Rev*, 1976, **2**, 17; *CA*, 1978, **88**, 146879g).

Root peel insecticide, 2-Ph-Et-isothiocyanate (*J Agric Food Chem*, 1964, **12**, 158). Contents of goitrogens in boiled and raw plants (*Endocrinol Exp*, 1970, **4**, 51; *CA*, **73**, 108433q).

Introduced into India and grown in Uttar Pradesh and Tamil Nadu.

*B. oleracea Linn. var. **botrytis** Linn. subvar. **cauliflora** DC.

Eng.–*Cauliflower*.

Leaves bitter stomch. Cauliflower, cardiotonic, antiinflam., antitussive and febge.; useful in bliousness and urinary diseases, rich in vit.C. Externally, leaves useful in gout, rheum., piles, skin diseases and on blistered surfaces (*Planta Med*, 1973, **23**, 381).

Growth of tissues *in vitro* and production of antimicrob. metabolites (*Can. J Microbiol*, 1965, **11**, 785). Seeds, antibact. substance (*Phytopathology*, 1966, **56**, 497).

Root peels contain 2-Ph-Et-isothiocyanate (*J Agric Food Chem*, 1964, **12**, 158). Cauliflower contains S-Me-*L*-cysteine sulfoxide; ulcer-preventing substance, vit. U(S-Me- methionine) [*Bitamin Kyoto*, 1960, **20**, 93; *CA*, 1964, **61**, 15093g; *Gig Sanit*, 1981, (6), 85]; contents of goitrogens, in raw and boiled (*Endocrinol Exp*, 1970, **4**, 51; *CA*, **73**, 108433q); volat. constituents (*Phytochemistry*, 1976, **15**, 763).

Cauliflower, folic acid content (*Philipp J Sci*, 1966, **95**, 311). Ca and P content of green leaves (*Indian J Med Res*, 1969,**57**, 204).

Introduced into India from UK and grown as vegetable.

*B. oleracea Linn. var. **capitata** Linn.f.

Eng.–*Cabbage.*

Cabbage—useful in Pb and Hg poisoning [*Vopr Pitan*, 1969, **28**(4), 76; 1976, (6), 69]; juice remedy against ulcer of stomach or duodenum; also useful in atherosclerosis [*Pharmaceutist*, 1965-66, **11**(1), 36]. Pharmacol. (*Turk Hik Tecr Biyol Derg*, 1971, **31**, 153; *BA*, 1973, **55**, 10073).

Seedling ext., fungistatic (*Curr Sci*, 1975, **44**, 279).

Cabbage head, indole-3-acetonitrile (*Plant Physiol*, 1964, **39**, 836); allyl isothiocyanate 0.36-20.19 mg/100 g, goitrogenic in rats in high doses (*Physiol Bohemslov*, 1964, **13**, 542; *CA*, 1965, **62**, 16870h); contents of goitrogens in raw and boiled (*Endocrinol Exp*, 1970, **4**, 51; *CA*, **73**, 108433q); mineral content (*Indian J Agric Sci*, 1971, **41**, 1084; *Indian J Med Res*, 1972, **60**, 1470). Rich source of ulcer-preventing substance vit. U (S-Me-methionine) (16.4-20.7 mg%); stable below 90°C [*Gig Sanit*, 1981, (6), 85]; S-Me- *L*-cysteine sulfoxide (*Bitamin*

Kyoto, 1960, **20**, 93; *CA*, 1964, **61**, 15093g); folate (*Can J Biochem*, 1973,**51**, 1617); mevalonic acid (*Phytochemistry*, 1975, **14**, 1643). Polyphenols (*Kaseigaku Zasshi*, 1966, **17**, 57; *CA*, **65**, 4543f; *Z Lebensm Unter Forsch*, 1966, **132**, 193; *CA*, 1967, **66**, 45594a). Vit. B6 detn. (*Indian J Nutr Diet*, 1981, **18**, 9).

Goitrogens and means to reduce their level in growing plant (*Bratisl Lek Listy*, 1966, **46**,-I, 9; *CA*, **64**, 18035g). Glucosinolates, rev. (*Planta Med*, 1972, **21**, 35); chem. and biol. effects, rev. (*J Agric Food Chem*, 1969, **17**, 483). Glucosinolates, potential toxicants; seeds contain 10 fold more than cabbage heads (*J Am Soc Hortic Sci*, 1980, **105**, 710; 714). Content and pattern of glucosinolates in seeds of *B. oleracea* vars. (*Cruciferae Newsl*, 1980, **5**, 43; *CA*, 1981, **94**, 80259v).

Seeds contain glucosamine (*Nature Lond*, 1964, **201**, 1328). Roots and leaves, glucobrassicin (*Biol Plant Acad Sci Bohemoslov*, 1964, **6**, 88; *CA*, **61**, 4883d); roots, I & F content (*Indian J Nutr Diet*, 1971, **8**, 66).

Introduced into India and cultivated in hills and plains.

*B. oleracea Linn. var. **gemmifera** DC.

Eng.–*Brussel sprouts.*

Leaves and roots, glucobrassicin (*Biol Plant Acad Sci Bohemoslov*, 1964, **6**, 88; *CA*, **61**, 4883d). Anal. for glucosinolates (*J Sci Food Agric*, 1980, **31**, 785; 593). Cooked plant, goitrogen, goitrin (*Z Lebensm Unters Forsch*, 1981, **172**, 90; *CA*, **94**, 101594t).

Cultivated in Maharashtra, Gujarat, W. Bengal and on hills of N. and S. India.

B. oleracea Linn. var. **gongylodes** Linn.

Eng.–*Knol-khol, kohlrabi.*

Tubers and so also steam distillate of peelings contain an antifung. substance (Wlth India, IIB, 293).

Content of goitrogens in raw and boiled plant (*Endocrinol Exp*, 1970, **4**, 51; *CA*, **73**, 108433q). Screening for alk. in different plant parts (*Lloydia*, 1974, **37**, 506). Plant contains ulcer-preventing vit.U [*Gig Saint,* 1981, (6), 85].

*B. oleracea Linn. var. **sabauda** Linn.

Eng.–*Savoy cabbage.*

Ointment prepared from leaves used in wart (*Lloydia,* 1969, **32,** 82).

Grown as vegetable in S. India, Maharashtra, Gujarat and Indo- Gangetic plains.

B. rapa Linn. syn. *B. campestris* Linn. var. *rapa* Hertm.

Eng.–*Field mustard, Indian colza, rape, turnip.*

Goitrogenic effect of turnip on rats (*Rev Esp Fisiol,* 1973, **29,** 21; *CA,* 1974, **80,** 10816m).

Tops (stems and leaves) may produce nitrate poisoning in cattle [*Indian Farming,* 1966, **16**(9), 46]. Stems, antibact. action on pathogenic bacteria (*J Sci Food Agric,* 1970, **21,** 110); ground fresh leaves applied to abscesses (*Planta Med,* 1973, **23,** 381).

Seed ext., fungitoxic; antifung. [*Nat Acad Sci Lett,* 1978, **1,** 187; *Environ India,* 1981, 4(I & II), 83]. Toxic effect of seed meals, rev., 54 refs. (*Br Vet J,* 1979, **135,** 3).

Turnip contains S-Me-*L*-cysteine sulfoxide (*Bitamin Kyoto,* 1960, **20,** 93; *CA,* 1964, **61,** 15093g). Stems and leaves, mineral content (*N Z J Exp Agric,* 1978, **6,** 151).

Seeds, quant. detn. of isothiocyanates and OZT; effect of var. and environment on glucosinolates (*J Sci Food Agric,* 1967, **18,** 510; 1968, **19,** 564); cyano compds. and goitrin (*Can J Physiol Pharmacol,* 1972, **50,** 373); glucosinolates, extn. (*Can Inst Food Sci Technol J* 1972, **5,** 149; *CA,* 1973, **78,** 41760b); alkenyl glucosinolates of *Brassica* spp. (*Z Pflanzenzuecht,* 1981, **87,** 96).

Seed, phenolics (*J Food Sci,* 1975, **40,** 820; 1980, **45,** 1669); also sinapine detn. (*J Agric Food Chem,* 1979, 27, 917; *Angew Bot,* 1980, **54,** 47).

BRAYERA (*Rosaceae*)

See **HAGENIA**

BREYNIA (*Euphorbiaceae*)

*B. cernua Muell.-Arg.

In Malaysia, leaves are ground and applied to swollen legs. Berries contain peonidin and cyanidin 3-pentose glycds. (Wlth India, IIB, 295).

Native of Polynesia, commonly grown in Indian gardens.

B. retusa Alston syn. *B. patens* Benth.

A constituent of many drugs, 'Leptaden', an ext. of *leptadenia reticulata* and *Breynia patens* effective galact. in humans and animals; its effect on smooth muscle pretreated with some antihistaminics and atropine (*Indian Pract,* 1965, **18,** 665; *Indian Vet J,* 1969, 46, 510; 1976, **53,** 345); indigenous drug, 'Aloes compd.' (vet.). useful in infertile brood-mares (*ibid,* 1980, **57,** 762); also useful in dysmenor., clin, trials (*Rajasthan Med J,* 1980, **19,** 29); of ayurvedic drug '*Ayapon*' used to check bleeding after medical termination of pregnancy [*Med Surg,* 1980, **20**(2), 26].

Leaves employed as poultice to hasten suppuration (Wlth India, IIB, 294).

B. vitis-idaea Fisch. syn. *B. rhamnoides* Muell.-Arg.

Eng.–*Indian snowberry.*

Pet. ether ext. of plant, poor sed. (*Naturwissenschaften,* 1964, **51,** 411). Heated leaves, as poultice applied to hasten suppuration; juice given to women after childbirth to prevent haemor.; bark also used for this purpose (Wlth India, IIB, 294).

In Philippines, decoct. of roots used as mouthwash for toothache.

Leaves, triacontane, penta- and triacontanoic acids, ceryl alc., lanosterol and cholesterol (*J Indian Chem Soc,* 1978, **55,** 964)

BRIDELIA (Euphorbiaceae)

B. airy-shawii Li syn. *B. retusa* Spreng.

Fruit used as laxt. (*Bull Bot Surv India*, 1973, **15**, 20).

EtOH(50%) ext. of stem bark, antivir., hypoten. and anticancer (*Indian J Exp Biol*, 1971, **9**, 91).

Stem bark decoct. with country liquor to prevent pregnancy (*Bull Bot Surv India*, 1980, **22**, 59); also for diar. and ear-ache. Paste of stem bark applied to wounds and bark juice taken internally in snake-bite (*Bull Med Ethno Bot Res*, 1980, **1**, 8).

Fruit pulp, β-sitosterol, gallic and ellagic acids; seeds, ellagic acid (*Acta Phytother*, 1971, **18**, 45).

Bark contains a new triterp. ketone (Wlth India, IIB, 296).

B.montana Willd.

Plant used in treatment of fractured bones (*Sri Lanka For*, 1980, **14**, 145).

Leaves and stems contain stigmasterol and friedelan-3-ol; leaves in addn. friedelin and β-sitosterol; its glucd., hexacosanol and triterp. (*Phytochemistry*, 1968, **7**, 2069; *Q J Crude Drug Res*, 1975, **13**, 127).

*B. scandeus Gehrm.

EtOH(50%) ext. of aerial parts, diur. (*Indian J Exp Biol*, 1974, **12**, 512).

Jogfall, Karnataka.

*B. squamosa Gehrm. syn. *B. retusa* Spreng. var. *squamosa* Muell.- Arg.

H.–*Khaja.*

EtOH(50%) ext. of aerial parts, antivir. (*Indian J Exp Biol*, 1973, **11**, 43).

Found in forests around Gorakhpur and in Western Ghats of Maharashtra.

*B. stipularis Blume

Ass.–*Mouhilika*; B.–*Harinhara*; H.–*Kangiabel*; Kan.–*Bisalballi*; Mal.–*Cheruka*; Mar.–*Asana*; Oriya–*Gaurkarsi*; Meghalaya–*U-mei-tong- krong.*

Plant used in pleur. and exudation (*Econ Bot*, 1970, **24**, 247). EtOH(50%) ext. of aerial parts, hypoten. (*Indian J Exp Biol*, 1971, **9**, 91). Seeds, haemagglutinating against human A, B & O red cells (*Indian J Med Res*, 1973, **61**, 1478).

Bark decoct. given to children for cough, fever and asthma, and as gargle for sores in mouth. Fresh tender leaves used for treatment of jaundice; emulsion for anaemia due to pregnancy (Wlth India, IIB, 296).

Bark, friedelin and β-sitosterol (*J Indian Chem Soc*, 1963, **40**, 247). Roots, taraxerone (*Indian J Chem*, 1973, **11**, 840).

Throughout hotter parts of India and along the foot-hills of Himalayas from Kashmir to Bhutan.

BRIZA (Poaceae)

*B. minor Linn.

Eng.–*Lesser* or *small quking grass.*

Grass contains CN glucd. (Fl Iraq, 1968, **9**, 58).

Native of Mediterranean region, found wild in Nilgiris and Palni hills of Tamil Nadu; occasionally cultivated for ornament.

BROMELIA (Bromeliaceae)

*B. pinguin Linn.

Eng.–*Pinguin, wild pineapple.*

Aq. MeOH ext. of stems and leaves, cytotoxic in KB assay [*J Cancer Chemother Rep*, 1972, 3(2), 1].

An enzyme, pinguinain from fruit juice (*Nature Lond*, 1964, **203**, 82; 1966, **210**, 527); isolation and purification of proteolytic enzyme (*Arch Biochem Biophys*, 1968, **126**, 91). Extn. of pinguinain from fruit (US Pat, 1968, 3384552; *CA*, **69**, 41450q); antioedematous (*Science*, 1975, **188**, 215).

Roots and basal stems contain flavons., penduletin, cirsimaritin and casticin, isoferulic acid and 3 new diterps. (two novel phyllocladane derivs. and 3-oxopimar-15-ene-7β, 8β-diol). Aq. MeOH ext. exhibit cytotoxic activity; activity due to flavons. (*J Org Chem*, 1981, **46**, 1094).

Introduced into IBG, Calcutta.

BROMUS (*Poaceae*)

*B. inermis Leyss.

Eng.–*Smooth bromegrass, Hangarian brome.*

Aq. ext. of root, stem, leaf and flower, active against Gram +ve bacteria and mycobacteria (*Econ Bot*, 1959, **13**, 287). In USA, in wild state, grass becoming highly ergotised dangerous under natural conditions (Kingsbury, 81).

Brome ergot resemble those of ergot caused by *Claviceps purpurea* on rye (*Secale cereale*) but fat and moisture content much lower; average alk. content slightly higher than official requirement and ergonorine content more than double; w.-insol. ext. contains ergotamine and ergotoxine (Kingsbury, 81; *J Am Pharm Assoc*, 1955, **44**, 480).

From Kashmir to Kumaun, at 1,500-3,900 m.

B. mollis Linn.

Grains reported to produce giddiness in men and quadrupeds and prove fatal to poultry (Chopra *et al*, II, 923).

Aerial parts contain an unknown alk. (*Phytochemistry*, 1965, **4**, 425).

B. unidoides H.B. & K. syn. *B. catharticus* Vahl

Eng.–*Prarie grass.*

Poisoning caused by high percentage of nitrates (Kingsbury, 420). Si (as SiO_2) as high as 45% of ash. Presence of *trans*-aconitic acid (large amt.) said to cause chelation of Ca and Mg in animal gut thereby inducing hypomagnesia, but this requires further confirmation (*N Z J Agric Bot*, 1972, **25**, 33).

BROUSSONETIA (*Moraceae*)

*B. papyrifera L' Herit. ex Vent.

Eng.–*Paper mulberry.*

In Hawaii, bark given to expectant mother; in Samoa, leaves used in indign. (*Econ Bot*, 1971, **25**, 245; 1974, **28**, 21). Preliminary pharmacol. (*Indian J Exp Biol*, 1974, **12**, 512). Seeds, tonic and diur.

Leaves, diaphor. Bark ext. recommended against eczema (Wlth India, IIB, 300).

Isolation and str. of 2 phytoalexins, broussonins A & B, produced by diseased plants; also isolation of antifung. compds. broussonin C and broussin from wounded xylem tissue of shoots (*Chem Lett*, 1980, 339; 1459).

Found from Punjab to Arunachal Pradesh and Meghalaya, W. Bengal and in peninsular India up to 1,000 m.

BRUCEA (*Simaroubaceae*)

B. javanica Merrill syn. *B. amarissima* Merrill; *B. sumatrana* Roxb.

Eng.–*Macassar kernels.*

Kernels, bitter; used in piles, intestinal haemor. accompanying dysen.; seeds and oil, in papilloma and verruca.

Fruits effective against fever and malaria, comparing favourably with atabrine and plasmoguin; more effective and less toxic than roots, stem and leaves of *Dichroa febrifuga* used for same purpose.

A poultice of leaves used over enlarged spleen, in fever and to cure mange in animals.

Roots valuable in bowel complaints, esp. dysen. Decoct., in colic and rheum. Chewed with betel for cough (Wlth India, IIB, 303)

Seeds extensively investigated abroad, contain brucenol, bruceolic acid, the glycds., brucellin, kosamine and yatanoside (probably identical with a new lactone, mp 258°) and alks., brucamarine and yatanine. Bruceoside A (bruceosin glycd.) & B (brusatol glycd.), potent antileukaemic quassinoid glycds. inhibitory against Ehrlich ascites carcinoma. Brucein D, significantly active against Walker 256 carcinosarcoma in rats. Kosamoside, a glycd. from seeds, emetocathartic, cholag., anthelm. and antimicrob.; also prevents coagulation of blood, in strong doses, causes vomiting, diar., coma and even death (Wlth India, IIB, 303). Pharmacol. action of 3 crystalline compds. (2 glucds. and a phenolic compd.) (*Nagasaki Igakki*

Zasshi, 1959, **34**, 1408; *CA*, 1965, **62**, 4493d).

Seeds also contain 4 bitter compds. including brucein A, B & C; also D, E & G; str. of D & E (*Experientia*, 1967, **23**, 424; 1968, **24**, 768; *C R Acad Sci Ser C*, 1968, **267**, 1346). Kernels, a phytotoxic protein, brutoxin (*Taiwan Yao Hsueh Tsa Chih*, 1977, **29**, 106; *CA*, 1979, **90**, 183160c). Quassinoids, bruceoside A (novel antileukemic agent); & B, in addn. to brucein D & E (*J Chem Soc Chem Commun*, 1977, 69; *J Org Chem*, 1979, **44**, 2180); str. of quassinoids, brucein C and bruceantinol; both antileukemic against murine P 388 lymphocytic leukemia (*Tetrahedron Lett*, 1980, **21**, 1853). Antitumour principles from seeds said to include oleic acid and triolein (*Chung Ts'ao Yao*, 1980, **11**, 529; 532; *CA*, 1981, **94**, 197464z).

Seeds and meal, brusatol; its str. (*Colloq Int C N R S*, 1966, No. 144, 205; *CA*, 1967, **67**, 88292p; *J Org Chem*, 1968, **33**, 429); non-lipophilic material of seeds yield a bitter lactone (*Tetrahedron Lett*, 1968, 6007). Main bitter principle of chinese seeds, brusatol (*J Chin Chem Soc Taipai*, 1971, **18**, 223); isolation of antidysen. compd., yatansin from seeds; identical with brusatol (*Agric Biol Chem*, 1980, **44**, 951). Chloroform ext. effective against malaria; contains bruceolide [*Duoc Hoc*, 1979, (4), 15; *CA*, 1980, **92**, 191396r].

Fruits, roots, as also stems contain brucein A (major compd.), 6 bruceolides, 2 dehydrobruceolides and a dihydrobruceolide; bruceolide fraction most cytotoxic; root ext. cytotoxic to TLX-5 mouse lymphoma cells; active fraction contains brucein A (*Planta Med*, 1980, **39**, 232; 1981, **41**, 209; 1979, **35**, 308); roots and fruits (from Fiji), brucein A, B & C; dehydrobrucein A & B; bruceantin and bruceantatin (*J Pharm Pharmacol*, 1979, **31**, Suppl., 10 P).

Brucein-E β-glucd. from plant (*Tzu Jan Tsa Chin*, 1980, **3**, 395; *CA*, 1981, **94**, 103758y). Bark triterp., rhuslactone (*J Chem Soc Chem Commun*, 1980, 909).

***B. mollis** Wall. ex Kurz

Ass.–*Koinine*.

Seeds useful in malaria, also act as stomch. (*Bull Bot Surv India*, 1976, **18**, 166).

EtOH(50%) ext. of aerial parts, anticancer (*Indian J Exp Biol*, 1977, **15**, 208).

Subtropical Eastern Himalayas, Sikkim, and Bhutan, up to 2,500 m.

BRUGMANSIA (*Solanaceae*)

***B. candida** Pers. syn. *Datura arborea* auct. non Linn.

Plant, highly poisonous and narcotic (Uphof, 174).

Alks. in flower, 0.42; leaves, 0.21; and stem, 0.16%. All parts contain higher percentage of scopolamine (hyoscine) than hyoscyamine. Aposcopolamine & meteloidine identified (*Planta Med*, 1966, **14**, 465). Roots, alk. estn. (*Indian J Pharm*, 1967, **29**, 199).

Grown in gardens on hills and it is common in Mahabaleshwar, Maharashtra.

***B. suaveolens** Bercht. & Presl syn. *Datura suaveolens* Humb. & Bonpl. ex Willd.

Eng.–*Angel's trumpet*.

EtOH(50%) ext. of plant, spasmog. and B.P. depress. (*Indian J Exp Biol*, 1969, **7**, 250).

Leaf alk. detn., 80% hyoscine [*Proc Nat Acad Sci India*, 1965, **34A**(Pt 3), 261]. Egyptian plant, alk. in stems (2.37%) and leaves (0.32%); scopolamine (hyoscine), meteloidine, hyoscyamine present (*J Pharm Sci UAR* 1969, **10**, 125; *CA*, 1970, **73**, 127727e). Distribution of alks. in different plant parts (*Phytochemistry*, 1972, **11**, 3293); pharmacognostic study [*An Farm Quim Sao Paulo*, 1977, **17**(2), 75; *CA*, 1978, **89**, 204070v].

Native of Mexico, grown in Indian gardens.

BRUGUIERA (*Rhizophoraceae*)

*B. cylindrica(Linn.) Blume syn. *B. caryophylloides* Blume; *B. malabarica* Arn.

Tam.–*Kakandan*, Tel.–*Varuda*.

Stem and bark, brugine, tropine 1,2-dithiolane-3- carboxylate, brugierol, isobrugierol and 4-OH-1, 2-dithiolane (*Phytochemistry*, 1975, **14**, 1458; 1976, **15**, 220).

Tidal forests of India.

*B. gymnorrhiza Lamk syn. *B. eriopetala* Hensl.; *B. conjugata* (Linn.) Merrill

B.–*Kankara*; Oriya–*Kekar*; Tam.–*Stgapukokandan*; Tel.– *Thuddaponna*.

EtOH(50%) ext. of aerial parts, hypoten. (*Indian J Exp Biol*, 1977, **15**, 208).

Stem and bark contain brugierol & isobrugierol (*Tetrahedron Lett*, 1972, 203). Extn. procedure of brugierol from bark (Jpn Kokai, 1973, 7310213; *CA*, **79**, 9883d). Leaves, a triterp. alc., gymnorhizol and sitosterol (*Indian J Chem*, 1978, **16B**, 742).

Found in littoral and estuarian forests of India including Andamans.

*B. sexangula Poir. syn. *B. eriopetala* Wight & Arn. ex Arn. Hensl. (FBI) in part.

Roots and leaves applied to burns (Wlth India, IIB, 306).

Bark ext., antitumour against Sarcoma 180 and Lewis lung carcinoma; activity partly due to tannin. Stem bark contains toxic alks. (0.08%) including brugine, tropine & its esters (*Tetrahedron Lett*, 1966, 6327; *Aust J Chem*, 1969, **22**, 1271).

Found in Orissa, Andhra Pradesh, Kerala and Tamil Nadu.

BRUNELLA (*Lamiaceae*)

See **PRUNELLA**

BRUNFELSIA (*Solanaceae*)

*B. americana Linn.

Eng.–*Lady of the night*.

Fruits, astrin.; used as tonic in chr. diar. and stomach disorders. In Dominica, plant employed as poison. Stem and leaves con-tain two unnamed alks. Leaves, flowers, stembark and roots, traces of cyanide; leaves, chlorogenic acid (Wlth India, IIB, 308).

Grown in gardens.

*B. grandiflora D. Don

Plant—antipyr., narcotic and hallucinogen.

Roots—antirheum., aphrodis., fish poison.

Rootbark, prunfelsamidine (pyrrole-3-carboxamidine) which induces convuls. in mice (Wlth India, IIB, 308).

Seeds yield scopoletin (*An Acad Bras Cienc*, 1964, **36**, 511; *CA*, 1966, **64**, 1007b).

Grown in gardens.

*B. nitida Benth.

Plant used for herbal bath. Fruits give +ve test for alk. [Wlth India, IIB, 308; *Lloydia*, 1970, **33**(3A), Suppl., 203].

Introduced into India.

*B. uniflora D. Don syn. *B. hopeana* Benth.

Eng.–*Manaca, vegetable mercury, rain tree*.

Roots—dried roots used as drug, official in Brazilian pharmacopoeia. Powd. root or its fluid ext., antiinflam., diur., antirheum., antisyphilitic, alter., narcotic and poisonous (Wlth India, IIB, 307). Ext., CNS depress., activity due to alk. fraction. Also effective in decreasing carrageenin-induced pedal oedema in rats (*Lloydia*, 1977, **40**, 356).

Fresh leaves also employed but less effective than roots. Bark and young shoots, resolv. and emetic (Wlth India, IIB, 307).

Roots contain alks. manacine and manaceine; bark, manacine (0.068%) which resembles strychnine in its physiological actions (Wlth India, IIB, 307); alk., hopeanine, str. detn. (*Symp Pap IUPAC Int Symp Chem Nat Prod*, 1978, **2**, 5; *CA*, 1980, **92**, 42210y). Seeds, scopoletin (*An Acad Bras Cienc*, 1964, **34**, 511; *CA*, 1966, **64**, 1007b).

Cultivated in India.

BRYONIA (*Cucurbitaceae*)

B. callosa Rottl.; see **Cucumis callosus**

B. lanciniosa Linn.; see **Diplocylos palmatus**

BRYONOPSIS (*Cucurbitaceae*)

B. lanciniosa auct. non Linn.; see **Diplocyclos palmatus**

BRYOPHYLLUM (*Crassulaceae*)

See **KALANCHOE**

BUCHANANIA (*Anacardiaceae*)

*B. axillaris (Desr.) Ramam. syn. *B. angustifolia* Roxb.

Eng.–*Bughanan's mango*; *cuddapah almond*; H.–*Piyala*; Kan.– *Murligidda*; Mal.–*Chaara paruppu*; Tam.–*Saraparuppu*; Tel.–*Pedda sara*.

EtOH(50%) ext. of aerial parts, CNS depress. (*Indian J Exp Biol*, 1980, **18**, 594).

Plant gum dissolved in goat milk, to this *Ragi* (*Eleusine coracana*) flour added, boiled till it becomes a paste; the paste applied on joints to alleviate pain (*Ancient Sci Life*, 1981-82, **1**, 117).

Commonly found in open scrub and dry deciduous forests of Peninsular India.

B. lanzan Spreng. syn. *B. latifolia* Roxb.

Kernels—oil in skin diseases caused by blood defects [*J Res Indian Med*, 1973, **8**(1), 82]; ointment used to cure itch and blemishes from face. Also applied to glandular swellings of neck (*Bull Bot Surv India*, 1980, **22**, 68); kernels as brain tonic (*J Econ Tax Bot*, 1981, **2**, 176).

Leaves—crushed or powd. leaves applied to wounds (*Econ Bot*, 1965, **19**, 24; *Bull Bot Surv India*, 1973, **15**, 15). EtOH(50%) ext. of aerial parts, anticancer (*Indian J Exp Biol*, 1969, **87**, 250). Leaves valued as tonic and cardiotonic (*Bull Med Ethno Bot Res*, 1980, **1**, 338).

Various plant parts used in inflam. of gums, in fever, burns, dysuria, cholera, phthisis, broncht. and asthma, consumption and as antid. (*Econ Bot*, 1970, **24**, 241).

Gum—stem exudate used in intercostal pains (Wlth India, IIB, 308); gum in cow's milk for rheum. pains (*Ancient Sci Life*, 1981- 82, **1**, 117).

BUCKLANDIA (*Hamamelidaceae*)

See **EXBUCKLANDIA**

BUDDLEJA (*Buddlejaceae*)

B. davidii Franch. syn. *B. variabilis* Hemsl.

Eng.–*Orange eye butterfly*, *summer lilac*.

Leaves yield glycds., catalpol & Mecatalpol having diur. properties (*Biochem J*, 1965, **96**, 1).

Leaves and flowers contain buddleoflavonoloside (linarin) (Wlth India, IIB,311).

Rootbark, 5 sesquiterps., buddledin A-E; all possess piscic. properties (*Tetrahedron Lett*, 1976, 3717; *Chem Pharm Bull*, 1978, **26**, 2535; 2543).

B. globosa Hoppe

An infusion of leaves used in callous ulcers and warts.

Leaves yield aucubin and lupeol (Wlth India, IIB, 312); iridoids, catalpol & Mecatalpol (*Biochem J*, 1965, **96**, 1); flavons., luteolin & 6-OH-luteolin (*Phytochemistry*, 1971, **10**, 367).

Flowers, linarin, cosmetin and rutin (Wlth India, IIB, 312).

*B. lindleyana Fort.

Plant, insectic.; crushed flowers employed to stupefy fish (Wlth India, IIB, 312).

Cultivated in gardens as ornamental.

*B. macrostachya Benth.

Khasi–*Jai-lenag- kren*; Nagaland–*Tikokra- molli*.

EtOH(50%) ext. of aerial parts, diur. (*Indian J Exp Biol*, 1974, **12**, 512).

Plant contains pectolinarigenin and salvigenin (*Phytochemistry*, 1980, **19**, 929).

Found in Sikkim Himalayas, Meghalaya and Nagaland.

*B. madagascariensis Lamk

Eng.–*Madagascar orange ball tree.*

In Malagsy, plant used as a remedy for broncht., cough and asthma.

Leaves contain *n*-alkanes, sterols and triterp. (*Fitoterapia*, 1981, **52**, 235).

Grown in gardens for ornament and hedges.

B. neemda Buch.- Ham. syn. *B. asiatica* Lour.

Eng.–*White butterfly bush.*

Leaves used for fomentation on inflam. and in preparation of domestic med. (*Econ Bot*, 1979, **33**, 52). EtOH ext. of leaves, hypoten.; mech. of action studied (*Q J Crude Drug Res*, 1980, **18**, 830).

Antibact. activity of essent. oil from flowers (0.95%) and buds [*Indian Perfum*, 1981, **25**(Pt. 3 & 4), 7].

Flowers, quercetin and linarin (*Indian J Chem*, 1963, **1**, 366).

*B. officinalis Maxim.

In Chinese med. used for eye ailments (Uphof, 89).

Found in Bihar.

BULBOSTYLIS (*Cyperaceae*)

*B. barbata C.B. Clarke syn. *Scirpus barbatus* Rottb.

H.–*Masa*; Kan.–*Chavuri*; Tam.–*Mukkutikorei.*

In Philippines, plant boiled in water and brew given in dysen. Pollen grains may cause allergy (Wlth India, IIB, 335).

Found throughout India as a weed.

BUNIUM (*Apiaceae*)

*B. persicum(Boiss.) Fedts. syn. *Carum bulbocastanum* Koch

H.–*Kala zira*; Kan.–*Shine jeerige*; Ladakh–*Umbhu.*

Essent.oil—from fruit(2.5%); constituents; cuminaldehyde, 40.6%; oil

increased level of w.-sol. protein in exp. animals and decreased EtOH and CCl4 toxicity (*Dokl Akad Nauk Tadzh SSR*, 1978, **21**, 33); blood vessel permeability, antid. and therapeutic application; oil increased hepatic protein content in rats; had remarkable antid. action against hepatotoxic substances (*Izv Akad Nauk Tadzh SSR Otd Biol Nauk*, 1978, 98; 101; *CA*, 1979, **90**, 133633p; 133796u).

Essent. oil of seeds (fruits), constituents (*Pak J Sci Ind Res*, 1977, **20**, 106; *CA*, 1979, **90**, 138033c).

BUPLEURUM (*Apiaceae*)

B. falcatum Linn.

Eng.–*Hare's ear.*

Roots—main therapeutic use in inflam., pyrexia, pain, muscle stiffness and neurosis. Important ingredient of various recipes in Chinese medicine (Plant known as *Chai-hu* in Chinese) to resolve tightness and resistance syndrome at the costal margin that might be related to inflam. of diaphragm and enlargement of liver caused by hepatitis (*in* Wagner & Wolff, 180-82). Useful in flatulence, as antipyr. and expect. (Wlth India, IIB, 336). Roots owe its activities to saikosides or saikosaponins (from *Saiko* in Japanese); yield from roots, 2.06-3.02%; saponin content varies with age (Wlth India, IIB, 336).

Cultivation and breeding effect on yield of root, content of saikosaponins, etc. (*Shoyakugaku Zasshi*, 1980, **34**, 209; 215; 221; *BA*, 1981, **71**, 63801-03).

Saikosaponins & their genins—major saikosaponins (triterps.) a, c and d; acetates of a & d. Steroid saponin, α-spinasteryl-β-glucd. (*Tetrahedron Lett*, 1968, 303); minor e; also f (*ibid*, 1977, 1227; 1976, 4167). Saikogenins, triterps, E, F & G as genuine sapogenins (of c, a & d resp.); A, C, D and B artefacts and longispinogenin (*Tetrahedron*, 1968, **24**, 675; 1967, **23**, 3333; 3353). Components of saikosaponin b (itself an artefact) (*J Chem Soc Perkin Trans I*, 1975, 2043). Extn., sepn., detn., etc. of saponins (*Planta*

Med, 1976, **29**, 247; 1978, **33**, 152; *Chem Pharm Bull*, 1979, **27**, 1836; 1980, **28**, 2367; *Shoyakugaku Zasshi*, 1975, **29**, 99; *CA*, 1976, **85**, 10342g).

Saikosaponins (characteristic, Δ^{11}, 13β, 28-epoxyoleanene system), extensive pharmacol. investigation; strong haemolytic and local irrit., CNS- suppressing effect while analg., antipyr., as well as antitussive; antipyr. action remarkable. Antiinflam. on oral administration; saikosaponins a & d (16 β-OH & 16 α-OH), their genuine genins (F & G) and artifact genin A (of a), with str.-activity relationship; no side effects like shrinking of adrenal gland that occurs quite often with exogenous prednisolone; reduces cholesterol and triglycerides level in plasma of cholesterol diet rats; exp. support for application in Chinese med. for inflam. and hepatobiliary diseases (*in* Wagner & Wolff, 181-83); antihepatotoxic in model galactosomine liver damage system (*in* Beal & Reinhard, 235-36; *Planta Med*, 1980, **40**, 366); stimulation of pituitary-adrenocortical axis by saikosaponins; str. and corticosterone-secretion inducing activities (*Chem Pharm Bull*, 1981, **29**, 495; 500); saikosaponin a, antivir. against influenza virus *in vitro*. Str. & various activities relationships (*J Pharm Sci*, 1974, **63**, 471; *Tetrahedron Lett*, 1976, 4163; *Planta Med*, 1978, **34**, 160; 287; 1980, **40**, 366; 1981, **42**, 356; 366).

Roots contain essent. oil, several sterols having metabolic activities and plasma cholesterol-lowering activity; α- and β-spinasterol, stigmasterol, stigmastenol and Δ^7- & Δ^{22}- stigmastenol, and bupleurumol (Wlth India, IIB, 337); also ribitol(adonitol); 10-nonacosanone, α-spinasterol and β-sitosterol (*Shoyakugaku Zasshi*, 1969, **23**, 96; 1972, **26**, 64; *CA*, 1970, **73**, 72845w; 1973, **78**, 1991w); coumarins (also in aerial parts) (*Rastit Resur*, 1970, **6**, 571; *CA*, 1971, **74**, 95441j); polyacetylenic compds. (*Yakhak Hoe Chi*, 1975, **19**, 16; *CA*, 1976, **84**, 71409k); khel-

lactone, (–)-anomalin (*Indian J Chem*, 1977, **15B**, 293).

Aerial parts, saponins (2.37% dry wt. basis). Leaves, rutin (0.3- 0.4%) (Wlth India, IIB, 337); rutin also in flowers (*Polez Rast Prir Flory Sib*, 1967, 92; *CA*, 1968, **69**, 93660c).

*B. falcatum Linn. var. **birarensis** Haines
Mundari–*Bir yambiri.*
Crushed herb given in headache (Wlth India, IIB, 338).
Found on mountains of Chota Nagpur.

*B. hamiltonii Balakr. syn. *B. tenue* Buch.-Ham. ex D. Don non Salisb.
Roots, as diaphor., antipyr. and in liver trouble (*Indian Drugs*, 1976-77, **14**, 47).
Kashmir to Sikkim from 300 to 2,700 m.

*B. lanceolatum Wall. ex DC.
J. & K.–*Sarpabuti.*
Fresh juice of herb mixed with *Piper longum* used as remedy for snake-bite (*Nagarjun*, 1979-80, **23**, 242).
Jammu & Kashmir.

*B. marginatum Wall. ex DC. syn. *B. falcatum* var. *marginatum* (Wall. ex DC.) C.B. Clarke
P.–*Kalizewar, silpil.*
Root, antipyr. and in amenor. (Wlth India, IIB, 338).
Some authors treat this species as *B. falcatum* var. *scorzoneraefolium* (Willd.) Ledeb, roots of which have same pattern of saponins though may not be as high in yield as *B. falcatum* (Wlth India, IIB, 338).
Himalayas and Meghalaya.

*B. wightii Mukherjee syn. *B.mucronatum* Wight & Arn. non Brouss. ex Spreng.
Eng.–*Common hare's ear.*
Crushed herb used for pain in legs and arms (Wlth India, IIB, 338).
Madhya Pradesh, Bihar, Orissa, Maharashtra and S. India.

BURSERA (*Burseraceae*)

*B. penicillata Engl. syn. *B. delpechiana* Poiss. ex. Engl.
Eng.–*Indian lavender tree.*

Essent. oil, antimicrob. (*Riechst Aromen Kosmet*, 1977, **27**, 303; *CA*, 1978, **88**, 99656v); insectic. against *Aedas aegypti* [*Pesticides*, 1980, **14**(9), 15].

Fruit and husk, essent. oil physicochem. properties (*Perfum Essent Oil Res*, 1965, **56**, 85); root bark contains essent. oil (*Curr Sci*, 1966, **35**, 152).

Native to Mexico, introduced and cultivated in S.India.

B. serrata Wall. ex Colebr.; see **Protium serratum**

BUTEA (*Fabaceae*)

*B. buteiformis Grierson & Long syn. *B. minor* Buch.-Ham.

Nagaland–*Fu*.

In Nagaland, seed paste mixed with water taken to kill intestinal worms (Wlth India, IIB, 347).

Found in Kumaun, C. India, Bihar, and E. India up to 1,200 m.

B. monosperma Taub. syn. *B. frondosa* Koenig ex Roxb.

Seeds—acrid, bitter, aper. and rubft. Decoct. given in gravel. Paste of powd. with lemon juice applied as cure for ringworm and herpes (Wlth India, IIB, 344); paste used for cooling effect (*Bull Med Ethno Bot Res*, 1980, **1**, 318); clin. use, as anthelm. not safe, it may cause nephrotoxicity (*Indian J Pharm*, 1965, **27**, 253). Freshly powd. seeds, effective against *Ascaris* (*J Agric Trop Bot Appl*, 1966, **13**, 268); ext., *in vitro*, anthelm. against *Ascaridia galli* worms, more effective than piperazine (*Indian J Physiol Pharmacol*, 1976, **20**, 64).

Seed powd., one of the ingredients of indigenous drug for hymenolepiasis (*Indian J Med Res*, 1970, **58**, 616); of 'Calcury' used against ureteric calculus, clin. trials [*Med Surg*, 1981, **21**(12), 15]. Finely powd. seeds alongwith *Acorus calamus* rhizome, or mixed with juice of *Cyperus rotundus* rhizome cure delirium [*J Res Indian Med*, 1978, **13**(4), 92; *Econ Bot*, 1981, **35**, 4].

Saline ext. of seeds agglutinates erythrocytes of animals (*Vox Sang*, 1964, **9**, 216; *CA*, **61**, 6205h).

Hot alc. ext. of seeds, antiimplantation and antiovulatory in animals (*Indian J Med Res*, 1968, **56**, 1575; *Indian J Exp Biol*, 1978, **16**, 1077; *Bull Med Ethno Bot Res*, 1980, **1**, 420). Dried alc. ext., abortif. in miçe and rats (*Indian J Physiol Pharmacol*, 1969, **13**, 239).

Plant—alc. ext. of whole plant produced persistent vesodepression in cats and showed activity against earth worms (*Sci Cult*, 1977, **43**, 344). An Ayurvedic preparation with other plant substances, anthelm. [*J Res Indian Med*, 1978, **13**(3), 130]. Various plant parts used in gravel, fever and menor.(*Econ Bot*, 1970, **24**, 247).

Flowers—used as emmen., and as poultice in orchitis and to reduce swellings, in bruises and sprains. Petals given to sheep for haemat. They are antifung. Decoct. given in diar. and to puerperal women (Wlth India, IIB, 344). Lotion prepared after distilling flowers used for certain eye diseases (*Econ Bot*, 1978, **32**, 278). Dried flowers for preventing sunstroke (*Bull Med Ethno Bot Res*, 1980, **1**, 318). Effective in leprosy, and gout [*Indian Drugs Pharmac Ind*, 1980, **15**(4), 14]. Alc. ext., antiestrogenic in mice (*Indian J Exp Biol*, 1966, **4**, 246). Aq. ext., antiimplantation in rats (*Indian J Med Res*, 1968, **56**, 1575). Pet. ether ext., very feeble antifert. in female rats [*J Res Indian Med*, 1976, **11**(1), 112]. Flowers alongwith *Hygrophila auriculata* leaves and roots taken with milk to cure leucor. [*ibid*, 1978, **13**(4), 92]. Juice given to women to induce sterility (*J Econ Tax Bot*, 1981, **2**, 68).

Bark—insectic. against house flies (*Bull RRL Jammu*, 1962-63 **1**, 156); astrin., pungent, alter., aphrodis. and anthelm. Useful in tumours, bleeding piles and ulcers. Decoct. given in cold, cough, fever, haemor. and menstrual disorders; alc. ext. of bark, as also of seeds inhibitory against *E. coli* and *Micrococcus pyogenes* var *aureus* (Wlth India, IIB, 344). Used in elixirs and tonics (*Q J Crude Drug Res*, 1970, **10**, 1555). Decoct. given in bloody diar. (*Bull Med Ethno Bot Res*, 1980, **1**, 8).

Gum—fresh from bark, applied to ulcers and septic sore throat. Given in phthisis, haemor. of stomach and bladder; its infusion as local application in leucor.

Gum sol. applied to bruises, erysipelatous inflams. and ringworm (Wlth India, IIB, 343). To check conception [*J Res Indian Med*, 1978, **13**(2), 104].

Leaves—diur. and aphrodis; used to cure boils, pimples, tumours, and haemor. Given in flatulent colic, worms and piles (Wlth India, IIB, 344). EtOH(50%) ext., spasmog. (*Indian J Exp Biol*, 1968, **6**,232); juice for skin diseases (*Bull Bot Surv India*, 1973, **15**, 15); with cow's milk, slow sterilizer (*Econ Bot*, 1980, **34**, 273).

Roots useful in night blindness, etc.; cause temporary sterility in women (Wlth India, IIB, 344). Root bark, aphrodis. (*Q J Crude Drug Res*, 1971, **11**, 1742); also in elephantiasis, as analg. and anthelm., applied in sprue, piles, ulcers, tumours and dropsy [*Indian Drugs Pharmac Ind*, 1980, **15**(4), 19].

Palasonin—anthelm. principle, isolation from seed and characterisation (*Indian J Chem*, 1967, **5**, 86); isolations; also of a new imide (*Chem Ind Lond*, 1970, 1376); configuration (*Helv Chim Acta*, 1974, **57**, 32). Hexahydro- 3α-Me-4,7-epoxyisobenzofuran-1,3-dione, 9Cl; de-Me-cantharidin (Dictionary Org. Compds., IV, 4475). Palasonin more effective than piperazine or santonin against round worms (*Ascaris lumbricoides*) in human (Wlth India, IIB, 344); stimulatory action on smooth muscles (*Indian J Physiol Pharmacol*, 1977, **21**, 247). Method for palasonin extn. (*Indian J Pharm Sci*, 1978, **40**, 97).

Unsap. matter of seed oil contains α-amyrin, β-sitosterol & its glucd. (*Indian J Pharm*, 1977, **39**,79). Seeds contain a new δ-lactone of *n*-heneicosanoic acid (*Planta Med*, 1979, **35**, 286); alk., monospermine (*Chem Ind Lond*, 1981, 98); new phytolec-

tin, its purification (*Indian J Biochem Biophys*, 1981, **18**, 166).

Plant flavon. glucds. butin, butrin, isobutrin and palastrin [*Pharmaceutist*, 1966-67, **12**(9), 12]; flowers, butrin, coreopsin, monospermoside & their iso-derivs. and sulphurein (*Phytochemistry*, 1970, **9**, 2231); chalcones (*J Food Sci*, 1980, **45**, 746).

B. parviflora Roxb. syn. *Spatholobus roxburghii* Benth.

Plant—insectic. and piscic.

Bark—decoct. used in dropsy and bowel complaints. Acetone ext., toxic to mosquito larvae (Wlth India, IIB, 346).

Ash of leaves given as vermifuge.

Seeds, friedelin (*J Indian Chem Soc*, 1970, **47**, 95); unsap. matter of seed oil, β-sitosterol (*Fette Seifen Anstrichm*, 1971, **23**, 437; *CA*, **75**, 106095y).

B. superba Roxb.

Seeds—sed. and anthelm.; decoct., emol. and used topically for piles (Wlth India, IIB, 347). Seed oil, anthelm. and hypoten. (*Indian J Pharm*, 1963, **25**,270). Seeds, haemagglutinating against human ABO red cells (*Indian J Med Res*, 1973, **61**, 1478).

Roots—rejuvenating. Also estrogenic substance and poisonous substance; hypoten. and cardiotonic. Root active against fungus *Helminthosporium sativum* (Wlth India, IIB, 347). Root bark, aphrodis. (*Q J Crude Drug Res*, 1971, **11**, 1742). Tuber paste in inflam. or ulcer of neck of oxen (*Bull Bot Surv India*, 1980, **22**, 201).

Decoct. of stem and leaves, emol. and sed.; topically used for piles (Wlth India, IIB, 347). Bark used in tonics, elixirs, etc. (*Q J Crude Drug Res*, 1970, **10**, 1555). Plant, in night fever, dysuria and gravel (*Econ Bot*, 1970, **24**, 247).

BUXUS (*Buxaceae*)

*B. papillosa Schneid.

Leaves, perhaps poisonous like European *B. sempervirens* causing deaths in camels and cattle in India (Chopra *et al*, II, 767).

Leaves and stems contain alks. buxpapine and buxapamine; also buxpapinine (*Pak J Sci Ind Res*, 1968, **11**, 253; 488); 4 alks. (–)-cyclobuxupaline C, (+)-cyclopapilosine D, (+)-buxamine C and desoxy-16-buxidienine (*Phytochemistry*, 1973, **12**, 2051).

Leaves and stems, also 2 steroid alcs., buxpapinol and buxpapininol (*Pak J Sci Ind Res*, 1970, **12**, 201). Plant, lupeol and lupenediol (*Phytochemistry*, 1973, **12**, 470).

Dry and arid slopes of Western Himalayas up to 1,200 m.

B. wallichiana Baill. syn. *B. sempervirens* Linn.

Eng.–*Himalayan boxwood tree*.

Leaves poisonous, causing death in camels and cattle in India (Chopra *et al*, II, 767).

Buxenine-G, cytotoxic (*Tetrahedron Lett*, 1966, 3815). European *B. sempervirens* (leaves) with its chief alk. cyclobuxine-D readily distinguishable from *B. wallichiana* (leaves) with buxtauine (cyclomicrobuxinine) as. chief alk. (*Pharmazie*, 1970, **15**, 363; *CA*, **73**, 127748n). Steroid alks., cyclovirobuxine-D, cyclobuxine-D, cycloprotobuxine-C, and buxtauine from New Jersy leaves (*Phytochemistry*, 1972, **11**, 1853).

Leaves contain several other alks., their isolation, str., etc. See also *Buxus* alks. (*in* Manske, IX, 378-406; *in* Manske, XVI, 60-61). Recent progress in *Veratrum* and *Buxus* alks. [*Symp Pap IUPAC Int Symp Chem Nat Prod*, 1978, **4**(Pt.1), 260]. Steroidal alks., rev., 59 refs. on *Buxus* and others (*Alkaloids Lond*, 1979, **9**, 238; *CA*, 1980, **92**, 147026w).

BYTTNERIA (*Sterculiaceae*)

*B. andamanesis Kurz
Bark used in hair-wash.
Middle and S. Andamans.

*B. aspera Colebr.
Ass.–*Tikoni-borua*.
Bark used in hair-wash (Wlth India, IIB, 350).
Bihar, Eastern parts of India up to 1,200 m; and in S. Andamans.

B. herbacea Roxb.
Rootstock used to treat cholera and diar. Plant contains steroids, alks. and saponins (Wlth India, IIB, 350).
Powd. stem applied to swellings (*Bull Bot Surv India*, 1973, **15**, 13).

*B. pilosa Roxb.
Leaf paste applied to sores of cattle (*Bull Bot Surv India*, 1976, **18**, 166).
Assam, and Khasi hills of Meghalaya.

CADABA (*Capparidaceae*)

C. fruticosa (Linn.) Druce syn. *C. farinosa* Forsk.; *C. indica* Lamk
H.–*Dabi*.
In Africa, infusion of leaves inhaled to clear head from colds (*Econ Bot*, 1979, **33**, 35).
Leaves, betaine-type base, cadabine; identical with stachydrine (*Pak J Sci Ind Res*, 1971, **14**, 343; 1975, **17**, 109; *Phytochemistry*, 1975, **14**, 292); also taxon. in relation to alks. (*ibid*, 1973, **12**, 2893). Pods, dilactone cadabalone (*Planta Med*, 1981, **43**, 293).

CAESALPINIA (*Caesalpiniaceae*)

C. bonduc (Linn.) Roxb. emend. Dandy & Exell syn. *C. bonducella* Flem.; *C. crista* Linn.; *C. nuga* Ait. f.
Seeds—in Hawaii, bean meat, as laxt., blood purifier and in congestion; fruit pulp, piscic. (*Econ Bot*, 1971, **25**, 245; 1970, **24**, 134). Powd., antidiar. in rat (*Indian J Pharm*, 1965, **27**, 307); purg. [*J Res Indian Med*, 1978, **13**(4), 92].
Root—decoct., in calculus and in honey cure leucor. [*J Res Indian Med*, 1978, **13**(4), 92]. EtOH(50%) ext. of root and stem, antivir. (*Indian J Exp Biol*, 1968, **6**, 232). Ext., antifung. (*Labdev*, 1971, **9B**, 136).

Plant—ext., antiinflam. in rats (*Indian J Pharm*, 1966, **28**, 341). In Samoa, used in hydrocile and as tonic (*Econ Bot*, 1974, **28**, 16). Ether ext. of leaves, antimicrob. (*Philipp J Sci*, 1976, **105**, 205). Powd. effective drug in blood dysen., clin. trials [*J Res Indian Med*, 1978, **13**(1), 140].

Seeds, 3 bitter compds., α-, β- & γ-caesalpin (*Tetrahedron Lett*, 1963, 2079); their str. (*Sci Res, Dacca*, 1964, **1**, 135; *CA*, **61**, 10718g; *Pak J Sci Ind Res*, 1963, **6**, 65; *CA*, 1966, **65**, 3681f; *Gazz Chim Ital*, 1966, **96**, 662; 687; *CA*, **65**, 8968a,h); also ε-caesalpin (*Tetrahedron Lett*, 1967, 5027).

New diterp., x-caesalpin (*Indian J Chem*, 1981, **20B**, 625).

*C. cacalaco Humb. & Bonpl.

Bark used in dentalgia (Hocking, 36); pods rich in tannin (Benthall, 167).

Native to S. America, cultivated in Indian gardens.

C. coriaria (Jacq.) Willd.

Eng.–*Divi-divi plant, American sumac.*

EtOH(50%) ext. of fruit, semen coagulant (*Indian J Exp Biol*, 1977, **15**, 208).

Fruits, a di-phenoylglucose named corilagin, chebulic acid, etc.(*Symp Phytochem Proc Meeting Univ Hong Kong*, 1961, 164; *CA*, 1964, **61**, 16443d).

C. decapetala Alston syn. *C. sepiaria* Roxb.

Eng.–*Mysore thorn.*

EtOH(50%) ext. of roots, antivir. and hypoten. (*Indian J Exp Biol*, 1969, **7**, 250).

C. digyna Rottl.

Eng.–*Teri pods.*

Roots—EtOH(50%) ext., active *in vitro* against *Mycobacterium tuberculosis* in guinea pigs (*Indian J Exp Biol*, 1966, **4**, 214). Plant, a minor constituent of indigenous drug 'Geriforte' (*Indian Drugs*, 1980-81, **18**, 346; *Rajasthan Med J*, 1980, **19**, 23).

*C. gilliesii Wall. ex Hook.

Eng.–*Bird of paradise.*

In Libya, leaves and flower used as purg. and reported to be poisonous; leaf, stem and flowers, unnamed alk. and leaves, +ve test for phenols, flavon., etc. (*Lloydia*, 1972, **35**, 70; 74). Total alks. in leaves, 0.63-0.70; and in stem, 0.40-0.45% [*Izuch i Ispol'z Lekarstv Rastit Resur SSSR* (Leningrad: Med) Sb, 1964, 198; *CA*, 1965, **62**, 10821b].

Cultivated in Indian gardens.

C. major Dandy & Exell syn. *C. glabra* Merrill; *C. jayabo* Maza

Seeds and leaves, in skin diseases and rheum. Seeds, in fever (*J Econ Tax Bot*, 1980, **1**, 140). Plant, in skeletal fractures (*Sri Lanka For*, 1980, **14**, 145).

*C. mimosoides Lamk

Mal.–*Kilansadu.*

Paste of young shoots and onion used in ulcer (*J Econ Tax Bot*, 1981, **2**, 68).

Reported from Kerala.

C. pulcherrima (Linn.) Swartz syn. *Poinciana pulcherrima* Linn.

Roots—acrid and even poisonous (Fl. Med., 264).

Leaves—decoct. and flowers, used against fevers of Tortola (Fl. Med., 260). Used as antipyr., tonic, abortif.; in liver disorder and for gargles (*Acta Phytother*, 1965, **12**, 81). Exts., anticancer (*Philipp J Sci*, 1967, **96**, 393); ext. fungitoxic (*Acta Bot Indica*, 1979, **7**, 147).

Plant—as laxt., in cold, fever, etc.; powd. in erysipelas (*Acta Phytother*, 1965, **12**, 81).

Seeds—in powd. form, a remedy for stomachache (Fl. Med., 264).

Leaves, myricitrqside (*C R Acad Sci*, 1965, **260**, 271; *Q J Crude Drug Res*, 1967, **7**, 964).

Bark, diterp. x-caesalpin (*Chem Ind Lond*, 1970, 534); β-sitosterol, sebacic acid, quercimeritrin and leucodelphinidin (*J Indian Chem Soc*, 1977, **54**, 646); 2 ellagitannins (*Phytochemistry*, 1980, **19**, 1995).

Flowers, cyanin (*J Indian Chem Soc*, 1977, **54**, 646). Chem. constituents of red and orange-flowers (*Indian J Pharm Sci*, 1978, **40**, 103). Seeds contain lectins (*Rev*

Colomb Quim, 1978, **8**, 25; *CA*, 1981, **94**, 45395q).

C. sappan Linn.

Essent. oil from leaves, antimicrob. (*Indian Perfum*, 1978, **22**, 73).

EtOH(50%) ext. of stem, semen coagulant and anticancer (*Indian J Exp Biol*, 1980, **18**, 594).

Heartwood MeOH ext., antiinflam. in rats; activity due to brazilin (*Planta Med*, 1971, **31**, 214). Heartwood, α-amyrin and amino acids (*Indian J Pharm*, 1977, **39**, 85); β-sitosterol [*J Res Indian Med*, 1978, **13**(3), 82].

CAESULIA (*Asteraceae*)

*C. axillaris Roxb.

H.–*Bangra*; Mar.–*Maka*; Tel.–*Guttikuncha*; Mundari–*Marang*.

Plant—used in baldness (*Econ Bot*, 1970, **24**, 241); fresh herb, crushed and applied to wounds (*Bull Bot Surv India*, 1971, **13**, 221). EtOH(50%) ext., diur. (*Indian J Exp Biol*, 1980, **18**, 594).

Essent. oil—from plant, antimicrob. (*Indian J Pharm*, 1975, **37**, 129; *Indian J Med Res*, 1976, **64**, 854); *in vitro* antimicrob. on human pathogenic bacteria and phytopathogenic fungi (*Indian Drugs*, 1977-78, **15**, 253); produced cardiac inhibition, in frog's isolated heart and fall of B.P. (*Curr Med Pract*, 1980, **24**, 161).

Essent. oil constituents; limonene, 34.4% (*Indian J Appl Chem*, 1967, **30**, 166); γ-asarone (*Aust J Chem*, 1968, **21**, 3001; *Nat Acad Sci Lett India*, 1979, **2**, 11).

Found throughout greater parts of India.

CAILLIEA (*Mimosaceae*)

C. cinerea Macb. syn. *Dichrostachys cinerea* Wight & Arn.

Roots—improve appetite, used in kidney stones, and in diseases of vagina, uterus, etc.; anal. of roots [*J Res Indian Med*, 1979, **14**(2), 80].

Roots, *n*-octacosanol, β-amyrin, friedelan-3 β-ol & 3-one and β-sitosterol (*J Indian Chem Soc*, 1977, **54**, 649); also

proanthocyanidin (*Proc Indian Acad Sci Pl Sci*, 1980, **89**, 73).

Seeds, dichrostachinic acid (*Phytochemistry*, 1973, **12**, 125). Bark contains friedelin, friedelan-3β-ol, α-amyrin and sitosterol; heartwood, octacosanol, and sitosterol; and leaves, hentriacontanol, β-amyrin and sitosterol (*ibid*, 1974, **13**, 2010).

CAJANUS (*Fabaceae*)

C. cajan (Linn.) Millsp. syn. *C. indicus* Spreng.

Seeds—EtOH(50%) ext., hypoglyc. (*Indian J Exp Biol*, 1968, **6**, 232). Seeds, enterokinase activity (*J Biosci*, 1981, **3**, 371); seeds with other vegetable ingredients used as abortif. (*J Sci Res Plants Med*, 1981, **2**, 39). Ext. of germinating seeds, virus inhibiting (*Indian Phytopathol*, 1981, **33**, 615).

Plant used in convuls., colic, and leprosy (*Econ Bot*, 1970, **24**, 241). Paste of leaves or flowers applied in sores of mouth and tongue (*Bull Bot Surv India*, 1976, **18**, 166). Dried plant with dried flowers of *Nymphaea alba* taken for asthma (*Nagarjun*, 1980-81, **24**, 242). Tribals use leaf decoct. for gargling (*J Econ Tax Bot*, 1981, **2**, 177).

Seed enzyme (*Biochim Biophys Acta*, 1973, **302**, 393). Oxalic acid, Ca and P contents of Indian seeds (*Qual Plant Mater Veg*, 1973, **22**, 335); also I, 0.27 and F, 3.07 ppm (*Indian J Nutr Diet*, 1971, **8**, 66). Hypolipidaemic activity of protein in rats (*Indian J Biochem Biophys*, 1973, **10**, 293); vit. B_6, 0.54 mg/100g (*Indian J Nutr Diet*, 1981, **18**, 9).

Essent. oil from plant contains α- ,β- & γ-selinenes, copaene and a mixt. of eudesmols (*Perfum Essent Oil Res*, 1969, **60**, 329).

Leaves, sterols, triterp. and other lipidic constituents (*Collect Czech Chem Commun*, 1977, **42**, 2448). Revised str. for phytoalexin, cajanol (*Z Naturforsch*, 1979, **34C**, 159; *CA*, **90**, 164736d). Leaves, 2 novel phytoalexins [*Indian J Biochem Biophys*, 1981, **18**(Suppl.), 177].

Roots, an antifung. isoflavon., cajanone. Rootbark, cajaflavanone; a new isoflavone glucd., genistein, lupeol, α- & β-amyrin, sitosterol & its glucd.; isoflavanone, 2'-O-Me-cajanone; prenylated isoflavon., cajaisoflavone (*Phytochemistry*, 1977, **16**, 143; 1978, **17**, 2045; 1979, **18**, 365; 693; 1254); a new anthraquinone deriv., cajaquinone (*Indian J Chem*, 1979, **17B**, 88).

Constituents of Indian seeds w.r.t. varietal difference, site, and seasonal variations (*Indian J Nutr Diet*, 1979, **16**, 440).

CALAMINTHA (*Lamiaceae*)

*C. graveolens Benth.

Seeds, stim. and aphrodis. (Wlth India, II, 11).

Reported to be imported from Iran.

C. hortensis Linn.; see **Satureja hortensis**

C. umbrosa Fisch. & Mey.; see **Clinopodium umbrosum**

C. vulgaris (Linn.) Druce syn. *C. clinopodium* Benth.

Eng.–*Wild basil.*

Aq. ext. of aerial parts, CNS depress. and sed. in mice (*Planta Med*, 1979, **36**, 259).

CALAMUS (*Arecaceae*)

C. draco Willd.; see **Daemonorops draco**

*C. floribundus Griff.

Ass.–*Bet.*

EtOH(50%) ext. of aerial parts, hypoten. and CNS depress. (*Indian J Exp Biol*, 1973, **11**, 43).

Found in Sibsagar, Assam.

C. rotang Linn.

EtOH(50%) ext. of aerial parts, spasmog. and anticancer (*Indian J Exp Biol*, 1968, **6**, 232). Plant used in convuls. and cramps (*Econ Bot*, 1970, **24**, 241).

*C. thwaitesii Becc. ex Hook. f.

EtOH(50%) ext. of aerial parts, hypoten. (*Indian J Exp Biol*, 1977, **15**, 208).

Found in Coorg, Karnataka.

CALANTHE (*Orchidaceae*)

*C. triplicata (Willem.) Ames syn. *C. veratrifolia* (Willd.) Lindl.

Eng.–*Australian christmas orchid.*

Herb used in diseases of stomach and intestine; roots chewed with betel-nuts in diar. Poultice of flowers used reduce pain due to ulcers (Burkill, I, 402; *Bul Kebun Raya*, 1979, **4**, 71).

Found in hilly parts of S. India at 1,800-2,400 m.

*C. vestita Lindl.

Pseudobulbs used in Vietnam for treating pain in legs (Uphof, 96).

Native of Burma and Malaysia, grown in Indian gardens.

CALENDULA (*Asteraceae*)

C. arvensis Linn.

Plant ext., antimicrob. (*Fitoterapia*, 1980, **51**, 281).

Plant contains isoquercitroside, rutoside and narcissoside (*C R Acad Sci Ser D*, 1975, **281**, 447; *CA*, 1976, **84**, 27994y).

C. officinalis Linn.

Eng.–*Marigold;* H.–*Zergul.*

Flower—ext., antimicrob. (*Farm Zh Kiev*, 1963, **18**, 56; *CA*, 1964, **60**, 3945h); various exts., estrogenic in mice (*Poznan Tow Przyi Nauk Wyd Lek Pr Kom Farm*, 1963, **1**, 53; *CA*, 1964, **61**, 2364h); aq. ext., sed. and hypoten. in animals (*Nauchni Tr Vissh Med Inst Sofia*, 1964, **43**, 15; *CA*, 1965, **63**, 1114a). Evaluation of antimicrob. activity.

Plant—homoeopathic mother tinctures (*Ann Pharm Fr*, 1970, **38**, 493); in Europe, tincture used in amenor. and after dilution, as lotion for pains and bruises (*Acta Phytother*, 1971, **18**, 21); aq. ext., antitumour against Crocker sarcoma 180 in mice (*Eksp Med Morfol*, 1964, **3**, 41; *CA*, 1965, **62**, 9652d). EtOH(50%) ext., antiprot. and spasmol.; also spermic. in rats (*Indian J Exp Biol*, 1968, **6**, 232; 1977, **15**, 231). Marigold as med. herb., rev., 37 refs.

(*Pharm Weekbl*, 1979, **114**, 1149; *CA*, 1980, **92**, 47157w).

Plant, rich in Mn and carotene; wound healing and antiinflam. properties said to be due to Mn and carotene (*Aptechn Delo*, 1963, **12**, 38; *CA*, 1964, **61**, 11001e); flavons. (*Farm Zh Kiev*, 1972, **27**, 44; *CA*, 77, 45484s). Oleanolic acid glycds. (*Izv Akad Nauk SSSR, Ser Khim*, 1973, 2713; *CA*, 1974, **80**, 96296b). Saponins effective as spermatocides, antiblastocyst and abortif., method of extn. (US Pat., 1975, 15125205; *CA*, **83**, 183387m). Saponosides decreased spontaneous motility and extended duration of hexobarbital narcosis in rats; also hypolipaemic (*Herba Pol*, 1980, **26**, 119; 233). Pentacyclic terps., reliantriols, manilladiol and longispinogenin (*Pol J Chem*, 1979, **53**, 2465). Antimicrob. principle from tissue culture (*Indian J Pharm Sci*, 1980, **42**, 113).

Leaves (and seedlings), distribution of sterols; of polyprenyl quinones, α-tocopherol, and triterp. alcs.; tocopherol (*Phytochemistry*, 1975, **14**,627; 1979, **18**,427; 1976,**15**,125;205; 1980, **19**,1391).

Flowers, glucd. fraction haemolytic (*Bull Acad Pol Sci Ser Sci Biol*, 1965, **13**, 77; *CA*, **63**, 11249h); distribution of triterp. alcs. and sterols (*ibid*, 1966, **14**, 645; *CA*, 1967, **66**, 62617c); 5 triterp. glycd. of oleanolic acid (*Phytochemistry*, 1967, **6**, 69; 1968, **7**, 1631). Method for detn. of oleanosides (*Herba Pol*, 1979, **25**, 107).

Petals, volat. oil, *n*-tricosane and triterp. glycds.; volat. oil, antibiot. (*Acta Pharm Hung*, 1968, **38**, 118; *CA*, **69**, 49756b). Extn. of inflorescence yields caryophyllene, 78% (*Farm Zh Kiev*, 1975, **30**, 72; *CA*, **83**, 152256q); carotenoids (*Herba Pol*, 1977, **23**, 191).

Sterols, triterps., etc. of flowers (*Rocz Chem*, 1967, **41** , 201; *CA* , **67**, 784s; *Chem Commun*, 1969, 107; *Bull Acad Pol Sci Ser Sci Chim*, 1969, **17**, 399; *CA*, 1970, **72**, 21802q; *Phytochemistry*, 1968, **7**, 1631; 1972, **11**, 1165; 1973, **12**, 157; 2299; 1979, **18**, 253; Fr. Demande, 1975, 2268518; *CA*,

1976, **84**, 155662a; *Rocz Chem*, 1977, **51**, 2493; *CA*, 1978, **89**, 39364j; *Pol J Chem*, 1979, **53**, 1071). Inflorescence, constituents (*Planta Med*, 1979, **36**, 286). Floral heads contain compd. similar to pyrethrins (*Pyrethrum Post*, 1979, **15**, 9).

Roots, 8 triterp. glycds; str. of calenduloside A & B; also str. of F; G & H; C & D (*Khim Prir Soedin*, 1969, **5**, 58; 1971, **7**, 22; 533; 1973, **9**, 560; 1974, **10**, 532; 1975, **11**, 366; *CA*, **71**, 773v; **74**, 112385p; **75**, 152042b; 1974, **80**, 15150z, 15151a; 1975, **82**, 54182x; 1976, **84**, 74566v); str. of glycds. of oleanolic acid (*Phytochemistry*, 1971, **10**, 1121); pharmacol. of calenduloside B; antiphl. and sed. (*Farmakol ToksikolMoscow*, 1978, **41**, 556; *BA*, 1979, **67**, 62623).

Seeds, haemagglutinins, isolation (*Univ Wyoming Agric Exp Sta Laramie Sci Monograph*, 1971, **24**, II, 1; *CA*, 1972, **76**, 70197n).

CALLA (*Araceae*)

See HOMALOMENA

CALLIANDRA (*Mimosaceae*)

*C. houstoniana Standl. syn. *C. houstonii* Benth.

Root bark used in Europe as an antipyr.; chewed to harden the gums; alk. reported to cause death by systolic arrest of heart (Uphof, 96; Hoppe, 162; Standley, I, 386; Gopalswamiengar, 263).

Grown in Indian gardens.

*C. portoricensis Benth.

Eng.–*Pink powderpuff.*

Roots—pungent and purg. In Ghana, with fresh ginger and water, given as an enema in lumbago with constip.; mixed with pepper and used for treating gonor. Dried and pulverized leaves used as sternutatory in relieving headache [Dalziel, 213; Irvine, 1961, 337; *Lloydia*, 1970, **33**(3A), Suppl., 104].

Cultivated in IBG, Calcutta.

CALLICARPA (Verbenaceae)

*C. americana Linn.

Eng.–*American beautiberry, French mulberry.*

Fruit, astrin.; juice reported to be used in dropsical conditions (Jacobs & Burlage, 221).

Cultivated in gardens.

C. arborea Roxb.

Paste of bark or leaf applied on scorpion sting (*Bull Bot Surv India*, 1976, **18**, 166). Bark used in various skin diseases (*Nagarjun*, 1980-81, **24**, 240).

Bark, Me-betulinate, baurenol and β-sitosterol-OAc (*J Indian Chem Soc*, 1974, **51**, 903). Leaves, β-sitosterol, maslinic, oleanolic and ursolic acids, last two also as Me-ester acetates, lupeol-OAc and β-amyrin-OAc; heartwood, β-sitosterol and oleanolic acid (*Curr Sci*, 1977, **46**, 667; *J Indian Chem Soc*, 1978, **55**, 744).

*C. arborea Roxb. var. **oblongifolia**

EtOH(50%) ext. of aerial parts, diur. (*Indian J Exp Biol*, 1971, **9**, 91).

Found in Nongoh, Meghalaya.

C. cana Linn. syn. *C. candicans* Hochr.

Callicarpone, a fish killing compd. isolated from leaves 10-fold more toxic against loach fish, than rotenone (*Tetrahedron Lett*, 1966, 3519); str. of callicarpone (*Agric Biol Chem*, 1967, **31**, 494, 498).

C. longifolia Lamk var. **lanceolata** C.B. Clarke

Leaves yield calliterpenone, its mono-OAc, ursolic acid, and same flavon. CMF 1, as in *C. macrophylla*(*Phytochemistry*, 1974, **13**, 306).

C. macrophylla Vahl

Plant used against dysen.; wood paste, in mouth and tongue sores (*Econ Bot*, 1970, **24**, 241; 1971, **25**, 419). Leaves, smoked to relieve headache (*Q J Crude Drug Res*, 1979, **17**, 65).

Seed paste used in stomatitis; also useful in leprosy and as diur. (*Khadi Gramodyog*, 1972-73, **19**, 273); fruit paste in treatment of boils and blisters on tongue (*Bull Med Ethno Bot Res*, 1980, **1**, 318).

Aerial parts, 2-tetracyclic diterp., calliterpenone & its mono- OAc(*Tetrahedron*, 1972, **28**, 4319); their str.; also configuration (*Tetrahedron Lett*, 1973, 2179; *Phytochemistry*, 1975, **14**, 2249). Leaves, sitosterol; calliterpenone & its mono-OAc, luteolin, apigenin & its 7-glucuronides (*ibid*, 1974, **13**, 306); ursolic acid, its 2-OH deriv., crategolic acid, etc.; seeds, calliterpenone & its -OAc (*J Indian Chem Soc*, 1976, **53**, 218; 1165). Str. of flavone CMF 1, from leaves (*ibid*, 1978, **55**, 628).

*C. rubella Lindl.

EtOH(50%) ext. of plant, anticancer and diur. (*Indian J Exp Biol*, 1974, **12**, 512).

Goalpara, Assam.

CALLIGONUM (Polygonaceae)

C. polygonoides Linn.

Leaf juice used for washing eyes as a cure against latex of *Calotropis procera* (*J Agric Trop Bot Appl*, 1966, **13**, 278).

Flowers have cooling effect and used in treating sunstroke (*Indian J Med Res*, 1962, **50**, 779).

CALLISTEMON (Myrtaceae)

C. citrinus Skeels syn. *C. citrinus* Stapf; *C. lanceolatus* DC.

Leaf ext., antibact. and antifung. [*Indian Drugs Pharmac Ind*, 1977, **12**(3), 21; **12**(5), 7].

Leaves yield essent. oil rich in cineol (Wlth India, II, 15); essent. oil, constituents and its commercial prospects (*Indian J Pharm*, 1975, **37**, 158); a terp., 1,8-expoxy-p-menthane, 60% (*Riechst Aromen Koerperflegem*, 1972, **22**, 113; 116; 118; 120; *CA*, **77**, 72527q).

Triterps. from leaves of Egyptian plant; also of Indian plant (*Aust J Chem*, 1975, **28**, 221; *Phytochemistry*, 1975, **14**, 592, 1675). Leaves phloroglucinol, myrtucommulone A (*ibid*, 1977, **16**, 1851).

Flowers, kaempferol and diglucds. of pelargonidin and cyanidin (*Naturwis-*

senschaften, 1970, **57**, 394); two triterp. acids including betulinic [*Proc Nat Acad Sci India*, 1972, **42A** (pt.1), 86]. Polyphenols of seeds and bark (*Indian J Chem*, 1972, **10**, 959).

CALLITRIS (*Cupressaceae*)

*C. rhomboidea R. Br. ex Rich. syn. *C. cupressiformis* F. Muell.
Eng.–*Coastal cypress, oyster bay pine*.
Properties of essent. oil from leaves as well as whole plant (*Perfum Essent Oil Rec*, 1967, **58**, 622). Leaves, 4- epiisocommunic acid and amentoflavone (*Phytochemistry*, 1977, **16**, 801).
Native of Australia, introduced into Nilgiris and elsewhere in Tamil Nadu.

*C. robusta R. Br. ex. Mirb.
EtOH(50%) ext. of aerial parts, semen coagulant, hypoten., and CNS depress. (*Indian J Exp Biol*, 1977, **15**, 208),
Found in Vishakhapatnam, A.P.

CALOCARPUM (*Sapotaceae*)

*C. sapota (Jacq.) Merrill
Ext. of leaves and stems, antitumour (*Rev Cubana Farm*, 1980, **14**, 311).
Reported to be cultivated in Indian gardens for its edible fruits.

CALONYCTION (*Convolvulaceae*)

See **IPOMOEA**

CALOPHYLLUM (*Clusiaceae*)

C. apetalum Willd. syn. *C. wightianum* T. Anders.
Nut, coumarin, aperalolide (*Indian J Chem*, 1967, **5**, 523). Kernel, an isomer of calophyllolide, apetalolide and β-sitosterol (*Planta Med*, 1968, **16**, 450).
Bark, friedelin and apetalic acid; its str. (*Tetrahedron Lett*, 1967, 4177; *Tetrahedron*, 1968, **24**, 6411); triterp. lactone, apetalactone (*J Chem Soc C*, 1968, 1323); friedelin, β-amyrin, betulinic acid, β-sitosterol and a xanthone (*Phytochemistry*, 1968, **8**, 323). Heartwood, a

clathrate composed of wightianone and palmitic acid (*J Chem Soc Chem Commun*, 1980, 283). Wood, mesoinositol (*Indian J Chem*, 1967, **5**, 523).

C. elatum Bedd. syn. *C. tomentosum* T. Anders. in part non Wight
Seed kernel, coumarin tomentolide A & B (*Tetrahedron Lett*, 1967, 2633); triterp. lactone, apetalactone (*J Chem Soc C*, 1968, 1323); tomentolide A & B, and β-sitosterol (*Planta Med*, 1968, **16**, 450).
Bark, tomentolide A & B and blancoic acid (*Indian J Chem*, 1969, **7**, 308); also friedelin, friedelan-3 β-ol and β-sitosterol (*Phytochemistry*, 1968, **8**, 323). 13 Xanthones and triterp. from branch-timbers, sapwood and heartwood from Sri Lanka plant (*ibid*, 1981, **20**, 1303).

C. inophyllum Linn.
Seeds—in Samoa, to treat skin rash, rheum. and as vermifuge.
Bark—in Samoa, as diur., emmen., and given to babies with fever and running stool.
Leaves—in Samoa, for chicken pox, skin inflam., scabies, sunburn, eye catarrh, debility, post natal lactation & sickness (*Econ Bot*, 1974, **28**, 15).
EtOH(50%) ext. of aerial parts, spasmol. and CNS depress. (*Indian J Exp Biol*, 1974, **12**, 512).
Seeds, chem. constituents, str. of new 4-Ph-coumarin; seed oil also contains 4-Ph-coumarin (*Bull Nat Inst Sci India*, No.31, 1965, 91; *Indian J Chem*, 1975, **13**, 746); coumarins from seeds, rev., 11 refs. (*Adv Mass Spectrom*, 1978, 7B, 1561). Seed auxin (*Sci Cult*, 1969, **35**, 581). Seeds, calophynic acid, str. (*Tetrahedron Lett*, 1972, 2715). Str. of new 4-alkyl-coumarin from plant (*C R Acad Sci Ser C*, 1972, **275**, 1105).
Calophyllolide, a complex 5-Ph-coumarin isolated from nuts antiarrhythmic (as effective as quinidine), bradicardiac coronary dilator, hyperten. and anticoagulant (*Life Sci*, 1962, 571); an-

tiinflam. and antiarthritic (*Indian J Med Res*, 1980, **72**, 762).

Flower pigments (*Bull Nat Inst Sci*, No.31, 1965, 39; *Phytochemistry*, 1971, **10**, 1679).

Bark yields resin containing brasiliensic and isophylloidic acid (*Tetrahedron Lett*, 1968, 3285). Root bark, antibact. principle (*Indian J Exp Biol*, 1970, **8**, 39).

Heartwood, measuaxanthone B and a new xanthone, calophyllin B (*Indian J Chem*, 1968, **6**, 57); also jacareubin, its 6-desoxy deriv. and a xanthone (*Phytochemistry*, 1969, **8**, 927). Sapwood γ-sitosterol and erythrodiol 3-OAc (*Indian J Chem*, 1970, **8**, 105). Heartwood xanthones of Australian plant; wood, xanthones and triterp. (*Phytochemistry*, 1971, **10**, 603; 1976, **15**, 2016); xanthones exhibited antiinflam. and CNS depress. activity in mice and rats; jacareubin & its 6-deoxy deriv., antiulcer in rats (*Indian J Pharmacol*, 1980, **12**, 181).

Leaves, amentoflavone (*Indian J Chem*, 1967, **5**, 523); friedelin and 3 new triterps., canophyllal, canophyllol and canophyllic acid (*Tetrahedron*, 1967, **23**, 1901); derivs. of (+)-inophyllolide, compds. with piscic. activity (*Tetrahedron Lett*, 1968, 2389); 5 piscic. compds., derivs. of inophyllolide designated as isophyllum A-E (*Bull Inst Chem Res Kyoto Univ*, 1972, **50**, 160; *CA*, 1973, **78**, 13744f).

CALOPOGONIUM (*Fabaceae*)

*C. mucunoides Desv.

In Tonga, leaves used as cure for filariasis (*Econ Bot*, 1971, **25**, 423). Plant ext., slightly estrogenic in mice (*Philipp Agric*, 1963, **46**, 673).

Seed, isoflavones (*Bull Soc R Sci Liege*, 1975, **44**, 306; 1976, **45**, 468; *CA*, 1976, **84**, 74136e; 1977, **86**, 152677q).

Introduced into India as cover crop in rubber and other plantations.

CALOTROPIS (*Asclepiadaceae*)

*C. acia Buch.-Ham.

H.–*Madar, auk.*

Milky juice from leaves excellent for cauterising sores in elephants (Cowan & Cowan, 92).

Found in W. Bengal.

C. gigantea (Linn.) Dryand.

Roots—preparations of roots and leaves in powds., balms, enemas and ghee or clarified butter used against abdominal tumours (*Lloydia*, 1967, **30**, 431); EtOH(50%) ext. anticancer and spasmol.; leaves ext., anticancer (*Indian J Exp Biol*, 1968, **6**, 232); powd. root with milk used for ear trouble and boils (*Econ Bot*, 1971, **25**, 418); ext., devoid of antiimplantation activity (*Indian J Med Res*, 1969, **57**, 893, 237); used in lupus, tuberculous leprosy, syphilis and syphilitic ulcerations and rheum. Useful in scorpion bites and night blindness (*Bull Bot Soc Bengal*, 1972, **26**, 27).

Leaves—EtOH(50%) ext. showed antiimplantation activity in albino rats (*Probe*, 1977-78, **17**, 315); warmed in *Lahi* oil and applied over inflamed parts of the body (*Bull Med Ethno Bot Res*, 1980, **1**, 318); used in external swellings. Juice highly poisonous, used for wounds (*J Econ Tax Bot*, 1980, **1**, 142). See roots also.

Plant—used in smallpox, leg and chest pains, ailments of spleen, dropsy and anasarca, boils, muscular pain, pain in loins, rheum., hemiplegia, epilepsy, tongue paralysis, tetanus, strangulation of intestine, convuls., postnatal complaints, delirium febris, scabies, ringworm, syphilis, carbuncle, hydrocele, cholera, dysen., neuralgia, pleur., pneum., protracted labour, bite of jackal or dog, and rabies and haemor. septicaemia (*Econ Bot*, 1970, **24**, 241). All parts used against bronch. asthma (*Nagarjun*, 1979-80, **23**, 9); skeletal fractures (*Sri Lanka For*, 1980, **14**, 145).

Flowers with black pepper useful in asthma, clin. study (*Sachitra Ayurveda*, 1980-81, **33**, 119, 210).

Latex—applied to teeth to remove worms; kills worms in ulcers of cattle. Also to cleanse and heal wounds (*Econ Bot*, 1965, **19**, 243); used as abortif. (*J Econ Tax Bot*, 1981, **2**, 187).

Leaves and stems, β-sitosterol (*Indian J Pharm*, 1965, **27**, 232). Root bark, triterp. (*Curr Sci*, 1968, **37**, 156). Flowers, β-amyrin and stigmasterol [*J Res Indian Med*, 1975, **10**(4), 162].

Latex, protease, calotropain FI (*J Chromatogr*, 1979, **168**, 284); calotropain FII (*Biochim Biophys Acta*, 1979, **568**, 111); TLC sepn. of constituents (*Chem Era*, 1978, **14**, 485; *CA*, 1980, **92**, 124956k);TLC sepn. and detection of constituents [*Met Miner Rev*, 1979, **18**(4), 24; *CA*, 1980, **92**, 193728z]; flip-flop chromatogr. for extn.-isolation of uscharine from sap (*J Chromatogr*, 1979, **186**, 15); calotropins DI & DII (*Arch Biochem Biophys*, 1980, **202**, 321); proteolytic enzymes [*Indian J Biochem Biophys*, 1981, **18**(Suppl), 178].

C. procera Ait. f. ssp. **hamittonii** Ali syn. *C. procera* auct. non Ait.

Roots—aq. and alc. ext. of roots, stimulate respiration and B.P. of dog; spasmog. to rabbit and rat, and vermicidal against earthworms (*Indian J Pharm*, 1965, **27**, 278). Root bark useful for treating chronic cases of dyspep., flatulance, constip., loss of appetite, indign. and mucus in stool; clin. trials [*J Res Indian Med*, 1979, **14**(3-4), 98].

Leaves—used against guinea worms (*J Agric Trop Bot Appl*, 1966, **13**, 252); EtOH(50%) ext. of root and leaves, anticancer and in cardiac arrythmia (*Indian J Exp Biol*, 1969, **7**, 250); used in rheum. (*Bull Bot Surv India*, 1973, **15**, 18); EtOH(50%) ext., shows antiimplantation activity in female albino rats (*Probe*, 1977-78, **17**, 315). Leaves, flower and root bark oil, antimicrob.; leaves possessed max. activity (*Pak J Sci*, 1979, **31**, 127). Powd.,

nematicidal (*Andhra Agric J*, 1980, **27**, 312).

Flowers—useful in asthma [*J Sci Res Plants Med*, 1979-80, **1**(1), 52]. Effect of flower ext. on testicular function of Indian desert male gerbil (*Indian J Exp Biol*, 1979, **17**, 859). Powd. flowers with black pepper and ash of barley seeds given in cholera (*J Econ Tax Bot*, 1981, **2**, 193).

Seed oil is geriatric and tonic. Green copra given in asthma (*Khadi Gramodyog*, 1972-73, **19**, 269).

Plant—used in spleen complaints, rheum., hemiplegia, epilepsy, sores, small pox and protracted labour (*Econ Bot*, 1970, **24**, 241). Plant ext., antifung. (*Geobios*, 1978, **5**, 49). Plant, anticancer in KB cell culture (*Fitoterapia*, 1981, **52**, 281).

Latex—crude latex and its protein fraction, highly fibrinolytic and anticoagulant in rats and human plasma (*Indian J Med Sci*, 1962, **16**, 873); irrit. and inflam. to eyes (*Isr J Med Sci*, 1977, **13**, 914). Effects of feeding sheep with plant; of administration of latex to sheep and goats (*J Comp Pathol*, 1979, **89**, 241; 251). Pharmacognostic study [*J Res Indian Med*, 1979, **14**(2), 134]; along with *gur* given orally, in bite of rabid dog (*Q J Crude Drug Res*, 1979, **17**, 64). Latex and leaves, nematicidal [*J Sci Res Plants Med*, 1979-80, **1**(2), 18].

Root bark, benzoyllineolone and benzoylisolineolone (*Aust J Chem*, 1968, **21**, 1625); alk. [*J Res Indian Med*, 1978, **13**(3), 120]. Root, stem and leaves, also latex, β-amyrin [*ibid*, 1979, **14**(2), 152].

Flowers contain evanidin 3-rhamnoglucd. (*Vijnana Parishad Anusandhan Patrika*, 1978, **21**, 177).

Plant contains o-pyrocatechuic acid (*Naturwissenschaften*, 1963, **50**, 734); cardenolides (calotropin, calotoxin, uscharin and uscharidin), and base, choline; calotropin has digitalis-like action (*Bull Fac Pharm Cairo Univ*, 1971, **10**, 1; *CA*, 1973, **78**, 156644j). NMR spectra of glycds. (*Phytochemistry*, 1972, **11**, 757). See also *Ascelpias*. Stem gave +ve test for alk. (*Lloydia*, 1972, **35**, 1).

Latex, chem. compn. (*Naturwissenschaften*, 1964, **51**, 109); sterols and triterps.; also in plant ext. (*Bull Fac Pharm Cairo Univ*, 1968, **7**, 91; *CA*, 1970, **73**, 63160e); uzarigenin, syriogenin and proceroside in addn. to calotropagenin & 6 of its glycds.; their str. (*Helv Chim Acta*, 1969, **52**, 2086; 2276). Cardenolides in latex and leaves (*Phytochemistry*, 1982, **21**, 2343).

CALPURNIA (*Fabaceae*)

*C. aurea (Ait.) Benth. syn. *C. lasiogyne* Mey.;*C. subdecandra* Schweick.

Eng.–*East-african laburnum, golden tussel.*

In Ethopia, ext. of plant used as insectic. and for treating scabies, amoebic dysen. and diar. in animals. Leaves, for killing lice in humans, and ticks in cattle (Watt & Breyer-Brandwijk, 565).

Seed agglutinins respond to antigen A of human erythrocytes (*Izv Akad Nauk Ser Biol*, 1968, 59; *CA*, **68**, 75726d).

Alk., calpurnine (*J Chem Soc*, 1963, 3067); also calpurmenin(ε) & its 13 α-(2'-pyrrolecarboxylic acid) ester (*Acta Crystallogr*, 1979, **35B**, 1839).

From Western Peninsula.

CALTHA (*Ranunculaceae*)

C. palustris Linn.

EtOH(50%) ext. of plant, CNS depress. and hypoten.; spermic. in rat and human (*Indian J Exp Biol*, 1977, **15**, 208; 231).

Plant, coumarins (*Farm Zh Kiev*, 1970, **25**, 57; *CA*, 1971, **74**, 20347z); pigment, calthaxanthin, a stereoisomer of lutein (*Z Pflanzenphysiol*, 1974, **72**, 177; *CA*, **81**, 87961h). Flowers, 3'-O-dihydrolutein (*Helv Chim Acta*, 1979, **62**, 2817).

Roots, alk. magnoflorine (*Pharm Weekbl*, 1963, **98**, 261; *CA*, **59**, 4208d); also triterp. glycds. which decreased serum cholesterol and total protein and increased blood sugar in rats; antiinflam., equivalent to butadion in rats; most triterp. glycds. located in internal layers of bark of adven-

titious roots (*Rastit Resur*, 1978, **14**, 93; 1979, **15**, 115; 1980, **16**, 235; *CA*, **88**, 115364f; **90**, 162170r; **93**, 41545v).

CALYCOPTERIS (*Combretaceae*)

C. floribunda (Roxb.) Poir.

Fruits used in jaundice (Wlth India, II, 23). Juice of leaves or bark given to cattle in distending stomach (*Indian For*, 1978, **104**, 676). Leaf juice, as a cure for fresh wounds and cuts (*J Econ Tax Bot*, 1981, **2**, 69). Flowers, as poultice for headache (Burkill, I, 416).

Leaves, flavanol calycopterin, str. (*Phytochemistry*, 1972, **11**, 2311); calycopterin-4'-Me ether & 3'-OMe-calycopterin (*Indian J Chem*, 1973, **11**, 403). Flowers, calycopterin and quercetin (*Curr Sci*, 1975, **44**, 888).

CAMELLIA (*Theaceae*)

*C. japonica Linn.

Eng.–*Japanese rose.*

Camellin, glycd. from seeds used as a cardiac stim. in endocarditis and pericarditis.

Cosmetic and dermopharm. beauty product comprising seed oil (Fr Demands, 1974, 2196147; *CA*, **81**, 82254v).

Seeds, saponins camelliagenin A, B & C; their str.; genins also in fruits (*Tetrahedron Lett*, 1967, 597; 591; *Yakugaku Zasshi*, 1968, **88**, 1463). Triterp. alc. of seed oil (*Lipids*, 1980, **15**, 407).

Leaves and flowers, theobromine (*Farm Vestn Ljubljana*, 1972, **23**, 219; *CA*, 1973, **78**, 156615a). Sterols, polyphenols, etc. of white flowers (*Acta Cient Compostelana*, 1971, **8**, 185; *CA*, 1973, **79**, 50729w).

Native of Japan, commonly cultivated in hill gardens.

C. sinensis (Linn.) Kuntze syn. *C. thea* Link; *C. theifera* Griff.; *Thea sinensis* Linn. including varieties, *sinensis & asamica* (Mast.) Kitamura

Leaves ext. in w. and alc., inhibitory against *Staphylococcus aureus* (*Nippon*

Shokuhin Kogyo Gakkaishi, 1963, **10**, 1; *CA*, 1965, **63**, 926a).

Antithiamine effects of tea (*Nutr Rep Int*, 1971, **4**, 223; *CA*, 1972, **76**, 12956y). Tea leaves among other constituents of an antiperspirant compn. (US Pat., 1973, 3743717; *CA*, **79**, 70094p; Ger. Offen, 1974, 2353087; *CA*, **81**, 29527k). Lyophilized aq. ext. of leaf, stem and twigs useful in cosmetic and dermo-pharmaceutical beauty products (Fr. Demande, 1974, 2196147; *CA*, **81**, 82254v). Effect of tea on serum cholesterol in a hypercholesteremic rat (*Nutr Rep Int*, 1977, **15**, 89; *CA*, **86**, 104804g). Leaves, inhibitor of *o*-diphenol oxidase and peroxidase (*Prikl Biokhim Mikrobiol*, 1977, **13**, 104; *CA*, **86**, 135488m). Effect of tea on alpha rhythm and physical fatigue on·human (*Indian J Physiol Allied Sci*, 1977, **31**, 36).

Cancer-promoting effects of phenols in fermented tea (*Cancer Philadelphia*, 1967, **20**, 614); carcinogenicity of tea and some tannin containing herbs administered sc in rats (*J Nat Cancer Inst*, 1976, **57**, 207). Also pharmaceuticals containing tea ext. and other ingredients useful against tumours, diabetes, arthritis, etc. (Jpn Kokai, 1978, 7829907; *CA*, **89**, 12190n).

Leaves contain theophylline and theobromine (*Inst Nac Pesqui Amazonia Publ Quim*, 1965, 17; *CA*, 1966, **65**, 4263f); caffeine (2-5%) and adenine (small amts.) (*Rev Fiz Chim Ser A*, 1974, **11**, 218; *CA*, 1975, **82**, 84684e). N-*p*-coumarylglutamic acid from black tea (*Chem Ind Lond*, 1980, 338). Theanine content of German tea (*Z Lebensm Unters Forsch*, 1974, **156**, 32; *CA*, **81**, 150685p).

Caffeine—extn. from leaves; also from tea waste (*Yakugaku Zasshi*, 1968, **88**, 729; *CA*, **69**, 61514s; *Sci Res Dacca*, 1969, **6**, 53; *CA*, 1970, **72**, 35717e). Conversion of caffeine into theophylline; the latter, diur. and its chloro deriv. used in motion sickness drug (*Annu Rep RRL Jorhat*, 1969-70, 23). See also *Coffea arabica*.

Med. compn. containing residual liquid left after extn. of caffeine, excellent astrin.

for gastrointestinal disease. Tea source of vit. P [*East Pharm*, 1961, 4(46), 15]; tannins of Indian tea, antibact. towards microorganism causing intestinal disorder (*J Indian Chem Soc*, 1962, **39**, 849). Tannic acid of tea, as incriminating factor for heart disease (*Indian J Nutr Diet*, 1979, **16**, 348). Microbiol. decaffeination of aq. sol. of tea (Can. Pat., 1980, 1086553; *CA*, 1981, **94**, 29080c).

Chem. of tea and tea manufacture, rev., 242 refs. (*Recent Adv Phytochem*, 1972, **5**, 247).

Persons drinking 6-9 cups of tea daily obtain required fluoride to prevent dental caries (*Tea Q*, 1973, **43**, 111). Leaves, Al (large amt. 5820 ppm) and F(1270 ppm) (*Kagaku To Seibutsu*, 1977, **15**, 362; *CA*, 1978, **88**, 135561w).

Tea catechol improves functioning of capillaries and very small blood vessels. Also used against poliomyelitis, rheum. and infection of respiratory organs; and radiation diseases (*Sci Cult*, 1965, **31**, 624). Inhibition of passive cutaneous anaphylaxis in mice by tea compds. (*Planta Med*, 1981, **42**, 75).

Sepn. of flavons. and detn. of their biol. activity (*Biochim Progr Tekhnol Chai Proizvod Akad Nauk SSSR Inst Biokhim*, 1966, 14; *CA*, 1967, **66**, 462v). Pharmacol. of black tea polyphenols (*Curr Sci*, 1972, **41**, 435; 1973, **42**, 540).

Flavons. (*Tetrahedron*, 1972, **28**, 2819; *Khim Prir Soedin*, 1971, 835; 1972, 803; 1974, 519; *CA*, 1972, **76**, 110314g; 1973, **78**, 94811a; 1975, **82**, 14008p; *Gazz Chim Ital*, 1976, **106**, 1117); phenolcarboxylic acid from leaves; tea coumarins (*Khim Prir Soedin*, 1975, 798; 1980, 409; 1972, 238; 1974, 84; *CA*, 1976, **84**, 102354v; **93**, 128774t; **77**, 45530d; **81**, 74195m).

Lead content of Indian tea (*Bull Environ Contam Toxicol*, 1973, **9**, 124); Indian green tea, sterol and lipid contents (*Phytochemistry*, 1974, **13**, 199); α-spinasterol gentiobioside from tea (*Curr Sci*, 1973, **42**, 720).

Black tea, vit.E (*Chem Ind Lond*, 1966, 1719). Nutr. & therapeutic value of tea, rev., 163 refs. (*J Sci Food Agric*, 1975, **26**, 1439).

Chem. of black & green tea (*Flavour Ind*, 1972, **3**, 23; 36). Relation of constituents with taste of green tea, rev., 24 refs. [*Chagyo KenKyu Hokoku*, 1973, (40), 1; *CA*, 1974, **80**, 119235x]. Tea flavour, rev., 83 refs. (*J Sci Ind Res*, 1975, **34**, 282); essent. oil constituents (*Agric Biol Chem*, 1971, **35**, 962; 1044; 1973, **37**, 1075; 1980, **44**, 2999; *Z Naturforsch*, 1981, **36B**, 755; *CA*, **95**, 76886a).

Str. of theasapogenol E isolated from tea (*Chem Ind Lond*, 1966, 2202). Str. and physiology of saponin from leaves and seeds, rev., 12 refs. [*Chagyo Kenkyu Hokoku*, 1970, (2), 52; *CA*, **73**, 43937k]; identn. (*Nippon Nogei Kagaku Kaishi*, 1973, **47**, 237; *CA*, 1974, **80**, 68381g).

Theasapogenol A & B (barringtogenol C) major triterp. alcs. of seeds; also camelliagenins A, B & C and their strs., present in fruits as well (*Tetrahedron Lett*, 1966, 5973; 1967, 1127; 5347; 597; 591; *Yakugaku Zasshi*, 1968, **88**, 1463; *CA*, 1969, **70**, 68563m). Seed saponins; antiexudative and antiinflam., str. similar to aescin (*Arzneim Forsch*, 1968, **18**, 1466; *CA*, 1969, **70**, 36279g). Genins (*Chem Pharm Bull*, 1970, **18**, 1610; 1971, **19**, 1186; *CA*, **73**, 109925p; '**75**, 77076k). Str. of theasaponins; also properties (*Khim Prir Soedin*, 1972, 654; *CA*, 1973, **78**, 84738t; *Tea Q*, 1973, **43**, 91).

Seed and seed oil constituents (*Lipids*, 1976, **11**, 434; 1980, **15**, 407; *Fette Seifen Anstrichm*, 1977, **79**, 115; *CA*, **87**, 20839e). Seed, haemagglutinin (*Shizuoka Daigaku Nogakubu Kenkyu Hokoku*, 1978, **28**, 51; *CA*, 1979, **91**, 18185c); two 3-oxo steroids (*Phytochemistry*, 1981, **20**, 175). Compn. of seed oil (*Bangladesh J Sci Ind Res*, 1980, **15**, 125; *CA*, 1981, **95**, 200606a).

Pollen flavons. (*Agric Biol Chem*, 1969, **33**, 818). Studies of white flower (*Acta Cient Compostelana*, 1971, **8**, 185; *CA*, 1973, **79**, 50729w). Leaves and flowers,

theobromine (*Farm Vestn Ljubljana*, 1972, **23**, 219; *CA*, 1973, **78**, 156615a).

CAMPSIS (*Bignoniaceae*)

*C. grandiflora (Thunb.) K. Schum. syn. *C. chinensis* Voss; *Tecoma grandiflora* Loisel.

Eng.–*Chinese trumpet creeper*.

Flowers, emmen. and in diabetes; pollen, harmful to human beings (Hoppe, 889).

Anthocyanins in taxon. in relation to (*Biochem Syst Ecol*, 1980, **8**, 273). Leaves, iridoid glucds. compenoside & its 5-OH deriv., detn. (*Heterocycles*, 1981, **16**, 1475; *CA*, **95**, 187598c).

Cultivated in Indian gardens.

*C. radicans Seem. ex Bur. syn. *Tecoma radicans* A. Juss. ex Spreng.

Eng.–*Trumpet vine*; Delhi–*Latkania*.

Root employed to induce sweating and for healing wounds. Vine, narcotic. Leaves and flowers may cause dermatitis in susceptible persons (Uphof, 513; Fl Missouri, 1370). Acidic ext. of plant active against Gram +ve bacteria; alkaline ext., against Gram–ve bacteria (*Econ Bot*, 1959, **13**, 307).

Petals, cyanidine 3-rutinoside; alk., boschniakine and lapachel (*Phytochemistry*, 1967, **6**, 1643; 1972, **11**, 2082); leaves, phenolic acids among others (*ibid*, 1976, **15**, 436).

Cultivated in Indian gardens.

CANANGA (*Annonaceae*)

C. odorata Hook.f. & Thoms. syn. *Canangium odoratum* Baill.

Eng.–*Ylang-ylang*.

In Tonga, bark infusion used in stomach troubles, leaves given to infants suffering from diar. and their decoct. used in boils (*Econ Bot*, 1971, **25**, 437). In Samoa, essent. oil, as carmin. (*Econ Bot*, 1974, **28**, 8).

Stem bark of Madagascar plant, alks., including canangine (*Ann Pharm Fr*, 1975, **33**, 43; *CA*, **83**, 111113x); canangine identical with alk. eupolauridine isolated from *Eupomatia laurina (Lloydia,* 1976, **39,** 459).

Compn. of essent. oil (*Helv Chim Acta,* 1964, **47,** 111); of oil from flowers of endemic plant in Fiji (*Int Flavours Food Addit,* 1975, **6,** 341).

CANANGIUM (*Annonaceae*)

See **CANANGA**

CANARIUM (*Burseraceae*)

C. strictum Roxb. syn. *C. sikkimense* King
Plant, canarone (*J Org Chem,* 1964, **29,** 2479); *epi*-ψ-taraxastanonol and *epi*-ψ-taraxastanediol (*Tetrahedron,* 1966, **22,** 2861).

Black dammar resin contains (+)-junenol, canarone and epikhusinal (*Tetrahedron,* 1965, **21,** 3197). Essent. oil from oleoresin, constituents (*Perfum Essent Oil Rec,* 1967, **58,** 622).

CANAVALIA (*Fabaceae*)

C. gladiata (Jacq.) DC. syn. *C. ensiformis* auct. non Linn. DC.
Eng.–*Jackbean.*
Bean toxic to rats, low haemagglutinin activity (*Nature Lond,* 1965, **22,** 827). Preparation of urease from jackbean seeds for clin. work [*Bull Calcutta Sch Trop Med,* 1966, **14**(1), 14]. Seeds show haemagglutinating activity for trypsin-treated and non-treated rabbit RBC [*Ryuku Daigaku Nogakubu Gakujustu Hokoku,* 1979, (26), 105; *CA,* 1980, **93,** 130339y].

EtOH(50%) ext. of aerial parts, diur. (*Indian J Exp Biol,* 1980, **18,** 594).

Seeds, sepn. of toxic constituents, concanavalin A (*Agroplantae,* 1971, **3,** 27; *CA,* 1972, **77,** 17847u). Canavanine sulphate; seed protein, canavanine; its str. (*Biochem Prep,* 1971, **13,** 41; *Phytochemistry,* 1972, **11,** 3533; *Arch Biochem Biophys,* 1975, **169,** 650). Convulsive toxin, mol. wt. 83,000; compd. strongly toxic to guinea pig [*Cienc Cult Sao Paulo,* 1980, **32** (Suppl.), 86; *CA,* 1981, **94,** 78067n]. Jack

beans, canatoxin (*Arch Biol Technol,* 1980, **23,** 234; *Field Crop Abstr,* 1981, **34,** 10273). Flavones (*Agric Biol Chem,* 1980, **44,** 1407).

Concanavaline A—purification of concanavaline A (& B and canavaline) from Japanese jackbeans (*Arch Biochem Biophys,* 1965, **111,** 499); chem. properties (*Biochemistry,* 1967, **6,** 105); haemagglutinin from jackbean (*Biochem Biophys Acta,* 1967, **133,** 376); method for isolation (*Indian J Biochem Biophys,* 1973, **10,** 145); production (*Rev Soc Quim Mex,* 1980, **24,** 35; *CA,* **93,** 146315y). Cytostatic proteins from seeds of *Abrus precatorius, C. ensiformis* and *Ricinus communis* (*Arzneim Forsch,* 1980, **30,** 759; *CA,* **93,** 128731b). Rev. (*in* Keeler *et al,* 583).

Seedlings, canaline (2-amino-4-aminoxybutyric acid) (*Naturwissenshaften,* 1967, **54,** 169). Hypocotyls contain antifung. compd., de-Me-homopterocarpin; seedling, 3-isoxazolidone (*Phytochemistry,* 1974, **13,** 291; 1981, **20,** 451).

CANNA (*Cannaceae*)

*C. edulis Ker-Gawl.
Rhizome, diur., diaphor., demulc.; used in fever and dropsy (*Indian Drugs,* 1976-77, **14,** 47).
S. India.

C. indica Linn. syn. *C. indica* Linn. var. *orientalis* Rosc.; *C. orientalis* Rosc.
In Samoa, plant used in inflam. (*Econ Bot,* 1974, **28,** 4). EtOH(50%) ext. of aerial parts, hypoten. (*Indian J Exp Biol,* 1977, **15,** 208).
Tubers exhibited enterokinase activity (*J Biosci,* 1981, **3,** 371).
Unsap. matter, molluscidal; triacontanol and mixt. of stigmasterol, β-sitosterol and campesterol (*J Afr Med Pl,* 1977, 107). β-lectin (*Aust J Plant Physiol,* 1979, **6,** 25).

CANNABIS (*Cannabidaceae*)

Monotypic, *C. sativa* with a large number of 'variants' and a wide variation of constituents as also in their contents (*in* Plant and Fungal Toxins, 474).

C. sativa Linn.

Eng.–*Indian hemp, marijuana, cannabis.*

Leaves—bigger leaves used in *bhang*; smaller ones in *ganja*; used in ear troubles; juice mixed with sugar applied to cuts; also anthelm. Crushed leaves in skin diseases (*Econ Bot*, 1971, **25**, 419; 1981, **35**, 4); ext., fungitoxic (*Acta Bot Indica*, 1979, **7**, 147).

In homoeopathy, flowering tops of freshly harvested plants used as diur., in gonor., for opaque cornea and in urethral carbuncle and phimosis (*Bull Bot Soc Bengal*, 1972, **26**, 25).

Plant—fresh, not poisonous; becomes poisonous when damaged on drying, heating, smoking, and/or aging of it or its exts. and plant parts (*in* Plant and Fungal Toxins, 491). Cannabis psychosis and paranoid schizophrenia (*Arch Gen Psychiatry*, 1976, **33**, 383). Therapeutic and human effect of cannabis, rev., 100 refs.; biol. aspects of cannabis uše, rev., 103 refs. (*NIDA Res Monogr*, 1977, **14**, 128; 1978, **19**, 149; *CA*, 1978, **87**, 193378g; 1979, **91**, 13274w). In hypochlorhydria and cholera; in cancer chemotherapy (*Lancet*, 1978, 859; 1980, 1187). Drugs from cannabis, rev., 47 refs. (*Naturwissenschaften*, 1978, **65**, 174). Cannabis in western med., rev., 73 refs. (*Ital J Biochem*, 1978, **27**, 378; *CA*, 1979, **90**, 179716w). Uses and abuses of narcotics including cannabis (*Dtsch Apoth Ztg*, 1981, **121**, 2067). Prolonged duration of surgical anaesthesia and sleeping time in dog (*Indian Vet J*, 1981, **58**, 731). Med. uses of opium and cannabis in medieval India (*Indian J Hist Sci*, 1981, **16**, 31). Biol. effects of chr. use of cannabis; useful in patients of diabetic hypertension (*Q J Crude Drug Res*, 1981, **19**, 81).

EtOH(50%) ext. of plant, spasmol., hypoten. and CNS depress.; on locomotor activity in rats and mices; cannabis-induced potentiation of hexabarbitone

hypnosis in mice; of hemp dust on lungs and lymphs of guinea pigs; on rat brain serotonin and Ac- choline; effect of cannabis ext. on testicular function of toad (*Bufo andersonii*); also of *Presbytis entellus entellus* (*Indian J Exp Biol*, 1968, **6**, 232; 1978, **16**, 82; 671; 1979, **17**, 1387; 1980, **18**, 393; 1977, **15**, 555; *Planta Med*, 1981, **41**, 288).

Marijuana—consists of leaves and flowering parts of female plant only. Teratogenic effect of ext. (*Toxicol Appl Pharmacol*, 1969, **14**, 276). Smoking causes myocardial infraction in human; beneficial in glaucoma and stomach cancer [*Clin Toxicol*, 1979, **14**, 433; *Am Pharm NS*, 1979, **19**(10), 25]. Neurohumoral responses to fume inhalation (*Indian J Exp Biol*, 1980, **18**, 513). Effect of cannabis smoke on brain function and ultrastructure in rhesus monkeys (*Biol Psychiatry*, 1980, **15**, 657; *CA*, **93**, 232388f).

A recent form of marihuana (a marijuana preparation item of illicit trade) with increased potency is 'Sinsemilla' comprising of flowering tops of female plant grown with great care to eliminate any male plants before pollination can occur, thus it contains no seeds; 7 times as potent as 'street' marihuana (*in* Plant and Fungal Toxins, 475-76).

A dangerous drug, may prove to have therapeutic value in med. practice but not a safe drug for recreational use; marihuana smoking and intraocular pressure; biol. effects (*J Am Med Assoc*, 1971, **217**, 1391; 1981, **246**, 1823).

Hashish—resin obtained from leaves and flowering parts of female plants or from marihuana (H.–*Charas*); extn. and pharmacol. of resin from different parts of Indian plant (*Arch Int Pharmacodyn*, 1963, **146**, 99; *CA*, 1964, **60**, 8528f). Advances in chem. research on resin [*Bull Narc*, 1964, **16**(4), 29; *CA*, 1966, **64**, 17529d]. Teratogen (*Lancet*, 1968, **2**, 406). Effect of resin and smoke condensate on oestrus cycle of rat [*Bull Narc*, 1981, **33**(3), 55].

Cannabis yields 421 chemicals of various classes broadly divided as i) cannabinoids, ii) cannabispirans, and iii) alks. (*J Natl Prod*, 1980, **43**, 169). Cannabis drugs owe their narcotic and psychotomimetic properties to cannabinoids.

Cannabinoids—a group of C_{21} dibenzopyran compds., their carboxylic acids, analogues and transformation products typical of, and present in cannabis plant. More than 60 cannabinoids isolated. Cannabinoids classified on the basis of str. are: a) cannabinol type; b) cannabidiol(CBD); c) Δ^9- *trans*-tetrahydrocannabinol; d) Δ^8- *trans*-tetrahydrocannabinol; e) cannabinodiol type; f) cannabigerol type; g) cannabichromene type; h) cannabielsoin type; and i) miscellaneous (*in* Plant and Fungal Toxins, 476-89).

Cannabinoids, therapeutics; cannabis and human cognition; their analg. and antitumour potential; antiepileptic potential; clin. pharmacol. of natural and synth.; heterocyclic analogues [*Ther Potential Marihuana Proc Conf*, 1975 (Pub'1976), 35; 271; 299; 383; 405; 419; *CA*, 1978, **88**, 69051b; 31753-55 u- w; 31856-57 xy].

Gas chromatogr. of constituents of Indian hemp (*Analyst*, 1967, **92**, 450). Chem. and pharmacol. of hallucinogenic plants, rev.; also clin. & psychological effects in man (*Science*, 1968, **162**, 1086; 1234). Chem. and pharmacol., rev., 7 refs. (*Indian Drugs*, 1976-77, **14**, 66); Indian variant, Pr- homologues of cannabinoids; chem. constituents (*J Pharm Sci*, 1972, **61**, 1476; *Planta Med*, 1979, **37**, 215); see also constituents of *C. sativa*, rev., 253 refs.;.leaves and stems of Indian variant grown in Mississippi, new cannabinoid, cannabiglendol (*J Natl Prod*, 1980, **43**, 169; 1981, **44**, 27; *Acta Univ Palacki Olomuc Fac Med*, 1981, **97**, 167; *CA*, **95**, 183883u).

Cannabinoids, advances in chem., 80 refs. (*Progr Org Chem*, 1973, **8**, 78; *CA*, 78, 148077m); chem. rev., 280 refs.; str.-activity relationships, rev., 50 refs.; in man, of cannabis constituents, and homologues and metabolites of Δ^9 -tetrahydrocannabinol (*Marijuana*, 1973, 1; 101; *CA*, 1974, **80**, 133633g; 127971z; *Pharmacology*, 1974, **11**, 3). Chem. and pharmacol. of cannabinoids, rev., 360 refs.; rev., 220 refs.; cannabis and health, rev., 170 refs. ; biochem. aspects of cannabis, rev., 74 refs. (*Cannabis Health*, 1976, 143; 43; 271; 77; *CA*, **85**, 171412v; 192904; 171413w; 171410t). Micromethod for estn. (*Sci Cult*, 1975, **41**, 492); contents during vegetation (*Chemosphere*, 1975, **41**, 299; *CA*, 1976, **84**, 715510a). EMIT detection in blood; assay (*J Anal Toxicol*, 1981, **5**, 165; 168).

Tetrahydrocannabinol, cannabidiolic acid and other cannabinoids; cannabidiolic acid, antibiot. (*Harokeach Haivri*, 1964, **10**, 96; *CA*, 1965, **63**, 3310c). Cannabinoids; cannabidiolic acid from Turkish var., antibact. (*C R Acad Sci Ser C*, 1973, **276**, 205; *CA*, **78**, 97431n; *Acta Univ Palacki Olomuc Fac Med*, 1975, **74**, 161; 167; *CA*, 1976, **85**, 177622k-23m). Effect of cannabinol on human behaviour (*Indian J Physiol Pharmacol*, 1978, **22**, 178).

Cannabinoids, rev. (*Med Pharmacol Toxicol*, 1979, **16**, 499; *CA*, **91**, 49044k); as analg., rev., 30 refs. (*Miles Int Symp Ser*, 1979, 467; *CA*, **91**, 150915v). Metabolic and psychophysiologic studies of cannabidiol (*Clin Pharmacol Ther*, 1980, **28**, 115). Cannabinoids as potential antiepileptic (*J Clin Pharmacol*, 1981, **21**, Suppl., 437; *CA*, **95**, 197573e).

Heterocyclic modifications of cannabinoids (*J Med Chem*, 1976, **19**, 445; 548). Active principles, as models of new drugs (*J Ethnopharmacol*, 1980, **2**, 145); cannabis, a possible source of new drugs (*Pharmacy Int*, 1980, **1**, 19).

Δ^9-*trans*-Tetrahydrocannabinol— Δ^9-THC (dibenzopyran–*CA* system; Δ^1 of terpenoid system of nomenclature); most active constituent in cannabis on CNS; not produced in biosynth. pathway, but through decarboxylation of Δ^9-THCA, readily on heating, smoking and more slowly by aging (*in* Plant and Fungal Toxins, 479-81).

CNS depressant, intoxication biphasic, euphoria followed by depression; chr. use by human causing "burnout" syndrome. CNS-activities; compd. causes physical dependence; mechanism of action in the brain still uncertain. Toxicity of (–)- Δ^9-*trans* THC; therapeutic index or safety ratio very great; lethal dose 4000 times behaviourally effective oral dose in human. Cardiovascular effect, heart beats increase; orthostatic hypotension (hypoten. in standing but not in supine position), in humans long-term effect on this system needs further research (*in* Plant and Fungal Toxins, 493); str.- activity relationships; relative cannabis activity of (–)- Δ^9-*trans*-THC, 100; Δ^8- THC(Δ^6- of terpenoid system), 75; CBD, 0; CBN, 0; and a metabolite 11-OH-Δ^9-THC, 100 times more potent; Δ^8 - THC have very low activities. Interactions of major cannabinoids, CBN, CBD and CBC with Δ^9-THC; CBN has no appreciable effect; CBD antagonizes behavioural effects; and CBC enhances activities of THC. THC and marihuana also affect reproductive systems and functions (*in* Plant and Fungal Toxins, 479-81; 490-96); teratogenic effects (*Toxicol Appl Pharmacol*, 1975, **33**, 333; 1976, **36**, 151).

Homogeneous enzyme immunoassay (EMIT) for cannabinoids in urine; radio immunoassay (RIA) of Δ^9-THC, in blood and plasma (*Clin Chem NY*, 1978, **24**, 95; 1981, **27**, 619); GLC-MS (mass spectrometry) validated RIA; detection in blood, RIA a forensic tool to detect usage of marihuana (*in* Plant and Fungal Toxins, 489).

Used totally synth. and not natural compd. in researches. Total synth.(*Helv Chim Acta*, 1967, **50**, 719; 1969, **59**, 1102); see also total synth. of cannabinoids (*in* Plant and Fungal Toxins, 482).

THC will probably have following major approved use areas: i) Antinauseant in cancer patients receiving chemotherapy. ii) In glaucoma, lowering of intraocular pressure, but with problems such as CNS effects and orthostatic hypotension (*Exp Eye Res*, 1978, **27**, 239; *J Clin Pharmacol*, 1981, **21**, 4725). iii) Bronchodilation in normal and asthmatic subjects; better dosage forms needed than oral capsules or marihuana cigarettes; still a lead for further study of new compds., without psychoactivity. iv) As analg.; but not morphine type, since narcotic antagonists do not block THC analgesia.

Compd. should not be considered antiepileptic drug because of CNS activity and provoking seizures in epileptic beagles.

It would be public service to differentiate medical usage of cannabis plant parts or marihuana from the potential of its constituents; cannabinoids, mainly Δ^9-THC, and CBD (anticonvuls. and therefore useful in epilepsy) viewed as chem. leads to new strs. in search of new med. agents (*in* Plant and Fungal Toxins, 496-500); see also therapeutic progress in cannabinoid research (*J Clin Pharmacol*, 1981, **21**, 1S-494S; *in* Plant and Fungal Toxins, 505).

Essent. oil from plant, constituents (*Can J Chem*, 1965, **43**, 3372; *Tetrahedron Lett*, 1973, 2841; *Phytochemistry*, 1975, **14**, 814; 1977, **16**, 719); its bacteriostatic action (*Ann Pharm Fr*, 1978, **36**, 603; *CA*, 1979, **91**, 50262m).

Seeds contain base, *l*-(+)-isolencine betaine (*Phytochemistry*, 1973, **12**, 2457). TLC detection of hashish substance in seeds; detection of cannabinols from seed resins (*Arch Krincinol*, 1977, **159**, 36; *CA*, 1980, **92**, 177414p; *Indian J Pharm Sci*, 1978, **40**, 166).

Root ext., cardiac activity in guinea pig (*J Pharm Sci*, 1974, **63**, 1167). Anticonvuls. effect of Δ^9- tetrahydrocannabinol and other cannabinoids from roots, in rodents (*Life Sci*, 1974, **15**, 931; *CA*, 1975, **82**, 106317s); cannabielsoic acid A & B (*Tetrahedron*, 1974, **30**, 2437). Root steroids (*Phytochemistry*, 1975, **14**, 580); triterps. and amide (*J Pharm Sci*, 1971, **60**, 1891); β-sitosterol, friedelin and epifriedelinol, carvone & dihydrocarvone and a basic substance (*Planta Med*, 1977,

32, 378). Roots and leaves, alk. cannabisativine (also hordenine and a β-arylethylamine in root) (*Tetrahedron Lett*, 1975, 2815; *Lloydia*, 1975, **38**, 540); those of Mexican variant, anhydrocannabisativine (*J Pharm Sci*, 1978, **67**, 124).

CANSCORA (*Gentianaceae*)

C. decussata Schult. & Schult.

Dried crude powd. of whole plant, anticonvuls. in albino rats (*Indian J Physiol Pharmacol*, 1972, **16**, 81).

Roots, β-amyrin, friedelin, gentianine and xanthones (*J Indian Chem Soc*, 1971, **48**, 589); also 16 xanthones including mangiferin (*Phytochemistry*, 1971, **10**, 2425). Mangiferin, CNS depress. and antiinflam. (*Indian J Pharm Sci*, 1979, **41**, 78); protective against induced liver- injury in albino rats (*Mediscope*, 1979, **22**, 65).

Aerial parts, 1-OMe-3,5-di-OH-xanthone & its 3-O-rutinosyl deriv. (*Phytochemistry*, 1976, **15**, 1041); (–)-loliolide (*J Pharm Sci*, 1976, **65**, 1549); xanthone glucds. & free xanthones (*J Chem Soc Perkin Trans I*, 1977, 1597); xanthones, active against *Mycobacterium tuberculosis* (*J Pharm Sci*, 1978, **67**, 721); 2 new xanthones from flowering tops (*Phytochemistry*, 1979, **18**, 1029).

CANSJERA (*Opiliaceae*)

*C. rheedii J.F. Gmel.

EtOH(50%) ext. of aerial parts, spasmol. (*Indian J Exp Biol*, 1971, **9**, 91).

Upper Gangetic Plain; and southwards to Peninsular India.

CANTHIUM (*Rubiaceae*)

*C. angustifolium Roxb.

EtOH(50%) ext. of aerial parts, spasmol. and diur. (*Indian J Exp Biol*, 1974, **12**, 512).

Jogfall, Karnataka.

C. dicoccum (Gaertn.) Teijsm. & Binn. syn. *C. didymum* Roxb.; *Plectronia didyma* Kurz

Leaves, 3-epibetulin (*Chem Ind Lond*, 1971, 1331); also *d*-mannitol (*Indian J Chem*, 1973, **11**, 840); and flavon. and tannins (*Lloydia*, 1975, **38**, 346).

Bark, triterps. including α-amyrin and oleanolic acid (*J Indian Chem Soc*, 1975, **52**, 1112); triterp. acid sapogenin, canthic acid [*Trans Bose Res Inst Calcutta*, 1979, **42**(3-4), 85]; sitosterol, scopoletin, quinovaic & Ac-quinovaic acids (*Phytochemistry*, 1979, **18**, 1385).

C. parviflorum Lamk syn. *Plectronia parviflora* Bedd.

EtOH(50%) ext. of aerial parts, hypoten. (*Indian J Exp Biol*, 1971, **9**, 91).

Leaves, *d*-mannitol (*J Indian Chem Soc*, 1966, **43**, 380).

CAPPARIS (*Capparidaceae*)

C. decidua Edgew. syn. *C. aphylla* Roth

Plant—aq. ext., anthelm.; that of root bark, purg. (*Indian J Hosp Pharm*, 1969, **6**, 153). Coal from wood, made into paste, applied to mascular injuries (*Sachitra Ayurveda*, 1977-78, **30**, 960). In Sudan, in swellings, jaundice and infections of joints (*Fitoterapia*, 1981, **52**, 243).

Leaves—in Unani system, shoots alongwith shoots of *Peganum hurmala* given as antifert. drug [*J Res Indian Med*, 1978, **13**(1), 106]. Leaf juice, as appetiser, helps in cardiac troubles (*J Econ Tax Bot*, 1981, **2**, 174; 192). Ground stem and leaves after boiling with water and forming a paste, applied during alveolaris and in pyorrhoea.

Fruit and seeds—in Ayurveda, used for urinary purulent discharges, cholera and dysen. Steam volat. fraction of flowers and seeds, highly antimicrob.; kinetics of antibact. activity of seed volatiles against *Vibrio cholerae* (*Indian J Pharm*, 1966, **28**, 343; 1972, **34**, 86). Prickled fruits used to kill intestinal worms (*J Econ Tax Bot*, 1981, **2**, 192).

Roots, alks., capparine, cappariline and capparinine (*Pak J Sci Ind Res*, 1968, **11**, 250). Rootbark, *n*-pentacosane, *n*-tricontanol, β-sitosterol and 2 alks. including *l*-stachydrine (*Planta Med*, 1969, **17**, 95).

Flowers and fruit husk, phthalic acid and *l*-stachydrine (*Indian J Pharm*, 1966, **28**, 338). Unsap. fraction of fruit husk and seed, *n*-triacontane (husk only), *n*- triacontanol, β-sitosterol and β- carotene. Seeds, glucocapparin; isothiocyanate aglycone of glucocapparin, highly antibact. [*Res Bull Panjab Univ Sci*, 1970, **21**(1-2), 67; (3-4), 519]. Chem. investigation of plant (*Proc Nat Acad Sci India*, 1972, **42A**, 24).

C. grandis Linn. f.

EtOH(50%) ext. of aerial parts, spasmol.; diur. and anticancer (*Indian J Exp Biol*, 1974, **12**, 512).

Roots, 4,5,6,7-tetra-OH-decyl isothiocyanate (*Phytochemistry*, 1975, **14**, 1415).

*C. longispina Hook. f.

EtOH(50%) ext. of aerial parts, antivir. and spasmol. (*Indian J Exp Biol*, 1968, **6**, 232).

Mahabaleswar, Maharashtra.

C. moonii Wight

Identity of plant, its value as drug (*J. Sci Ind Res*, 1964, **23**, 53).

EtOH(50%) ext. of aerial parts, CNS depress. (*Indian J Exp Biol*, 1973, **11**, 43). Fruits eaten in weakness, cough and T.B. (*Bull Bot Surv India*, 1980, **22**, 201).

*C. rotundifolia Rottl.

EtOH(50%) ext. of aerial parts, CNS depress. and hypoten. (*Indian J Exp Biol*, 1973, **11**, 43).

Ratnagiri, Maharashtra.

C. sepiaria Linn.

Leaves, taraxasterol, α- & β- amyrin and β-sitosterol (*Phytochemistry*, 1970, **9**, 1885); erythrodiol (*J Indian Chem Soc*, 1970, **47**, 751). Chem. investigation of various plant parts; leaves, betulin [*Res Bull Panjab Univ Sci*, 1970, **21**(Pt.1-2), 23].

C. spinosa Linn.

Eng.–*Caper.*

Juice and volat. fraction of plant, anticystic, fungicidal and bactericidal; leaves and fruits, alk. (*Azerb Med Zh*, 1978, **55**, 70; *CA*, **89**, 87180t).

Major constituent of Liv-52 useful in steatorrhoea of cirrhosis of liver [*J Res Indian Med*, 1973, **8**(3), 28]; drug for acute viral hepatitis (*Indian J Med Res*, 1976, **64**, 738). Ingredient of indigenous drug 'Geriforte' (*Rajasthan Med J*, 1980, **19**, 23; *Probe*, 1979-80, **19**, 99; *Indian Drugs*, 1979-80, **18**, 346).

Root bark, alk. stachydrine which increased coagulation of blood in animals, shortened bleeding time and reduced loss of blood (*Farmakol Toksikol Moscow*, 1972, **35**, 715). Aq. ext. of cortex and leaves, stachydrine (*Khim Prir Soedin*, 1969, **5**, 67; *CA*, **70**, 112377e).

Todzhkistanian plant, coumarin derivs. (*Dokl Akad Nauk Tadzh SSR*, 1965, **8**, 22; *CA*, 1966, **65**, 10960f).

Buds, glucosinolates glucocapparin, sinigrin, glucoiberin and glucocleomin (*Phytochemistry*, 1972, **11**, 251); flavons. of floral buds (*Rev Agroquim Technol Aliment*, 1976, **16**, 252; 568; 1978, **18**, 232; *CA*, **85**, 190887v; 1977, **86**, 185906s; 1979, **90**, 100117v); of aerial parts (*Izv Akad Nauk Turkm SSR Ser Fiz Tekh Khim Geol Nauk*, 1981, 123; *CA*, **95**, 12930w).

C. zeylanica Linn. syn. *C. horrida* Linn. f.

Various plant parts used in pain, swelling, rheum., hemiplegia, sores, colic, cholera, neuralgia, pleur., pheum., pleuritis, breast pain and dropsy (*Econ Bot*, 1970, **24**, 241). EtOH(50%) ext. of aerial parts, spasmol. (*Indian J Exp Biol*, 1971, **9**, 91). Paste of rootbark applied to boils and swelling of testicles (*Bull Med Ethno Bot Res*, 1980, **1**, 318).

Seeds and leaves, thioglucd. glucocapparin, *n*-tricontane, α-amyrin and fixed oil (*Indian J Pharm Sci*, 1978, **40**, 225).

CAPSELLA (*Brassicaceae*)

C. bursa-pastoris (Linn.) Medic.

Plant used against ulcers, tumours and uterine cancer (*Lloydia*, 1969, **32**, 83). Plant, haemostatic; good substitute for ergot of rye to arrest bleeding from the lungs, uterus and kidney (*Indian J Hosp Pharm*, 1969, **6**, 102).

Pharmacol. investigations(*Life Sci*, 1969, **8**, 151). One of the constituents of antihaemor. herb exts., stabilization (*Farm Pol*, 1970, **26**, 739; *CA*, 1971, **75**, 40336u). Leaves ext. shows antifert. activity in animals (*Lloydia*, 1975, **38**, 135).

Herb, constituents (*Rocz Chem*, 1964, **38**, 29; *CA*, **60**, 14565c); flavons. (*Diss Pharm*, 1965, **17**, 389; *CA*, 1966, **64**, 10086c).

Pharmacognostic study by flavon. detn.; rutin present (*Gyogyszereszet*, 1967, **11**, 179; *CA*, 1968, **68**, 6223a; *Dtsch Apoth Ztg*, 1972, **112**, 1158; *CA*, **77**, 137346b); hesperidin, rutin, etc.; flavon. reduced permeability of blood vessel walls in white mice (*Farmatsiya Moscow*, 1973, **22**, 34; *CA*, 1974, **80**, 24822x).

Aerial parts, alk. (*Pak J Sci Ind Res*, 1963, **6**, 53). Choline (*Aptechn Delo*, 1966, **15**, 36; *CA*, **65**, 14091g). Isolation of physiologically active substances (*Nature Lond*, 1968, **220**, 707). Identn. of choline, histamine and 2 crystalline alks. (*Tartu Rikliku Ulik Toim*, 1971, No.270, 71; *CA*, 1972, **76**, 23018v).

Sinigrin (*Aust J Chem*, 1967, **20**, 2799). Essent. oil from plant, major compd. camphor (*Yakugaku Zasshi*, 1979, **99**, 1041).

Proteolytic enzyme (*Restit Resur*, 1968, **4**, 356; *CA*, 1969, **70**, 17566g). Stigmasterol (*Indian J Chem*, 1975, **13**, 97). Isolation of neoplasm inhibitor; identified as fumaric acid (Jpn Kokai, 1977, 7741207; *CA*, **87**, 122792b). Constituents of Egyptian plant (*Egypt J Pharm Sci*, 1975, **16**, 521; *CA*, 1978, **89**, 160097c).

Seeds, quercetin derivs. (*Khim Prir Soedin*, 1973, 800; *CA*, 1974, **81**, 132874v). Seed mucilage trapped and killed *Aedes albopictus* larvae (*Eisei*

Dobustu, 1978, **29**, 345; *CA*, 1979, **90**, 146344v). Detn. of *L*-canaline (*Anal Biochem*, 1979, **92**, 265).

CAPSICUM (*Solanaceae*)

Capsicum spp., various aspects (Parry, 12-22; 185-86; *in* Purseglove *et al*, 331-439).

C. annuum Linn.

Eng.–*Sweet pepper, paprika.*

Paprika is whole or ground dried ripe fruit; in mainly 3 categories — sweet, semisweet, and pungent (Parry, 14).

Fruit—effect on blood glucose level in rat (*Asian Symp Med Plants and Spices, IV*, 1980, 143); ext., hypoglyc. in rat (*Q J Crude Drug Res*, 1980, **18**, 1); powder, increased acid secretion in patients with duodenal ulcer (*Indian J Med Res*, 1977, **66**, 440). Gargle effective against sore throat; paste used as rubft. and as local stim. for tonsils. Decoct. with opium and fried asafoetida given in cholera; infusion with cinnamon and sugar, in delirium.

Leaves steeped in milk applied to reduce swellings and hardened tumours [*Indian Frms Dig*, 1978, **11**(6&7), 73].

Fruit, quercetin deriv., as principal flavon. (*J Food Sci*, 1964, **29**, 27; *CA*, **61**, 1180h). Flavone glycds., apiin and luteolin 7-glucd. (*Naturwissenschaften*, 1967, **54**, 368); principal colouring matter, carotenoid pigment, capsanthin, carotene, capsorubin, etc. (Parry, 186); colour and carotenoid changes in heated paprika; capsanthin & derivs.; pungency by GLC; pungent principles (*J Food Sci*, 1973, **38**, 25; 1971, **36**, 823; 858; 1977, **42**, 660). Fruit enzyme *L*-asparaginase, in two forms, one of which, antitumour (*J Biosci*, 1980, **2**, 291).

Oleoresin—obtained by ether, alc. or acetone extn., a thick, dark reddish-brown coloured liquid intensely pungent; chief active principle capsaicin (Parry, 186). Used in topical analg. compn. (US Pat., 1975, 3880996; *CA*, **83**, 65485v); rev. (*Flavour Ind*, 1971, **2**, 23).

Capsaicin(e)—pungent principle, constitution (*Nippon Nogei Kagaku Kaishi*, 1961, **35**, 596; 923; *CA*, 1964, **60**, 1807f; 9827g); constitution & biosynth. (*J Chem Soc C*, 1968, 442). Quantity varies in fruits, greatest in hot, slight or nil in mild or sweet fruits (Parry, 186). Capsaicin and nonanoic acid vanillyl amide; latter extremely pungent and also available as a synth. substitute (*Naturwissenschaften*, 1965, **52**, 514; *in* Purseglove *et al*, 374-76). Endo capsaicin a & b (*Acta Agron Budapest*, 1969, **18**, 113). Antibact.; more effective than capsicidin (*Z Lebensm Unters Forsch*, 1968, **138**, 86; *CA*, **69**, 104148v); chem., rev., 82 refs. (*Flavour Ind*, 1971, **2**, 691). Hypocholesterolemic effect of red pepper and capasicin (*Indian J Exp Biol*, 1980, **18**, 898). No hallucinogenic property (*in* Beal & Reinhard, 345).

Seed aleurone granules and root cortex contain saponin capsicidin (*Experientia*, 1965, **21**, 383). Endosperm and embryo of seeds, alks. solanine and solanidine (*Diss Pharm Pharmacol*, 1966, **18**, 61; *CA*, **65**, 3665h).

Capsicidine—antibiot. compd. from Hungarian paprika; capsicidin, mixt. of capsicidine A, B & C (*Elelmiszervizsgalati Kozl*, 1966, **12**, 229; *CA*, 1967, **66**, 76275b); extn. from seeds (*Z Lebensm Unters Forsch*, 1964, **124**, 333; 1972, **148**, 286; *CA*, **61**, 8630f; 77, 72319y).

Seeds, glycd. capsicoside (*Chem Ber*, 1975, **108**, 265; *CA*, **82**, 121686c); sterols (*Steroids*, 1977, **29**, 569; **30**, 425; *CA*, **87**, 130505a; 1978, **88**, 47524f; *Lipids*, 1980, **15**, 20).

Leaves, luteolin glycds. (*Afinidad*, 1980, **37**, 517; *CA*, 1980, **94**, 136132t).

C. frutescens Linn. syn. *C. minimum* Roxb.

Eng.–*Chilli, bird chilli, cayenne pepper, red pepper.*

Fruit—crude juice of pepper, antimicrob. (*Qual Plant Mater Veg*, 1972, **22**, 29); in stomach and backache, for chest trouble and cough (*Econ Bot*, 1974, **28**, 27); ext., insectic. (*Indian J Agric Sci*, 1980, **50**, 510).

Leaves—used in headache (*Econ Bot*, 1965, **19**, 244). Used in night blindness, pain, adenitis, sores, dysuria, broncht. crocodile bite (*ibid*, 1970, **24**, 241). In Samoa, used as an ingredient in remedies for heatstroke and inflam.; in chest troubles and cough; bark and leaves, in difficult breathing and plant, in gonor. (*ibid*, 1974, **28**, 27). EtOH(50%) ext. of aerial parts, diur. (*Indian J Exp Biol*, 1977, **15**, 208).

Fruit, capsaicin & dihydrocapsaicin in equal proportions; in another sample (2:1 ratio) together with homodihydrocapsaicin as minor compd.; capsaicin (major), dihydro- & nordihydrocapsaicin and nonanoic acid vanillylamide (*in* Purseglove *et al*, 377); capsaicin a & b (*J Food Sci*, 1971, **36**, 823); pungent principles, see capsaicinoids; also capsaicin under *C. annuum* (*in* Purseglove *et al*, 375-82). Vit. C and capsaicin content of 10 different chilli varieties (*Coll Agric Nagpur Magazine*, 1969-70, **42**, 53; *HA*, 1971, **41**, 9130); in frozen green peppers (*J Food Sci*, 1978, **43**, 532).

Plant, sesquiterp. capsidiol, principal phytoalexin; one of the most fungitoxic compds.; exocyclic double bond seems to increase fungitoxicity; derivs. less active (*Can J Bot*, 1974, **52**, 2481; *Phytopathology*, 1972, **62**, 1186).

In cell cultures, progesterone converted to 4-pregnen-20 α-ol-3-one (yield, 60-90%) with very little byproducts (*Appl Environ Microbiol*, 1978, **36**, 213; *in* Beal & Reinhard, 488).

CARAGANA (*Fabaceae*)

*C. brevispina Royle

EtOH(50%) ext. of aerial parts, hypoglyc. (*Indian J Exp Biol*, 1980, **18**, 594).

Chamoli, U.P.

CARALLIA (*Rhizophoraceae*)

C. brachiata (Lour.) Merrill syn. *C. integerrima* DC.; *C. lucida* Roxb. ex Kurz

Leaves, alk. (+)-hygroline (*Aust J Chem*, 1965, **18**, 589).

CARAPA (*Meliaceae*)

C. granatum (Koenig) Alston syn. *C. obovata* Blume; *C. moluccensis* Hiern non Lamk

In Philippines, decoct. of fruit and seeds used as antidiar. (*Econ Bot*, 1971, **25**, 442).

Seeds, limonoid, xylocarpin (*J Chem Soc C*, 1970, 211); 7 α-OAc-dihydronomilin and mexicanolide (*Can J Chem*, 1979, **57**, 3088).

Wood, gedunin (*J Chem Soc*, 1965, 3495). Gedunin, antifung. (*Curr Sci*, 1977, **46**, 714).

Heartwood, β-sitosterol (*ibid*, 1976, **45**, 293). Bark, triacontanol, friedelin, β-sitosterol, stigmasterol and 2 meliacate derivs.; leaves, β-sitosterol, stigmasterol and 2 tetratriterps. (*Indian J Chem Soc*, 1976, **53**, 947).

Rootbark, insect antifeedant N-Me-flindersine compd. antimicrob., other alks. also present (*Heterocycles*, 1977, **7**, 969).

C. moluccensis (Lamk) M. Roem. syn. *Xylocarpus moluccensis* Hiren non Linn.

Dried fruit peel as appetiser. Unripe fruit of African tree, an antifeedant, xylomollin (*J Am Chem Soc*, 1976, **98**, 6704). Seeds and timbers, xyloccensins A-F and Me-angolensate (*J Chem Soc Perkin Trans I*, 1976, 1993).

CARDAMINE (*Brassicaceae*)

C. laxostemonoides Schultz syn. *C. pratensis* auct. non Linn.

Plant juice used against tumours (*Lloydia*, 1969, **32**, 83).

Flowers, kaempferol glycd. (*C R Acad Sci Ser C*, 1970, **271**, 769).

CARDARIA (*Brassicaceae*)

C. draba Desv. syn. *Lepidium draba* Linn.

MeOH and aq. ext. of plant, antidiur. (*Fitoterapia*, 1981, **52**, 195).

Plant, isothiocyanates, erysoline and sulphoraphane; both compds. active against Gram +ve and –ve bacteria, fungi, yeasts and protozoa, broad antivir., marked nematocide action and strong inhibitors of tumour growth (Ehrlich ascites carcinoma) (*Pharmazie*, 1975, **30**, 792; *CA*, 1976, **84**, 100072c);also 2 alks. [*Med Zh Uzb*, 1976, (2), 61; *CA*, **85**, 30605y].

CARDIOSPERMUM (*Sapindaceae*)

C. halicacabum Linn.

Eng.–*Balloon vine, heartseed.*

Plant—EtOH(50%) ext., spasmol. and hypoten. (*Indian J Exp Biol*, 1968, **6**, 232). Powd. leaves used externally for healing wounds (*Bull Bot Surv India*, 1973, **15**, 13); used in fever (*J Econ Tax Bot*, 1980, **1**, 140); against skeletal fractures (*Sri Lanka For*, 1980, **14**, 145).

Roots—used for abortion (*Ancient Sci Life*, 1981-82, **1**, 72). Ext., diur. in male albino rats (*J Sci Res Plants Med*, 1981, **2**, 32).

Essent. oil—from seeds, B.P. depress.; w.-sol. fraction of ext., hypoten. in animals; alk. fraction of seeds, *in vitro* antibact., hypoten. and cardiac inhibitory (*Indian J Pharm*, 1972, **34**, 76; 1973, **35**, 40).

Seed oil ester (*Phytochemistry*, 1968, **7**, 619). Seeds, cyanogenic glycd. (*Lloydia*, 1972, **35**, 69). Leaves, phytochem. (*Indian J Pharm Sci*, 1981, **43**, 68).

CARDUUS (*Asteraceae*)

C. nutans Linn.

Plant, kaempferol 3-α-*L*-rhamnofuranoside and acacetin-7-β-D-glucd. (*Khim Prir Soedin*, 1975, 654; *CA*, 1976, **84**, 71427q).

CAREX (*Cyperaceae*)

*C. fedia Nees

EtOH(50%) ext. of plant, CNS depress. (*Indian J Exp Biol*, 1980, **18**, 594).

Kheri, U.P.

*C. japonica Thunb.

EtOH(50%) ext. of plant, CNS depress. and anticancer (*Indian J Exp Biol*, 1980, **18**, 594).

Panchmari, M.P.

CAREYA (*Barringtoniaceae*)

C. arborea Roxb.

Bark decoct. in diar. and as eyewash (*Econ Bot*, 1965, **19**, 242); powd., to cure skin diseases (*Bull Bot Surv India*, 1973, **15**, 17).

Plant used in *prolapsus ani* and *fistula ani* and snake-bite (*Econ Bot*, 1970, **24**, 241); Root useful in T.B. (*Nagarjun*, 1980-81, **24**, 1); in skeletal fractures (*Sri Lanka For*, 1980, **14**, 145).

Bark, lupeol and betulin (*Indian J Chem*, 1964, **2**, 510).

Leaves, hexacosanol, quercetin, ellagic acid, taraxerol, its-OAc, β-sitosterol and α-spinasterol, (*Indian J Pharm*, 1975, **37**, 161); and valoneic acid dilactone as its Me deriv.; also ellagic acid-4,4′-di-Me- ether, triterp. ester, careaborin and β-amyrin (*J Indian Chem Soc*, 1976, **53**, 639; 1981, **58**, 814).

Seeds, α-spinasterol & α-spinasterone (*Phytochemistry*, 1972, **11**, 2116). Acid hydrolyzate of seed saponin yields barringtogenol-C (with its 16-deoxy deriv.) & D, and careyagenol D (*J Indian Chem Soc*, 1973, **50**, 254); careyagenol E, str. (*Indian J Chem*, 1964, **12**, 888); revised str. of barringtogenol B (*Trans Bose Res Inst Calcutta*, 1976, **39**, 29).

*C. herbacea Roxb.

EtOH(50%) ext. of plant, hypoten. (*Indian J Exp Biol*, 1980, **18**, 594).

Kheri, U.P.

CARICA (*Caricaceae*)

C. papaya Linn.

Latex—proteolytic activity (*Curr Sci*, 1966, **35**, 42).

Biochem. rev. (*J Sci Ind Res*, 1971, **30**, 640). Preservation (*Hua Hsueh*, 1976, 19; *CA*, 1977, **87**, 49283c). Milky juice, against ringworm and leaves to expel guinea worm. Ripe fruit, in digest. troubles; unripe, in excretory troubles of children. Latex, as antipruritic and in ulcer (*Indian Drugs*, 1977-78, **15**, 145; 1981-82, **19**, 406). One of the constituents of indigenous drug 'Gasex', useful in post operative period to relieve distension (*Probe*, 1977-78, **17**, 330). Latex inhibitory against *Candida* spp. (*Bull Brew Sci*, 1980, **26**, 47; *CA*, 1981, **95**, 215728n). Latex used in abortion (*J Econ Tax Bot*, 1981, **2**, 69).

Unripe fruit—pulp, antifert. in albino rats (*Indian J Med Res*, 1970, **59**, 302; 1974, **62**, 831; 1225).

Shampoos or detergents containing papaya ext., beneficial for skin (Jpn Kokai, 1978, 7854207; *CA*, **89**, 135678k). Ripe fruit, digest. (*Q J Crude Drug Res*, 1979, **5**, 163; *CA*, **93**, 44259n). Chem. of essent. oil from fruit (*Flavour Ind*, 1971, **2**, 305).

Seeds—agglutinate human red cells (*J Chem UAR*, 1963, **6**, 191). Anthelm. activity; active constituent benzyl isothiocyanate (*Indian J Pharm*, 1965, **27**, 335); as source of reliable antibiot. (*Planta Med*, 1974, **26**, 79). Oral administration of powd. of ripe fruit showed antifert. activity in male rats (*Indian J Exp Biol*, 1980, **18**, 408). In Panama, seeds used as laxt.; fruit beverage for diar. and dysen. (*Q J Crude Drug Res*, 1979, **17**, 115); β- sitosterol (*Indian Drugs*, 1981-82, **19**, 406).

Antibact. and antineoplasmic activity (*Rev Cubana Farm*, 1980, **14**, 303; 1981, **15**, 71).

Plant—antifert. agents from plants, rev. [*J Res Indian Med*, 1973, **8**(3), 79]. Ext., *in vitro*, anthelm. against *Ascaridia galli* worms (*Indian J Physiol Pharmacol*, 1976, **20**, 64). Leaves of red var., in fractures (*Bull Bot Surv India*, 1976, **18**, 247).

Bark—in Samoa, inner bark applied to sore tooth (*Econ Bot*, 1974, **28**, 10); ext., antihaemolytic, in jaundiced rat (*Dakar Med*, 1979, **24**, 255); antihaemolytic effect of xylitol, isolated from bark (*Planta Med*, 1981, **41**, 40).

Papain—active principle from latex, pharmacol. effects (*Arch Int Pharmacodyn*, 1963, **145**, 166; *CA*, 1964, **60**, 2221f). Papain inactivates Gram –ve bacterial endotoxins; in wound healing of rats (*Proc Soc Expl Biol Med*, 1964, **115**, 140; 1010). Induction of aetherosclerosis in rabbits by enzyme (*Arch Pathol*, 1965, **79**, 144; *CA*, **62**, 13636g). 'Fibrin-to-clot' clotting time after oral papain (*Life Sci*, 1965, **4**, 1301). Constituent of antiinflam. compn. (Brit. Pat., 1965, 1005985; Fr. M., 1967, 4624; *CA*, 1966, **64**, 535c; 1969, **70**, 99634q). Diur. effect in rats (*Life Sci*, 1965, **4**, 2115); papain, antidiur. in rats (*Exp Med Surg Suppl Issue*, 1966, **23**, 36). Analg. and antiinflam. in rats (*Arch Int Pharmacodyn*, 1966, **159**, 126; *CA*, **64**, 16481e). Constituent of dentifrices (Brit. Pat., 1966, 1033229; *CA*, **65**, 10437g). Str. and activity of papain and other thiol proteinases (*Hakko Kyokaishi*, 1968, **26**, 53; *CA*, **69**, 199w). Checks growth of pathogenic yeast, *Candida albicans* (*Boll Soc Ital Biol Sper*, 1968, **44**, 729; 731; *CA*, **69**, 65358s; 65359t). Dissolves kidney stones (*Z Urol Nephrol*, 1968, **61**, 295; *CA*, **69**, 75386p). Enzyme used as drugs, rev., 45 refs. (*Bull Soc Pharm Lille*, 1970, 135; *CA*, 1971, **74**, 83281u); may cause asthma [*Chem Ind News*, 1977, **55**(10), 12]. Teratogenic and embryotoxic effects in rat; changes in rat foetal brain; also in liver and kidney (*Indian J Med Res*, 1978, **67**, 499; 1979, **69**, 671; 1980, **72**, 300). Changes in placenta of rat fetuses induced by maternal administration of papain; also on peritoneal mast cells (*Indian J Exp Biol*, 1978, **16**, 1256; 1979, **17**, 591).

Papain purification (US Pat., 1965, 3210257; *CA*, **63**, 16138h). Str. and activity of proteolytic enzymes, rev., 221 refs. (*Tampakushitsu Kakusan Koso*, 1967,

12, 539; *CA*, 1970, **73**, 83980a). Papain, rev., 59 refs. (*Methods Enzymol*, 1970, **19**, 226). Isolation of med. enzymes from latexes (Ger Offen, 1976, 2605576; *CA*, **85**, 173514d; Fr. Demande, 1976, 2301267; *CA*, 1977, **86**, 161286p); production (*Biochem Soc Trans*, 1978, **6**, 255). Papain, yield dependence on isolation procedure from latex (*J Sci Food Agric*, 1980, **31**, 279). Papain & other enzymes of papaya, rev., 274 refs. (*Top Enzyme Ferment Biotechnol*, 1981, **5**, 262; *CA*, **94**, 20422s).

Chymopapain—chymopapain C, an immunosuppressive enzyme from plant ext. (*Proc Soc Exp Biol Med*, 1974, **145**, 1250). Chymopapain, extn. from latex, useful as topical and systematic antiinflam. agent (Fr Demande, 1975, 2235702; *CA*, **83**, 152325m). Sepn. of chymopapain from latex (*J Chromatogr*, 1976, **121**, 65). Enzyme injected into intervertebral disks of patients with herniated disk syndrome; chemonucleolysis as it is called, liquifies slipped disk that pinches a patient's spinal nerve. Injection effective but controversial (*in* Plant and Fungal Toxins, 791-92).

Plant contains alk. (*Rev Biol Trop Univ Costa Rica*, 1965, **13**, 207; *CA*, 1966, **65**, 10963h). Plant, 4 alks., including nicotine, continine and myosmine (*Tydskr Natuurwet*, 1968, **8**, 156; *CA*, 1969, **71**, 36405r).

Carpaines—carpaine ext. from plant (US Pat., 1966, 3248300; *CA*, **64**, 19329f); anti-T.B. (*Indian J Pharm*, 1967, **29**, 157); chem. and pharmacol. rev., 16 refs. (*Econ Bot*, 1971, **25**, 363). Chief alk., bispiperidine, amoebicidal, antibact., possesses pharmacol. activity which is digitalis-like on one hand and emetine-like on other; needs further study (*in* Wagner & Wolff, 110; 207); from leaves, alk. carpaine (*Phytochemistry*, 1971, **10**, 2544); antitumour, *in vitro*, against mouse lymphoid leukemia L 1210; lymphocytic leukemia 388 and Ehrlich ascites tumour cells [*Asian J Pharm*, 1972, **2**(2), 26; *CA*, 1974, **80**, 33710m]; effective on circulatory function in rat, decreases B.P. (*Res Commun Chem Pathol Pharmacol*,

1978, **22**, 227). Leaves alks., dehydrocarpaine I & II (*Phytochemistry*, 1979, **18**, 651).

CARISSA (*Apocynaceae*)

C. carandas Linn.

Roots—histamine-releasing (*Jpn J Pharmacol*, 1970, **20**, 367; *CA*, 1971, **74**, 97321m); their paste, insect-repellent (*Nagarjun*, 1979-80, **23**, 177); paste of root bark useful in diabetic ulcer (*Indian For*, 1978, **104**, 676). Alc. ext. of roots, hypoten. in cats (*Bull Calcutta Sch Trop Med*, 1965, **13**, 14).

A fraction of mature fruit, cytotoxic (*Indian J Med Res*, 1968, **56**, 445). Various plant parts, used in dropsy, anasarca, madness, rheum., hemiplegia, epilepsy, convuls., postnatal complaints, sores and bite of rabid jackal or dog (*Econ Bot*, 1970, **24**, 241).

Roots yield 4 cardioactive compds., carissone, β-sitosterol and w.-sol. polyglyceride fraction (*Indian J Chem*, 1966, **4**, 132); enzymic and mild acid hydrolysis of polar glycds., afforded adoroside H, digitoxigenin, its 14,15-anhydro compd. and *D*-digitalose; cardiotonic activity due to glucd. of odoroside H (*ibid*, 1967, **5**, 215). Root, str. of triterp., carindone (*Phytochemistry*, 1972, **11**, 1797). Root, new lignan, carinol (*ibid*, 1975, **14**, 2302).

Fruits, ascorbic acid (915 mg/100g) (*Indian J Appl Chem*, 1965, **28**, 119).

*C. conjesta Wight
G.–Bel.

Root decoct. in diar. (*Bull Med Ethno Bot Res*, 1980, **1**, 8). Pharmacol. [*J Sci Ind Res*, 1961, **20A** (Suppl.), 1].

Dungs, Gujarat.

*C. inermis Vahl syn. C. macrophylla Wall.
Mar.–*Karanja*.

EtOH(50%) ext. of aerial parts, CNS depress. and hypoten. (*Indian J Exp Biol*, 1973, **11**, 43).

Ratnagiri, Maharashtra.

*C. opaca Stapf ex Haines

EtOH(50%) ext. of aerial parts, CNS depress. and hypoten. (*Indian J Exp Biol*, 1971, **9**, 91).

Mirzapur, U.P.

C. spinarum Linn.

Alc. ext. of roots lowered B.P. in cats (*Bull Calcutta Sch Trop Med*, 1965, **13**, 14). Rootbark useful in malignant ulcers as antibiot. [*J Res Indian Med*, 1973, **8**(1), 83]. Root paste taken orally in fever; also used in inflam., body pain and in cut injury (*Bull Bot Surv India*, 1976, **18**, 247).

Cardiotonic activity of root, leaves and stems 4-6 times greater than that of *C. carandas* (*Indian J Med Res*, 1963, **51**, 937).

EtOH(50%) ext. of aerial parts, diur. and hypoten. (*Indian J Exp Biol*, 1964, **12**, 512).

Roots, 5 cardiac glycds. including evomonoside, odoroside G & H (*Indian J Chem*, 1969, **7**, 1102); caffeic acid (0.017%) (*Indian J Pharm*, 1971, **33**, 76).

Berries, coumarin (*Indian J Pharm*, 1965, **27**, 90). Stems and leaves gave +ve test for alk. (*Lloydia*, 1974, **37**, 506).

CARMONA (*Ehretiaceae*)

C. retusa Masu. syn. C. microphylla G. Don; Ehretia buxifolia Roxb.; E. microphylla Lamk

EtOH(50%) ext. of aerial parts show low antiinflam. and cardiovascular activities (*Indian J Exp Biol*, 1977, **15**, 208).

Plant, microphyllone (*Tetrahedron*, 1980, **36**, 1435).

CARPESIUM (*Asteraceae*)

C. abrotanoides Linn.

Fruits, sesquiterp. lactone, carabone; its str. (*Proc Chem Soc Lond*, 1964, 120; *J Chem Soc*, Suppl 1, 1964, 5503). Plant, antibact. substance, granilin; ψ-guaianolides carpesiolin and carabone, as antifung. and antibact. substances resp.; stems, leaves and flowers, ivalin (eudesmanolide)(*Phytochemistry*, 1975, **14**, 2247; 1977, **16**, 782; 1976, **15**, 2026).

CARPINUS (*Carpinaceae*)

*C. viminea Wall. ex Lindl.

H.P.–*Cakri.*

EtOH(50%) ext. of aerial parts, CNS depress. (*Indian J Exp Biol*, 1973, **11**, 43).

Dalhousie, H.P.

CARTHAMUS (*Asteraceae*)

C. lanatus Linn.

Isolation method of substances with interferon-inducing activity (Ger. Offen., 1980, 3004018; *CA*, 1981, **94**, 52920k).

C. oxyacantha Bieb.

EtOH(50%) ext. of plant, diur. (*Indian J Exp Biol*, 1980, **18**, 594).

Plants—luteolin-7-glucd. (*Indian J Appl Chem*, 1970, **33**, 262). Aerial parts, sesquiterp. glycd., hinesol-β-*D*-fucopyranoside (*Chem Ber*, 1976, **109**, 3953).

C. tinctorius Linn.

Eng.–*Safflower.*

EtOH(50%) ext. of seeds, spasmol. (*Indian J Exp Biol*, 1969, **7**, 250).

Seed oil—favours development of cirrhosis in rat (*Arch Pathol*, 1968, **86**, 545; *CA*, 1969, **70**, 9674a). Mixt. of oil with rice bran oil lowered blood cholesterol in human (*Eiyogaku Zasshi*, 1970, **28**, 194; *CA*, 1971, **75**, 60711r). Oil increased plasma insulin in human (*Diabetes*, 1972, **21**, 923; *CA*, 1973, **78**, 24754k). *C. tinctorius* as a med. oil-producing plant, rev. with 25 refs. (*Gyogyszereszet*, 1973, 17, 411; *CA*, 1974, **81**, 41297t). Beneficial in aetherosclerosis in dogs (*Lab Invest*, 1976, **34**, 394; *CA*, **84**, 148913e). Oil enhanced bile flow with increased amts. of cholesterol, in animals (*Chem Phys Lipids*, 1976, **17**, 315; *CA*, 1977, **86**, 54221s). Oil, in anticholesteremic compn. (Jpn Kokai Tokyo Koho, 1978, 78126089; *CA*, 1979, **90**, 92440c). Med. uses (*Planta Med*, 1974, **26**, 65).

Flowers—one of the minor constituents of compns. for poliomyelitis, paralysis of brain and spine, heart disease and other nerve diseases (Fr. Demande, 1973, 2160297; *CA*, 1974, **80**, 6956q). Corolla ext. affective in coronary occlusion in animals; also as mixt. with other plant drugs (*Acta Pharm Sin*, 1979, **14**, 474; 461).

Seeds, matairesinol monoglucd. as bitter principle (*Phytochemistry*, 1970, **9**, 2407). Steroid glycd.; str. of steroid diglucd., aellobioside, tracheloside; cathartic lignan glycd., 2-OH-arctiin (*ibid*, 1972, **11**, 819; 2327; 2629; 2871). Fruit contains alk. (*Lloydia*, 1974, **37**, 522). Seeds, 1,8,11,14-heptadecatetraene; polyacetylenes (*Phytochemistry*, 1975, **14**, 2085; 1978, **17**, 315). Conjugated serotonins related to cathartic activity in seeds; also phenolic constituents (*Agric Biol Chem*, 1978, **42**, 1805; 1980, **44**, 2951). Extn. of milk coagulating enzyme from seeds (*J Agric Food Chem*, 1979, **27**, 190).

Fatty acid compn. of oil (*Fette Seifen Anstrichm*, 1969, **71**, 446; *CA*, **71**, 79901s). Oil, Δ^7- avenasterols (*Riv Ital Sostanze Grasse*, 1974, **51**, 50; *CA*, **81**, 148446t); sterols (*J Am Oil Chem Soc*, 1973, **50**, 122; *Fette Seifen Anstrichm*, 1976, **78**, 301; *CA*, **85**, 141510h). Oil, α-tocopherol (300 ppm) (*An Bromatol*, 1975, **27**, 287; *CA*, 1976, **85**, 4046x).

Removal of deleterious glucds., cath. 2-OH-arctiin and bitter matairesinol monoglucd. from seed meal (*J Am Oil Chem Soc*, 1979, **56**, 560).

Aerial parts, acetylenic compds. (*Chem Ber*, 1970, **103**, 2853). Flowers, yellow pigment safflomin A (*Chem Lett*, 1981, 433).

CARUM (*Apiaceae*)

C. bulbocastanum Koch; see **Bunium persicum**

C. carvi Linn.

Eng.–*Caraway.*

Seed ext. agglutinate human blood cells (*Acta Univ Palacki Olomuc Fac Med*, 1965, **38**, 199; *CA*, 1969, **70**, 95015r). Fruit, antisep. (*Q J Crude Drug Res*, 1972, **12**, 1922). In Europe, used in flatulence and stomach disorder (*Acta Phytother*, 1971, **18**, 21). Alc. ext. of seeds, antisp. (*Planta Med*, 1980, **40**, 309).

Essent. oil—from seed, antibact. [*Indian Drugs*, 1979- 80, **17**, 394; *Pak J Sci Res*, 1974, **26**, 25; *CA*, 1977, **86**, 84191z; *Indian Drugs Pharmac Ind*, 1980, **15**(6), 7]; antifung. [*ibid*, 1979, **14**(1), 3; *Fitoterapia*, 1980, **51**, 201].

Various plant parts used in venereal sores, syphilis, constip., cholera, *prolapsus ani* and *fistula ani* (*Econ Bot*, 1970, **24**, 241).

Fruits, lipids, umbelliferone, scopoletin and herniarin (*Fette Seifen Anstrichm*, 1969, **71**, 276; *CA*, **71**, 57561d). Seeds flavons. (*Phytochemistry*, 1972, **11**, 1741). Fruits, abscisic acid (*Z Pflansenphysiol*, 1978, **86**, 61). Aflatoxin detn. in caraway (*Fleischwirtschaft*, 1981, **61**, 1034; *CA*, **95**, 113542h).

Effect of pH and temp. on volat. constituents (*J Food Sci*, 1970, **35**, 531). Romanian caraway oil, *trans-* & *cis-* carveol (*Pharmazie*, 1972, **27**, 340). Essent. oil constituents (*Planta Med*, 1975, **28**, 112; 1976, **30**, 93). Gas chromatogr. sepn. of essent. oil of various origin for O- containing monoterps. (*Sci Pharm*, 1978, **46**, 93; *CA*, **89**, 160134n). Colorim. detn. of carvone, menthone and pulegone in essent. oil (*J Assoc Anal Chem*, 1979, **62**, 250).

Leaves, flavon. glycds. (*Z Lebensm Unters Forsch*, 1977, **164**, 194; *CA*, **87**, 166146y).

C. copticum Benth. & Hook. f.; see **Pteroselinum crispum**

C. roxburghianum Benth. & Hook. f.; see **Trachyspermum roxburghianum**

CARVIA (*Acanthaceae*)

C. callosa (Wall.) Bremek. syn. *Strobilanthes callosus* Nees

EtOH(50%) ext. of aerial parts, CNS depress. and diur. (*Indian J Exp Biol*, 1977, **15**, 208).

Roots, lupeol (*Indian J Chem*, 1970, **8**, 851). Flowers, *n*-alkanes, alcs., sterols, etc. (*J Indian Chem Soc*, 1979, **56**, 115).

CARYA (*Juglandaceae*)

*C. illinoinesis (Wang.) Koch syn. *C. pecan* Engl. & Graebn.; *C. oliviformis* Nutt.

Leaves, essent. oil (*Rastit Resur*, 1980, **16**, 441); juglone, antifung. (*J Agric Food Chem*, 1980, **28**, 340); 3- glucd., 3-diglycd. and 3-rhamnoside of azaleatin, and caryatin- 3′-(or 4′-)-rhamnoglucd. (*Phytochemistry*, 1980, **19**, 2512). Stembark, a new 2H- pyran, caryapyran (*Proc Sci Program Am Soc Pharmacog Sec Econ Bot*, 1981, abstr. 10).

Native of Mexico, grown in N. India.

CARYOPHYLLUS (*Myrtaceae*)

See **SYZYGIUM**

CARYOTA (*Arecaceae*)

C. mitis Lour.

Mature fruits, Ca oxalate in toxic amt. (*Toxicol Appl Pharmacol*, 1979, **48**, 287).

C. urens Linn.

Charred fruit used in hemicrania; juice, as tonic (*Nagarjun*, 1980-81, **24**, 243).

CASEARIA (*Flacourtiaceae*)

C. elliptica Willd. syn. *C. tomentosa* Roxb. H.–*Kirci*; Oriya–*Khokaray*.

Tribals of Bastar consider rootbark as a tonic for anaemia (*Econ Bot*, 1965, **19**, 242). Fruits, edible and hypoglyc.

EtOH(50%) ext. of aerial parts, antivir., hypoten and spasmol. (*Indian J Exp Biol*, 1969, **7**, 250). Various plant parts used in fever, spleen complaints, scabies, ringworm, sores, colic, neuralgia, pleur., pneum., diar., breast pain, bite of rabid jackal or dog and snakebite (*Econ Bot*, 1970, **24**, 241).

C. graveolens Dalz.

B.–*Chur-chur.*

EtOH(50%) ext. of plant, anticancer (*Indian J Exp Biol*, 1971, **9**, 91). Fruit, fish poison (*Nagarjun*, 1979-80, **23**, 177). Decoct. of stembark and roots given in stomach pain (*Bull Med Ethno Bot Res*, 1980, **1**, 8).

Bark, new coumarindiol, casegravol (*Chem Ind Lond*, 1980, 154).

C. ovata Willd. syn. *C. esculata* Roxb.

H.–*Saptarangi.*

Antidiabetic effects of root ext. in rats and rabbits (*Indian J Med Res*, 1967, **55**, 754); hypoglyc. investigation of plant exts. (*J Pharm Sci*, 1967, **56**, 1404; *CA*, 1968, **68**, 10209t). Pharmacognosy of bark (*Indian J Pharm*, 1967, **29**, 341).

Roots, leucopelargonidin (*Curr Sci*, 1965, **34**, 634); also β-sitosterol (*Indian J Chem*, 1971, **9**, 611). Isolation procedure of polypeptide-like antibiot. substances, α-, β- & γ- casercidin (S. Afr. Pat., 1968, 680867; *CA*, 1969, **71**, 33429r).

*C. verca Roxb.

EtOH(50%) ext. of aerial parts, antiprot. and anticancer (*Indian J Exp Biol*, 1971, **9**, 91).

Nongph, Meghalaya.

CASIMIROA (*Rutaceae*)

*C. edulis Leave & Lex.

Eng.–*White sapota.*

Leaves used in diar. and as anthelm. (Wlth India, II, 93). Drug aspects of fruit, of white sapotas, rev., 64 refs. (*Econ Bot*, 1962, **16**, 288).

Seeds, alks. casimiroine and casimiroedine (Wlth India, II, 93); constituents (*J Chem Soc*, 1956, 4163); str. of casimiroine (*J Am Chem Soc*, 1957, **79**, 6328); partial str. of casimiroedine (*Tetrahedron*, 1958, **2**, 1680; *Tetrahedron Lett*, 1962, 357); a hypoten. principle, N', N'-di-Me-histamine (*J Org Chem*, 1958,

23, 1564); lactone obacunone (*ibid*, 1959, **24**, 870); casimiroine, anti-TB (*Indian J Pharm*, 1967, **29**, 157); 5- MeO-8-geranyloxypsoralen, phellopterin, zapotin, zapoterin, eduline, edulein, casimiroine, 1-Me-2-Ph-4-quinolone, 7α-obacunol and de-Ac-nomilin (*J Org Chem*, 1968, **33**, 3577); str. of zapoterin (*Tetrahedron Lett*, 1968, 5153). Histamine-like compd. hypoten. in dogs (*Arch Invest Med*, 1978, **9**, 565; *CA*, 1979, **90**, 97588s).

Bark constituents (*J Chem Soc*, 1956, 4170); edulien (*J Org Chem*, 1958, **23**, 762).

Rootbark, flavones, zapotin & zapotinin (*Tetrahedron*, 1960, **9**, 139).

Native of C. America, cultivated in gardens.

CASSIA (*Caesalpiniaceae*)

C. absus Linn.

Powd. leaves in ulcer dressing (*J Econ Tax Bot*, 1981, **2**, 178). One of the constituents of Unani drug for leprosy (*J Nat Integ Med Assoc*, 1981, **23**, 43).

Seeds, sitosterol glycd. (*Pak J Sci Ind Res*, 1964, **7**, 219); Pharmacol. of alk. chaksine (*Bull Calcutta Sch Trop Med*, 1962, **12**, 378); of alk. isochaksine (*Pak J Sci Ind Res*, 1963, **6**, 97; 285; *Arch Int Pharmacodyn*, 1965, **158**, 307; *CA*, 1966, **64**, 102541); galactomannan compn. (*Phytochemistry*, 1971, **10**, 621; *Indian J Chem*, 1972, **10**, 155; 1973, **11**, 13); mucilage, active ingredient for medicaments useful in soothing digest., mucous tissues (Fr Demande, 1973, 2167219; *CA*, 1974, **80**, 52362r); flavons., triterps., etc. (*Indian J Chem*, 1977, **15**, 764).

Roots, anthroquinones chrysophanol, aloe-emodin; alks. chaksine & isochaksine; leaves, same alks., quercetin and rutin (*J Natl Prod*, 1979, **42**, 299).

C. alata Linn.

In Samoa, leaves used among others as poultice and purg.; bark to treat skin diseases (*Econ Bot*, 1974, **28**, 16). Leaf ext., antifung. [*J Res Indian Med*, 1976, **11**(2), 70].

Med. uses in Spain (*Science*, 1975, **188**, 215). EtOH (50%) ext. of aerial parts, CNS depress., diur., and antiinflam. (*Indian J Exp Biol*, 1977, **15**, 208). Leaf juice used against eczema (*Q J Crude Drug Res*, 1979, **17**, 66). Plant ext., antiinflam. and antitumour (*Fitoterapia*, 1981, **52**, 195).

Plant, xanthone cassiollin (pinselin) (*J Chem Soc Chem Commun*, 1971, 423); chrysophanol, emodin, rhein and aloe-emodin (*Asian J Pharm*, 1976, **3**, 10, 17; *CA*, 1977, **86**, 40173r). Leaves, kaempferol and aloe-emodin (*Curr Sci*, 1975, **44**, 790); anthraquinone derivs. (*Rev Peru Bioquim*, 1977, **1**, 31; *CA*, 1978, **88**, 101586t); leaves and fruits, anthraquinones (*Curr Sci*, 1978, **47**, 271); also of Fiji plant (*N Z J Sci*, 1979, **22**, 123); 6-OH-musizin glycd. and tinnevellin glycd. (*Planta Med*, 1981, **43**, 11).

Leaves contain volat. oil (sesquiterps. and phenolic compds), volat. oil active against Gram +ve and –ve bacteria (*Q J Crude Drug Res*, 1981, **19**, 93).

Root, quinone pigments, str. (*Planta Med*, 1970-71, **19**, 299).

C. angustifolia Vahl

Standardized tablets useful against constip. in patients in postpartum period; no effect on breast-fed baby if taken by mother (*S Afr Med J*, 1980, **57**, 78).

Resin, one of the constituents of Unani drug '*Itrifal Ustukhudus*', used for purging viscid matter from brain and stomach (*Nagarjun*, 1978-79, **22**, 237).

Pods, glycds. of rhein, chrysophanic acid and sennosides A & B; extn. and sepn. of anthraquinone glycds. (*J Pharm Sci*, 1964, **53**, 110).

Leaves contain sennoside C (*Helv Chim Acta*, 1965, **48**, 1911); also diglucd. of aloe-emodin dianthrone (*Pharm Acta Helv*, 1967, **42**, 37; *Int Pharm Abstr*, **4**, 906c); anthraquinones (*Rev Peru Bioquim*, 1977, **1**, 31; *CA*, 1978, **88**, 101586t). Naphthalene glucd. (*Planta Med*, 1981, **43**, 11). Anthronic heterosides during development (*Phytochemistry*, 1975, **14**, 1397).

Sennosides—production of concentrate from leaves and pods (*Res Ind*, 1975, **20**, 124). Effect of plant growth regulator on yield from leaves (*Planta Med*, 1978, **34**, 437). Leaflets, highest sennoside content on 50th day (*Indian J Pharm Sci*, 1979, **41**, 157); leaf spot disease and content (*Indian Drugs*, 1979-80, **17**, 1). Spectrophotom. detn. of sennoside and related compds. (*J Natl Prod*, 1980, **43**, 452). Inhibition of intestinal water and electrolyte absorption by senna derivs. in rats (*J Pharm Pharmacol*, 1979, **32**, 330). From leaflets and fruits (*Planta Med Phytother*, 1979, **13**, 34). Potentiating effect of sennoside C on purg. action of sennoside A in mice (*Planta Med*, 1981, **42**, 302).

C. auriculata Linn.

Flower and seed exts., hypoglyc.; seed ext. more effective (*Indian J Med Res*, 1963, **51**, 464); flowers useful in diabetes and urinary disorders (*J Agric Trop Bot Appl*, 1966, **13**, 255). Seed ext. used in cough and asthma (*J Econ Tax Bot*, 1980, **1**, 140).

EtOH(50%) ext. of plant, antivir. (*Indian J Exp Biol*, 1968, **6**, 232).

Plant produced liver lesions and histopathology in lungs and kidneys of rats; contains pyrrolizidine alk. (*J Ethnopharmacol*, 1981, **4**, 159).

Flowers, β-sitosterol and kaempferol (*Vijnana Parishad Anusandhan Patrika*, 1972, **15**, 85); proanthocyanidin dimer (*Indian J Chem*, 1972, **10**, 956). Leaves, 3 keto alcs., β-sitosterol and emodin (*Planta Med*, 1973, **23**, 363). Pod husk, β-sitosterol, chrysophanol, emodin, rubiadin; and nonacosan-6-one (*J Indian Chem Soc*, 1981, **58**, 820; 989).

C. fistula Linn.

In Ayurveda, used in haematemesis, pruritus, leucoderma and diabetes (*Acta Phytother*, 1972, **19**, 141). EtOH (50%) ext. of pod and stem bark, hypoglyc., antivir.and anticancer (*Indian J Exp Biol*, 1968, **6**, 232). Used in cancer, epilepsy, convuls. and delirium febris, pimples, bums, syphilis, dysuria, haemat., gravel and diar. (*Econ Bot*, 1970, **24**, 241). Plant used in skeletal fractures (*Sri Lanka For*, 1980, **14**, 145). Ayurvedic preparation '*Aragwatha Kwatham*' (containing decoct. of bark) useful in scabies, clin. study [*J Sci Res Plants Med*, 1980, **1**(3-4), 29].

Fruit—abortif. (*Q J Crude Drug Res*, 1972, **12**, 1922). Fruit pulp useful in chest and heart disease (*Indian Drugs*, 1977-78, **15**, 145). EtOH ext., showed antifert. activity in female albino rats; estrogenic (*Comp Physiol Ecol*, 1979, **4**, 277; *BA*, 1980, **69**, 32736; *Bull Med Ethno Bot Res*, 1980, **1**, 281). Heated fruits applied on the neck to allay swellings due to cold; pulp used as tonic and in chest infection; with sugar taken in constip.; fruit powd. mixed with brassica oil and powd. turmeric given orally to cattles suffering from cough and as stomch. (*J Econ Tax Bot*, 1981, **2**, 178; 193; 1980, **1**, 140); pulp, in liver disorder. Seeds in jaundice. Bark paste given internally in blindness (*Bull Med Ethno Bot Res*, 1980, **1**, 8; 318).

Leaves, in ringworm. Flowers effective in fungal infection (*Indian Drugs*, 1977-78, **15**, 145).

Leaves sennoside A & B (*Curr Sci*, 1964, **33**, 462); flavons. (*Shoyakugaku Zasshi*, 1977, **31**, 172; *CA*, 1978, **88**, 148947b). Production of interferon-like factor due to infection of cells of callus by an animal virus (*Indian J Exp Biol*, 1981, **19**, 349).

Bark, leucoanthocyanidin, fistucacidin (*Bull Nat Inst Sci India*, 1965, No. 31, 28). Bark and heartwood, flavons., fistucacidin, barbaloin and rhein (*Tetrahedron*, 1967, **23**, 515). Sennosides (*Indian J Pharm*, 1968, **30**, 8). Stembark ext., antivir.; contains lupeol, β-sitosterol and hexacosanol (*J Indian Chem Soc*, 1968, **45**, 744).

Rootbark flavon. glycd. fraction, antifung. activity [*J Res Indian Med*, 1975, **10**(4), 110]; fistucacidin; a preparation useful in pyoderma, clin. trials; hydroxyflavones active constituents [*ibid*, 1977, **12**(1), 77; **12**(4), 16].

Flower, ceryl alc., kaempferol and fistulin; also proanthocyanidins (*Indian J Chem*, 1966, **4**, 460; 1972, **10**, 379).

Pods, aloeemodin, emodin, chrysophanol, rhein, sennidin A & B (*Indian J Pharm*, 1965, **27**, 71). Pod wax constituents (*Proc Nat Acad Sci India*, 1970, **40A**, 338). Seeds, galactomannan (*Planta Med*, 1972, **22**, 71).

*C. hirsuta Linn.

EtOH(50%) ext. of aerial parts, CNS depress. and hypoten. (*Indian J Exp Biol*, 1974, **12**, 512).

Irrutupalyam, T.N.

C. javanica Linn.

EtOH(50%) ext. of aerial parts, semen coagulant, CNS depress. and hypoten. (*Indian J Exp Biol*, 1977, **15**, 208).

Root bark, emodin & its 5-OH deriv. (*Phytochemistry*, 1979, **18**, 906); 2 new lucoanthocyanins (*J Indian Chem Soc*, 1980, **57**, 566); and chalcone (*Symp Pap IUPAC Int Symt Chem Natl Prod 11th*, 1978, **2**, 180; *CA*, 1980, **92**, 55042v).

Flowers, flavons. (*Phytochemistry*, 1971, **10**, 2256); constituents (*J Indian Chem Soc*, 1979, **56**, 746).

Seed mucilage, chem. anal. (*Indian For*, 1980, **106**, 810); seeds, anthraquinone pigments (*Planta Med*, 1981, **43**, 381).

Wood, ceryl alc., chrysophanol, piceatannol and (–)-epiafzelechin (*Indian J Chem*, 1978, **16B**, 437). Variation of anthraquinone deriv. with season (*Indian J Pharm*, 1965, **27**, 338). Leaves, flavons. and anthraquinones (*Curr Sci*, 1966, **35**, 364). Constituents of heartwood, stembark and leaves (*Planta Med*, 1975, **28**, 190).

*C. lavigata Willd.

EtOH(50%) ext. of aerial parts, hypoten. (*Indian J Exp Biol*, 1974, **12**, 512).

Pods, 2 flavon. glycds. (*Planta Med*, 1978, **34**, 319); also new anthraquinone digalactoside; leaves, flavons. (*Phytochemistry*, 1979, **18**, 347; 2060). Seeds, 2 anthraquinones and a flavon. (*J Indian Chem Soc*, 1979, **56**, 942). Roots, anthraquinones and flavons. (*Phytochemistry*, 1980, **19**, 1253). Pithoragarh, U.P.

C. mimosoides Linn.

Roots given in stomach spasm (*Indian Drugs*, 1976-77, **14**, 47).

Leaves contain emodin, its glycds and luteolin-7-glucd., also free emodic acid; roots and leaves, physcion (*Indian J Pharm*, **31**, 110; 1970, **32**, 70).

Seeds—used to prepare a stimulating drink (*Econ Bot*, 1965, **19**, 241). Seed, laxt. compn. (Fr. M., 1967, 5549; *CA*, 1969, **71**, 42291s). Seed and leaves ext., anthelm. (*Indian J Pharm*, 1973, **35**, 44). Ext., fungitoxic against *Helminthosporium oryzae* (*Nat Acad Sci Lett*, 1978, **1**, 287). Minor constituent of indigenous drug 'Geriforte' (*Probe*, 1978-80, **19**, 99; *Rajasthan Med J*, 1980, **19**, 23; *Indian Drugs*, 1980-81, **18**, 346). Ext. of roots and seeds useful in whooping cough (*J Econ Tax Bot*, 1980, **1**, 140).

Leaves—in Samoa, used to treat asthma, typhoid and stomach trouble (*Econ Bot*, 1974, **28**, 17); aphrodis. (*Indian Drugs*, 1977-78, **15**, 145); in foot and mouth diseases in cattle (*J Econ Tax Bot*, 1980, **1**, 140).

C. occidentalis Linn.

Antibiot. activity (*Indian J Pharm*, 1966, **28**, 248). One of the ingredients of 'Liv-52' used in hepatitis, clin. study [*J Res Indian Med*, 1973, **8**(3), 28; *Indian J Med Res*, 1976, **64**, 738]. Senna toxicity in cattle, rev., 8 refs. (*Southwest Vet*, 1977, **30**, 165; *CA*, 1978, **88**, 32605j).

Sennosides from Senna pods (Brit., 1968, 1135528; *CA*, 1969, **70**, 40626k); action on human colon and rectum (*Gut*, 1970, **11**, 1038; *CA*, 1971, **74**, 123593f). Seeds, N-Me- morpholine (*J Agric Food Chem*, 1971, **19**, 198); anthraquinone glycd.; anthraquinones (*Experientia*, 1973, **29**, 141; 1974, **30**, 850; *Shoyakugaku Zasshi*, 1979, **33**, 72). Seed polysaccharides; str. of galactomannan (*Indian J Chem*, 1973, **11**, 505; 1134; 1975, **13**, 1152).

Leaves contain dianthronic heteroside; pericarp, apigenin; and roots, emodol (*Ann Pharm Fr*, 1968, **26**, 673; *CA*, 1969, **70**, 84918m). Chem. anal. and uses of *Cassia* spp., rev., 49 refs. (*Planta Med Phytother*, 1968, **2**, 255; *CA*, 1969, **70**, 84909j). Leaves, constituents; also anthraquinone pigments (*Planta Med*, 1973, **23**, 74; 1977, **32**, 375); flavons. (*Phytochemistry*, 1977, **16**, 1107); constituents (*Yakugaku Zasshi*, 1978, **98**, 1288; *CA*, **89**, 193900n).

Plant, xanthone casiolline (*J Chem Soc C*, 1970, 1285; *Chem Commun D*, 1971, 423); islandicin, helminthosporin, and xanthorin (*Indian J Chem*, 1974, **12**, 1042).

Roots, constituents (*An Fac Farm Porto*, 1964, **24**, 65; *CA*, 1965, **63**, 17797b); physcion and phytosterol (*Phytochemistry*, 1973, **12**, 1186). Flowers, physcion, and its glucd., emodin, and β-sitosterol (*Planta Med*, 1973, **23**, 298).

C. pumila Lamk

EtOH(50%) ext. of plant, spasmol., CNS depress. and diur. (*Indian J Exp Biol*, 1980, **18**, 594).

C. siamea Lamk

Trunk bark, dianthraquinones and triterp. (*J Indian Chem Soc*, 1964, **41**, 415); lupenone (*ibid*, 1966, **43**, 63); str. of siameanin, a dianthraquinone (*Bull Nat Inst Sci India*, 1965, No. 31, 141). Trunk bark and root bark, cassiamin A, B & C (*Indian J Chem*, 1970, **8**, 109); constituents of bark and flowers (*J Indian Chem Soc*, 1977, **54**, 548). Anthraquinones from bark and leaves (*Curr Sci*, 1977, **46**, 814).

Heartwood, stilbene deriv. (*Indian J Appl Chem*, 1968, **31**, 239). Leaves, dioxaphenalene deriv., barakol (*J Chem Soc C*, 1970, 1686). Plant, isoquinolone deriv., siamin (*Tetrahedron Lett*, 1976, 821). Leaves, cassiachromone and other compds. (*Planta Med*, 1978, **33**, 258); flavons. and β-sitosterol (*Curr Sci*, 1978, **47**, 621).

Flowers, chromone (*Tetrahedron*, 1971, **27**, 981); β-sorbitol and lupeol (*Indian J Pharm*, 1978, **40**, 15). Constituents of flowers and leaves (*Arch Pharm Wein*, 1978, **311**, 569; *CA*, 1979, **90**, 83580w).

Polysaccharides of mucilage isolated from endosperms (*Sci Cult*, 1977, **43**, 316). Isolation procedure of Na salt of a natural 2-Me-chromone from pods (Indian Pat., 1976, 140032; *CA*, 1980, **92**, 107613d). Seed, new anthraquinone (*Proc Indian Sci Congr*, 1980, Pt.III,91); flavons. (*ibid*, 1981, Pt. III, 99).

C. sophera Linn.

EtOH(50%) ext. of plant, spasmol. (*Indian J Exp Biol*, 1968, **6**, 232). In Samoa, bark said to cause dermatitis, used for skin diseases. Leaves in coughs (*Econ Bot*, 1974, **28**, 17).

Flowers, anthraquinone and flavonol glycd. (*Planta Med*, 1975, **28**, 182). Leaves, new flavonol-8-C-glycd. (*Indian J Chem*, 1981, **20B**, 437).

*C. surrattensis Burm. f. var. **suffruticosa** Chatterjee

EtOH(50%) ext. of aerial parts, CNS depress. and diur. (*Indian J Exp Biol*, 1977, **15**, 208).

Kheri, U.P.

C. tora Linn.

Leaves—pounded and applied on cuts, act like tincture of iodine; applied against eczema. Tender, taken internally to prevent skin diseases; infusion, vermicidal (*Econ Bot*, 1965, **19**, 241; 1978, **32**, 278). Curative effect in ringworm in cattle, clin. study (*Indian J Vet Sci Anim Husb*, 1968, **38**, 160); ext., used in laxt.-hypnotic drug compn. (Ger. Offen, 1972, 2128447; *CA*, 1973, **78**, 62189n). Toxicity of ext. in mice (*Indian Drugs*, 1977-78, **15**, 49).

Plant—EtOH(50%) ext., antivir; spasmol. and diur. (*Indian J Exp Biol*, 1968, **6**, 232; *ibid*, 1969, **7**, 250); used against epilepsy, scabies and sores (*Econ Bot*, 1970, **24**, 241). Alc. ext., active *in vivo* against P388 lymphocytic leukemia in mice; isolation of several compds. (*Rev Latinoam Quim*, 1973, **4**, 8; *CA*, 1979, 123630u).

Seeds—EtOH ext., spasmol. (*Indian J Exp Biol*, 1974, **12**, 512). Boiled with tea taken for cold (*Econ Bot*, 1971, **25**, 418); seeds, antibact. [*J Res Indian Med*, 1974, **9**(2), 65]. Powd. given in abnormal delivery (*Bull Med Ethno Bot Res*, 1980, **1**, 8). Seeds with turmeric and brassica oil used against eczema (*J Econ Tax Bot*, 1981, **2**, 193). Water sol. senna ext. for constip. (Fr. M., 1969, 6611; *CA*, 1971, **74**, 45601r).

Powd. seeds, and active constituent chrysophanic acid, useful in ringworm (*Agric Res Delhi*, 1965, **5**, 208); content of rhein-like aglycones in seeds (*Indian J Pharm*, 1967, **29**, 342); anthraquinones; also anthraquinone glucds., glucoobtusifolin and glucoaurantioobtusin (*Shoyakugaku Zasshi*, 1979, **33**, 72; 1963, **17**, 43; *CA*, 1965, **62**, 5326e); glucd. cassiaside and other known anthraquinones (*Yakugaku Zasshi*, 1966, **86**, 1087; *BA*, 1967, **48**, 46188); components (*Pharm Zentralhalle*, 1968, **107**, 571; *CA*, **69**, 109773e); rubrofusarin glycd. (*Chem Pharm Bull*, 1969, **17**, 458; *CA*, **71**, 13323y); yellow pigment, torachrysone (*ibid*, 1969, **17**, 454; *Int Pharm Abstr*, **6**, 2786); polysaccharide str. (*J Agric Food Chem*, 1973, **21**, 222); 2 antifung. compds., isolation procedure (Indian Pat, 13552¹; *Indian Sci Abstr*, 1974, **10**, 4094); chrysophanol- β-gentiobioside (*Indian J Chem*, 1974, **12**, 1251); chrysophanic acid-9-anthrone, antifung. (*Lloydia*, 1975, **38**, 218; *Sci Cult*, 1974, **40**, 316). Seed oil, chrysophanic acid (*Gujarat Agric Univ Res J*, 1978, **4**, 60). Seed, torosachrysone, questin & its analog; questin analog, antibact. (*Nihon Daigaku Yakugaku Kenkyu Hohoku*, 1980, **19**, 30; *CA*, 1981, **94**, 20287t); naphthalenic lactones, isotoralactone and cassialactone, str., (*Phytochemistry*, 1981, **20**, 1951).

Sennosides—recovery of sennoside-rich concentrates from pods (Ger., 1970, 1617667; *CA*, **73**, 117395f). Estn. in leaves, pods, etc. (*Planta Med*, 1972, **21**, 304). Preparation of concentrates (Hung.

Teljes, 1973, 6006; *CA*, **79**, 83457j). Production for drug (*Herba Hung*, 1973, **12**, 129; *CA*, 1975, **83**, 65368j); extn. from leaves (Jpn Kokai, 1973, 7441524; *CA*, 1974, **81**, 82370e). Quant. anal. of leaves and fruits (*Planta Med*, 1974, **25**, 342); content of various Indian spp. (*Curr Sci*, 1975, **44**, 67). Extn. (Jpn Kokai, 1974, 74118820; *CA*, 1975, **82**, 103135v). Solid concentrates of sennoside A & B (Hung. Teljis, 1975, 9961; *CA*, **83**, 183390h).

Leaves and stems contain *d*-mannitol, myricyl alc. and β-sitosterol (*Curr Sci*, 1965, **34**, 481). Roots, anthraquinones and β-sitosterol (*Planta Med*, 1972, **21**, 393).

CASSINE (*Celastraceae*)

C. glauca (Rottb.) Kuntze syn. *Elaeodendron glaucum* Pers.

Trunk bark, triterp. canophyllal (*Indian J Chem*, 1967, **5**, 523); 6 known and 2 new nortriterps., elaeodendrol and elaeodendradiol (*Phytochemistry*, 1980, **19**, 1163); octacosanol, dulcitol, friedelin, betulonic acid, 23-OH betulin, β-sitosterol & its glucd. (*J Indian Chem Soc*, 1980, **57**, 1042). Bark, cardiac glycd., elaeodendradiol B (*Indian J Chem*, 1980, **19B**, 944).

Seeds, cytotoxic cardiac glycd., elaeodendroside A (*J Chem Soc Chem Commun*, 1977, 255); elaeodendrogenin, elaeodendroside B & C; elaeodendroside, D, E, H, I & J (*Heterocycles*, 1979, **12**, 1445; 1981, **15**, 355; *CA*, 1980, **92**, 164168m; **94**, 157182z).

Leaves, luperol and β-sitosterol; heartwood, β-sitosterol (*Indian J Chem*, 1979, **18B**, 292).

CASSYTHA (*Cassythaceae*)

C. filiformis Linn.

Plant used in dropsy and anasarca; also in conjestion (*Econ Bot*, 1970, **24**, 241; *ibid*, 1971, **25**, 245). In Exumas and Long Islands, plant used in rheum., waist pain and as aphrodis. (*ibid*, 1975, **29**, 316). Pharmacognosy (*Bull Med Ethno Bot Res*, 1980, **1**, 478).

Stem alk., cassyfiline (*Yakugaku Zasshi*, 1965, **85**, 827; *CA*, **63**, 18187e). Plant, alks., cassythine, cassythidine and its -OMe deriv. (*Aust J Chem*, 1966, **19**, 297); nantenine (*Indian J Chem*, 1973, **11**, 342).

CASTANEA (*Fagaceae*)

C. sativa Mill. syn. *C. vulgaris* Lamk
Eng.–*Spanish chestnut.*

EtOH(50%) ext. of stem bark, antivir. and spasmol. (*Indian J Exp Biol*, 1968, **6**, 232).

Nuts—crushed with vinegar and barley flour used against indurations of breast (*Lloydia*, 1969, **32**, 176). Ext. may be used as platelet inhibitors in thrombosis and aetherosclerosis [*Bibl Haematol Basel*, 1971, **38**(Pt.2), 221]. Tobacco aroma and flavour enhancement by arom. substance (US Pat., 1972, 3651815; *CA*, **77**, 149833w).

Leaves as tobacco substitute (Brit. Pat., 1973, 1315086; US Pat., 1975, 3854485; *CA*, **79**, 63641m; **83**, 40392z).

Leaves, inhibitors of pectinolytic enzymes (*Przem Spozyw*, 1966, **20**, 743; *CA*, 1969, **71**, 10311g); ursolic acid, lupeol, beutlin, waxes and fatty acids (*Phytochemistry*, 1972, **11**, 2733); paraffins and triterps. (*Yakugaku Zasshi*, 1978, **98**, 349; *CA*, **88**, 166742k); flavons., 3-O-*p*- coumarylquinic acid and β-sitosterol glucd. (*Pharmazie*, 1980, **35**, 647); flavons. (*Liebigs Ann Chem*, 1981, 761; *CA*, **95**, 58092j).

Wood, vanillin, quercetin and a triterp. acid (*Cuoio Pelli Mater Concianti*, 1961, **36**, 398; *CA*, 1962, **56**, 3817b). Galls, 5 phenolic glycds. (*Agric Biol Chem*, 1978, **42**, 1213).

CASTANOPSIS (*Fagaceae*)

*C. indica (Roxb.) DC.

B.–*Dalne-katus*; Eng.–*Indian chestnut*; Meghalaya–*Chakko.*

EtOH(50%) ext. of stem bark, antivir., CNS depress., hypoten., spasmol., diur. and anticancer (*Indian J Exp Biol*, 1974,

12, 512). In Meghalaya, paste of leaves applied to forehead to cure headache (*Bull Bot Surv India*, 1980, **22**, 161).

Plant, triterps., castanopsone and castanopsol; castanopsin (*Phytochemistry*, 1977, **16**, 1787; 1978, **17**, 575).

Meghalaya.

*C. tribuloides DC.

B.–*Mushre katus.*

EtOH(50%) ext. of aerial parts, CNS depress. (*Indian J Exp Biol*, 1973, **11**, 43).

W. Bengal.

CASTANOSPERMUM (*Fabaceae*)

C. australe A. Cunn. & Fraser

Bark, bayogenin and triterp. sapogenin castanogenol (*Indian J Chem*, 1969, **7**, 1203).

Wood, castanogenin and bayogenin; also bavin; minor sapogenins and koparin (*Aust J Chem*, 1963, **16**, 900; 1966, **19**, 1717; 1973, **21**, 629; 1977, **30**, 1827).

Seeds, alk. castanospermine (*Phytochemistry*, 1981, **20**, 811).

CASTILLA (*Moraceae*)

*C. elastica Cerv.

Bark, bitter; its decoct. good for dysen. (Standley, I, 214).

Seeds, cardiac glycds., cymarin, periplocymarin or cymarol (Brit. Pat., 1964, 972917; *CA*, 1965, **62**, 5149c).

Cultivated in Karnataka and in W. Bengal.

CASUARINA (*Casuarinaceae*)

C. equisetifolia J.R. & G. Forst.

Leaves—ext. in acetic acid(1%) and sodium bicarbonate(50%), anticancer (*Philipp J Sci*, 1967, **96**, 393).

Bark—in Tonga, infusion, in nervous disorder, coughs, ulcers, stomachache and constip. Philippinians use decoct. as emmen. and infusion of branch as diur. (*Econ Bot*, 1971, **35**, 437).

Leaves, kaempferol and isoquercitrin (*J Indian Chem Soc*, 1970, **47**, 179); also glycds. of kaempferol and quercetin (*Z Naturforsch*, 1977, **32C**, 444).

Bark, polyols, alicyclic and amino acids; also polyphenols (*Leath Sci Madras*, 1978, **25**, 369; 1979, **26**, 196).

CATABROSA (*Poaceae*)

*C. aquatica (Linn.) Beauv. syn. *C. sikkimensis* Stapf

Eng.–*Box grass.*

Grass, hydrocyanic and cyanogenetic glycd. (Chopra *et al*, 1958, 593).

Ladakh.

CATAMBIUM (*Zingiberaceae*)

C. speciosum Holttum syn. *Alpinia nutans* Rosc.; *A. speciosa* K. Schum.

Aq. ext. of plant, spasmog. on guinea pig ileum (*Rev Bras Farm*, 1968, **49**, 67; *CA*, **69**, 95034a). Ext. of herb showed antiulcer activity, tested in adrenalectomized rats with stress-induced ulcers (*Taiwan I Hsueh Hui Tsa Chih*, 1972, **71**, 256; *CA*, **77**, 96972g).

Rhizomes yield dihydro-5, 6- & 5, 6-dehydrokawain (*Yakugaku Zasshi*, 1966, **86**, 1184); labdane and disnorlabdane type diterpenes (*Chem Pharm Bull*, 1980, **28**, 3452); a new dihydrochalcone, dihydroflackawin B and 6 known phenolic compds. (*Phytochemistry*, 1981, **20**, 2503).

Seeds yield cardamonin and alpinetin (*ibid*, 1973, **12**, 238).

CATENARIA (*Fabaceae*)

*C. caudata Schindl. syn. *C. laburnifolia* Benth.; *Desmodium caudatum* DC.

Ass.–*Biyonihaputa*; B.–*Bhuter-chira*; Miri– *Tangamasing.*

Shrub used as a drug known as 'Moh-Ts'ao, in China. It is toxic and insectic. Root ext., for treatment of eye ailments; stem and leaf exts. prevent haemor.; used to cure sarcoma and to relieve stomachache (*J Chin Chem Soc*, 1965, **12**, 61).

Roots crude alks. (0.12%) including N,N-di-Me-tryptamine, bufotenine & its N-oxide. Stems and roots, flavone desmodol, and leaves, swertisin; also alks. (*Chem Pharm Bull*, 1968, **16**, 1842; 1978, **26**, 2411).

Found in tropical Himalayas from Kumaun to Bhutan, Assam and Arunachal Pradesh (Mishmi hills) up to 1,200 m.

CATHA (*Celastraceae*)

C. edulis Forsk.

Eng.–*Kat, kath.*

Aq. ext. of leaves, sympathomimetic in dogs (*C R Acad Sci*, 1965, **260**, 1020). Kat(h), rev., med. properties and constituents of drug (*Acta Phytother*, 1963, **10**, 161). Physiological properties and chem. constituents (*Lloydia*, 1966, **29**, 275). Kat, rev., 59 refs. covering chem., and pharmacol. (*Can J Pharm Sci*, 1974, **9**, 64; *CA*, **81**, 148435p). Identn. of kat (*Medd Nor Farm Selsk*, 1978, **40**, 1; *CA*, **89**, 54186w).

Leaves, kaempferol, quercetin, myricetin and dulcitol (*Planta Med*, 1966, **14**, 76); of Egyptian plant, alks. cathine, cathinine and ephidrine; total alks. in leaves 20-28% > in stems; content in young leaves 24% > mature ones (*J Pharm Sci UAR*, 1968, **9**, 147; 159; *CA*, 1970, **73**, 117169 k-70 l); leaves and young shoots, norpseudoephedrine (*Planta Med*, 1973, **24**, 61); str. of cathidine (*Tetrahedron*, 1974, **30**, 2577); cathine, cathidine A, B, C & D (*ibid*, 1975, **31**, 2727); 6 alks.; str. of cathedulin-3, -4, -5 & -6; str. of cathedulin alks. from Kenyan and Ethopian plants (*J Chem Soc Chem Commun*, 1976, 463, 465; 1978, 107); str. of alks. cathedulins; K_1, K_2, K_6 &' K_{16}; also of E_{3-6} and K_{12}; E_2 & E_8 (*J Chem Soc Perkin Trans I*, 1979, 2976, 2982; 2972). Leaves contain norephedrine, 1-Ph- 1,2-propanedione, 1-cinnamoyl-Et-amine and a dimer of cathinone (*Planta Med*, 1979, **36**, 264). Rev. on chem., pharmacognosy, pharmacol. and alks. of kat [*Bull Narc*, 1980, **32**(3), 5; 37; 51; 65; 67; 843]. Leaves, ampelopsin and its rhamnoside (*Phytochemistry*, 1981, **20**, 1759).

Cathinone—plant contains CNS-active Ph-Pr-amines viz., cathinone, (+)-nor- ψ-and norephedrines (*Experientia*, 1979, **35**, 572). Cathinone from leaves major CNS-active compd.; alk. showed amphetamine-like properties (*Life Sci*, 1980, **27**, 2143; *Eur J Pharmacol*, 1980, **68**, 213). Chem. of kat, (–)- α-aminopropiophenone (cathinone), its CNS-stimulating action [*Bull Narc*, 1980, **32**(3), 5]; psychopharmacol. in CNS (*Planta Med*, 1980, **39**, 194; 244). Effect in lipolysis (*Pharmacol Res Commun*, 1980, **12**, 855); cardiovascular effects of *l*-form in dog (*J Pharm Pharmacol*, 1981, **34**, 338).

CATHARANTHUS (*Apocynaceae*)

Catharanthus alks., bot., chem., pharmacol. and clin. (*in* Taylor & Farnsworth, 1-323).

C. pusillus (Murr.) G. Don syn. *Lochnera pusilla* K. Schum.; *Vinca pusilla* Murr.

Plant, oncolytic, contains 0.49% crude alks., ajmalicine and vindorosine isolated; vindoline detected; alk. fractions, hypoten. (*Lloydia*, 1965, **28**, 354; 259). Leaves, crude alks. (0.6%) including lochnerinine, active against Eagle's 9 KB carcinoma (*J Pharm Sci*, 1968, **57**, 2167); ursolic acid, and leurosine with high degree of activity against P-1534 leukemia in mice and cytotoxic effect against Eagle's 9 KB carcinoma (*Lloydia*, 1970, **33**, 261). Whole plant, a new base-A and rauwolscine besides known alks.; leaves, a monoterp. pyridine base, vinoterpine and roots, alk. lochnericine (*Indian J Chem*, 1973, **11**, 7; 1979, **17B**, 175). Chem. (*in* Taylor & Farnsworth, 108-10). Roots and leaves, vincapusine, a minor alk.; also lochnericine, vindorosine and venoterpine (*Phytochemistry*, 1981, **20**, 865).

Whole plant, N-benzoyl-*l*-Ph-alaninol (*Tetrahedron Lett*, 1965, 3529). Usual triterps. and stigmast-4-en-3-one, stigmast-4,22-dien-3-one, β-sitosterol, etc. (*Indian J Chem*, 1980, **19B**, 331).

C. roseus (Linn.) G. Don syn. *Lochnera rosea* Reichb.; *Vinca rosea* Hook.f.; non Murr.

Eng.–*Madagascan periwinkle, red periwinkle, old maid.*

Plant shot into prominence for its anticancer activity (*Planta Med*, 1979, **36**, 150). Three distinct vars.; var. *rosea* (pink-flowered), var. *alba* (white-flowered) and var. *oceallatus* (white with a pink or yellow ring in orifice region); commercial roots a free admixt. from said vars. (*Curr Sci*, 1979, **48**, 80). Commercial cultivation in Tamil Nadu, Karnataka and West Bengal [*Indian Farming NS*, 1977- 78, **27**(4), 11; 1981-82, **31**(6), 18].

Some of the several review on anticancer drugs or alks. (*Sci Ind Karachi*, 1967, **5**, 137; *CA*, 1968, **68**, 93467z; *Curr Topics Plant Sci*, 1969, 303; *CA*, 1972, **76**, 80919p; *Planta Med*, 1972, **22**, 324; *Lloydia*, 1977, **40**, 107; *Indian Drugs*, 1977-78, **15**, 231; *Med Chem Academic*, 1980, **16**, 271; *CA*, 1981, **94**, 76387t; *J Ethnopharmacol*, 1980, **2**, 149).

Monograph on *Catharanthus* alks. (*in* Taylor & Farrsworth, 323); alks. (*in* Manske, VIII, 269-78; XI, 99-108; *in* Rodrigo, XX, 192-239). 61 Alks., status of research, antitumour effect of *Vinca rosea* alks. [*Proc Symp GECA*, 1965 (Pub., 1966) 9-28; *CA*, 1968, **68**, 58398f]. Antivir. activity of 36 alks., pericalline most effective (*J Pharm Sci*, 1968, **57**, 2174). Vincamine, vincarine, vinervine, tombozine, etc., analeptic, sed., hypoten. and emet. (*Aktual Probl Farmakol Farm Vses Nauch Konf*, 1971, 159; *CA*, 1972, **76**, 111f).

Plant alks., vincarodine (*Heterocycles*, 1974, **2**, 73; *CA*, **81**, 2583f); vincoline; new antimitotic dimeric alks., leurocolombine and vinamidine (*J Pharm Sci*, 1974, **63**, 536; 1975, **64**, 1953); leurocolombine, antimitotic agent (US Pat., 1975, 3890325; *CA*, **83**, 183388p); vincathicine (*J Org Chem*, 1976, **41**, 1001); vincubine; its str. (*Rev Cubana Farm*, 1975, **9**, 139; 1976, **10**, 19; *CA*, 1976, **84**, 161765c; 1977, **86**,

167891d); isositsirikine str. (*J Chem Soc Chem Commun*, 1979, 1081).

Synth. of antitumour alks. from *Catharanthus* spp.; also biosynth. (*J Natl Prod*, 1980, **43**, 72; *J Chem Soc Chem Commun*, 1980, 452).

Plant, 2 secoiridoid glucds., secologanic acid and secologanoside (*J Am Chem Soc*, 1971, **93**, 6320); monoterp. glycds. loganin, deoxy- & dehydrologanin, sweroside with iridoid-like str., intermediates in synth. of indole alks. (*Indian J Chem*, 1972, **10**, 454).

Roots, alks. (0.13%) and smaller roots (lateral, 0.08%) (*Indian J Pharm*, 1971, **33**, 126); roots from acclimatized plant in Romania, 0.85% (as against cultivated roots in Vietnam, 0.83%); leaves 0.37% (*Farmacia Buc*, 1965, **13**, 273; *CA*, **63**, 6784h). Fluorim. detn. of VLB., in healthy roots, 0.23; aster yellow virus-infected, 0; and δ-yohimbine, in healthy, 0.55%; in infected, 2.45% (*Stud Cercet Biochim*, 1968, **11**, 153; *CA*, **69**, 65154x).

Rootbark, alks. vincaline I & II (*J Indian Chem Soc*, 1964, **41**, 552). Root, ajmalicine and alstonine (*Pharmazie*, 1965, **20**, 522; *CA*, **63**, 16775e); floral parts, vindoline and leurozine; roots, ajmalizine (*Farmatsiya Moscow*, 1969, **18**, 42; *CA*, 1970, **72**, 136335g). Extn. of alks. (Rom. Pat., 1970, 52178; *CA*, 1971, **74**, 52258x); 5 alks. including new alk. venalstonine (*Rev Cubana Farm*, 1976, **10**, 3; *CA*, 1977, **86**, 185876g); tetrahydro-alstonine (Fr. Demande, 1979, 2397415; *CA*, **91**, 198925a). See vinblastine & vincristine, as also ajmalicine.

Roots, ursolic acid; oleanolic acid (*Rastit Resur*, 1966, **2**, 513; *Bangladesh J Sci Ind Res*, 1979, **14**, 354; *CA*, 1967, **66**, 102493t; 1981, **94**, 2032b); bornesitol (*Phytochemistry*, 1973, **12**, 1177).

Total alks.—antivir. (*J Pharm Sci*, 1968, **57**, 2174); also spermic. in male rats (*Indian J Exp Biol*, 1968, **6**, 256); offer scope for insect/pest control by chem. sterilization of male population (*Curr Sci*, 1981, **50**, 552; 555; *CSIR News*, 1979, **29**, 105;

Indian J Agric Sci, 1978, **48**, 306; 1980, **50**, 781).

Leaves, diur. alks. (*Lloydia*, 1964, **27**, 203); leurosine, vindoline, catharanthine, lochnerine and tetrahydroalstonine, hypoglyc. (*Abh Dtsch Akad Wiss Berlin Kl Chem Geol Biol*, 1966, 465; *CA*, 1967, **67**, 10249k); first 2 alks. and vindolinine, more potent than tolbutamide in rats (*J Ethnopharmacol*, 1980, **2**, 119); dihydrovindolinine and coronaridine, diur. and hypoglyc.; coronaridine, isolation and identn. [*Proc Symp GECA*, 1965 (Pub. 1966), 9-28; *CA*, 1968, **68**, 58398f; *Bull Soc Chim Belg*, 1981, **91**, 83]; vincarodine (*J Org Chem*, 1974, **39**, 431). Catharanthamine; 21-oxo-leurosine; leurosidine-N'b-oxide; pericyclivine and 5 alks. (*J Natl Prod*, 1980, **43**, 157; 1981, **44**, 611; 335); see also vinblastine & vincristine.

Leaves, nonalks., essent. oil (0.01-0.03%) with constants and constituents (*Perfum Essent Oil Rec*, 1965, **56**, 214); leaves and stems, roseoside, a C_{13} glycd., str. (*Phytochemistry*, 1974, **13**, 2541); stem, α- amyrin-OAc (*J Indian Chem Soc*, 1981, **58**, 628).

Flower, alks. (20) and non-alk. constituents (*Diss Pharm Pharmacol*, 1967, **19**, 403; *CA*, **67**, 114334a); hypoglyc. studies of alk. mixt. (*Pak J Sci Res*, 1975, **27**, 101).

Seed alks., vinsedine and vinsedicine but vindoline (major alk. of leaves) not detected (*Lloydia*, 1965, **28**, 259); tabersonine from ripe seed (*Acta Chim Acad Sci Hung*, 1971, **69**, 241); nonalk., loganic acid (1%) in indole-alk. biosynth. (*J Am Chem Soc*, 1970, **92**, 6098).

Tissue culture—antimitotic activities of *C. roseus*, extensive attention to alk. production of substances with desirable therapeutic properties; potential of cell culture for pharmaceutical production (*in* Beal & Reinhard, 448-69; 484-86); alk. production in cell culture (*Phytochemistry*, 1980, **19**, 2583; 2589; *Planta Med*, 1980, **40**, 22; *J Natl Prod*, 1981, **44**, 536; *Heterocycles*, 1981, **16**, 1169; *CA*, **95**, 58166m; *Z Natur-*

forsch, 1981, **36B**, 1153; *Helv Chim Acta*, 1981, **64**, 1837); (–)-tabersonine (*Physiol Veg*, 1980, **18**, 771; *CA*, 1981, **94**, 117838m).

Vinblastine & vincristine—also known as vinleukoblastine or VLB & (vin)leurocristine or VCR; 2 clinically most important bisindole alks. (2 monomeric units, velbanamine and vindoline). VLB & VCR confirmation of strs. (*J Am Chem Soc*, 1965, **87**, 4963); absolute configurations of stereo centres (*Acta Crystallogr*, 1966, **21**, 322); they differ only in substituents on nitrogen of vindoline unit; N-Me in VLB; and N-CHO in VCR; slight str. difference but markedly different therapeutic profile.

VLB, in treatment of Hodgkin's disease; in testicular cancer, breast cancer, bladder cancer and non-small cell lung cancer. VCR, most useful and highly active agent but with neurotoxicity as side effect; rarely used alone; used as a critical component of all major combinations in treatment of childhood leukemia, Wilm's tumour, embryonal rhabdomyosarcoma, non-Hodgkin's lymphomas; melanoma, small cell lung cancer (*in* Wagner & Wolff, 124-25; 73). Usefulness of VLB & VCR sulphates in malignant tumours, clin. study (*Oncology*, 1967, **21**, 214); alks. as anticancer drugs with biol. activity (*J Sci Ind Res*, 1973, **32**, 382); chemotherapy of cancer, rev.; also for VLB production [*J Ethnopharmacol*, 1980, **2**, 149; *Med Chem Academic*, 1980, **16**, 271; *CA*, 1981, **94**, 76387t; *East Pharm*, 1980, **23**(272), 71; 128]. Mech. of action in tumour, of VCR, VLB and vindesine, rev., 36 refs. (*Bordeaux Med*, 1980, **13**, 607; *CA*, **93**, 88307j).

VCR, as also VLB in nonmalignant diseases as well as thrombotic thrombocytopenic purpura and drug-induced microangiopathic haemolytic anaemia (*N Engl J Med*, 1974, **291**, 376; *Blood*, 1981, **57**, 431).

VCR active *in vivo* against a virus infection; VLB completely inactive (*Ann NY Acad Sci*, 1965-66, **130**, 52).

Therapeutic history, uses, etc., rev. (*Q J Crude Drug Res*, 1965, **5**, 701). Both effective against a variety of human neoplasms (*Abh Dtsch Akad Wiss Berlin Kl Chem Geol Biol*, 1966, 465; *CA*, 1967, **67**, 10249k). Pharmacol. studies; effect of VLB on intestinal lactase and sucrase of rats [*J Shivaji Univ*, 1971, **4**(8), 121; 129; 1972, **5**(10), 5; *Indian J Med Res*, 1980, **72**, 97]. VLB & VCR; root and leaf total alks., sterilant against *Dysdercus cingulatus*, the red cotton bug (*Sci Cult*, 1981, **47**, 395; *Curr Sci*, 1981, **50**, 555).

VCR, a suspected teratogen; VLB, a suspected carcinogen (*in* Plant and Fungal Toxins, 165-66; 262).

Assay of VLB; bioassay of antimitotic alks. (*Lloydia*, 1968, **31**, 202; *Planta Med*, 1979, **36**, 87).

Purification of alks. from crude ext. by gradient *p*H extn. technique using preparative-TLC and of VLB by HPLC (*Indian J Pharm Sci*, 1979, **41**, 207); isolation of VLB sulphate by defatting leaves; solvent extn., fractionation and crystallization, NCL, Pune method (*Sci Cult*, 1980, **46**, 251).

Naturally occurring cogeners of VLB are: de-Ac [*J Pharm Sci*, 1964, **53**, 1227; *Proc Symp GECA*, 1965, (Pub. 1966), 9-28; *CA*, 1968, **68**, 58398f]; 4-deoxy (*Tetrahedron Lett*, 1968, 783); de-OAc (*Experientia*, 1975, **31**, 18); anhydro (*J Am Chem Soc*, 1976, **98**, 7017; 1978, **100**, 6253; *J Chem Soc Chem Commun*, 1975, 670; 1979, 582); synth. of congeners (*Lloydia*, 1977, **40**, 107); HPLC for sepn. and detn. of VLB and its congeners, also detection (*J Chromatogr*, 1977, **139**, 203); anhydro - 16 - decarboMeO-16-CONHMe (*Can J Chem*, 1978, **56**, 2560). Str.-activity relationship of dimeric (rather bisindole) alks., de-Ac-VLB amide (vindesine) sulphate; of N-substituted (*J Med Chem*, 1978, **21**, 88; 1979, **22**, 391).

Isolation and sepn. of VLB from VCR; VCR yield can be increased by formylating alk. mixt. before sepn. and purification (Ger. Pat., 1974, 2259388; 1975, 2442245; Br. Pat., 1975, 1382460; Neth. Pat., 1974, 7217069; Fr. Pat., 1974, 2210392; *CA*, 1974, **81**, 82369m; **83**, 120821d; 79459b; 84848g; **82**, 116076b).

VCR of greater clin. importance than VLB, but present in very small amt. (0.0003% yield, the lowest level of any med. useful alk. produced on commercial basis); important to convert VLB to VCR; intensive research; also on preparation of dimeric alks. from monomeric units (*in* Wagner & Wolff, 125-26; Markets Selected Med. Plants, 89). Exts. contain N-de-Me-VLB and formylating alk. mixt. before sepn. and purification, increases VCR yield. Microbial method of N-demethylation of VLB by *Streptomyces albogriseolus*, followed by N-formylation (*Helv Chim Acta*, 1974, **57**, 1886; Ger. Offen., 1975, 2440931; *CA*, **83**, 7184k); Chem. methods of utilizing Pd/C and formic acid in oxygen atmosphere (Belg. Pat., 1975, 823560; *CA*, 1976, **84**, 59835p); a low temp. (–70°) chromic acid oxidation followed by formylation (Fr. Demande, 1974, 2210393; US Pat., 1975, 3899493; *CA*, 1975, **82**, 73294b; **83**, 179360f); chromic acid, not satisfactory with anhydro-VLB & its deriv., oxidation of N-formyl compds. in better yield by Jones' reagent in large excess at –78° (*Can J Chem*, 1978, **56**, 2560). VCR, large scale isolation (Belg. Pat., 1978, 867670; *CA*, 1979, **90**, 61230e).

See also latest rev. on antitumour bisindole alks. from *C. roseus* (*in* Brossi & Suffness, XXXVII, 1- 250).

Ajmalicine—also known as raubasine, extracted from root (*Pharmazie*, 1965, **20**, 522; *CA*, **63**, 16775e). Used as vasodilator and hypoten. agent. Serpentine also obtained from root and converted into ajmalicine by catalytic hydrogenation or reduction; may also be obtained from *Rauwolfia* (Markets Selected Med. Plants,

8; 89). Raubasine reduces cerebral blood flow (in Beal & Reinhard, 259); chromatogr. sepn. of 4 alks. raubasine, serpentine, alstonine & tetrahydroalstonine [Fitoterapia, 1966, **37**(4), 98; CA, 1968, **69**, 65104f]. Extn. (Pol. Pat., 1975, 74439; CA, 1976, **84**, 28213e); estn. (Indian J Pharm, 1977, **39**, 62); recovery (Res Ind, 1978, **23**, 1166); isolation (S. African Pat., 1979, 7802537; CA, **91**, 163048q); from roots (Fr. Demande, 1980, 2442338; CA, 1981, **94**, 71476m). Plant tissue culture; potential of plant cell cultures for pharmaceutical production (in Beal & Reinhard, 447-49; 484-86).

Leurosine—alk. useful in exp. study of origin and mech. of cancer; extn. from leaf alks. of Polish plant; extn. (US Pat., 1968, 3370057; S. African Pat., 1979, 7802537; CA, **68**, 81400j; **91**, 163048q); antileukemic and cytotoxic (Lloydia, 1970, **33**, 261); hypoglyc. (Abh Dtsch Akad Wiss Berlin Kl Chem Geol Biol, 1966, 465; CA, 1967, **67**, 10249k).

Str. (J Pharm Sci, 1969, **58**, 694). Production (Acta Pharm Hung, 1964, **34**, 36; CA, **61**, 2906a); isolation from aerial parts (Hung. Pat., 1966, 153200; 1968, 154715; Hung. Teljes, 1972, 3317; CA, 1967, **66**, 118854x; **69**, 38732c; **76**, 131476b); extn. (Rev Cubana Farm, 1975, **9**, 183; CA, 1976, **85**, 25307y); sepn. of leurosine and VLB from alk. mixt. (Ger. Offen, 1977, 2648284; CA, **87**, 90720h); of leurosine, VLB and coronaridine; also 17-de-OAc. deriv. of leurosine (Bull Soc Chim Belg, 1981, **90**, 185; 1982, **91**, 75).

CAUTLEYA (Zingiberaceae)

*C. spicata Baker

H.–Jangli adua.

EtOH(50%) ext. of rhizomes and roots, antivir., spasmol. and hypoten. (Indian J Exp Biol, 1968, **6**, 232).

Darjeeling, W.Bengal

CAYRATIA (Vitaceae)

C. carnosa (wall.) Gagnep. syn. Vitis carnosa Wall.

B.–Chota-goale.

EtOH(50%) ext. of aerial parts, CNS depress. (Indian J Exp Biol, 1971, **9**, 91). Roots given in anaemic conditions (Bull Med Ethno Bot Res, 1980, **1**, 8).

*C. trifolia (Linn.) Domin

Seeds and roots used for treatment of yoke sores of bullocks (J Econ Tax Bot, 1980, **1**, 140).

Eastern Rajasthan.

CEDRELA (Meliaceae)

See TOONA

CEDRUS (Pinaceae)

C. deodara (Roxb.) G. Don syn. C. libani A. Rich. var. deodara Hook. f.; Pinus deodara Roxb.

Eng.–Cedarwood.

Aq. ext. of bark, exceptionally effective in reducing sugar content of diabetic patient's urine and blood to normal levels (Can. Pat., 1967, 767079; CA, 1968, **68**, 16149v). EtOH(50%) ext. of stem, spasmol. and anticancer (Indian J Exp Biol, 1968, **6**, 232).

Essent. oil—from wood, called 'deodara oil' or 'cedarwood oil' 20% soln. of processed deodara oil in castor oil, on external application, very effective against sarcoptic mange in buffalo-calves; also in sheep (Indian J Vet Sci, 1968, **38**, 203; 1976, **53**, 543). Effective insect repellant (Khadi Gramodyog, 1972-73, **19**, 269); in vitro antibact. efficacy against nine pathogenic Gram +ve and Gram –ve microorganisms (Parfuem Kosmet, 1980, **61**, 219); fungitoxicity [Indian Perfum, 1981, **25** (3 & 4), 1]; vascular permeability-increasing action (Indian Vet J, 1978, **55**, 963); some toxicol. effect (Annu Conf Indian Pharmacol Soc, 1980, abstr. 15); clin. study of toxicol. (Clin Toxicol, 1981, **18**, 1485).

Essent. oil, constituents and characteristics, rev. (*Perfum Essent Oil Rec*, 1967, **58**, 622). Oleoresin sesquiterp. hydrocarbons (*Izv Sib Otd Akad Nauk SSSR Ser Khim Nauk*, 1968, 114; *CA*, **69**, 84075p); chem. characteristics, of essent. oil from kumaun plant (*Indian Perfum*, 1978, **22**, 16); of Indian cedar wood oil used in skin diseases (*Parfuem Kosmet*, 1979, **60**, 247). Extn. (*Indian J Technol*, 1980, **18**, 42).

Alc. portion of essent. oil, longiborneol and sesquiterp. alcs., himachalol and allohimachalol; and its stereochem.; deodarone (*Tetrahedron Lett*, 1964, 3761; 1980, **21**, 325; 1973, 427); strs. of himachalenes; himachalol; and allohimachalol (*Tetrahedron*, 1968, **24**, 3809; 3861; 3869). Hexane ext. of wood, allohimachalol and sesquiterps. himadarol, centdarol & isocentdarol; allohimachalol most active *in vitro* spasmol. while centdarol most active *in vivo* (*Indian J Exp Biol*, 1975, **13**, 369). Himachalol and centdarol major antisp. constituents of wood, similar to papaverine; such activity not noted for sesquiterps. earlier (*J Pharm Sci*, 1975, **64**, 258; *in* Wagner & Wolff, 217). Strs. of centdarol; isocentdarol (*Phytochemistry*, 1975, **14**, 2237; 1976, **15**, 557).

Stem bark, dihydroflavonol, deodarin; taxifolin and other flavons. (*Tetrahedron*, 1965, **21**, 3727; *Curr Sci*, 1971, **40**, 464); β-sitosterol in unsap. matter (*Indian Oil Soap J*, 1970-71, **36**, 311).

Alc. ext. of flakes, nonvolat. dewardiol and dewarenol (*Pak J Sci Ind Res*, 1964, **7**, 86). Diterp. of cones (*Phytochemistry*, 1971, **10**, 2818). Flavons. of needles (*Z Naturforsch*, 1980, **35C**, 342).

Triterp. as insect attractant (*C R Acad Sci Ser D*, 1978, **287**, 285). Constituents of essent. oil from leaves and twigs [*Kinki Daigaku Rikogakubu Kenkyu Hokoku*, 1980, (51), 61; *CA*, **93**, 91890z].

Wood, novel dihydroflavons., cedeodarin, dihydromyricetin, cedrin and cedrinoside; neolignan, cedrusin and other phenolic constituents; himasecolone and isopimaric acid (*Phytochemistry*, 1980, **19**, 893; 1260; 1981, **20**, 1319). Phenolic constituents of alc. ext. (*Indian J Pharm Sci*, 1979, **41**, 251). [13]NMR of dihydroflavonols (*Planta Med*, 1981, **43**, 82).

CEIBA (*Bombacaceae*)

C. pentandra (Linn.) Gaertn. syn. *Eriodendron anfractuosum* DC.

EtOH(50%) ext. of aerial parts, CNS depress. and diur. (*Indian J Exp Biol*, 1974, **12**, 512). Natives of Egypt use root in diabetes [*Hamdard*, 1982, **25** (1-4), 37].

Plant, linarin (acacetin 7-rutinoside) (*C R Acad Sci Ser D*, 1966, **262**, 1368); w.-sol. antigen (Brit. Amended, 1969, 978262; *CA*, 1971, **75**, 132986j).

CELASTRUS (*Celastraceae*)

*C. monosperma Roxb.

Ass.–*Bhumlati*.

EtOH(50%) ext. of aerial parts, CNS depress. and hypoten. (*Indian J Exp Biol*, 1973, **11**, 43).

Sibsagar, Assam.

C. paniculatus Willd.

Leaves and roots used as poultice to cure headache (*Econ Bot*, 1965, **19**, 240). Various plant parts used in sore throat, anaemia, colic, syphilis and carbuncle (*ibid*, 1970, **24**, 241); EtOH(50%) ext. of aerial parts, antivir. (*Indian J Exp Biol*, 1969, **7**, 250). Leaves, emmen. (*Q J Crude Drug Res*, 1970, **12**, 1922); bark decoct. in bronch. (*Bull Med Ethno Bot Res*, 1980, **1**, 8). Plant, minor constituent of indigenous drug 'Geriforte' (*Rajasthan Med J*, 1980, **19**, 23; *Indian Drugs*, 1980-81, **18**, 346).

Seed oil—crude malkanguni oil, sed. and tranquillizing in rats (*Arch Int Pharmacodyn*, 1963, **144**, 34; *CA*, 1963, **59**, 15813a); drug combination containing *C. paniculata* as chief ingredient, useful as depress. especially in hysteria, clin. trial (*Indian J Psychiatry*, 1964, **6**, 142). Resin from seed oil, lowers B.P. of dogs. Oil, vasoconstrictor and spasmol. in rats uterus

(J Sci Res BHU, 1964-65, **15**, 135). Tranquillizing on CNS. In higher doses stim. Alongwith benzoin, clove, nutmeg and mace, it is powerful stim. (*Q J Crude Drug Res*, 1971, **11**, 1742). Relieves body pain and used in cut wounds (*Bull Bot Surv India*, 1978, **18**, 247; *Econ Bot*, 1978, **32**, 281). Oil massage in rheum.; as hair tonic (*Bull Med Ethno Bot Res*, 1980, **1**, 8; 318). In doses of one or two drops internally in pneum. in children; also used externally in scabies (*Nagarjun*, 1980-81, **24**, 1). Seed oil administered to rats improved their learning and memory (*Arogya*, 1981, **7**, 83).

Seeds, polyhydric alc., malkanguniol; 4 related alcs. (*Tetrahedron Lett*, 1973, 845; 1974, 2219). Sesquiterp. ester, malangunin, and alks. celapanine and celapanigine; their strs. and of celapagine (*ibid*, 1974, 213; 2219; *Tetrahedron*, 1975, **31**, 1949). Seeds, triterps. paniculatadiol, malkanguniol, alongwith polyesters, β-amyrin and β-sitosterol; short rev. of biochem. and pharmacol. of plant [*J Oil Technol Assoc India*, 1975, **7**(2), 51; 1977, **9**(1),1].

CELOSIA (*Amaranthaceae*)

C. argentea Linn. var. **cristata** Kuntze syn. *C. cristata* Linn.

EtOH(50%) ext. of plant, antiprot. and spasmol. (*Indian J Exp Biol*, 1969, **7**, 250). Seeds useful in diar. and seminal diseases (*Nagarjun*, 1980-81, **24**, 263).

Sepn. of hyaluronic acid (Jpn Kokai, 1977, 77145594; *CA* 1978, **88**, 126347d).

CELSIA (*Scrophulariaceae*)

See **VERBASCUM**

CELTIS (*Ulmaceae*)

C. caucasica Willd. syn.*C.australis* auct. non Linn.

Bark and heartwood, betulin, di-Me-ellagic acid, gallic acid, quebrachitol and leucocyanidin glycd. (*Indian J Chem*, 1968, **6**, 231).

CENTAUREA (*Asteraceae*)

C. behen Linn.

Roots, taraxasterol, its -OAc & myristic ester (*Phytochemistry*, 1972, **11**, 2267). Aerial parts, lactones including a new deriv. of solistitialin A (*ibid*, 1981, **20**, 2427).

C. calcitrapa Linn.

Leaves contain sesquiterp. lactone cnicin (*Diss Pharm Pharmacol*, 1967, **19**, 223; *CA*, **67**, 41013h); cytostatic activity of cnicin (*Planta Med*, 1978, **33**, 356); also of sesquiterp. lactones, (*Arch Farmacol Toxicol*, 1977, **3**, 241;*CA*, 1978, **89**, 36469m). Cnicin, hypoglyc. and antibiot. against *Brucella abortus, Staphylococcus aureus* and *Pseudomonas aeruginosa* (*Egypt J Pharm Sci*, 1975, **16**, 445; *CA*, 1978, **89**, 160096b). Chem. and pharmacol. of *Centaurea* spp. (*Plant Med Phytother*, 1979, **13**, 41).

C. cyanus Linn.

Antifung. activity of seed ext. [*Environment India*, 1981, **4**(I & II), 83].

Flowers contain *n*-nonacosane, triterp. and steroidal compds. (*Poznan Two Przyj Nauk Wyd Lek Pr Kom Farm*, 1966, **5**, 65; *CA*, 1967, **66**, 112955j); pigments (*Phytochemistry*, 1974, **13**, 1219).

C. moschata Linn.; see **Amberboa moschata**

C. picris Pall.

Ladakh–*Basaka*.

Used as purifier and also in fever and skin diseases (*in* Atal & Kapur, Med. Plants, 519).

CENTELLA (*Apiaceae*)

C. asiatica (Linn.) Urban syn. *Hydrocotyle asiatica* Linn.

Plant—EtOH(50%) ext., antiprot. and spasmol.(*Indian J Exp Biol*, 1968, **6**, 232). Alter and astrin. (*Q J Crude Drug Res*, 1970, **10**, 1555).

In homeopathy, employed in ulceration of womb, eczema, elephantiasis, ascariasis and in granular cervicitis (*Bull Bot Soc Bengal*, 1972, **26**, 29).

Leaves—juice useful in cataract and other eye troubles, also given in fever (*ibid*, 1971, **25**, 419); in diar. among children (*Khadi Gramodyog*, 1972-73, **19**, 271). Leaves, to cure severe headaches (*Nagarjun*, 1979-80, **23**, 217). Psychedelic drug hoaxes, contains 2 saponin glycosides with sed. effect but no psychoactive principles (*in* Beal & Reinhard, 347-48).

Asiatic acid & asiaticoside—alc. ext. containing these 2 triterps., used as cream to improve skin texture; regenerates skin of old people; alc. ext. of herb with other ingredients, useful in pruritis and other skin disorders (Fr. Pat., 1966, 143383; M4209; *CA*, **65**, 1845b; 1967, **67**, 938982t); w.-insol. fraction of herb, two triterps., and madegascaric or madecassic acid (*C R Acad Sci Ser D*, 1967, **264**, 407). Topical application of asiaticoside dissolved in carcinogen(benzene), weak tumour-promoting activity in hairless mice (*Cancer Res*, 1972, **32**, 1463). Herb ext., madecassic acid, asiatic acid & asiaticoside, effective locally on wounds in rats (*Oyo Yakuri*, 1973, **7**, 833;*CA*, 1974, **80**, 66674f; *C R Acad Sci Ser D*, 1978, **286**, 789); isolation (*Diss Pharm Pharmacol*, 1968, **20**, 69; *CA*, **69**, 16790r; *Chung Ts' ao Yao*, 1980, **11**, 244;*CA*, 1981, **94**, 71287a); asiatic acid (*Indian J Chem*, 1967, **5**, 586); str. of heteroside, asiaticoside; treatment of ulceration, wounds and leprosy, attributed to it (*Cienc Cult Sao Paulo*, 1968, **20**, 19; *CA*, 1969, **70**, 830r). Variation in chem. compn. of Indian samples of herb (*Curr Sci*, 1969, **38**, 77); asiatic acid, asiaticoside, etc., from an Indian variety (*Phytochemistry*, 1969, **8**, 917).

Str. of madecassic acid (*Bull Soc Chim Fr*, 1967, 1890); extn. of madecassoside and madecassic acid; both antiinflam. (Brit. Pat., 1968, 1123288; *CA*, **69**, 87240z).

Crude ext. of herb and product derived from it, isothankuniside and BK compd., oral antifert. agents in albino mice (*Indian J Exp Biol*, 1968, **6**, 181); isothankuniside (*Bull Nat Inst Sci India*, 1968, No. 37, 178).

Str. of brahmic acid (*Phytochemistry*, 1968, **7**, 1385). Herb, polyacetylenes (*Arch Pharm Wein*, 1973, **306**, 197; *CA*, **78**, 156633e).

CENTIPEDA (*Asteraceae*)

C. minima (Linn.) A. Br. & Aschers. syn. *C. orbicularis* Lour.; *Myriogyne minuta* Less.

EtOH(50%) ext. of plant, antiprot. and spasmol.; CNS depress. and diur. (*Indian J Exp Biol*, 1969, **7**, 250; 1977, **15**, 208). Plant used in epilepsy and epidydimitis or hydrocele (*Econ Bot*, 1970, **24**, 241).

Plant ext. yields, lupeol, its -OAc, hexacosanol, β- sitosterol and stigmasterol (*J Indian Chem Soc*, 1970, **47**, 96); taraxasterol, its -OAc and palmitate stigmasterol, β-sitosterol, arnidiol and a pentacyclic triterp.diol (*Yakugaku Zasshi*, 1970, **90**, 846; *CA*, **73**, 106344n); diterp. acid, centipedaoic acid and flavons. (*Phytochemistry*, 1979, **18**, 1067).

CENTRATHERUM (*Asteraceae*)

C. anthelminticum (Willd.) Kuntze syn. *Serratula anthelmintica* Roxb.; *Vernonia anthelmintica* Willd.

Seeds—EtOH(50%) ext., antivir.; also spermic. in rats (*Indian J Exp Biol*, 1969, **7**, 250; 1977, **15**, 231). Seeds used in asthma (*Econ Bot*, 1978, **32**, 282). EtOH ext. of achenes exhibited good results in giardiasis patients [*J Sci Res Plants Med*, 1981, 2(3), 47].

Various plant parts used in syphilis, constip., and against cholera (*Econ Bot*, 1970, **24**, 241). Drug, anthelm. against earthworms and tapeworms. Also smooth muscle-relaxant, hypoten. in animals [*J Res Indian Med*, 1979, 14(1), 133]. Plant, insect-repellent and insectic. (*Nagarjun*, 1979-80, **23**, 177). Clin. study on vicarcika eczema (*Ancient Sci Life*, 1981-82, **1**, 221).

Seeds, extn. of (+)-threo-12, 13-di-OH-oleic acid (US Pat., 1964, 3139387; *CA*,

61, 5963f); Δ^7-avenasterol (main) (*Tetrahedron Lett*, 1968, 3779); sterols (*Recl Trav Chim Pays Bas*, 1970, **89,** 186; 1054; *CA*, **72**, 100984d; *CA*, 1971, **74**, 28864m); seed oil, vernosterol (*Tetrahedron Lett*, 1970, 2971). Seeds, a bitter principal as elemanolide lactone (*Phytochemistry*, 1977, **16**, 1838).

Leaves, abscisic acid (*Planta*, 1970, **92**, 282). Essent. oil, antibact. [*Indian Drug Pharmac Ind*, 1979, **14**(2), 29]. Str. of centratherin, germacranolide from leaves and stem (*Phytochemistry*, 1979, **18**, 681).

CEPHAELIS (*Rubiaceae*)

C. ipecacuanha (Brot.) A. Rich. syn.
Psychotria ipecacuanha Stokes
Eng.–*Ipecac.*

Root—concentrate stable up to 4 months under normal temp. (*Farm Pol*, 1968, **24,** 1; *CA*, **69**, 46024p). Ipecac syrup, emetic in cat (*J Am Vet Med Assoc*, 1972, **161,** 1677; *CA*, 1973, **78**, 67078k); origin and uses, rev., 5 refs. (*Econ Bot*, 1973, **27**, 231); combined effects with other drugs in antitussive activity and acute toxicity (*Oyo Yakuri*, 1975, **10,** 407; *CA*, 1978, **88**, 115366h). Toxicol. rev., 94 refs. (*Clin Toxicol*, 1977, **10**, 221; *Toxicol Annu*, 1977, **2**, 221).

Ipecacuanha alks., mass spectra (*Tetrahedron*, 1964, **20**, 399). Str. and synth. of alks., rev., 164 refs. & rev., 181 refs. (*Magy Tud Akad Kem Tud Oszt Kozl*, 1965, **23**, 109; 191; *Recent Dev Chem Natl Carbon Compd*, 1967, **2**, 63; *CA*, 1968, **68**, 98662u).

Alk. content of cultivated ipecac (*Bull Calcutta Sch Trop Med*, 1966, **14**, 91). Roots, chem. evaluations of various infusions and decoct. according to Polish pharmacopoeia (*Acta Pol Pharm*, 1966, **23**, 531; *CA*, 1967, **66**, 108189v).

Estn. of nonphenolic and total alks. in Dover's powd. and its pharm. preparation (*Labdev*, 1969, **7B**, 207). Rev., 45 refs. (*Chem Alkaloids*, 1970, 31; *CA*, 1971, **74**, 64327x); rev., 97 refs. (*Alkaloids*, 1971, **13**, 189; *CA*, 1972, **76**, 59810m). Estn. of

alk. by TLC and spectrophotom. (*Planta Med*, 1975, **27**, 294). Assay of ipecac and its compn.; colorim. and spectrophotom. detn. of total nonphenolic alks. and compn. (*J Assoc Off Anal Chem*, 1971, **54**, 614; 609; 1979, **62**, 1113).

Emetine & cephaeline—both have 2 tetrahydroisoquinoline nuclei; while emetine has four OMe groups, cephaelin has three OMe and one phenolic OH group; both alks. emetic from irritating effect on stomach; of the two, cephaeline more toxic. In smaller doses, both expect. (Sim, 66-68); emetine, standard antiamoebic principal in pharmacol. It is anticancer but without any clin. efficacy; 2, 3-dihydroemetine may be more promising (*in* Wagner & Wolff, 5, 63); detn., colorim., in roots and pharmaceuticals (*Acta Pol Pharm*, 1963, **20**, 43; 1967, **24**, 393; *CA*, 1964, **61**, 9355c; 1968, **68**, 16174z); quant. detn. (*J Pharm Pharmacol*, 1969, **21**, Suppl., 57); cephaeline in roots (*Arch Pharm Wein*, 1970, **303**, 209; *Acta Pol Pharm*, 1970, **27**, 469; *CA*, **73**, 28950r; 1971, **74**, 79726a); emetine, spectrophotom. (*Planta Med*, 1978, **34**, 430).

Plant, neutral glycd., ipecoside (*J Chem Soc Chem Commun*, 1967, 219). Root, *d*-mannitol (*Phytochemistry*, 1971, **10**, 2125).

CEPHALANDRA (*Cucurbitaceae*)

See **COCCINIA**

CEPHALOTAXUS (*Cephalotaxaceae*)

*C. manni Hook. f.

Plant from Shillong forests, a new alk. cephalomannine, taxol and an unident. alk.; cephalomannine, cytotoxic to KB cell culture and inhibitory to P388 leukemia in mice. Baccatin III and other diterps. of taxane series also present but usual alk. of genus absent (*Lloydia*, 1978, **41**, 655). Stems and roots, cephalomannine, taxol and beccatin III (*J Chem Soc Chem Commun*, 1979, 102). Str. and antileukemic

activity of cephalomannine (US Pat. Appl., 1979, 073903; US Pat., 1980, 4206221; *CA*, 1980, **92**, 28557k; **93**, 168465z).
Khasi hills, Meghalaya.

CERASTIUM (*Caryophyllaceae*)

*C. cerastoides (Linn.) Britton syn. *C. trigynum* Villars
Ladakh–*Spengyankarpo.*
Used in renal colic and headache (*in* Atal & Kapur, Med. Plants, 521).
Western Himalayas at 3,000-5,000 m.

CERATONIA (*Caesalpinaceae*)

C. silliqua Linn.
Eng.–*Carob, caroa bean tree, locust bean.*
Hydrocolloides in cosmetic drug; rev. of application of carob in cosmetic and pharm. compn. (*Drug Cosmet Ind*, 1964, **95**, 337). Effects of plant ext. on autonomic and CNS in dogs and rats (*Plant Med Phytother*, 1978, **12**, 248).
Pods, leucoanthocyanins and related phenolics (*J Sci Food Agric*, 1968, **19**, 543); hydrocarbons (*Acta Pharm Jugosl*, 1979, **29**, 97). Egyptian seeds, mucilagenous content (*Planta Med*, 1980, **38**, 73).
Leaves, catechols (*Prikl Biokhim Microbiol*, 1972, **8**, 207).

CERATOPHYLLUM (*Ceratophyllaceae*)

C. demersum Linn.
Plant, purg. (*Nagarjun*, 1979-80, **23**, 217).
EtOH(50%) ext., antimicrob. (*Lloydia*, 1973, **36**, 80).
Source of pro-vit. A for turkey poult (*Nutr Rep Int*, 1971, 4, 197; *CA*, 1972, **76**, 13036k). Plant gave +ve test for alk., flavon. and steroid (*Lloydia*, 1973, **36**, 72).

CERBERA (*Apocynaceae*)

C. manghas Linn. syn. *C. odollam* Gaertn.
Seeds, poisonous. In Samoa, plant used to treat wounds and yaws. Roots, laxt. (*Econ Bot*, 1974, **28**, 9).

Str. of cerbertin (*Tetrahedron Lett*, 1964, 3783). Seed kernels, cardiac glycds. cerbertin and cerbertatin; str. of cerbertin & Ac-cerbertin; thevetin B & its mono-Ac-deriv. (*Aust J Chem*, 1964, **17**, 1423; 1965, **18**, 1079; *Indian J Pharm*, 1974, **36**, 75). Kernel, cerberin and di-Ac-neriifolin (*Phytochemistry*, 1976, **15**, 848); seed, thevetin B, Ac- thevetin B, neriifolin, and glycds. of tanghinigenin and digitoxigenin (*Chem Pharm Bull*, 1977, **25**, 2744). Four cardiac glycds., mono-Ac-thevetin B, thevetin B, tanghinoside & de-Ac-tanghinoside and four monoglycds. cerberin, neriifolin, tanghinin and de-Ac-tanghinin (*Acta Pharm Sin*, 1981, **16**, 361).

Estn. of cardenolide contents of various plant parts (*Egypt J Pharm Sci*, 1972, **13**, 309; *CA*, 1975, **82**, 28503h). Cardiac glycds. of *Thevetia peruviana* and *C. odollam*, their pharmacol. and clin. aspects, rev., 62 refs. (*Indian J Pharm*, 1973, **35**, 107).

Leaves and fruits, iridoid glucds., theviridoside and theveside (*Phytochemistry*, 1972, **11**, 1852). Each plant part, 5 compds. including neriifolin, thevetin B and a non-cardenolidal substance (may be responsible for cath. effect of bark) (*Bull Fac Pharm Cairo Univ*, 1973, **12**, 91). Root and stem bark, cardiac glycds. gentiobiosyl thevetoside, glucosyl thevetoside and thevetosides of tanghinigenin. Leaves, cardenolides varied with season, 17-βH-neriifolin major (*Chem Pharm Bull*, 1977, **25**, 2744).

Roots, β-sitosterol (*Indian J Chem*, 1970, **8**, 851). Leaves, succinic acid, nicotiflorin, rutin and L-(+)-bornesitol (*Yakugaku Zasshi*, 1976, **96**, 1046); flavon. triglycds., manghaslin and clitorin (*Chem Pharm Bull*, 1980, **28**, 1219); new flavon. glycds. (*Phytochemistry*, 1980, **19**, 712).

C. thevetia Linn.; see Thevetia peruviana

CEREUS (*Cactaceae*)

C. grandiflorus Mill.
Flowers, flavon. glycds., cacticin and narcissin (*Chem Ber*, 1966, **99**, 1384; *CA*, **65**, 791d). Plant, alk. (*Phytochemistry*, 1968, **7**, 2031).

CERIOPS (*Rhizophoraceae*)

*C. decandra (Griff.) Ding Hou syn. *C. roxburghiana* Arn.
B.–*Baragoran*; H.–*Goran*; Oriya–*Gortah*; Tam.– *Chiru*; Tel.–*Gatharu.*

EtOH(50%) ext. of aerial parts, hypoten., diur. and antiinflam. (*Indian J Exp Biol*, 1977, **15**, 208).

Bark tannins, catechin and several leucoanthocyanidins; purification of bark tannin (*Leath Sci*, 1963, **10**, 403; 1965, **12**, 119).

Leaves, endogenous gibberellins (*Trans Bose Res Inst Calcutta*, 1979, **42**, 35).

From tidal forests of E. coasts and Sunderbans.

C. tagal (Perr.) C.B. Robins. syn. *C. candolleana* Arn.
EtOH(50%) ext. of stem bark, hypoglyc. (*Indian J Exp Biol*, 1971, **9**, 91).

CERISCOIDES (*Rubiaceae*)

C. turgida (Roxb.) Tirvengadum syn. *Gardenia turgida* Roxb.
Fruit—used against eye ailments of cattles; pulp pounded and applied to forehead in fever (*Econ Bot*, 1965, **19**, 242); as lep in abdominal colic (*Nagarjun*, 1980-81, **24**, 1).

EtOH(50%) ext., antivir., hypoten. and anticancer (*Indian J Exp Biol*, 1968, **6**, 232).

Plant—various plant parts used in fever, epilepsy, pimples, tubercular fistula, ringworm, haemat., cholera, smallpox, dysen., neuraligia, pleur., pneum., snakebite, etc. (*Econ Bot*, 1974, **24**, 241).

Saponin from bark decreased formation of histamine, and inhibited spasmogenic effects of slow-reacting substance of anaphylaxis in guinea pigs; saponin may find use as antiasthmic drug (*Curr Sci*, 1972, **41**, 614); market drug, not effective in asthma, good expect. and weak spasmol. [*J Res Indian Med*, 1976, **11**(4), 100].

Bark and wood, β-sitosterol, hederagenin, Me-esters of oleanolic and gypsogenic acids (*Phytochemistry*, 1973, **12**, 1831).

Roots, gardenin A, B & E, oleanolic acid, α- amyrin, β-sitosterol and *d*-mannitol (*J Indian Chem Soc*, 1979, **56**, 327).

CEROPEGIA (*Asclepiadaceae*)

C. bulbosa Roxb.
Tuberous roots, refrig. (*Econ Bot*, 1978, **32**, 282).

*C. macrantha Wight
B.–*Man-lata.*
EtOH(50%) ext. of aerial parts, diur. (*Indian J Exp Biol*, 1974, **12**, 512).
Burdwan, W.Bengal.

CESTRUM (*Solanaceae*)

*C. aurantiacum Lindl.
B.–*Gandephul.*
EtOH(50%) ext. of aerial parts, smasmol. (*Indian J Exp Biol*, 1969, **7**, 250).
Fruits contain alks. (*Biol Soc Quim Peru*, 1961, **27**, 161; *CA*, 1964, **61**, 15032a).
Commonly cultivated in Indian gardens as ornamental.

C. diurnum Linn.
EtOH(50%) ext. of aerial parts, spasmol. and CNS-depress. (*Indian J Exp Biol*, 1969, **7**, 250). Leaf meal caused hypercalcemia and hypophosphatasemia in pigs (*Cornell Vet*, 1977, **67**, 190; *CA*, **87**, 16851k). Leaves and their essent. oil, fungitoxic (*Naturwissenschaften*, 1980, **67**, 150). Aq., alc. and acetone exts. of plant, antibact. and antitumour (*Rev Cubana Farm*, 1980, **14**, 311).

Leaves, ursolic acid; saponin, tigonin (*Bull Calcutta Sch Trop Med*, 1963, **11**, 20; 1962, **10**, 123); pharmacol. of saponin mixt. (yuccanin, 90% and tigonin, 10%) (*ibid*, 1964, **12**, 58); saponin, cardiotonic and cardiotoxic (*Indian J Exp Biol*, 1968, **6**, 160); tigogenin (*Experientia*, 1964, **20**, 200). Alk. nornicotine and nicotine (*Planta Med*, 1971, **20**, 44); plant possesses 1,25-di-OH-cholecalciferol-like activity (*Biochem Biophys Res Commun*, 1975, **62**, 85); presence of 1, 25-di-OH-vit. D$_3$-glycd. (*Nature Lond*, 1977, **268**, 347).

C. nocturnum Linn.

Eng.–*Night jesmine.*

EtOH(50%) ext. of aerial parts, spasmol., diur. and hypoten. (*Indian J Exp Biol*, 1977, **15**, 208).

Leaves, tigogenin and yuccagenin (*Bull Calcutta Sch Trop Med*, 1963, **11**, 56). Saponin, cardiotonic and cardiotoxic (*Indian J Exp Biol*, 1968, **6**, 160). Leaves, alk. nornicotine, cotinine and myosmine (*Planta Med*, 1971, **20**, 44).

*C. parqui L'Herit.

Eng.–*Willow-leaved jesmine.*

In Chile, leaves used as sudorific and in skin troubles (*Planta Med*, 1974, **25**, 183).

Leaves contain 0.8% of toxic alk., paraquine which resembles atropine and strychnine in activity (Wlth India, II, 125).

Isolation of solasonin and digitogenin (*J Pharm Sci*, 1962, **51**, 289). Leaves, tigogenin, digallogenin, digitogenin and ursolic acid; same compds. from bark alongwith 3 unknown alks. (*Ann Chim Paris*, 1963, **53**, 1761; *CA*, **60**, 12370f); 0.34% tigogenin and a mono-OH-sapogenin (*Khim Prir Soedin*, 1970, **6**, 379; *CA*, **73**, 117182j).

Cultivated in Indian gardens.

CETERACH (*Aspleniaceae*)

C. officinarum DC. ex Lamk syn. *Asplenium caterach* Linn.; *Hemidictyum ceterach* Linn.

In Europe, decoct. of plant used in melancholia. Plant diur., astrin. and used in disease of spleen [*J Res Indian Med*, 1974, **9**(4), 62].

Leaves, chlorogenic acid, a flavonol heteroside and quercetin glucd., 0.25% (dry basis); whole plant, caffeic acid, neohesperidin, etc. (*Sci Pharm*, 1971, **39**, 170; 1980, **48**, 51; *CA*, 1972, **76**, 1811w; **93**, 41535s); estn. of trace elements and their relation to diur. action of whole plant (*J Radioanal Chem*, 1979, **54**, 103; *CA*, 1980, **92**, 152946p).

CHAEROPHYLLUM (*Apiaceae*)

*C. villosa Wall.

Eng.–*Wild carrot*; Kash.–*Jangli gazar.*

Plant yields essent. oil 0.98% (*Perfum Essent Oil Rec*, 1967, **58**, 622). Aerial parts, sitosterol (*Indian J Chem*, 1976, **14B**, 475).

Kashmir to Sikkim, Arunachal Pradesh and Meghalaya, at 1200-4,000 m.

CHAETACHME (*Ulmaceae*)

*C. aristata Planch. syn. *C. microcarpa* Rendle

Eng.–*Elephant's lime tree.*

Bark used in haemorrhoides. Powd. roots, dental anodyne (Watt & Breyer-Brandwijk, 1032).

Introduced into IBG, Calcutta.

CHAMAECYPARIS (*Cupressaceae*)

*C. lawsoniana (Murr.) Parl.

Leaves, sterols and other components (*Diss Pharm Pharmacol*, 1972, **24**, 401; *CA*, **77**, 149656r).

Grown in hill gardens for ornament.

CHAMAESYCE (*Euphorbiaceae*)

C. hirta Millsp. syn. *Euphorbia hirta* Linn.

Plant—used in postnatal complaints, failure of lactation, breast pain and bone fracture in cattle; skin eruptions (*Econ Bot*, 1970, **24**, 241; 1974, **28**, 1).

EtOH (50%) ext. antiprot., antivir., spasmog. and anticancer (*Indian J Exp Biol*, 1968, **6**, 232); both plant and leaf exts., antibact. [*Bull Bot Surv India*, 1976, **18**, 161; *Indian Drugs Pharmac Ind*, 1979, **14**(4), 27]. Plant ext., *in vitro*, antidysen.

similar to emetine chlorohydrate (*Plant Med Phytother*, 1981, **15**, 113).

Latex, vermifuge and used in diseases of urinogenitory tract (*J Agric Trop Bot Appl*, 1966, **13**, 245).

Plant, an alk., effective in respiratory system and produces dilatation of bronchi (*J Agric Trop Bot Appl*, 1966, **13**, 245). Herb, leucocyanidol, compol, etc. (*Plant Med Phytother*, 1972, **6**, 106; *CA*, **77**, 98756p); aerial parts, choline, shikimic acid, *l*-inositol and sugars (*Lloydia*, 1978, **41**, 73); 1-hexacosanol, 24-Me-enacycloartenol, tenol, cycloartenol, β-sitosterol, euphorbol hexacosonate, β-amyrin-OAc, tinyatoxin, 2 derivs. of deoxyphorbol-OAc and ingenol-tri-OAc (*Curr Sci*, 1980, **49**, 311).

Stem, hentriacontane, myricyl alc., taraxerol, etc., flowers, ellagic acid (*Bull Chem Soc Jpn*, 1966, **39**, 2532). Leaves and stems, triterps. and usual sterols (*Phytochemistry*, 1972, **11**, 1860).

Roots, 2 derivs. of deoxyphorbol-OAc, ingenol-tri-OAc and taraxerone (*Indian J Chem*, 1980, **19B**, 717).

CHEILANTHES (*Cheilanthaceae*)

*C. farinosa Kaulf.

Eng.–*Silver fern*; H.–*Shankhpushpi*; Pachmarhi hills– *Chhota hansraj.*

In Pachmarhi hills, fronds used in seasonal cold fever (*J Sci Res BHU*, 1969-70, **20**, 227). EtOH(50%) ext. of fern, spasmol. and CNS depress. (*Indian J Exp Biol*, 1973, **11**, 43).

Fern, sesquiterp., cheilanthatriol (*Tetrahedron Lett*, 1971, 4443); also cheilarinosin (*Indian J Chem*, 1972, **10**, 482).

Found in Uttar Pradesh and Madhya Pradesh.

C. tenuifolia Swartz

In Ranchi hills, root used in sickness (*J Sci Res BHU*, 1972-73, **23**, 137).

Fern contains 2 ecdysone analogues, cheilanthones A & B (*J Chem Soc D*, 1970, 243).

CHEIRANTHUS (*Brassicaceae*)

C. cheiri Linn.

Eng.–*Wall flower.*

Root with vinegar used in scirrhous inflam. Oil of wall flower in tumours of uterus and joints, indurations and scirrhous of sinews. Decoct. for sitz-bath in indurated uterine tumours. Wax salve in protracted tumours. Emol. in scirrhous and indurations. Balsam in tumours. Boiled flowers in scirrhous or hard imposthumes of uterus (*Lloydia*, 1969, **32**, 83).

Production of cardioactive substances by plant tissue culture, screening for cardiovascular activity (*J Pharm Pharmacol*, 1967, **19**, 760). Tissue culture ext., antimicrob. (*Lloydia*, 1968, **31**, 180). Leaves, fungicide antagonist (*Phytopathol Z*, 1969, **64**, 213).

Pharmacol. study of plant ext. effects on autonomic and CNS activities effect in dogs and rats (*Plant Med Phytother*, 1978, **12**, 248).

Seeds contain high levels of cardiac aglycones (*Diss Pharm*, 1963, **15**, 65; *CA*, **59**, 14297g). Seeds, stem and rhizome, glucoiberin (*Naturwissenschaften*, 1966, **53**, 200). Seeds yield 30 cardiac glycds. on paper chromatogr. (*Khim Prir Soedin*, 1975, 662; *CA*, 1976, **84**, 102279z); 5 cardiac glycds. (*ibid*, 1980, 424; *CA*, **93**, 128778x).

Leaves, volat. constituents (*Phytochemistry*, 1976, **15**, 763). Flowers, volat. constituents including 3-Me-thio-Pr isothiocyanate [*Dev Plant Biol*, 1978 (Pub'1979), **3**, 263; *CA*, 1979, **91**, 136413y]; flavons. (*Herba Pol*, 1979, **25**, 183).

CHENOPODIUM (*Chenopodiaceae*)

C. album Linn.

Plant—blood-purifier; oil kills stomach worms (*Labdev*, 1969, **7B**, 195). EtOH(50%) ext., CNS depress. (*Indian J Exp Biol*, 1969, **7**, 250). Plant, in Indigan. [*J Res Indian Med*, 1973, **8**(2), 67].

Leaves—powd. useful externally as an antisep. around genitalia of children. Among Zulu tribes of Africa, infusion used for curing intestinal ulcers; considered useful in piles and throat, and eye troubles; decoct., aper., tonic, diur. and aphrodis.; given in biliousness, hepatic disorders and spleen enlargement (*Planta Med*, 1972, **23**, 381).

In Hawaii, flowers and buds used in stomach trouble, weakness in children, and for fattening (*Econ Bot*, 1971, **25**, 245); Seeds, for abortion (*J Sci Res Plants Med*, 1981, **2**, 39).

Roots, ecdysteroids; β-ecdysone and polypodine B (*Fitoterapia*, 1981, **52**, 77).

C. ambrosioides Linn.

In Mexico, powd. seeds used against intestinal worms (*Econ Bot*, 1971, **25**, 234); produced tumour in rats (*Lloydia*, 1977, **40**, 619).

Leaves, ext., anthelm. (*Econ Bot*, 1975, **29**, 316). Shoot and root ext., nematicidal (*Geobios*, 1978, **5**, 116). Essent. oil from leaves, antimicrob. (*Herba Pol*, 1980, **26**, 245; *Fitoterapia*, 1980, **51**, 201); strong antifung. against human pathogenic fungi [*Indian Perfum*, 1981, **25**(3 & 4), 1].

Leaves, kaempferol-7-rhamnoside and ambroside (*Yakugaku Zasshi*, 1971, **91**, 552; *CA*, **75**, 59801p). Contents of Ca, P and oxalates in Indian plant (*Qual Plant Mater Veg*, 1973, **22**, 335). Screening for alk., steroid, triterp., etc. (*An Fac Farm Univ Fed Pernambuco*, 1976, **15**, 45; *CA*, 1979, **91**, 35717v).

Characteristics and constituents of essent. oil from shrub (*J Indian Chem Soc*, 1972, **49**, 317).

C. botrys Linn.

Eng.–*Jerusalem oak.*

Plant used in liver and stomach diseases, as diur. and laxt. (*in* Atal & Kapur, Med. Plants, 519).

Pharmacol. of alks. (*Tr Alma-At Zootekh Vet Inst*, 1968, **15**, 21; *CA*, 1971, **74**, 41007d). Plant used as antiasthmatic, antisp. and anticatar.; 2 bases including

betaine in all parts (*Khim Prir Soedin*, 1973, **9**, 569; *BA*, 1975, **59**, 4153). Aerial parts, chrysoeriol and quercetin pyranosides (*ibid*, 1974, **10**, 403; *CA*, 1975, **82**, 13990r); flavon., hispidulin, 7-Me-eupatulin, sinensetin, salvigenin & 5-salvigenin (*Planta Med*, 1981, **41**, 389).

Essent. oil, 26 compds. including chenopodic acid (*Izv Akad Nauk Turkm SSR Ser Biol Nauk*, 1973, 88; *CA*, 1974, **80**, 96169n). New and known sesquiterps.; 3 new eudesmane-type (*An Quim*, 1978, **74**, 91; 1575; *CA*, **89**, 197737n; 1979, **91**, 57205d). 12 New polyoxygenated sesquiterps. from aerial parts (*Tetrahedron*, 1980, **36**, 371).

Fruit, new alk. (*Rastit Resur*, 1978, **14**, 385; *CA*, **89**, 126150e).

*C. murale Linn.

Rajasthan–*Goyalo.*

Aq. ext. of plant, anthelm., B.P. lowering in dogs (*Nagarjun*, 1980-81, **24**, 126); antidiur. (*Fitoterapia*, 1981, **52**, 195).

Native of Europe and Asia, found almost throughout India.

CHIONACHNE (*Poaceae*)

C. koenigii (Spreng.) Thw. syn. *Polytoca barbata* Stapf

In Ayurvedic system, plant considered useful in painful urination, in constip., headache and anorexia due to excess of bile (*Bull Bot Soc Bengal*, 1968, **22**, 69).

CHLORANTHUS (*Chloranthaceae*)

C. erectus (Buch.-Ham.) Verdc. syn. *C. elatior* R. Br. ex Sims; *C. officinalis* Blume

Plant used in skin diseases and V.D. Poultice of root recommended in boils and carbuncle. In Java, infusion of root mixed with bark of *Cinnamomum culilowan* used to treat puerperal eclampsia (Quisumbing, 220; Burkill, I, 529).

C. glaber Makino syn. *C. brachystachys* Blume

Fruits, pelargonidin-3-rhamnosylglucd. (*Experientia*, 1971, **27**, 1006). Plant, 2 new sesquiterps., chloranthalactone A & B (*Heterocycles*, 1978, **9**, 139; *CA*, **88**, 170325x). Succinic acid, linalool-OAc and isofraxidin; all 3 compds., antitumour in animals (*Chung Ts'ao Yao*, 1981, **12**, 9; *CA*, **95**, 103209r). Aerial parts, isofraxidin, β-sitosterol glucd., astilbin, etc. (*Shoyakugaku Zasshi*, 1981, **35**, 217).

CHLORIS (*Poaceae*)

*C. gayana Kunth
Eng.–*Rhodes grass.*
Grass, estrogenic (*Indian Vet J*, 1974, **51**, 610).
Seed sterols including campesterol, β-sitosterol & stigmasterol (*Phytochemistry*, 1971, **10**, 3135). Grass, phytotoxic substances (*J Chem Ecol*, 1975, **1**, 183).
Introduced into India.

CHLOROPHORA (*Moraceae*)

C. excelsa Benth. & Hook. f.
Handling of wood may cause acute contact eczema; sensitising agent being chlorophorine (*Berufs-Dermatosen*, 1962, **10**, 17; *CA*, **56**, 13195e). Chlorophorine toxic to subterranean termite, *Reticulitermes* (*Holzforschung*, 1968, **22**, 104; *CA*, 1969, **70**, 46373x).

CHLOROPHYTUM (*Liliaceae*)

C. arundinaceum Baker
Root powd., fried in ghee, chewed in case of aphthae in mouth and throat (*Nagarjun*, 1980-81, **24**, 1).
Fruits, new galactoglucan (*Planta Med*, 1979, **37**, 94).

*C. tubersosum (Roxb.) Baker
Roots used as vegetable and tonic (*Econ Bot*, 1978, **32**, 284).
C. India and Western Peninsula.

CHLOROXYLON (*Rutaceae*)

C. swietenia DC.
EtOH(50%) ext. of stem bark and leaves, spasmol. (*Indian J Exp Biol*, 1971, **9**, 91).

Str. of gum (*Indian J Chem*, 1963, **1**, 324; 1968, **6**, 428).

Indian bark, *tert*-Bu-ketone, swietenone (*Tetrahedron Lett*, 1975, 867); coumarin, rutamarin; also 9 new coumarins and 2 new alks. (*Indian J Chem*, 1972, **10**, 674; 1977, **15**, 440); 3 new swietenocoumarins G, H & I (*ibid*, 1980, **19B**, 1046).

Heartwood, 5 coumarins xanthoxyletin, 7-de-Me-suberosin, luvangetin, aesculetin-di-Me-ether and nodakenetin (no xanthyletin); and alks. skimmianine and γ-fagarine (*Phytochemistry*, 1972, **11**, 2647); 2, 4-di-OH-5-Ph-cinnamic acid and coumarin, swietenol, xanthyletin, xanthoxyletin, alloxanthoxyletin, and 7-de-Me-suberosin (*Indian J Chem*, 1977, **15B**, 200).

CHONEMORPHA (*Apocynaceae*)

*C. macrophylla (Roxb.) G. Don syn. *C. fragrans* (Moon) Alston; *Echites fragrans* Moon
EtOH(50%) ext. of stem bark and leaves, spasmol. (*Indian J Exp Biol*, 1980, **18**, 594). Crushed roots with salt taken with boiled water for stomach disorders (*Bull Bot Surv India*, 1980, **22**, 161).

Roots, steroid alk., chonemorphine (*Indian J Chem*, 1967, **5**, 146). Funtumafrine-C from roots, identical with deaminochonemorphinone (*ibid*, 1972, **10**, 1197). Root bark, several steroid alks., including N-formylchonemorphine and japindine. Leaves, a triterp. baurenol-OAc and β- sitosterol (*ibid*, 1978, **16B**, 346).

In moist forests of India.

CHREMANTHOPODIUM (*Asteraceae*)

*C. arnicoides (DC.) Good var. **trigida**
Ladakh–*Reskunsemar.*
Flowers used in peptic ulcer, dysen. and liver diseases (*in* Atal & Kapur, Med. Plants, 519).
Found in Ladakh.

CHROMOLAENA (*Asteraceae*)

C. odorata King & Robinson syn. *Eupatorium odoratum* Linn.

EtOH(50%) ext. of aerial parts, spasmol. (*Indian J Exp Biol*, 1969, **7**, 250). Leaf and shoot used as fish poison (*Curr Sci*, 1980, **49**, 251). Crushed leaves stop bleeding from cuts and wounds (*Bull Med Ethno Bot Res*, 1980, **1**, 447).

Leaves, ceryl alc. and sterols; trihydric alc. and anisic acid (*Sci Res Dacca*, 1967, **4**, 154; 1969, **6**, 37; *CA*, 1968, **68**, 57405u; *Trans Bose Res Inst Calcutta*, 1974, **37**, 25); isosakuranetin and chalcone, odoratin; aerial parts, flavons., scutellarein tetra-Me-ether, sinensetin, chalcones, etc. (*Phytochemistry*, 1973, **12**, 667; 1978, **17**, 1807).

Plant, lupeol, β-amyrin and flavone, salvigenin (*Phytochemistry*, 1974, **13**, 284); epoxylupeol alongwith known terps. (*Indian J Chem*, 1977, **15B**, 806); flavons., kaempferide, tamarixetin, sakuranetin & its iso deriv. (*Planta Med*, 1981, **42**, 403).

CHROZOPHORA (*Euphorbiaceae*)

C. prostrata Dalz.

Aq. ext. of leaves and branches of plant alongwith flower heads of *Sphaeranthus indicus* and leaves of *Grewia tiliaefolia* given orally to persons suffering from dermatitis (*Ancient Sci Life*, 1981-82, **1**, 236).

EtOH(50%) ext. of plant, spasmol. (*Indian J Exp Biol*, 1969, **7**, 250).

Plant, pyridinium salt oxidizing enzyme (*Phytochemistry*, 1970, **9**, 2443). Seed fatty acid compn., linoleate-rich oil (*Fette Seifen Anstrichm*, 1980, **82**, 204; *CA*, 1980, **93**, 44317h).

C. rotteri A. Juss. ex Spreng. syn. *C. tinctoria* Hook. f.

Roots used in cough (*J Econ Tax Bot*, 1980, **1**, 144).

Seed sterols (*C R Acad Sci Ser D*, 1967, **265**, 409).

CHRYSANTHEMUM (*Asteraceae*)

C. cinerariifolium Vis. syn. *Pyrethrum cinerariifolium* Trev.

Flowers—fresh and dry, insectic. activity (*J Sci Food Agric*, 1965, **16**, 186). Manufacture of pyrethrum powder (*Pyrethrum Post*, 1965, **8**, 14). Production of concentrated ext. (*Chem Ind Lond* 1969, 756). Uses and cultivation in India (*Perfum Essent Oil Rec*, 1969, **60**, 19); highly concentrated exts. of Dalmatian pyrethrum (Jpn Kokai, 1976, 7648425; *CA*, **85**, 43836z); its preparation (Jpn Tokkyo Koho, 1979, 7900920; *CA*, **90**, 134016b).

Oleoresin—from flowers in combination with *neem* seed, toxic against housefly [*Pesticides*, 1980, **14**(3), 11].

Flowers contain pyrethrosin, pyrethrol, lupeol, α- & β-amyrol and taraxasterol (*Acta Farm*, 1966, **32**, 121; *Phytochemistry*, 1972, **11**, 2267); sesquiterp. (+)-sesamin and β-cyclopyrethrosin; its dihydro deriv., chrysanin and chrysanolide (*Can J Chem*, 1969, **47**, 1139; 1971, **49**, 2103).

Flowers, insecticidal constituents pyrethrin I & II, alongwith cinerin I & II and jasmolin II (*Chem Ind Lond*, 1964, 371). Plant, jasmolin II, activity (*J Econ Entomol*, 1965, **58**, 548); jasmolins I & II from flower heads (*J Chem Soc C*, 1966, 332). Pyrethrin content of plant organs grown in Egypt; in Central Anatolia (*Egypt J Pharm Sci*, 1974, **15**, 21; *Commun Fac Sci Univ Ankara Ser B*, 1980, **26**, 3; *CA*, 1981, **95**, 58097q); identn. of 6 pyrethrins (*Pestic Sci*, 1976, **7**, 225). Petals, pyrethrins (*Prax Naturwiss Biol*, 1979, **28**, 309; *CA*, 1980, **92**, 158811z).

Pyrethroids—chem. & biochem. of pyrethrins, rev., 35 refs. (*Pyrethrum Post*, 1966, No. 4, 27). Extn. of pure pyrethrins (*Med Prom SSSR*, 1966, **20**, 35; *CA*, **65**, 20510a). Yield of flowers and active principle (*Indian J Pharm*, 1968, **30**, 120). Chrysanthemum insecticides, rev. covering cultivation, chem. compn., assay, uses and synthetic analogues (*Plant Med Phytother*,

1969, **3**, 296; *CA*, 1970, **73**, 54912z); pyrethroids (*in* Jacobson & Crosby, 3-70).

Aerial parts, flavons.; flowers, polyphenols (*Pyrethrum Post*, 1972, **11**, 82; *Curr Sci*, 1973, **42**, 811). Cultivation aspects in Meghalaya; in hills; crop yield [*Pesticides*, 1980, **14**(6), 27; *J Res Indian Med*, 1974, **9**(1), 73; *Indian Farming*, 1974-75, **24**(12), 7].

C. coronarium Linn.

Plant, 4 lyratol esters and a S-containing alkenyne (*Phytochemistry*, 1979, **18**, 1888).

C. indicum Linn. syn. *Pyrethrum indicum* Linn.

Pharmacol. of aerial parts; EtOH ext. of blossoms and stems, antiinflam. (*C R Acad Bulg Sci*, 1981, **34**, 1029).

Plant, yejuhua lactone (*Yao Hsueh Hsueh Pao*, 1963, **10**, 129; *CA*, **59**, 15326b); asteglasine A, sesquiterp. alk. which causes contact dermatitis in man (*Naturwissenschaften*, 1975, **62**, 585; *Phytochemistry*, 1976, **15**, 1573).

Essent. oil, extn. (*Nauchni Tr Vissh Inst Khranit Vkusova Prom St Plovdiv*, 1972, **19**, 129; *CA*, 1975, **83**, 168306s); constituents (*Phytochemistry*, 1981, **20**, 2691).

Flowers, acacetin glycd. (*Phytochemistry*, 1981, **20**, 1760).

*C.leucanthemum Linn.

EtOH(50%) ext. of plant, spasmol. and CNS depress. (*Indian J Exp Biol*, 1968, **6**, 232). Estrogenic and toxic effects of plant on mouse (*Can J Zool*, 1980, **58**, 1575).

Plant, cyclitol, leucanthemitol and viburnitol (*C R Acad Sci*, 1962, **255**, 360). Aerial parts from Siberia, esculetin, scopoletin and 3 alks. (*Farmatsiya Moscow*, 1977, **26**, 33).

Nainital, U.P.

*C. morifolium Ramat.

Screening for antitumour activity (*Shoyakugaku Zasshi*, 1979, **33**, 95). Essent. oil from leaves, antibact. (*Herba Pol*, 1980, **26**, 245).

Plant, sesquiterps. chrysartemins A & B; lactone chlorochrymorin; and chrysandiol

(*Agric Biol Chem*, 1971, **35**, 1966; *Tetrahedron Lett*, 1973, 5135; 1977, 1169).

Native of Asia, cultivated as ornamental.

CHRYSOPHYLLUM (*Sapotaceae*)

*C. cainito Linn.

Leaves ext. in 1% HCl, MeOH, EtOH and pet. ether, anticancer (*Philipp J Sci*, 1967, **96**, 393).

Milky fruits avoided by pregnant, Choco Indians, in belief that foetus will grow too large (*Econ Bot*, 1970, **24**, 357).

Leaves, myricetin glycds. (*Curr Sci*, 1973, **42**, 746).

Native of W. Indies, cultivated mainly in Vadodara, Gujarat and in Maharashtra for edible fruits.

CHRYSOPOGON (*Poaceae*)

*C. aciculatus (Retz.) Trin.

Eng.–*Lesser spear grass*; B.–*Chorlanta*; H.–*Lampa*; Tam.–*Tuttiri*; Tel.–*Putthigadi*.

EtOH(50%) ext. of plant, diur. (*Indian J Exp Biol*, 1977, **15**, 208). Roots crushed with water and juice taken as stomch. (*Bull Bot Surv India*, 1980, **22**, 161).

Throughout India.

CHRYSOSPLENIUM (*Saxifragaceae*)

*C. trichospermum Edgew. ex Hook. f.

EtOH(50%) ext. of plant, antiinflam. (*Indian J Exp Biol*, 1977, **15**, 208).

Temperate Western Himalayas at *c*.3,000 m.

CHUKRASIA (*Meliaceae*)

C. tabularis A. Juss.

EtOH(50%) ext. of stembark, hypoten.; spasmol., and diur. (*Indian J Exp Biol*, 1971, **9**, 91; 1974, **12**, 512). Plant used in skeletal fractures (*Sri Lanka For*, 1980, **14**, 145). Seed ext., agglutinating (*Aust J Exp Biol Med Sci*, 1981, **59**, 195).

Bark, sitosterol, melianone, scopoletin and 6,7-di-MeO-coumarin (*Phytochemistry*, 1974, **13**, 2012). Strs. of tetranorterps. from bark, tabularin; and from timber, bussein homologue and chukrasin (*J Chem Res S*, 1978, 20; *CA*, **88**, 191164f). Wood, chukrasins A, B, C,D & F (*Helv Chim Acta*, 1978, **61**, 1914).

Roots, a triterp. cedrelone (*Indian J Chem*, 1969, **7**, 308). Leaves, guercetin galactoside, galloyl glucd. and tannic acid [*J Res Indian Med*, 1975, **10**(1), 29]; also a flavone (*Phytochemistry*, 1977, **16**, 398).

Seeds, new tetranorterps., phragmalin esters and 12 α-OAc-phyramalin (*J Chem Soc Perkin Trans I*, 1978, 285).

CIBOTIUM (*Cyatheaceae*)

C. barometz Smith

Fern, pterosin deriv. (*Phytochemistry*, 1980, **19**, 1743).

CICCA (*Euphorbiaceae*)

See PHYLLANTHUS

CICER (*Fabaceae*)

C. arietinum Linn.

Eng.–*Bengal gram.*

Seeds—Seed and its lipid ext., hypocholesterolemic in human (*Proc Asian-Pacific Congr Cardiol 3rd Kyoto*, 1964, **1**, 575; *CA*, 1966, **65**, 2709f); white var., hypocholesterolemic in albino rats (*Indian J Biochem Biophys*, 1979, **16**, 444). Germinated seeds more effective. Lipid fraction from ungerminated and carbohydrate fraction of both type of seeds more effective in lowering lever and serum cholesterol than whole legume (*Nutr Rep Int*, 1979, **20**, 371; 383; *CA*, **91**, 191864w-65x).

EtOH(50%) ext. of seeds, spasmol. (*Indian J Exp Biol*, 1968, **6**, 232). Pet. ether ext. of husks showed 20% antiimplantation in albino rats (*Probe*, 1977-78, **17**, 315). Seed ext., agglutinating with *Pseudomonas aeruginosa* (*Jpn J Exp Med*, 1980, **50**, 263). Seeds reduced postprandial plasma glucose in human (*Am J Clin Nutr*, 1981, **34**, 2450); seed coat, diur. [*Indian Drugs Pharmac Ind*, 1981, **16**(1), 39].

Seeds, activated carbon for Argentine pharmaceutical requirements (*Rev Asoc Bioquim Argent*, 1964, **29**, 179; *CA*, 1965, **62**, 15989d). Lipid , sterol compn. (*Riv Soc Ital Sci Aliment*, 1975, **4**, 257; *CA*, 1976, **84**, 102304 d). Gram, hypolipidemic isoflavons., biochanin-A and formononetin (*Lipids*, 1976, **11**, 243). Development and distribution of isoflavone-7-O-β-glycd. specific β-glycosidases (*Planta Med*, 1976, **30**, 97); germinated seeds, α-galactosidases (*Phytochemistry*, 1977, **16**, 1053). Seeds, new disaccharide, galactopinitol (*J Sci Food Agric*, 1978, **29**, 148). Levels of phenolic substance in leachates at different stages (*Indian J Exp Biol*, 1979, **17**, 116).

Isoflavones, biochanin A and formonetin, hypolipidermic in rats (*Lipids*, 1979, **14**, 535). Total flavons. reduced rat serum and lever cholesterol, triglycerides, when given orally prevented hyperlipidemia (*Vopr Med Khim*, 1979, **25**, 444; *CA*, **91**, 117409k). Isolation and estn. of phytoestrogens (*Indian J Anim Sci* 1975, **45**, 622).

Seedlings, flavons.; aerial parts, kaempferol, quercetin, isorhamnetin and pratensein (*Phytochemistry*, 1965, **4**, 89; 1970, **9**, 2053); phytoalexin, cicerin (*Plant Dis Probl Proc Int Symp*, 1966-67, 724; *CA*, 1972, **76**, 110294a). Vanillic and *p*-OH-benzoic acids, major compds. in leaf leachates (*Indian J Exp Biol*, 1978, **16**, 1213).

Roots, medicagol and 12-OMe-coumesterol (*Phytochemistry*, 1969, **8**, 2261). Stems and roots, coniferin-specific glucosidases (*Z Pflanzenphysiol*, 1981, **101**, 207; *CA*, **95**, 75946h).

CICHORIUM (*Cichoriaceae*)

C. endivia Linn.

Eng.–*Endive.*

Plant, OH-flavone glycds. and D-(+)-dicaffeoyltartaric acid (*Z Naturforsch*, 1974, **29C**, 355; 360). Flavonols and flavones; detn. of OH-cinnamic acids (*Z Lebensm Unters Forsch*, 1974, **156**, 153;

1975, **159**, 255; *CA*, 1975, **82**, 2980m; 1976, **84**, 57534r).

C. intybus Linn.

Eng.–*Chicory.*

Plant—wild and cultivated for food, fodder and med. Chicory fed to cattle in large quant., imparts bitter flavour to milk and butter (Chopra, *et al*, I, 469). In Europe, considered as diur. and laxt. (*Acta Phytother*, 1971, **18**, 21). Alc. ext. useful against exp.-induced chlorpromazine hepatic damage in albino rats (*J Res Ayur Siddha*, 1980, **1**, 77). Ext., a major component of indigenous drug 'Liv-52' (*Indian J Med Res*, 1976, **64**, 738); also of 'Geriforte' (*Probe*, 1979-80, **19**, 99; *Rajasthan Med J*, 1980, **19**, 23; *Indian Drugs*, 1980-81, **18**, 346).

Root—decoct. given in jaundice, liver enlargement, gout and rheum. In India, roots used as blood purifier, emmen. and in asthma (*Acta Phytother*, 1971, **18**, 21); hot beverage, as coffee or its extender (Herbal Med., 51); alc. ext., antimicrob. against micro-organisms causing gingival inflam. (*J Indian Dent Assoc*, 1981, **53**, 25).

Seeds—carmin. and cordial [*East Pharm*, 1980, **23**(272), 39]; ext., agglutinating (*Acta Pol Pharm*, 1963, **20**, 83; *CA*, 1964, **61**, 9898h).

Flowers picked early in the day, soaked in fresh water in the sun, and strained liquid or essence stored; a few drops of this essence act as a unique remedy when added to tea of those who are on a crying jag, or unduly possessive and overcritical of others (Herbal Med., 51).

Detn. of caffeine (*Analyst Lond*, 1964, **89**, 146). Potent carcinogen 3,4-benzpyrene detected (*in* Plant and Fungal Toxins, 257-58). Flowers, a glucd. cichoriin; milky juice, 2 bitter principles, lactucin and lactucopicrin (Chopra *et al*, I, 469); chem. of bitter substances esculetin, esculin, cichoriin, lactucin and lactucopicrin, rev., 26 refs. (*Ann Gembloux*, 1965, **71**, 211; *CA*, 1967, **66**, 35364m). Cichoriin, esculin, umbelliferone, scopoletin and 6,7- dihydrocoumarin from

racemes; shoot flavons. (*Khim Prir Soedin*, 1971, **7**, 115; 1973, **9**, 119; *CA*, **74**, 136458r; **79**, 2751a). Aerial parts yield derivs. of OH-cinnamic acid; their detn. (*ibid*, 1972, **8**, 796; *Z Lebensm Unters Forsch*, 1975, **159**, 255; *CA*, 1973, **78**, 94815e; 1976, **84**, 57534n). Sepn. of coumarins; cichoriin, esculetin and esculin (*Herba Pol*, 1974, **20**, 339; *CA*, 1975, **83**, 120711t). Aerial parts valuable sources of esculetin; highest in leaves and flowers (*Rastit Rasur*, 1974, **10**, 573; *CA*, 1975, **82**, 90001w).

Extn. of chicory for polyphenols with cholagogue activity (USSR Pat., 1977, 577033; *CA*, 1978, **88**, 27793q); grain not toxic up to 60g/day, in human for 6 months (*Aliment Vie*, 1979, **67**, 24; *CA*, **91**, 173491t). Plant contains a substance with prostaglandin-like activity (*Khim Prir Soedin*, 1980, 825; *CA*, 1981, **94**, 180557j).

CICUTA *(Apiaceae)*

C. virosa Linn.

Eng.–*Water hemlock.*

In Homoeopathy, fresh root used in convuls. with loss of consciousness; in epilepsy, lock jaw, and in cerebro-spinal meningitis. Also used in somnonbulism (*Bull Bot Soc Bengal*, 1972, **26**, 25).

Water hemlock poisoning; roots and leaves very toxic even fatal when taken as a food, rev. with testing for toxic principle cicutoxin and alk., cicutine (*Dtsch Z Gesamte Gerichtl Med*, 1962, **53**, 87; *CA*, 1963, **58**, 8347d); cicutoxin, isolation and str., a highly unsaturated higher alcohol, *trans*-heptadeca-8:10:12- triene-4:6-diyne-1:4-diol, isomeric with oenanthotoxin from the related genus *Oenanthe* proven poisonous (Kingsbury, 377). Cicutoxin, cicutol and poly-ynes (*Chem Ber*, 1969, **102**, 3293). Fruits contain 7 flavon. glucds. (*Acta Pol Pharm*, 1972, **29**, 417; *CA*, 1973, **78**, 94864v). Plant, umbelliferone and scopoletin (*Khim Prir Soedin*, 1973, **9**, 112; *CA*, **79**, 2765h).

CIMICIFUGA (Ranunculaceae)

C. foetida Linn.

Eng.—*Fetid bugbane.*

Plant ext., with other ingredients, effective compn. for bad breath; and as skin cosmetics (Jpn Kokai, 1975, 7588243; 7588238; *CA*, **83**, 136738t; 152208a).

Root, alks. (?) (*in* Jacobson & Crosby, 222).

*C. racemosa (Linn.) Nutt.

In Homoeopathy, fresh roots a valuable remedy in all rheumatic diseases, in nervous hysterical women arising from irritation of uterus. Useful in cererospinal meningitis, locomotor ataxia, sciatica and angina pectoris (*Bull Bot Soc Bengal*, 1972, **26**, 25).

Glycds. from roots (*Arzneim Forsch*, 1964, **14**, 1037; *CA*, 1965, **62**, 815h). Seeds, alk. (*Proc W Va Acad Sci*, 1965, **37**, 143; *CA*, 1966, **65**, 4265e). Str. of actein; roots, 27-de-OAc-aceteol (*Corsi Semin Chim*, 1968, **11**, 61; *Arch Pharm Wein*, 1968, **301**, 335; *CA*, 1970, **72**, 55835t; 67559g). Rhizomes contain triterp., actinea, and cimicifugoside (*Gazz Chim Ital*, 1971, **101**, 139). NMR of cimigoside, actein, and cycloartenol (*Tetrahedron Lett*, 1975, 4287).

Pharmacol. of constituents, rev., 42 refs. (*Erfahrungsheilkunde*, 1981, **30**, 439; *CA*, **95**, 72960x).

Temperate Himalayas from Kashmir to Bhutan up to 2,000 m.

CINCHONA (Rubiaceae)

C. alks.; antimalarials (Sim, 75-82; *in* Manske, III, 1-64; XIV, 181-224; V, 141-56).

C. ledgeriana Moens ex Trimen syn. *C. calisaya* Wedd. var. *ledgeriana* Howard
Trade–*Yellow cinchona.*

EtOH(50%) ext. of leaves, antivir. (*Indian J Exp Biol*, 1973, **11**, 43).

Leaves, alk. cinchophyllamine & its iso. deriv. (*Ann Pharm Fr*, 1965, **23**, 691; *CA*, **64**, 13085a); their strs, (*Bull Soc Chim Fr*, 1966, 2309); alks. quinchophylline and quinchophyllamine, both analg. (Neth. Appl., 1965, 6413518; *CA*, **63**, 18193a); their pharmacol. effects (*C R Acad Sci Ser D*, 1969, **268**, 441; *Ann Pharm Fr*, 1969, **27**, 397; *CA*, 1970, **72**, 65061b); five monomeric and 7 quasi-dimeric indole alks.; also bisindole monoterp. alk.[*Phytochemistry*, 1980, **19**, 2451; *Bull Soc Chim Fr*, 1981, (1- 2, Pt 2), 75].

Leaves, quinone (*J Pharm Pharmacol*, 1970, **22**, 469); Flavon. (*Curr Sci*, 1974, **43**, 479); phenolic acids, anthocyanins and flavons. (*Ann Pharm Fr*, 1975, **33**, 73; *CA*, **83**, 160770t).

Heartwood, a glycd. and alks. (*Indian J Chem*, 1968, **6**, 566).

Quinine & quinidine — alks. of quinoline group from bark. Quinine antimalarial, commonly used as sulphate; weak increase in uterine contraction and local anaesthetic effect observed (Sim, 80); may be teratogenic (*in* Plant and Fungal Toxins, 172). Quinidine used principally for restoring certain types of cardiac arrhythmia; antiarrhythmic drugs (Sim, 82; *in* Goodwin & Gilman, 699-710). Quinine & quinidine production by leaf, root and unorganised cultures (*Phytochemistry*, 1981, **20**, 2495).

C. officinalis Linn. f.

Bark—in Homoeopathy, in catar. jaundice, useful in debility of anaemia due to loss of fluids, in gallstone colic, gastric trouble in children, one of the best remedies for chr. liver trouble (*Bull Bot Soc Bengal*, 1972, **26**, 25).

Leaves, flavon. avicularin (*Curr Sci*, 1976, **45**, 21).

C. robusta Howard

Leaves, flavon. avicularin (*Curr Sci*, 1976, **45**, 21).

C. succirubra Pavon ex Klotz.

Trade–*Red cinchona.*

Bark—cinchona; antimal. and antiarrhythmic in immature rats (*Med Exp*, 1969, **19**, 79). Tincture, a constituent of hair lotion (Rom. Pat., 1968, 50627; *CA*, **69**, 109753y). Powd., in compn. useful in capillary treatment for hair; tincture, a constituent of capillary-lotion for alopecia (Fr. Demande, 1971, 2112085; 1974, 2216987; *CA*, 1973, **78**, 62194k; 1975, **82**, 160229c).

Alks. cinchonine extn. from bark (*Trav Soc Pharm Montpellier*, 1967, **27**, 227; *CA*, 1968, **68**, 117108m); chromatogr. and spectrophotom. sepn. of main alks. & other alks. from cortex (*Acta Pharm Hung*, 1973, **43**, 25; 49; 1977, **47**, 249; *CA*, **78**, 133371d; **79**, 5481y; 1978, **88**, 158517a).

Quinine and quinidine production by leaf, root and unorganised cultures (*Phytochemistry*, 1981, **20**, 2495); see *C. ledgeriana* also.

Leaves phenolic acids, anthocyanins and flavons. (*Ann Pharm Fr*, 1975, **33**, 73; *CA*, **83**, 160770t).

CINNAMOMUM (*Lauraceae*)

C. camphora (Linn.) Presl

In Europe, used in cold, chills and diar. (*Acta Phytother*, 1971, **18**, 21). EtOH(50%) ext. of aerial parts, hypoten. and CNS depress. (*Indian J Exp Biol*, 1977, **15**, 208); bark, minor fradulent hallucinogen, see *C. cassia*. Camphor useful in chr. pulmonary inflam. [*Farm Zh Kiev*, 1972, **27**(6), 78; *BA*, 1973, **56**, 56516]. Camphor used against carbuncles (*Nagarjun*, 1979-80, **23**, 10).

Essent. oil—*in vitro* antimicrob. activity [*Indian Drugs Pharmac Ind*, 1978, **13**(6), 25]; antifung. [*Indian Perfum*, 1979, **23**, 138; *East Pharm*, 1979, **22**(257), 109].

Chem. of Indian essent. oils, rev. (*Perfum Essent Oil Rec*, 1967, **58**, 622). Essent. oil sesquiterps. campherenone and campherenol (*Tetrahedron Lett*, 1967, 5069); constituents (*Bull Chem Soc Jpn*, 1968, **41**, 1465; *Perfum Essent Oil Rec*, 1968, **59**, 914).

Roots, alks. laurolitsine and reticuliene (*Yakugaku Zasshi*, 1964, **84**, 365; *Int Pharm Abstr*, **1**, 1296 b). Leaves, palmitone (*J Indian Chem Soc*, 1971, **48**, 288). Heartwood, cyclopentenone (*Phytochemistry*, 1979, **18**, 488).

C. cassia Nees ex Eberm. ex Blume syn.

C. aromaticum Nees

Eng.–*China cassia*.

In Yemenite folk med., plant as an ingredient of compn. against headache and melancholy (*Q J Crude Drug Res* 1963, **3**, 395). A mixt. of exts. of *C. cassia, Zinziber officinale* and *Bupleurum falcatum* decreased blood urea and increased blood cholesterol, in rats (*Yakugaku Zasshi*, 1978, **98**, 1642). Preparation of a mixt. containing *Ephedra distachya*, apricot, *C. cassia* and licorice, useful chinese drug in cough and fever (*Jpn Kokai Tokkyo Koho*, 1979, 79163830; *CA*, 1980, **92**, 220721a).

Bark, minor constituent of Unani compn., '*Jawarish Jalinoos*' useful drug for gastro-enterological complaint [*J Res Indian Med*, 1979, **14**(3 & 4), 34]; a minor fradulent hallucinogen, no appreciable CNS activity (*in* Beal & Reinhard, 347).

Essent. oil, from bark of Nigerian plant, 70% cinnamaldehyde and 13% eugenol; leaves oil, 92% benzyl benzoate and 4% cinnamaldehyde (*Indian J Pharm*, 1976, **38**, 158); cinnamaldehyde, major constituent of both bark oil and leaf oil; 'Cassia oil' of commerce is derived from leaf and twigs, constituents, rev. covering all aspects (Purseglove *et al*, I, 100-73). Oil of Nigerian plant (*J Pharm Pharmacol*, 1979, **31**, Suppl., 8p); oil from bark, constituents (*Planta Med*, 1979, **36**, 380). Effect of essent. oil on digest. enzymes (*Chem Pharm Bull*, 1981, **29**, 2966).

Aq. ext. of bark, anticomplement, 10 compds.; diterp. cinncassiol C_1; compd. antiallergic; cinncassiol B & its glucd. (*ibid*, 1980, **28**, 1432; 1969, 2682); also cinncassiol C & its glucd., C_2, C_3; root bark ext. also anticomplement, contains cinncassiol D_1, D_2 & D_3, as also glucds. of D_1 & D_2 (*ibid*, 1981, **29**, 2686;,2451). Pentacyclic diterp. cinncassiol D_1 & its glucd. from aq. ext. of bark exhibiting anticomplement activity (*Tetrahedron Lett*, 1980, **21**, 2647).

C. cecidodaphne Meissn.

Fruit essent. oil, α- & β-pinene, 22.5; cineole, 10.1; Me-cinnamate, 16.0% and others [*Indian Perfum*, 1967, **11**(Pt.2), 21]. Fruits, trilaurin (major) (*Indian Oil Soap J*, 1968, **34**, 117).

C. tamala Nees & Eberm.

Leaves and bark mixed with tea cures coughs and colds. Used in many Ayurvedic recipes, '*Sudarshan Choorna*', '*Chanderprabhavati*', '*Yograj Guggul*', '*Ashwaganghrishta*', '*Dasmoolarishta*', etc. [*Indian Perfum*, 1970, **14**(Pt.1), 41]. Hypoglyc. in rabbits [*J Res Indian Med*, 1979, **14**(3-4), 159]; plant, hypoglyc. in patients of insulin-independent diabetes (*J Res Ayur Siddha*, 1980, **1**, 275). Used in the preparation of Ayurvedic drug '*Vyaghri Haritaki*', as minor constituent (*J Nat Integ Med Assoc*, 1980, **22**, 229).

Leaves, arom., in dyspep., cough and scorpion sting. Bark, carmin. (*Khadi Gramodyog*, 1980-81, **27**, 401).

Essent. oil, antibact.; that from leaves, antifung. (*Curr Sci*, 1978, **47**, 454; *Indian Drugs*, 1978-79, **16**, 24).

Essent oil, Indian, chem., rev. (*Perfum Essent Oil Rec*, 1967, **58**, 622). Production of leaf oil, eugenol & isoeugenol [*Ind Bull Bombay*, 1969, **10**(12), 10]. Chem. and uses; oil from leaves of different places (*Indian Perfum*, 1977, **21**, 15; 1979, **23**, 75).

C. verum Presl syn. *C. zeylancium* Blume

Eng.–*Ceylon cinnamon, true cinnamon* or *cinnamon*.

Leaves and stem ext., inhibitory against Ehrlich ascites tumour cells (*Philipp J Sci*, 1964, **93**, 57).

Bark—minor constituent of Unani compn. '*Jawarish Jalinoos*' used in gastro-enterological complaints [*J Res Indian Med*, 1979, **14**(3 & 4), 34]; and of Ayurvedic drug '*Vyaghri Haritaki*'(*J Nat Integ Med Assoc*, 1980, **22**, 229); cinnamon (inner bark of shoots) used in med. preparation as flu-preventive, indig. and flatulence control, etc. Bark, used in mouthwashes, gargles, combination of herbal teas for taste and antisep. ability; tincture (diluted) to control profuse menstrual flow (Herbal Med., 46-48, 144; 120, 165).

Essent. oil—from bark, known as 'Cinnamon oil' of commerce inhibitory to aflatoxin production (*J Food Sci*, 1977, **42**, 1107); inhibitory effect on pathogenic and nonpathogenic fungi. Leaf oil, antifung.; in combination with other essent. oils, active against *Salmonella typhi* [*Indian Drugs Pharmac Ind*, 1978, **13**(1), 7; 1979, **14**(4), 29; 1980, **15**(6), 7]; oil from leaves, antimicrob. (*Indian Perfum*, 1978, **22**, 118; 1979, **23**, 205); also from seed; and from bark (*Indian J Hosp Pharm*, 1978, **15**, 166; *Indian Drugs*, 1979-80, **17**, 360).

Essent. oil, Indian, chem., rev. (*Perfum Essent Oil Rec*, 1967, **58**, 622); from plant grown in Ghana, constituents (*Planta Med*, 1972, **21**, 416); from leaves, essent. oil, yield 0.49-0.87% with eugenol content, 28-98% (*Indian Perfum*, 1978, **22**, 187); volat. compds. from leaf, stembark, and rootbark oils (*J Agric Food Chem*, 1978, **26**, 822). In steam volatile bark oils, cinnamaldehyde as major constituent; in leaf oils, eugenol as major; root bark oil, camphor as major, Chem. compn. of individual oils vary with geographical origin, harvesting practice, distillation method and in case of bark, and its quality; constituents; rev. (Purseglove *et al*, I, 100-73).

Str. of polyhyroxylated pentacyclic diterp. cinnzeylanine & cinnzeylanol from bark; both compds. insectic. (*Agric Biol Chem*, 1976, **40**, 2305; 1977, **41**, 1779); str. of latter; cinnzeylanine-OAc, isolation and str. (*Chem Pharm Bull*, 1980, **28**, 1432; *Acta Crystallogr*, 1977, **33B**, 623).

CIPADESSA (*Meliaceae*)

*****C. baccifera** (Roth.) Miq. syn. *C. fruticosa* Blume

H.–*Nalbila*; Kan.–*Chitundi*; Oriya–*Nahalbeli*.

Roots for killing tapeworms (Bressers, 27). EtOH(50%) ext. of aerial parts, spasmol.(*Indian J Exp Biol*, 1969, **7**, 250).

Found in Peninsular India, Bihar, Orissa and in Eastern Himalayas up to 1,500 m.

CIRSIUM (*Asteraceae*)

C. arvense (Linn.) Scop. syn. *Cnicus arvensis* Hoffm.

EtOH(50%) ext. of plant, spasmol. and hypoten. (*Indian J Exp Biol*, 1969, **7**, 250). Root paste used as diur. (*Bull Med Ethno Bot Res*, 1980, **1**, 318).

Plant, alkanes, triterp. and hydrocarbon (*Trans Ill State Acad Sci*, 1971, **64**, 300; *CA*, 1972, **77**, 16569t); glucuronides of apigenin and acacetin; leaves, flavon., linarin (*Khim Prir Soedin*, 1972, **8**, 240; 1977, **13**, 282; *CA*, **77**, 58854n; **87**, 114617h); plant taraxasterol, its -OAc and stigmasterol (*Phytochemistry*, 1972, **11**, 2267); tricin- 5-O-glucd. and other flavons. (*ibid*, 1974, **13**, 2320). Coagulating and proteolytic properties of papainase (*Rocz Inst Przem Mlecz*, 1974, **16**, 47; *CA*, 1975, **83**, 95044t).

Flowers, Me-kaempferol (*Khim Prir Soedin*, 1972, **8**, 118; *CA*, **77**, 85580b); kaempferol, apigenin and luteolin (*Fitokhim Izuch Flory BSSR Issled Lek Prep*, 1975, 95; *CA*, 1978, **88**, 186100c).

Root contains phototoxic compd. (*Phytochemistry*, 1975, **14**, 2007).

*C. wallichii Hook.f. syn. *Cnicus wallichii* Hook.f.

EtOH(50%) ext. of flowers, spasmol. and antivir. (*Indian J Exp Biol*, 1968, **6**, 232).

Cnicin, bitter principle present in plant is a sesquiterp. lactone of germacrane type (*Tetrahedron Lett*, 1969, 293; *J Chem Soc Chem Commun*, 1970, 148); cnicin & its hydrolysis products; test for cytotoxic and antibiot. activity (*Planta Med*, 1976, **29**, 179).

Ranikhet, U.P.

*C. wallichii DC. var. wightii Hook.f. syn. *Cnicus wallichii* DC. var. *wightii* Host. EtOH(50%) ext. of aerial parts, effect on CNS (*Indian J Exp Biol*, 1971, **9**, 91). Found in Himachal Pradesh.

CISSAMPELOS (*Menispermaceae*)

C. pareira Linn. var. **hirsuta** Forman syn. *C. hirsuta* Buch.-Ham. ex DC.

Root—employed in leucor., gonor.; also in chr. inflam. of bladder. Decoct. given in enlarged spleen; in Paraguay, for abortion (*Econ Bot*, 1965, **19**, 239; 1977, **31**, 302); lowers B.P. (*Q J Crude Drug Res*, 1970, **10**, 1555); ext., hypoglyc. in animals [*J Res Indian Med*, 1979, **14**(3 & 4), 159]. Pounded root internally in indign. and headache (*Nagarjun*, 1980-81, **24**, 1).

Leaves—juice in eye troubles; plaster of crushed leaves, applied on various skin ailments, burns and wounds (*Econ Bot*, 1971, **25**, 421; *J Econ Tax Bot*, 1980, **1**, 138); purific. (*Khadi Gramodyog*, 1972-73, **19**, 271); chewed in fever; crushed ones applied on forehead in cold and fever (*Bull Med Ethno Bot Res*, 1980, **1**, 8; *J Econ Tax Bot*, 1981, **2**, 184).

Plant—various plant parts in fever, epilepsy, mad convuls., delirium febris, haemat., gravel, cholera and broncht.; decoct., in colic and dysen. (*Econ Bot*, 1970, **24**, 241; *Bull Med Ethno Bot Res*, 1980, **1**, 8).

Hayatine (*dl*-bebeerine) — as methiodide isolated from roots, a potent neuromuscular blocking agent; estn. in blood and urine; nontoxic under tested conditions; extensive pharmacol. of metho salts (*Indian J Exp Biol*, 1964, **2**, 129; 134; 1973, **11**, 89). Action of hayatine deriv. on CNS of cats and dogs (*Arch Int Pharmacodyn*, 1964, **152**, 106; *CA*, 1965, **62**, 8275b); major component of alk. fraction in roots collected from Kashmir. Clin studies showed that it is *c*. one-third as potent as tubocurarine and duration of activity was of equal extent, at equipotent doses (*in* Wagner & Wolff, 216). Str. & stereochem. of hayatine (*J Org Chem* 1967, **32**, 819).

Rootbark contains in its aq. ext. 11 quaternary alks. including menismine, cissamine, pareirine, *d*-isochondrodendrine, *l*-bebeerine, hayatine; and hayatinine, str. & stereochem. (*Chem Ber*, 1964, **97**, 2732; *Indian J Chem*, 1967, **5**, 102).

Roots, *l*-curine (*Lloydia*, 1965, **28**, 191). Spectroscopic detn. of str. of cissamine chloride obtained from roots; identical with cyclanoline chloride (*Experientia*, 1968, **24**, 999). Alks. of *Menispermaceae*, rev.; roots from Ghana plant, alks., dicentrine, its dihydro deriv., cycleanine, insularine and isochondodendrine (*Phytochemistry*, 1968, **9**, 157; 1975, **14**, 2520).

Roots, essent. oil (0.2%) containing thymol (*Perfum Essent Oil Rec*, 1967, **58**, 622).

Plant yields alk. cissampareine; alk. inhibitory against human carcinoma cells of the nasopharynx in cell culture (*J Pharm Sci*, 1965, **54**, 580); str. of cissampareine (*J Am Chem Soc*, 1966, **88**, 4212). Plant, (+)-4"-OMe-curine (*J Chem Soc C*, 1966, 615). Leaves yield cycleanine, *l*-bebeerine, hayatidine, hayatinine, hayatine and *d*-quercitol (*Sci Cult*, 1972, **38**, 358). Alk. *dl*-curine dimethiodide (Daijisong) from plant, effective as muscle relaxant, clin. use (*Huo Hsueh Hsueh Pao*, 1980, **38**, 567; *CA*, 1981, **94**, 127204r).

CISSUS (*Vitaceae*)

C. adnata Roxb. syn. *Vitis adnata* Wall.

Various plant parts used in bone fracture, swelling, sores, wounds, syphilis, ulcer, diar. and dysen., and menor. (*Econ Bot*, 1970, **24**, 241).

*C. discolor Blume syn. *Vitis discolor* Dalz.

EtOH(50%) ext. of plant, diur. (*Indian J Exp Biol*, 1974, **12**, 512).

Maharashtra.

C. quadrangula Linn. syn. *Vitis quadrangula* Wall.

EtOH(50%) ext. of aerial parts. hypoten.; of stem, diur. (*Indian J Exp Biol*, 1969, **7**, 250; 1980, **18**, 594). Stem pulp

useful in eye diseases and chr. ulcers (*Indian Drugs*, 1977-78, **15**, 145). Herb, antifung. (*Acta Bot Indica*, 1979, **7**, 147). Root decoct. useful in dysen. and in digest. disorders (*J Econ Tax Bot*, 1981, **2**, 176).

Healing of bone fractures in humans (*Indian J Pharm*, 1962, **24**, 190). Herb ext. on parenteral administration neutralized antianabolic effect of cortisone in healing of fractures of rabbits; beneficial in bone fractures; biochem. and histopathological studies of bone healing properties (*Indian J Med Res*, 1963, **51**, 667; 1964, **52**, 480; 1975, **63**, 824; 1976, **64**, 1365).

Herb yields an anabolic oxo-steroid which accelerated fracture healing in rats; action similar to durabolin; mode of action in bone fractures [*Life Sci*, 1965, **4**, 317; *J Res Indian Med*, 1970, 4(2), 132; 1972, 7(4), 29]. Plant, β- sitosterol (*Indian J Chem*, 1966, **4**, 457); study of steroids (*Curr Sci*, 1966, **35**, 317).

*C. repanda Vahl

Tuber is pounded fine and applied to folliculosis (*Econ Bot*, 1965, **19**, 240). Paste of bark applied externally in fractures (*Bull Med Ethno Bot Res*, 1980, **1**, 8).

Bastar, M.P. and Pithoragarh, U.P.

C. repens Lamk syn. *Vitis repens* Wight & Arn.

EtOH(50%) ext. of plant, diur. (*Indian J Exp Biol*, 1977, **15**, 208). Root paste, and also leaf juice given in dog bites (*Bull Bot Surv India*, 1980, **22**, 164).

C. setosa Roxb. syn. *Vitis setosa* Wall.

Tel.–*Barubutsali.*

Every plant part, exceedingly acrid (Lindley, 65). EtOH(50%) ext. of aerial parts, antibiot. hypoten. and spasmol. (*Indian J Exp Biol*, 1968, **6**, 232).

*C. trilobata Lamk

EtOH(50%) ext. of aerial parts, diur. (*Indian J Exp Biol*, 1974, **12**, 512).

Reported from Maharashtra.

CISTANCHE (*Orobanchaceae*)

C. tubulosa Wight syn. *Phelipaea calotropidis* Walp.

Aq. ext. of plant used against piles (*J Agric Trop Bot Appl*, 1966, **13**, 277). EtOH(50%) ext., anticancer and hyperten. (*Indian J Exp Biol*, 1980, **18**, 594).

CITHAREXYLUM (*Verbenaceae*)

*C. subserratum Sweet

Flowers, very fragrant (Santapau & Henry, 40).

EtOH(50%) ext. of aerial parts, antiinflam. (*Indian J Exp Biol*, 1977, **15**, 208).

A flavone glucd. from leaves (*Phytochemistry*, 1976, **15**, 838).

Native of America, planted in Indian gardens for ornament.

CITRULLUS (*Cucurbitaceae*)

C. colocynthis Schrad.

Eng.–*Colosynth, bitter apple.*

Fruits—dried pulp of ripe fruit forms commercial drug colosynth, freed from rind, drastic hydrogogue, cath. and providing large watery evacuation; in large doses, causes violent gripping, prostration and sometimes bloody discharges. In moderate doses, as an adjuvant to other cath. Small fruits taken out during rainy season and stuffed with common salt and *Ajwain*, a cure for acute stomach-ache (*J Agric Trop Bot Appl*, 1966, **13**, 274). In Unani med., used in *kala-azar* (*J Nat Integ Med Assoc*, 1978, **20**, 19). Hypoglyc. in rabbits [*J Res Indian Med*, 1979, **14**, (3-4), 159].

Elaterin glucd. (*Bombay Technol*, 1962, **12**, 133). Fruits, elaterin (cucurbitacin E), elatericin B (cucurbitacin I) & dihydroelatericin B (cucurbitacin L). Smooth muscle and cardiovascular pharmacol. of α-elaterin 2-*d*- glucopyranoside (coloside A) from fruit pulp (*J Pharm Sci*, 1967, **56**, 1665). Estn. of cucurbitacins (*Indian J Pharm*, 1970, **32**, 10). Choline and 2 alks. from different plant parts; also glycd. (*Planta Med*, 1973, **24**, 260; 1974, **26**,

293). Cucurbitacins from fruit and leaves (*Indian J Chem*, 1979, **17B**, 417).

Fruit peal, hepatacosan-1-ol (*J Chem Soc*, 1965, 3488); alkanes, ketone, etc.; waxes and essent. oil; their constituents (*Dokl Bolg Akad Nauk*, 1980, **33**, 811; 1981, **34**, 529; 55; *CA*, 1981, **94**, 61790v; **95**, 93822u; 3434s; *C R Acad Bulg Sci*, 1981, **34**, 55; 529); constituents (*Fitoterapia*, 1981, **52**, 9; 13; 17; 19).

Seed oil, citrullonal and a OH-ketotetracyclic triterp. (*Dokl Bolg Akad Nauk*, 1975, **28**, 1641; *CA*, 1976, **85**, 33212d).

C. lanatus (Thunb.) Mats. & Nakai var. **fistulosus** V.J. Nair syn. *C. vulgaris* Schrad.

Eng.–*Watermelon.*

Fruits, laxt.; seed, diur. (*Econ Bot*, 1971, **25**, 245; 1975, **28**, 324). Seeds given in impotency [*J Res Indian Med*, 1977, **12**(4), 53]. Fruit antisep. in typhus fever; useful in gonor. and other urinary affections, hepatic congestion and intestinal catarrah [*Indian Fmrs Dig*, 1978, **11**(6 & 7), 80].

Fruit, detn. of ferulic, caffeic and chlorogenic acids (*Z Lebensm Unters Forsch*, 1966, **132**, 193; *CA*, 1967, **66**, 45594a); cucurbitacins (*Tetrahedron*, 1975, **31**, 1561); characteristics of cucurbitin (*Eur J Biochem*, 1980, **103**, 577); folic acid content (*Invest Clin Suppl*, 1979, **3**, 50; *CA*, 1980, **93**, 219570q); epicarp, serine-OAc (*Chem Pharm Bull*, 1979, **27**, 2484).

Essent. oil from pulp and peelings, characteristics (*Flavour Ind*, 1971, **2**, 305). Volat. constituents (*Nippon Shokuhin Kogyo Gakkai-Shi*, 1969, **16**, 474; *CA*, 1971, **74**, 2847h); 3,6-nonadien-1-ol; volat. constituents (*Phytochemistry*, 1974, **13**, 1167; 1975, **14**, 2637).

Pollen flavons. (*Experientia*, 1980, **36**, 1136).

CITRUS (*Rutaceae*)

Biflavons.—from *Citrus* spp., most commonly encountered higher plant exts. used in 1973 (*in* Wagner & Wolff, 4). Med.

aspects , rev., 97 refs. (*ACS Symp Ser*, 1980, **143**, 43; *CA*, 1981, **94**, 45870r).

C. aurantifolia(Christm.) Swingle syn. *C. medica* Linn. var. *acida* Hook.f.

Eng.–*Lime.*

Plant—used against syphilis (*Econ Bot*, 1970, **24**, 241). EtOH(50%) ext. of aerial parts, CNS depress. and diur. (*Indian J Exp Biol*, 1977, **15**, 208). Used in fractures (*Sri Lanka For*, 1980, **14**, 145).

Leaves—used in filariasis; a constituent of tea for cold (*Econ Bot*, 1974, **28**, 26; 1975, **29**, 318).

Fruit—in Samoa, used against skin irrit. and in nausea; juice for sores in throat, and in eye complaints. Decoct. to alleviate cough (*ibid*, 1977, **31**, 354). Exts. of skin and seeds, antibact. [*Indian Drugs Pharmac Ind*, 1980, **15**(3), 39].

Essent. oil—from peel, highly toxic to eggs and larvae of Caribbean fruit fly [*Agric Res USDA*, 1978, **27**(4), 3]; antimicrob. (*Herba Pol*, 1980, **26**, 245; *Fitoterapia*, 1980, **51**, 201).

Essent. oils, Indian, chem., rev. (*Perfum Essent Oil Rec*, 1967, **58**, 622); psoralens and substituted coumarins from oil (*Phytochemistry*, 1967, **6**, 585); constituents (*J Agric Food Chem*, 1972, **20**, 1029).

Seeds contain bitter compd. limonin (*Phytochemistry*, 1966, **5**, 367).

Citrus fungistatic flavones, tangeretin & nobiletin absent from leaves (*ibid*, 1971, **10**, 2657).

C. aurantium Linn.

Eng.–*Sour/bitter orange, Seville* or *bigarade orange.*

Plant—used against enlarged spleen, stomachache and menor. (*Econ Bot*, 1970, **24**, 241); ext., antisp. (*Planta Med*, 1980, **40**, 309). Screening for antitumour activity (*Shoyakugaku Zasshi*, 1979, **33**, 95). Used in fractures (*Sri Lanka For*, 1980, **14**, 145). Boiled aq. ext., carcinogenic (*J Nat Cancer Inst*, 1971, **46**, 1131).

Leaves—used as tea in headache and stomach pain (*Econ Bot*, 1971, **25**, 240).

Ext., antibact. [*Indian Drugs Pharmac Ind*, 1977, **12**(3), 21].

Essent. oil—antifung.; antimicrob. (*Flavour Ind*, 1972, **3**, 368; 1970, **1**, 725; *Herba Pol*, 1980, **26**, 245; *Fitoterapia*, 1980, **51**, 201; *Parfuem Kosmet*, 1980, **61**, 255).

Pharmacol. of pressor action; of active principles (*Kexue Tongbao*, 1978, **23**, 58; 1980, **25**, 616). Crude ext. of plant and its active principles synephrine and N-Metyramine, mech. of hyperten. and antishock effects (*Acta Pharm Sin*, 1980, **15**, 71); effect on cardiovascular receptors (*ibid*, 1981, **16**, 253).

Dried peels, nobiletin (*Indian J Chem*, 1964, **2**, 562); fungistatic flavones tangeretin & nobiletin present in leaves yet *C. aurantium* susceptible to fungal attack (*Phytochemistry*, 1971, **10**, 2657); naringin (*Ann Chem Warsaw*, 1966, **691**, 186; *CA*, **64**, 14582d).

Peel, cirantin, identical with hesperidin, antifert. activity [*Phytochemistry*, 1968, **7**, 1881; *J Res Indian Med*, 1973, **8**(3), 79]; methoxylated flavones, max. in peel (*Arch Pharm Wein*, 1968, **301**, 785; *CA*, 1969, **70**, 22862e). Flavons. of fruits (*Tr Prikl Bot Genet Sel*, 1972, **48**, 114). Hesperidin extn. from rind (Fr Pat., 1973, 2165213; *CA*, 1974, **80**, 68524f); source of neohesperidin (*Econ Bot*, 1976, **30**, 38).

Essent. oil constituents (*Bioquim Quim Farm*, 1977, **20**, 69; *CA*, 1979, **91**, 181256k). HPLC of peel oil (*J Agric Food Chem*, 1979, **27**, 1334).

Flowers, flavon. glycds, neohesperidin and naringin (*Nippon Nogei Kagaku Kaishi*, 1961, **35**, 942; *CA*, 1964, **60**, 11044a); β-sitosterol (32.74% of nonsap. matter) (*Fitoterapia*, 1980, **51**, 207).

Seeds, bitter compds. limonin and de-Ac-nomilin; isolimonic acid and other compds. (*Phytochemistry*, 1966, **5**, 367; 1980, **19**, 2417).

Roots, xanthyletin (*ibid*, 1969, **9**, 2069).

C. bergamia Risso & Poit. syn. *C. aurantium* Linn. var. *bergamia*
Eng.–*Bergamot orange.*

Steroid fraction from citrus fruit, cortisone like antiinflam. in rats and guinea pigs (*Rend Accad Sci Fis Mat Naples*, 1968, **35**, 121; *CA*, 1971, **75**, 3655b).

Bergamot and its oil, rev., 41 refs. (*Perfum Essent Oil Rec*, 1966, **57**, 18). Bergamot essence, minor constituents of antibaldness scalp-treating lotions (Fr. Demande, 1971, 2070045; *CA*, 1972, **77**, 9595v). Citral, antibact. and antifung. [*J Sci Res Bhopal* 1980, **2**(2), 83].

Leaf, essent. oil compn. (*Proc Natl Sci Counc Repub China*, 1981, **5**, 278; *CA*, **95**, 111798x).

C. grandis (Linn.) Osbeck syn. *C. decumana* Linn. syn. *C. maxima* (Burm.) Merrill

Peel flavons. (*Bull Nat Inst Sci India*, 1965, No. 31, 63).

C. hystrix DC.

Eng.–*Mauritius papeda, porcupine papeda.*

Seeds yield limonin and de-Ac-nomilin (*Phytochemistry*, 1966, **5**, 367). Leaf and peel oil, constituents (*ibid*, 1971, **10**, 1404).

C. japonica Thunb.; see **Fortunella japonica**

C. limetta Risco syn. *C. limettioides* Tanaka; *C. medica* Linn. var. *limetta* Wight & Arn.

Essent. oil, antimicrob. (*Herba Pol*, 1980, **26**, 245; *Fitoterapia*, 1980, **51**, 201).

Bitter principle, rutaevin (*J Org Chem*, 1967, **32**, 3442). Xanthyletin from roots (*Phytochemistry*, 1970, **9**, 2069).

C. limon (Linn.) Burm.f.syn. *C. medica* Linn. var. *limonum*; *C. jambhiri* Lush.; *C. limonis* (Linn.) Burm. f.

Eng.–*Lemon.*

In Europe, used in cough, cold and febrile diseases (*Acta Phytother*, 1971, **18**, 21). Leaves and stems, antibact.; antitumour activity test (*Rev Cuban Farm*, 1980, **14**, 311; 1981, **15**, 71).

Fruit juice, minor constituent of compn. for capillary treatment for hair combating loss and stimulating growth and regrowth

(Fr. Demande, 1971, 2112085; 1972, 2130046; *CA*, 1973, **78**, 62194k; 140404v).

Essent. oil, antimicrob. (*Flavour Ind*, 1970, **1**, 725; *Herba Pol*, 1980, **26**, 245; *Fitoterapia*, 1980, **51**, 201; 1980, **61**, 255).

Peel flavons. (*Bull Nat Inst Sci India*, 1965, No. 31, 63); limocitrol & iso deriv.; tangeretin, as also β-sitosterol (*Tetrahedron*, 1964, **20**, 2312; 1965, **21**, 1441); naringin (*Ann Chem*, 1966, **691**, 186; *CA*, **64**, 14582d). Analg. effect of lemoran in rats (*Farmakol Toksikol Moscow*, 1966, **29**, 394). Peel, hesperidin (1.06-2.84 g/kg); fruit, flavons. (*Rev Agroquim Technol Aliment*, 1970, **10**, 150; 1974, **14**, 100; *CA*, **73**, 63219g; **81**, 134795u); juice, flavonone glycd.(*J Agric Food Chem*, 1971, **19**, 513).

Essent. oil from fruit peel, bergamotine (*Plant Med Phytother*, 1978, **12**, 112). HPLC of peel oils for coumarins and psoralens (*J Agric Food Chem*, 1979, **27**, 1334). Distribution of coumarins in plant parts (*Pharmazie*, 1981, **36**, 569).

Leaf essent. oil, compn. (*Bull Brew Sci*, 1970, **16**, 1; *CA*, **75**, 16080k); oil components (*Rev Bras Frutic*, 1978, **1**, 63; *CA*, 1979, **90**, 200357s); major compds., limonene, 32.4 and β-ocimene, 7.3% (*Khim Prir Soedin*, 1981, 803; *J Agric Food Chem*, 1981, **29**, 490).

Seeds, bitter principles, obacunone and limonin (*Phytochemistry*, 1966, **5**, 367).

Roots contain xanthyletin, stigmasterol & β- sitosterol (*Phytochemistry*, 1970, **9**, 2069; *Taiwan Yao Hsuesh Tsa Chih*, 1972, **24**, 6; *CA*, 1974, **81**, 23072m).

C. medica Linn. syn. *C. medica* var. *medica* Watt

Eng.–*Citron.*

Fruit, astrin. (*Q J Crude Drug Res*, 1972, **12**, 1922); given in whooping cough and broncht. to children; juice alongwith other plant ingredients used in insanity (*Nagarjun*, 1979-80, **23**, 10; 1980-81, **24**, 242). Seeds used as antifert. (*Econ Bot*, 1980, **34**, 273).

Plant used against colic and vomiting (*Econ Bot*, 1970, **24**, 241). Med. uses (*J Sci*

Ind Res, 1975, **34**, 644). EtOH(50%) ext. of aerial parts, anticancer (*Indian J Exp Biol*, 1980, **18**, 594).

Fruit juice constituents, rev., 30 refs. (*J Agric Food Chem*, 1966, **14**, 450). Seeds contain obacunone and limonin (*Phytochemistry*, 1966, **5**, 367).

Citrus fungistatic flavones, tangeretin & nobiletin absent from leaves (*ibid*, 1971, **10**, 2657).

Essent. oil, antimicrob. (*Parfuem Kosmet*, 1980, **61**, 255); leaves essent. oil, GLC anal.; ocimene, 17.1, linalool, 11.4, citral B, 49.3%, etc. (*Indian J Pharm*, 1976, **38**, 159).

C. paradisi Macf.

Eng.–*Grapefruit*.

Plant. ext., anticancer in mice (*Chim Acta Turc*, 1981, **9**, 525).

Press residue of seed oil contains toxic factor limonin when mixed with meal may prove toxic to fowl, swine and chicks (Kingsbury, 205-06).

Nootkatone, flavour constituent; from Florida, coumarins (*J Food Sci*, 1964, **29**, 565; 1965, **30**, 869). Coumarins (*Tetrahedron*, 1966, **22**, 1489; 1967, **23**, 2523). Sesquiterp. alc., paradisiol from grapefruit peel oil (*J Org Chem*, 1971, **36**, 2422). Peel oil, coumarins and psoralens; HPLC anal. (*Phytochemistry*, 1979, **18**, 500; (*J Agric Food Chem*, 1972, **20**, 100; 1979, **27**, 1334). Essent. oil constituents, rev. [*Perfum Flav Int*, 1979-80, 4(1), 48].

Fruit juice and pulp, bitter principle, limonin (*J Food Sci*, 1965, **30**, 8740; limonoic acid, nonbitter (*Phytochemistry*, 1969, **8**, 243).

Apigenin-7 glucd. (*J Food Sci*, 1963, **28**, 195). Seasonal variation of naringin and other flavones (*ibid*, 1966, **31**, 542); extn. of naringin (USSR Pat., 1970, 261166; *CA*, **73**, 2838k); fruits and leaves, dihydrokaempferol; twigs, naringenin and kaempferol; leaves, apigenin-7-rutinoside (*Phytochemistry*, 1967, **6**, 763; 1968, **7**, 1653). Flavons., tangeretin & nobiletin from leaves, fungistatic probably due to high degree of methylation (*ibid*, 1971, **10**, 2657).

Peel, triterps. (*Biochem J*, 1965, **96**, 31P). Principal flavon. glycds.; and sterol of endocarp and peel (*Phytochemistry*, 1967, **6**, 1127; 1137). Peel pectin as plasma substitute (*Yao Hsueh Tung Pao*, 1981, **16**, 54; *CA*, **95**, 138467a).

Seeds, obacunone, limonin and de-Acnomilin; isolimonic acid (*Phytochemistry*, 1966, **5**, 367; 1980, **19**, 2417). Seed oil sterols (*J Am Oil Chem Soc*, 1972, **49**, 85).

Roots contain xanthyletin (*Phytochemistry*, 1970, **9**, 2069).

C. reticulata Blanco syn. *C. aurantium* var. *aurantium*, proper (in part).

Eng.–*Mandarin orange, orange*.

Exts. of fruit skin and seeds, antibact. [*Indian Drugs Pharmac Ind*, 1980, **15**(3), 39]. Essent. oil, antimicrob. (*Herba Pol*, 1980, **26**, 245; *Fitoterapia*, 1980, **51**, 201).

Leaf essent. oil of 3 vars. growth in Egypt [*Perfum Flav Int*, 1979-80, 4(2), 27].

Peels, flavons., tangeretin, hesperidin, citromitin, etc. (*Bull Nat Inst Sci India*, 1965, No. 31, 63; *Indian J Chem*, 1967, **5**; 239). Chem. of citrus flavons., rev., 56 refs (*Nippon Shokuhin Kogyo Gakkai-Shi*, 1971, **18**, 38; *CA*, 1972, **76**, 125472f). Peel, 13 flavons. (*Chem Pharm Bull*, 1980, **28**, 717). *Citrus* biflavonoids, most commonly used plant ext. (*in* Wagner & Wolff, 5).

Peels, nobiletin, 5-de-Me-nobiletin, ponkanetin, esculetin deriv., limonin, sterols, etc. (*Taiwan Yao Hsueh Tsa Chih*, 1977, **29**, 1; *CA*, 1979, **90**, 148494t).

Seeds yield obacunone, limonin and de-Ac-nomilin; isolimonic acid (*Phytochemistry*, 1966, **5**, 367; 1980, 19, 2417). Leaves, fungistatic flavones, tangeretin and nobiletin (*ibid*, 1971, **10**, 2657).

C. sinensis (Linn.) Osbeck

Eng.–*Sweet orange*.

Plant used in fractures (*Sri Lanka For*, 1980, **14**, 145).

Essent. oil—of sweet orange, possible carcinogen (*Br J Cancer*, 1959, **13**, 92);

from fruit peel, detergent constituent (Jpn Kokai, 1974, 74109404; *CA*, 1975, **82**, 100611m); antimicrob. [*Herba Pol*, 1980, **26**, 245; *Fitoterapia*, 1980, **51**, 201; *Indian Drugs Pharmac Ind*, 1980, **15**(3), 39]; against keratinophilic microorganism (*Indian Drugs*, 1978- 79, **16**, 43).

Press residue from seed oil extn. when used in meal proves toxic at certain levels to certain fowl, swine and chicks due to a toxic factor, a carbohydrate (?) (Kingsbury, 205-06).

Seeds, bitter compds., obacunone, limonin, and de-Ac-nomilin (*Phytochemistry*, 1966, **5**, 367). Fruits, nonbitter lactone limonoic acid (*ibid*, 1969, **8**, 243); coumarins (*Dokl Akad Nauk SSSR*, 1973, **208**, 1484; *CA*, **78**, 15018g); peel oil, HPLC (*J Agric Food Chem*, 1979, **27**, 1334).

Peel flavone, rutinosides (*Bull Nat Inst Sci India*, 1965, No.31, 78); naringin (*Ann Chem Warsaw*, 1966, **691**, 86; *CA*, **64**, 14582d). Sap flavons.; fruit flavons. of different vars. (*Rev Agroquim Technol Aliment*, 1970, **10**, 571; 1974, **14**, 271; 561; *CA*, 1971, **74**, 121341y; 1975, **82**, 2986t; **83**, 4974g). Flavones tangeretin & nobiletin, fungistatic; plant flavons. (*Phytochemistry*, 1971, **10**, 2657; 1972, **11**, 2283).

Roots xanthyletin, stigmasterol & β-sitosterol (*ibid*, 1970, **9**, 2069; *Taiwan Yao Hsueh Tsa Chih*, 1972, **24**, 6; *CA*, 1974, **81**, 23072m).

CLADIUM (*Cyperaceae*)

*C. jamaicense Crantz

Tribals of Exumas and Long Island use plant ext. for bathing solution, in chicken pox (*Econ Bot*, 1975, **29**, 324).

Found in Kashmir.

CLAUSENA (*Rutaceae*)

C. excavata Burm. f.

Sap of leaves rubbed on all kinds of muscular pain (*Bull Bot Surv India*, 1976,

18, 166). In traditional use, root decoct. given in malarial fever (*ibid*, 1980, **22**, 59).

Coumarins, clausenin and clausenidin from root and stembark (*J Indian Chem Soc*, 1973, **50**, 753).

*C. heptaphylla Wight & Arn.

Roots contain carbazole alk., heptaphylline (*Tetrahedron Lett*, 1967, 4019); also 2 pyranocoumarins, clausenin & clausenidin (*Tetrahedron*,1967, **23**, 4785); β- sitosterol (*Indian J Chem*, 1967, **5**, 523); root alk. murrayanine and coumarin dentatin; 3-Me-carbazone; alk. murrayacine (*Phytochemistry*, 1973, **12**, 1831; 1974, **13**, 1017; 1976, **15**, 356).

Stem bark contains alk. heptazoline (*J Indian Chem Soc*, 1970, **47**, 1197); isolation and str. of heptazolidine (*Chem Ind Lond*, 1974, 303); 2-Me-anthraquinone (*Phytochemistry*, 1978, **17**, 2043).

Str. of clausenolide isolated from plant (*J Chem Soc Chem Commun*, 1979, 246).

Near Calcutta and in Khasi hills ascending to 1,600 m.

*C. indica Oliv.

EtOH(50%) ext. of aerial parts, hypoten. and spasmol. (*Indian J Exp Biol*, 1974, **12**, 512).

Roots, β-sitosterol; also alk. indizoline (*Indian J Chem*, 1970, **8**, 851; 1974, **12**, 437); furanocoumarins; imperatorin, phellopterin, chalepensin and dihydrofuranocoumarin, chalepin; coumarins including indicolaclonediol (*Phytochemistry*, 1971, **10**, 480; 1978, **17**, 1194); also coumarin, clausindin identical to rutolide (*Experientia*, 1974, **30**, 2231; *J Chem Soc Perkin Trans I*, 1974, 1561). Plant, sesquiterp. clausantalene (*Experientia*, 1975, **13**, 138).

From Western Ghats of Maharashtra to Anaimalai hills.

C. lansium (Lour.) Skeels syn. *C. wampi* Blanco

Leaves contain, β-sitosterol, heptaphylline, lansamide-I and lansine (*Indian J Chem*, 1980, **19B**, 1075).

211

C. pentaphylla (Roxb.) DC.

EtOH(50%) ext. of aerial, spasmol. (*Indian J Exp Biol*, 1977, **15**, 208). Leaf decoct. in cough and cold; root paste in ulcers and liver disorders (*Bull Med Ethno Bot Res*, 1980, **1**, 318).

Aerial parts, a C_{33} terp., OMe-clausenol; roots, clausarin, Me- linolenate, dentatin, clausenidin, β-sitosterol and heptaphylline (*Experientia*, 1977, **33**, 153; 412). Spasmol. terpinic coumarins, clausmarins A & B (*J Chem Soc Chem Commun*, 1978, 281). Aerial parts, method of isolation of coumarin having spasmol. properties (Indian Pat, 1977, 145322; *CA*, 1980, **92**, 153133v).

*C. willdenowii Wight & Arn.

Leaves and twigs, essent. oil; its physicochem. characteristics and constituents (*Perfum Essent Oil Rec*, 1967, **58**, 622). Diclausenan from leaves resolved into 2 isomers diclausenan A & B (*Tetrahedron Lett*, 1976, 1019).

Rootbark, coumarins, imperatorin, dentatin & nordentatin (*Tetrahedron*, 1968, **24**, 753). Root and bark, also 3-(1, 1- di-Me- allyl) xanthyletin (*Indian J Chem*, 1981, **20B**, 88).

Common in Western Peninsula ascending to 1,200 m, and also in Sikkim Himalayas.

CLAVICEPS (*Clavicipitaceae*)

Several alk.-producing strains from *Claviceps* spp. have been isolated; their classification given w.r.t. their biochemical capacities (*in* Atal & Kapur, Med. Plants, 188). See ergot alks (*in* Brossi, XXXVIII, 1-156).

*C. fusiformis Loveless

Feeding in mice inhibited lactation; alk. agroclavine, active principle (*Proc Roy Soc Ser B*, 1968, **170**, 423; *CA*, **69**, 25958f); tryptophan deriv.; clavicipitic acid, its str. (*Tetrahedron Lett*, 1975, 4269; 1973, 215; *J Chem Soc Perkin Trans I*, 1977, 2099); production of tumour-inhibiting clavicepamines (Hung Telges, 1978, 14568; *CA*, **89**, 74205e).

Clavine, chanoclavine and other clavine alkaloides (*in* Atal & Kapur, Med. Plants, 188).

Spotted on grasses and on millets in Bihar and Maharashtra, Mysore (Karnataka) and Hissar (Haryana).

*C. paspali Stev. & Holler

Tremorgenic metabolites from sclerotia (*J Agric Food Chem*, 1977, **25**, 1197).

Ergot alks.—production; indole alks. (US Pat., 1965, 3224945; Ger. Offen. 1972, 2207553; *CA*, 1966, **64**, 7330f; **77**, 156333m; *Helv Chim Acta*, 1966, **49**, 1907; 1974, **57**, 113); production of tumour- inhibiting clavicepamines (Hung. Teljes, 1978, 14568; *CA*, **89**, 74205e); of alks. by submerged fermentation; effect of micronutrients (*Indian Drugs*, 1978-79, **16**, 88; 250). Type of alk. in sclerotia (*Folia Microbiol Prague*, 1969, **14**, 602).

Lysergic acid & its derivs.—formation during development of *C. paspali* (*Nature Lond*, 1964, **202**, 312); lysergic acid-α - OH-Et-amide (*Chim Ind Milan*, 1965, **47**, 611). From submerged culture; production; effect of surfactants; from cultures of fungal stems; by fermentation (*Mikrobiologiya*, 1966, **35**, 606; *CA*, **65**, 17658b; *Appl Microbiol*, 1967, **15**, 1270; *Lloydia*, 1969, **32**, 327; Fr. Pat., 1966, 1463426; Fr. Addn., 1968, 91948; *CA*, 1967, **67**, 84858e; 1969, **71**, 69351y); biogenesis (*Experientia*, 1969, **25**, 926).

A fungus parasitic on grasses and millets.

C. purpurea (Fr.) Tul.

Eng.-*Ergot.*

Ergot—chem. and pharmacol. of ergot, rev., 68 refs.; pharmacol. and its preparations, rev. (*J Soc Cosmet Chem*, 1965, **16**, 369; *CA*, **63**, 8119d; *Pharm Weekbl* 1965, **100**, 1261; *CA*, 1966, **64**, 5662a). Haemostatic; they stimulate contractions of uterus. In high doses, very toxic causing gangrene, violent pains, delirium and death, disease known as St. Anthony's fire in previous centuries (Med. Plants, 21). Ergot, a chameleon among drugs, rev., 47 refs. (*Dtsch Apoth Ztg*, 1980, **120**, 319; *CA*, **92**, 169085a).

Ergot alks.—pharmacol., in migraine, effective drug [*Background Migraine Symp*, *2nd*, 1967, (Pub., 1969), 53; *CA*, 1971, **75**, 97177x]. Ingredients in compn., useful against chr. kidney infection; in treatment of nephrosis (Ger. Offen, 1974, 2311071; Neth. Appl., 1974, 7303795; *CA*, 1975, **82**, 47747g; **83**, 33051j; U.S. Pat., 1974, 3849562; *CA*, 1975, **83**, 152345t; 152387h). Toxicity to young and growing pigs (*Res Vet Sci*, 1977, **22**, 146; *CA*, **87**, 965q). Protective against hypoxic hypoxia in rats (*Gerontology Basel*, 1978, **24**, Suppl. 1, 6; *CA*, **88**, 130859q). Hyperprolactinemia; also parkinsonism treatment (*Fed Proc Fed Am Soc Exp Biol*, 1978, **37**, 2192; 2207). Pharmacol. of ergot alks. in clin. use, rev., 171 refs; clin. pharmacol. rev., 20 refs. [*Pharmacology*, 1978, **16**, Suppl.1, 12; *Med J Aust*, 1978, 2(3 Special Suppls.), 3; *Farumashia*, 1979, **15**, 703; *CA*, **91**, 186249v]. Importance in med., rev., 100 refs. (*Ther Hung*, 1979, **27**, 108). Antiepileptic activity (*Psychropharmacology Berlin*, 1978, **57**, 57). Therapeutic value of brain dopamine receptor agonists including ergot derivs., rev., 15 refs. (*Indian Drugs*, 1980-81, **18**, 240).

Ergot alks. in hypertension and heart rate; in peripheral vascular diseases of atherosclerotic nature, clin. study (*Settim Med*, 1978, **66**, 87; 133; *CA*, 1979, **91**, 49660h; 49663m). Dextro-rotatory alks. more effective in arterial hyperten., heart insufficiency, arrhythmia and cephalalgia (Brit. UK Pat. Appl., 1980, 2025960; *CA*, **93**, 101472f). Antiadrenergic effect (*Acta Pharm Jugosl*, 1981, **31**, 1).

Ergot alks. including chem. (Sim, 88-113; *in* Manske, VIII, 725- 83; XV, 1-40). Biosynth.; tryptophan (*J Org Chem*, 1973, **38**, 2249; *Tetrahedron Lett*, 1974, 2107); rev., 127 ref. (*Alkaloids*, 1975, **15**, 1; *CA*, 1976, **84**, 59796b). Mech. of action, rev.,

33 refs. (*Acta Med Port*, 1980, **2**, 149; *CA*, 1981, **94**, 10777p).

Ergotamine—the peptide alk., still used as uterocontracting in gynaecology; its dihydro deriv. (nongenuine alk.), in migraine (*in* Wagner & Wolff, 272-73; *in* Manske & Holmes, VIII, 774-75); administration of ergotamine & related alks. and clavine alks., causing foetal death/abortion in rats (*in* Plant and Fungal Toxins, 215-16). Production, along with other alks. (Brit. Pat., 1965, 998254; 1969, 1158380; Indian Pat., 1975, 126456; *CA*, **63**, 9026g; **71**, 69349d; 1980, **92**, 135403d); in submerged cultures, also physiology (*Appl Microbiol*, 1967, **15**, 597). Biosynth. (*Biochem J*, 1971, **122**, 58p); sepn. (US Pat., 1975, 3880734; *CA*, **83**, 183386n); simple method of extn. of alk. of ergotamine and ergotoxine group (Eur. Pat. Appl., 1981, 22418; *CA*, **94**, 16274j).

Ergotoxine—group of alks. well-defined mixt. of ergocornine, ergokryptine and ergocristine by combined fermentation (Swiss Pat., 1976, 577556; *CA*, 1977, **86**, 41798k). Hydergine (dihydroergotoxine), used in treatment of cerebral insufficiency. 2-Bromo- α-ergocryptine, new deriv.; used as a prolactin inhibitor; regarded as international standard for dopaminergic stim. and successful in treatment of galactorrhoea and morbus Parkinson (*in* Wagner & Wolff, 273).

Ergolines—unlike peptide alks., do not yield lysergic or isolysergic acid on alkaline hydrolysis (Sim, 104); as potential prolactin and mammary tumour inhibitors (*Lloydia*, 1977, **40**, 90); derivs., biosynth.; their production; by fermentation; derivs., production (Hung. Pat., 1965, 152238; Ger. Offen, 1978, 2637764; Jpn Kokai, 1978, 7838696; US Pat., 1978, 4086141; Ger. East Pat., 1978, 130421; *CA*, **63**, 15509f; **88**, 168514m; **89**, 1954422g; 105907t; 1979, **91**, 18360f). Sepn. of clavine alks. and stabilization of alk. yield from saprophyte cultures (*Acta Pharm Hung*, 1964, **34**, 131; *CA*, **61**, 7082c;

Herba Hung, 1965, **4**, 89); alk. chanoclavine isomers (*Helv Chim Acta*, 1964, **47**, 2186). By virtue of tryptamine particle in its str. on one hand and Ph-Et-amine, eg. dopamine on another, ergoline derivs. can have tryptaminergic (serotoninergic) as well as a dopaminergic effects (*in* Wagner & Wolff, 279).

CLEISTANTHUS (*Euphorbiaceae*)

C. collinus (Roxb.) Benth. & Hook.f.

EtOH(50%) ext. of aerial parts, anticancer (*Indian J Exp Biol*, 1969, **7**, 250).

Bark, lupeol and β-sitosterol (*Leath Sci*, 1965, **12**, 438); glycd. cleristanthin B (*Curr Sci*, 1970, **39**, 395); triterp., lignan lactones and other compds. (*Proc Indian Sci Congr*, 1980, Pt III, 72).

Leaves, lignan lactone collinusin, diphyllin and ellagic acid (*Tetrahedron Lett*, 1967, 3517; 4183); str. of collinusin and cleistanthin (*Tetrahedron* 1969, **25**, 2815); cleistanthin induces significant increase in neutrophilic granulocyte count (NGC) in animals through oral, ip, iv, im and sc routes (*Pharmacology*, 1970, **4**, 347). TLC detection of lignan lactones (*J Chromatogr*, 1975, **107**, 230). A new hydroxy-lignan, wodeshiol, also dihydrocubebin and glucopyranoside of diphyllin (*Tetrahedron Lett*, 1975, 2961).

Heartwood, new diphyllin glycd.; named cleistanthin C (*Phytochemistry*, 1975, **14**, 1875; *Indian J Chem*, 1977, **15B**, 10).

Unsap. fraction of fruits, lupeol and β-sitosterol (*Curr Sci*, 1965, **34**, 179). Seed oil compn. [*J Oil Technol Assoc India*, 1977, **9**(4), 156].

*C. malabaricus Muell.-Arg.

EtOH(50%) ext. of aerial parts, hypoten. and diur. (*Indian J Exp Biol*, 1974, **12**, 512).

Jogfall, Karnataka.

CLEMATIS (*Ranunculaceae*)

Spp. of genus, generally acrid and raise blisters when applied in fresh state but not on drying or exposure to heat (Lindley, 1).

*C. buchaniana DC.

EtOH(50%) ext. of aerial parts, antivir. and spasmol. (*Indian J Exp Biol*, 1969, **7**, 250).

Shimla, H. P.

C. gouriana Roxb. ex DC.

EtOH(50%) ext of aerial parts, antivir. (*Indian J Exp Biol*, 1968, **6**, 232). Fungitoxic properties of plant ext. (*Geobios*, 1978, **5**, 49). Volat. vapours from leaves, antifung. (*Indian Perfum*, 1979, **23**, 61; *Indian J Mycol Plant Pathol*, 1979, **9**, 250; *Acta Bot Indica*, 1979, **7**, 147).

Leaf ext. yields protoanemonin; compd. more active than several commercial fungicides; also a strong fungitoxic compd. (*Indian Phytopathol*, 1976, **29**, 488; 1977, **30**, 577).

*C. hedysarifolia DC.

Root decoct. given in worms. Leaf paste applied on head in hemicrania (*Bull Med Ethno Bot Res*, 1980, **1**, 8).

Gujarat.

*C. montana Buch.-Ham. ex DC.

EtOH(50%) ext. of aerial parts, spasmol., diur. and antiinflam. (*Indian J Exp Biol*, 1977, **15**, 208).

Chamoli, U.P.

C. napaulensis DC.

Leaves, deleterious to skin, vesic.; used in blood diseases, and leprosy (*Indian Drugs*, 1976-77, **14**, 47).

C. orientalis Linn. syn. *C. graveolens* Lindl.

Aerial parts, ranunculin and an aglycone (*Farm Zh Kiev*, 1964, **19**, 59; *CA*, **61**, 8625a). Plant, 10 triterp. glycds. including vitalboside F, as major one (*Khim Prir Soedin*, 1974, **10**, 256; *CA*, **81**, 74891k). Triterp. saponins, flavon., coumarin deriv. of γ -lactone, etc. detected in aerial parts and also in roots; roots contain 5 or more glycds. of oleanolic acid and hederagenin

(*Izv Akad Nauk Gruz SSR Ser Khim*, 1979, **5**, 307; *CA*, 1980, **93**, 3920f).

C. triloba Heyne ex Roth

EtOH(50%) ext. of plant, hypoten. and spasmol. (*Indian J Exp Biol*, 1973, **11**, 43).

CLEOME (*Cleomaceae*)

C. chelidonii Linn. f.

Fresh flowers, rutin (*Curr Sci*, 1965, **34**, 246).

C. gynandra Linn. syn. *C. pentaphylla* Linn. *Gynandropsis gynandra* Briq. *G. pentaphylla* DC.

Leaves—remedy for muscular pain, headache and intestinal wounds (*J Agric Trop Bot Appl*, 1966, **13**, 256). Leaf juice, and seed oil used to cure skin diseases (*Econ Bot*, 1978, **32**, 280).

Seeds—applied as poultice to sores having maggots; and given as infusion in cough (*J Agric Trop Bot Appl*, 1966, **13**, 256); powd., good remedy for piles, clin. study [*J Res Indian Med*, 1978, **13**(3), 104].

Plant—EtOH(50%) ext., anticancer and spasmol. (*Indian J Exp Biol*, 1968, **6**, 232); in eye complaints and wounds (*Econ Bot*, 1970, **24**, 241). Used in skeletal fractures (*Sri Lanka For*, 1980, **14**, 145).

Seeds, unsaturated viscosic acid (0.1%), a flavone, viscosin (0.04%), etc. Herb and seeds yield essent. oil similar to garlic or mustard oil (Chopra *et al*, I, 173-74).

Seeds contain glucocapparin (*Phytochemistry*, 1963, **2**, 29); and hexacosanol, kaempferol, β-sitosterol & its glucd. (*Indian J Pharm*, 1968, **30**, 127).

C. vahliana Farsen syn. *C. brachycarpa* Vahl ex DC.

Plant used to cure worms in camel's nose (*J Econ Tax Bot*, 1980, **1**, 138).

C. viscosa Linn. syn. *C. icosandra* Linn.; *Polanisia icosandra* Wight & Arn.

Eng.–*Wild mustard.*

Leaves—useful in fever (also plant juice or pulp), paratyphoid, dysen., broncht., gonor., etc. (*J Agric Trop Bot Appl*, 1966,

13, 257). Leaf ext., strong antifung. (*Indian Phytopathol*, 1968, **21**, 445). Juice to remove pus esp. from ear (*Econ Bot*, 1978, **32**, 280); infusion with garlic, poured into nostrils as a cure for headache (*J Econ Tax Bot*, 1981, **2**, 184).

Plant pulp, beneficial in plague and fever (*J Agric Trop Bot Appl*, 1966, **13**, 257); juice in fever (*Sachitra Ayurveda*, 1977-78, **30**, 960); plant used in fractures (*Sri Lanka For*, 1980, **14**, 145).

Seeds—used in piles and for removing round worms and other worms (*J Agric Trop Bot Appl*, 1966, **13**, 257); used internally in fever and diar. (*Bull Bot Surv India*, 1973, **15**, 13); also used in infantile convuls. (*Nagarjun*, 1980- 81, **24**, 263).

Bark, irrit., acrid, rubft., vesic. (*Nagarjun*, 1980-81, **24**, 263). In USA, roots used as vermifuge (*Bull Bot Soc Bengal*, 1975, **29**, 97).

Whole plant, new glycoflavanone (*Curr Sci*, 1979, **48**, 430); new naringenin glycd. (*Phytochemistry*, 1979, **18**, 2057). A novel diterp. lactone, eleomeolide; its str. (*J Am Chem Soc*, 1979, **101**, 4720; *Tetrahedron*, 1980, **36**, 3489).

Chem., nutritional and toxicol. evaluation of seed oil (*Indian J Med Res*, 1978, **67**, 604).

Seeds contain novel umbelliferone deriv., cleosandrin (*Indian J Chem*, 1979, **17B**, 438); coumarinolignoid, cleomiscosin A (*Tetrahedron Lett*, 1980, **21**, 4477).

Roots, 3-glucuronides of kaempferide & dihydro and docasanoic (*Phytochemistry*, 1979, **18**, 691; *Chem Scr*, 1979, **13**, 24); naringenin 4'-galactoside and dihydrokaempferol - 4' - xyloside; dihyerorobinetin pyranoside (*Indian J Chem*, 1979, **17B**, 300; 1980, **19B**, 715); new glycd., xyloside of OH-yethanoic acid, lupeol, betulin, betulinic acid, β-amyrin and β- sitosterol (*Proc Indian Sci Congr*, 1981, Pt. III, 77).

CLERODENDRON (*Verbenaceae*)

See CLERODENDRUM

CLERODENDRUM (*Verbenaceae*)

*C. colebrookianum Walp.

Nagaland–*Hinchang.*

Young leaves useful anthelm. (*Bull Bot Surv India*, 1976, **18**, 166).

Roots contain triacontane, clerodin, (24*S*)-Et-cholesta-5, 22, 25- triene-3 β-ol, α-amyrin, β-sitosterol and clerodolone (*Planta Med*, 1979, **37**, 64).

Found in Mikir hills of Assam, and also in Nagaland.

C. indicum (Linn.) Kuntze syn. *C. lerodendron siphonanthus* C.B. Clarke

Used in fever, atrophy, emaciation of cachexy, gravel, cholera, consumption, cough, broncht. and blindness (*Econ Bot,* 1970, **24**, 241). Fruit decoct. alongwith other ingredients used as antifert. drug (*ibid*, 1980, **34**, 274).

Flowers contain β-sitosterol and triterp. (*Proc Indian Sci Congr*, 1980, Pt. III,, 73).

Stems, (24*S*)-Et-cholesta-5,22,25-triene -3β-ol and β-sitosterol (*J Indian Chem Soc*, 1981, **58**, 726).

Leaves, scutellarin (0.5%), hispidulin (0.1%) & their 7-0- glucuronides; also sterol (*Phytochemistry*, 1973, **12**, 1195; 2078).

C. inerme (Linn.f.) Gaertn.

Plant—EtOH(50%) ext., hypoten. (*Indian J Exp Biol*, 1969, **7**, 250). Used in stomachache, and wounds.

In Samoa, bark as laxt; seeds, as poultice. Leaves, as ingredient in remedies for vomiting of blood, fever and as anticoagulant (*Econ Bot*, 1974, **28**, 28); pharmacol. studies (*Qual Plant Mater Veg*, 1969, **17**, 293).

Essent. oil, antifung. [*Indian Drugs Pharmac Ind*, 1979, **14**(1), 3].

Leaves, aq. ext., chem. study (*Planta Med*, 1971,**19**, 318); (24*S*)- Et-cholesta-5,22,25-triene-3β-ol; the said compd. isolated from *C. campbelli*, hypoten.; other flavons. (*Tetrahedron Lett*, 1970, 1883; *Indian J Pharm*, 1973,**35**,191; *Phytochemistry*, 1973, **12**, 1195; 1977, **16**, 294); 3-epicaryoptin (*J Chem Soc Chem Commun*, 1979, 97). Seeds, neolignan (*Phytochemistry*, 1981, **20**, 2757).

C. multiflorum (Burm.f.) Kuntze syn. *C. phlomoides* Linn.f.

Leaves applied against guinea worms. Root decoct., in gonor. as demulc. (*J Agric Trop Bot Appl*, 1966, **13**, 286). Root and bark bitter tonic, used in nervous disorders and debility [*J Res Indian Med*, 1973, **8**(2), 67].

Plant parts used in fever, postnatal complaints, dyspep., stomachache, colic, cholera, dysen. and anthrax (*Econ Bot*, 1970, **24**, 241). Plant given to cattles in diar. and green leaves applied to wounds [*Nagarjun*, 1975-76, **19**(12), 20]. Herb ext., hypoglyc., clin. trial; juice given in ear pain [*J Res Indian Med*, 1975, **10**(4), 1; 1978, **13**(4), 92]. Leaf juice, anthelm. for cow and goat. Plant decoct. in dyspep. of buffalo, and paste in diar. (*Bull Bot Surv India*, 1980, **22**, 96).

Scutellarein and pectolinaringenin from leaves (*Phytochemistry*, 1972, **11**, 3095). Roots contain ceryl alc., clerodin, clerosterol and clerodendrin A (*Planta Med*, 1979, **37**, 64).

Stems, *d*-mannitol, β-sitosterol, its glucd. and ceryl alc. (*Indian J Pharm*, 1967, **29**, 102).

*C. nutans Wall.

EtOH(50%) ext. of aerial parts, diur. (*Indian J Exp Biol*, 1974, **12**, 512).

Found in Assam.

C. philippinum Schauer syn. *C. fragrans* Vent.

Roots and stems, triacontane, α-amyrin, β-sitosterol, its glucd., clerosterol and (24*S*)- Et-cholesta-5, 22,25-triene-3 β-ol (*J Indian Chem Soc*, 1981, **58**, 626).

C. serratum (Linn.) Moon

Plant—used in fever, dropsy, anasarca, rheum., hemiplegia, sores, *prolapsus ani*, *fistula ani*, cholera, and rinderpest (*Econ Bot*, 1970, **24**, 241). EtOH(50%) ext. of aerial parts, spermic. and CNS depress. (*Indian J Exp Biol*, 1974, **12**, 512; 1977, **15**, 231).

Root—decoct. as appetizer (*Bull Bot Surv India*, 1973, **15**, 19). Rootbark ext., antihistaminic (*Indian J Pharm*, 1964, **26**, 105). Polyhydric alc. fraction from root useful as hypoten. and bronchoconstrictor (*Curr Sci*, 1967, **36**, 42).

Saponin from roots, antihistaminic and antiallergic (*J Pharm Pharmacol*, 1968, **20**, 801). Root, source of mannitol (*Curr Sci*, 1967, **36**, 126). Root bark, a saponin, mannitol and stigmasterol (*Phytochemistry*, 1969, **8**, 515).

Bark sapogenins, oleanolic, queretaroic and serratogenic acids (*Tetrahedron*, 1969, **25**, 3701). Leaves contain (+)- catechin, α-spinasterol, luteoline & its glucuronide (*Curr Sci*, 1976, **45**, 391); polyphenolic components (*ibid*, 1979, **48**, 440).

*C. serratum (Linn.) Moon var. **wallichii** C.B.Clarke

EtOH(50%) ext. of plant, hypoten. and spasmol. (*Indian J Exp Biol*, 1973, **11**, 43).
W. Bengal.

*C. splendens G. Don

EtOH(50%) ext. of aerial parts, CNS depress. (*Indian J Exp Biol*, 1980, **18**, 594).
Bihar.

*C. squamatum Vahl

EtOH(50%) ext. of leaves, flowers and roots, spasmol. (*Indian J Exp Biol*, 1968, **6**, 232).
W. Bengal.

CLINOPODIUM (*Lamiaceae*)

*C. umbrosum Koch syn. *Calamintha umbrosa* Fisch. & Mey.

Eng.–*Catmint*.

EtOH(50%) ext. of plant, anthelm., hypoglyc. and spasmog.; also spermic. in rats (*Indian J Exp Biol* 1968, **6**, 232; 1977, **15**, 231).

Pet. ether ext. (0.05%) yielding eugenol, 12.5%; 3-octanol, 30% among others [*Indian Perfum*, 1969, **13**(Pt I), 26].

In temperate Himalayas from Kashmir to Bhutan, Arunachal Pradesh, Khasi hills up to 1,300 m and in hills of S. India.

CLITORIA (*Fabaceae*)

C. ternatea Linn.

Roots—emetic (Lindley, 243). Roots used by tribals to cause abortion; paste applied on cattle stomach for curing abdominal swellings (*J Econ Tax Bot*, 1981, **2**, 68; 185).

Seed ext., insectic. against European cornborer (*J Econ Entomol*, 1979, **72**, 541).

Roots, taraxerol and taraxerone (*Bull Calcutta Sch Trop Med*, 1963, **11**, 106; 1964, **12**, 23).

Seeds, cinnamic acid, flavonol glycd., etc. (*Curr Sci*, 1967, **36**, 124; *Chem Ber*, 1968, **101**, 2096); hexacosanol, β-sitosterol and an anthoxanthin glucd. (*Indian J Pharm*, 1968, **30**, 167).

Leaves, glycds. of kaempferol (*Indian J Chem*, 1973, **11**, 89; *Yakugaku Zasshi*, 1977, **97**, 649); also stigmast-4-ene- 3,6-dione (*Pharmazie*, 1978, **33**, 82; *CA*, **88**, 186110f).

Certain studies on *Aparajita*, rev.; 11 refs. (*J Nat Integ Med Assoc*, 1980, **22**, 140).

CNICUS (*Asteraceae*)

See CIRSIUM

COCCINIA (*Cucurbitaceae*)

C. grandis (Linn.) Voigt syn. *C. cordifolia* Cogn.; *C. indica* Wight & Arn.; *Cephalandra indica* Naud.

Root—EtOH and aq. exts. of sun-dried and defatted root powd.,orally hypoglyc. in rabbits; comparable to tolbutamide (*J Pharm Pharmacol*, 1963, **15**, 411). Hypoglyc. activity in glucose-fed albino rats (*Indian J Med Res*, 1963, **51**, 716). EtOH(50%) ext., antiprot. (*Indian J Exp Biol*, 1969, **7**, 250); powd. taken with water to stop vomiting; paste applied to forehead in headache (*Bull Bot Surv India*, 1980, **22**, 161).

Leaves—w.-sol. alk. fraction of leaves and whole plant show hypoglyc. activity of short duration (*Indian J Exp Biol*, 1972, **10**, 347). Leaves useful in diabetes in human patients (*Br Med J*, 1980, **280**, 1044; *Bangladesh Med Res Counc Bull*, 1979, **5**, 60). Juice and decoct. of leaves and stem, and decoct. of fruits, hypoglyc. in rabbits (*Bull Med Ethno Bot Res*, 1980, **1**, 234).

Fruits—useful in diabetes (*J Econ Tax Bot*, 1980, **1**, 141); of *C. indica* var. *palmata* more potent (*Bull Med Ethno Bot Res*, 1980, **1**, 234).

Various plant parts used in slow pulse, convuls., scrofulosa colli, sores, syphilis and gravel (*Econ Bot*, 1970, **24**, 241). Plant juice cures ear pain [*J Res Indian Med*, 1978, **13**(4), 92].

Aerial parts yield alc. cephalandrol, tritriacontane, β-sitosterol, and 2 alks. cephalandrine A & B; also heptacosane [*Sci Res Dacca*, 1965, **2**(1/2), 27; 1968, **5**(1), 71; *CA*, **63**, 12004g; **69**, 65149z].

Young green immature fruits of bitter variety, a glycd. of cucurbitacin B, β-amyrin and lupeol (*J Sci Ind Res*, 1962, **21B**, 237). Fruits, β-sitosterol and taraxerol (*Trans Bose Res Inst Calcutta*, 1972, **35**, 43). Ripe fruit carotenoids (*Curr Sci*, 1979, **48**, 630).

COCCULUS (*Menispermaceae*)

C. hirsutus (Linn). Diels syn. *C. villosus* DC.

Roots—used to allay irritation, fever and rheum; leaves for same purpose; roots substitute for sarsaparilla. Aq. ext. of stem and root, sed., hypoten., bradycardiac, cardiotonic and spasmol. (*Indian Drugs*, 1977-78, **15**, 145).

Leaves—decoct., as laxt. (*Bull Bot Surv India*, 1973, **15**, 13); see root also. Powd. mixed with water and applied to eyes, gives cooling effect (*Econ Bot*, 1978, **32**, 280). EtOH(50%) ext. of aerial parts, diur. (*Indian J Exp Biol*, 1977, **15**, 208).

Roots and stems alk., coclaurine, magnoflorine, trilobine & its iso deriv. (*Indian J Chem*, 1976, **14B**, 62). Leaves, alk. (*Pak J Sci Res*, 1979, **31**, 79).

C. laurifolius DC.

EtOH(50%) ext. of roots, neuromuscular blocking (*Indian J Exp Biol*, 1969, **7**, 250).

Leaves, oily alk., erythroculine (*Tetrahedron Lett*, 1969, 153); str. of erythroculine (*Chem Pharm Bull*, 1970, **18**, 1951; *CA*, 1971, **74**, 23052k); known alks., reticuline, laurifoline and magnoflorine (*Yakugaku Zasshi*, 1970, **90**, 92).

Str. of cocculine (*Khim Prir Soedin*, 1970, **6**, 74; *CA*, **73**, 35585d); str. of cocculine and cocculidine; belong to erythrina alks. (*Izv Akad Nauk SSSR Ser Khim*, 1972, 500; *J Chem Soc Chem Commun*, 1974, 150). Nitrates of alks., hypoten. in dogs; but no detectable CNS activity (*Farmakol Alkaloidov Serdech Glikozidov*, 1971, 197; *CA*, 1972, **77**, 135092 m).

Spanish plant, alk. coclaurine (*Rev Acad Farm Barcelona*, 1973, No.7, 29; *CA*, 1974, **80**, 45643e). Leaves, alks. laurifonine, laurifine and laurifinine; their strs. (*Tetrahedron Lett*, 1975, 1201; *J Chem Soc Perkin Trans I*, 1976, 2197); cocculine, isococculine, cocculidine and coccoline (*Phytochemistry*, 1976, **16**, 739); coccuvinine; lactam alk., coccolinine (*Indian J Chem*, 1977, **15B**, 288; 1976, **14B**, 366); coccuvine (*Experientia*, 1976, **32**, 1368); cocculitine (*Lloydia*, 1977, **40**, 322); isococculine (*Nat Acad Sci Lett India*, 1978, **1**, 93); new alks. erythlaurine and erythramide (*Heterocycles*, 1981, **16**, 555).

Leaves, alk. isococculidine; str.; alk. powerful neuromuscular- blocking agent (*in* Wagner & Wolff, 216); w.-sol. fraction yields quaternary aporphine bases laurifoline and magnoflorine chlorides and isocorydine, its -OMe deriv. and boletine methochlorides, responsible for neuromuscular blocking and hypoten. action of w.-sol. fraction (*J Indian Chem Soc*, 1979, **56**, 1020).

C. macrocarpus Wight & Arn.; see **Diploclisia glaucescens**

C. pendulus (Forsk.) Diels syn. *C. leaeba* DC.

EtOH(50%) ext. of aerial parts, antivir., spasmol., hypoten. and anticancer (*Indian J Exp Biol*, 1969, **7**, 250).

Stems and leaves, biscoclaurine alk., penduline; and bisbenzylisoquinoline alk., cocsuline (*Experientia*, 1970, **26**, 12; 241); alk. cocsulinine, active against the cells derived from human epidermoid carcinoma of nasopharynx (9KB), *in vitro* (*Indian J Chem*, 1974, **12**, 517);biscoclaurine alks. cocsuline, cocsoline, cocsulinine, pendulinine, pendine and penduline (*Tetrahedron*, 1975, **31**, 2575). Leaves, hentriacontanol, β-sitosterol, and choline, penduline and cocsuline (*Curr Sci*, 1978, **47**, 768).

COCHLEARIA (*Brassicaceae*)

C. armoracia Linn.; see **Armoracia rusticana**

COCHLOSPERMUM (*Cochlospermaceae*)

C. religiosum (Linn.) Alston syn. *C. gossypium* DC.

Pounded bark applied to broken limbs of cattle (*Econ Bot*, 1965, **19**, 239). Plant used in sores and T.B. (*ibid*, 1970, **24**, 241). EtOH(50%) ext. of stem bark, hypoten. (*Indian J Exp Biol*, 1971, **9**, 91).

Str. of plant gum (*J Chem Soc*, 1965, 4325). Leaves, terps., saponins and tannins (*Econ Bot*, 1969, **23**, 274).

COCOS (*Arecaceae*)

C. nucifera Linn.

Fruit—ripe coconut, antibiot. [*East Pharm*, 1968, **11**(122), 36]. In Hawai, shoots, and ashes of dry meat used in deep cuts, general debility and swollen womb; in Samoa, meat and spongy interior of sprouting nut, ingredient in remedy for fever; and in Bahamas, grated meat to treat burns and abscesses (*Econ Bot*, 1971, **25**, 245; 1974,

28, 6; 1975, **29**, 314). In java, nut milk as contracep. (*Planta Med*, 1972, **23**, 167).

Oil—clin. use, for elevating glycogen level in human heart (*Surg Forum*, 1978, **29**, 318). Chaco Indians use with chicken fat and honey to treat asthma. In Bahamas, taken for chest colds (*Econ Bot*, 1971, **24**, 344; 1975, **29**, 314); in stomach troubles, as laxt., applied to open sores and wound (*ibid*, 1974, **28**, 6). Oil, used against cancer (*Lloydia*, 1970, **33**, 316); cancer curing studies (*Kansai Ika Daigaku Zasshi*, 1974, **26**, 72; *CA*, 1975, **82**, 110772d); *J Nat Cancer Inst*, 1979, **62**, 1009).

Oil constituent of many hair compns. (Span. Pat., 1969, 348229; Ger. Offen, 1974, 2361080-081; US Pat., 1974, 3824304; *CA*, 1969, **71**, 53471b; 1974, **81**, 82242q-43r; 1975, **83**, 15494b); also of med. useful skin compds. (Ger Offen, 1977, 2532693; 1978, 2654743; 2658723; Jpn Kokoi Tokkyo Koho, 1979, 7936306; *CA*, **86**, 111203p; **89**, 80243g; 95015h; **91**, 78764a).

Oil, aetherosclerosis producing, studies in animals (*Prog Biochem Pharmacol*, 1968, **4**, 482; *J Atheroscler Res*, 1967, **7**, 59; 1969, **9**, 319; *Atherosclerosis*, 1975, **21**, 115; 1980, **35**, 189); hypercholesteramic in monkeys (*Exp Mol Pathol*, 1971, **15**, 281). Unsupplemented hydrogenated oil, produced ventricular necrosis in albino mice (*Am J Anat*, 1969, **124**, 481).

Green coconut water—source of K for cholera patient (*Bull Calcutta Sch Trop Med*, 1964, **12**, 20). Clin. study of tender coconut water in gastroenteritis (*Ceylon Coconut Q*, 1970, **21**, 113).

Husk—Chaco Indians use resin extd. by heating inner husk to treat toothaches; husk of green nut as purg. (*Econ Bot*, 1971, **24**, 344; 1974, **28**, 6).

Shell & fibre—compn. of antimicrob. product from shell fibres (*Curr Sci*, 1973, **42**, 841). EtOH ext. of shell, antifung. (*J Ethnopharmacol*, 1980, **2**, 291).

Flowers mixed with oil applied to swellings; leaves to treat abscesses; roots in wounds and gonor. (*Econ Bot*, 1974, **28**, 6); EtOH(50%) ext. of leaves, diur. (*Indian J Exp Biol*, 1977, **15**, 208). Plant in skeletal fractures (*Sri Linka For*, 1980, **14**, 145).

Oil, pharmacodynamics of 18-ethoxylated fatty alc. (*Rev Fac Farm Bioquim Univ Sao Paulo*, 1969, 7, 33; *CA*,1970, **72**, 65226j); triterp. alc., sterols & Me-sterols (*J Am Oil Chem Soc*, 1966, **43**, 254; 1973, **50**, 300; *Lipids*, 1981, **16**, 306). α-tocopherol, 2.2 mg/100g (*Int J Vitam Nutr Res*, 1980, **50**, 242).

Aflatoxins in coconut products, rev., 41 refs. (*Ceylon Coconut Q*, 1972,**23**, 108). Detn. of penicillic acid (*Z Lebensm Unters Forsch*, 1981, **172**, 110; *CA*, **94**, 101463z).

Plant ext., pharmacol. of GABA (*J Pharm Pharmacol*, 1962, **14**, 556; 562).

C.plumosa Hook. f.; see **Arecastrum romanzoffianum**

C.romanzoffiana Cham.; see **Arecastrum romanzoffianum**

CODIAEUM (*Euphorbiaceae*)

C. variegatum Blume

Leaves, ext. in 5% Na-bicarbonate, anticancer (*Philipp J Sci*, 1967,**96**, 393). EtOH(50%) ext. of aerial parts, anticancer (*Indian J Exp Biol*, 1980, **18**, 594).

Leaves, polyphenols (*Acta Biochim Pol*, 1973, **20**, 343; *CA*, 1974, **80**, 68409t). Plant releases volat. Hg (*Org Geochem*, 1980, **2**, 99; *CA*, **92**, 194777b).

COELOGYNE (*Orchidaceae*)

*C. ochracea Lindl.

EtOH(50%) ext. of plant, diur. (*Indian J Exp Biol*, 1980, **18**, 594).

Gangtok, Sikkim.

COFFEA (*Rubiaceae*)

C. arabica Linn.

Coffee—effect on functions of sympathoadrenomedullary system in man (*Acta Med Scand*, 1967, **181**, 431). Med. for varied heart troubles (*Indian Coffee*, 1970, **34**, 239); but heavy consumption with infrequent eating habits, heart disease-risk factor in men (*Experientia*, 1978, **34**, 1182); tannic acid, as incriminating factor for heart disease (*Indian J Nutr Diet*, 1979, **16**, 348). Antithiamine action (*Probl Ernaedr Lebensmittelwiss*, 1977, **4**, 75; *CA*, 1978, **89**, 1445580m). Coffee in prevention and control of pellagra (*Indian Coffee*, 1979, **43**, 204). Hypoglyc. effect of raw beans and β-sitosterol, in mice (*Rev Med Univ Fed Ceara*, 1979, **19**, 49; *CA*, 1981, **95**, 91690a). A bath on coffee grounds warmed by fomentation heat may have therapeutic effect on diabetes, neuralgia, rheum. and poor blood circulation (*Chem Ind Lond*, 1979, 293). Coffee (beverage), cause of cancer of pancreas (*N Engl J Med*, 1981, **304**, 630); powd. coffee bean, anticarcinogenic in stomach tumours in mice (*Chem Ind Lond*, 1981, 581).

EtOH(50%) ext. of aerial parts, spasmol. (*Indian J Exp Biol*, 1971, **9**, 91).

Caffeine—distribution of chlorogenic acid and caffeine in various plant parts (*Planta*, 1964, **61**, 90). Extn. from green coffee (*Indian J Technol*, 1965, **3**, 225). Major purine constituent of coffee and teas, increases CNS activity, mainly affecting cerebral cortex, respiratory stim., used in headache compns. Chemosterilant activity against stored-grain pests reported, rev., 170 refs.; see also purine alks. and their biol. activity (*Adv Heterocycl Chem*, 1966, **6**, 1; *CA*, 1967, **67**, 10871g; in Brossy, XXXVIII, 225-310, 311-23). Xanthine alks. including caffeine harmful during pregnancy [*Pharmatimes*, 1979, **11**(12), 28]; may be a teratogen (*in* Plant and Fungal Toxins, 169-70). Extn. (Fr. 1965, 1389634; *CA*, **63**, 1159c); from crude coffee (Ger. Offen., 1972, 2221560; *CA*, 1973, **78**, 41878w). From tissue culture (*Lloydia*, 1971, **34**, 170). Detn. of caffeine and trigonelline by reflection spectrophotom. (*Z Lebensm Unters Forsch*, 1973, **152**, 145; *CA*, **79**, 90557 v). Distribution (*J Food Sci*, 1974, **39**, 1055).

Chem. & technol. of coffee, rev., 220 refs [*Colloq Int Chim Cafes C R*, 1973, (Pub'1974), **6**, 18; *CA*, 1975, **83**, 176754b].

Chlorogenic acid—content in coffee products (*Dtsch Lebensm Rundsch*, 1967, **63**, 273; *CA*, **67**, 115936t); see caffeine; physiol. and pharmacol. (*Ann Nutr Aliment*, 1969, **23**, 1R; *CA*, **70**, 113486b); possible cocarcinogen (*Nature Lond*, 1975, **254**, 532).

Caffeoylquinic acid (*Ann Chim Paris*, 1963, **53**, 1315); str. of 3 di-caffeoylquinic acid (*Tetrahedron Lett*, 1964, 2851); 4,5-di-O- deriv. (*Chem Pharm Bull*, 1965, **13**, 101; *CA*, **62**, 11894g); estn. of feruloylquinic and caffeoylquinic acids (*J Sci Food Agric*, 1976, **27**, 73). Chem. of coffee [*New Sci*, 1965, **26**, 380; *Indian Coffee*, 1965, **29**(7), 19]. F content of coffee bean (*Nippon Shokuhin Kogyo Gakkaishi*, 1965, **12**, 59; *CA*, 1966, **64**, 18320a). Roasted coffee polysaccharides (*J Food Sci Technol*, 1966, **2**, 7). Raw coffee, scopoletin (*Z Lebensm Unters Forsch*, 1968, **137**, 1; *CA*, **69**, 18153m). Mn toxicity of coffee (*Indian Coffee*, 1971, **35**, 316). Antimitotic or cytostatic effects on human blood lymphocytes in culture with proposal for lack of mutagenic activity (*Mutat Res*, 1972, **15**, 197; *CA*, **77**, 84051t).

Theobromine and theophylline—content in raw coffee (*Pharmazie*, 1968, **23**, 502; *CA*, 1969, **70**, 27769 q). Pharmaceuticals based on coffee include theophylline & its deriv. (*Annu Rep RRL Jorhat*, 1969-70, **23**). Theobromine detn., spectrophotom. (*J Food Sci*, 1970, **41**, 458). Theophylline reduces cerebral blood flow by 20- 30% or 15% for short duration (*in* Beal & Reinhard, 259). Theophylline & caffeine, teratogenic in animals; in humans, conflicting view (*in* Plant and Fungal Toxins, 169). Theobromine (xanthine deriv.) and theophylline (1,3-di-Me-xanthine), powerful diur., as salts of org. acids, in oral use. Former, a cardiac stim. and arterial dilator; latter, in treatment of bronchial conditions. 7-Amino- Et-theophylline derivs., spasmol. similar to papaverine; some other derivs., potential new antiatherosclerosis agents. *p*-Xanthine (1,7-di-Me), efficient diur. and possesses antithyroid properties (*in* Brossy, XXXVIII, 311-23).

Brazilian coffee, trigonelline and nicotinic acid content (*Rev IBPT Curitiba*, 1970, No. 15, 11, 14; *CA*, 1971, **74**, 139678-79y-z); choline, microbioassay (*Rev Microbiol*, 1972, **3**, 173; *CA*, 1974, **81**, 150585f); free & combined vit B6 (*Arq Biol Technol*, 1979, **22**, 183; *CA*, 1980, **93**, 41553w). Madagascar wild coffee, chem. compn. (*Cafe Cacao The*, 1972, **16**, 161).

Roasted bean, atractyligenin; str. of atractylosides (*Chem Ber*, 1974, **107**, 2409; 1976, **109**, 3450). Compds., hypoglyc. (*in* Liener, 436).

Str. of kahweofuran, constituent of coffee aroma (*J Org Chem*, 1971, **36**, 199). Cycloalkapyrazines in aroma (*J Agric Food Chem*, 1975, **23**, 510).

Beans, sterols (*Phytochemistry*, 1971, **10**, 1101); sterols from seed oil (*Rev Ital Sostanze Grasse*, 1979, **56**, 283; *CA*, 1980, **92**, 90899b). Tocopherol from coffee bean oil (*J Agric Food Chem*, 1977, **25**, 283).

Husk suitable for furfural production (*Rev Univ Ind Santander*, 1966, **8**, 59; *CA*, 1967, **66**, 56862 n).

Aflatoxins of green coffee (*J Assoc Off Anal Chem*, 1968, **51**, 609); content survey (*Ann Nutr Aliment*, 1977, **31**, 477; *CA*, 1978, **89**, 41037y); content (*Hrana Ishrana*, 1978, **19**, 451; *CA*, 1979, **90**, 185047v). 11 Phytotoxins; isolation from different plant parts (*Bot Bull Acad Sin*, 1980, **21**, 25). Coffee contains 1,3,7-tri-Me-xanthine; antifung. compd. (*Naturwissenschaften*, 1980, **67**, 459).

*C. bengalensis Roxb.

EtOH(50%) ext. of aerial parts, hypoten. (*Indian J Exp Biol*, 1971, **9**, 91). Leaf ext., bath for infants suffering from fever (*Bull Bot Surv India*, 1976, **18**, 116).

Meghalaya.

COIX (*Poaceae*)

C. lachryma-jobi Linn. syn. *C. lachryma* Linn.

In China, plant used as diur. and laxt. (*Q J Crude Drug Res*, 1963, **3**, 437). Plant and its juice used in tumours and cancers (*Lloydia*, 1969, **32**, 191). Various plant parts used in fever, smallpox, dysen. and anthrax (*Econ Bot*, 1970, **24**, 241). In Hawaii, leaves, in diabetes (*ibid*, 1971, **25**, 245). Fruit decoct. as tonic (*Bull Bot Surv India*, 1973, **15**, 21). Med. evaluation, rev. on med. uses in China; aq. ext. lowered B.P. in rabbits (*Chanyonmul Hwahak Yonguso Yongu Pogo*, 1974, **2**, 7; 19; *CA*, 1977, **87**, 145423 w; 177652m). EtOH(50%) ext. of aerial parts, spasmol. (*Indian J Exp Biol*, 1977, **15**, 208).

Seedlings yield glucds. of 1,4-benzoxazine derivs. (*Eur J Biochem*, 1969, **8**, 109). Gas chromatogr. detn. of benzoxazolinones (*Phytochemistry*, 1975, **14**, 2077). Roots, benzoxazolinones (*Yakugaku Zasshi*, 1981, **101**, 1156).

Seeds, coixenolide, a mixed ester of palmitoleinic and vaccenic acids (*Khim Prir Soedin*, 1970, **6**, 170; *CA*, **73**, 55595k). Coixenolide, anticancer agent (*Chanyonmul Hwahak Yonguso Yongu Pogo*, 1974, **2**, 13; *CA*, 1977, **87**, 130483s).

Triterps., taxonomy (*Yakugaku Zasshi*, 1969, **89**, 814; *Phytochemistry*, 1970, **9**, 2085).

COLA (*Sterculiaceae*)

*C. acuminata (Beauv.) Schott & Endl.

Nut contains oxalic acid, 6.4% (dry basis) (*Indian J Nutr Diet*, 1970, **7**, 119).

Cola nuts chewed for 14 or 28 days did not alter antipyrine, in male subjects (*Clin Pharmacol Ther*, 1979, **26**, 287). In Amerindian and African traditional med., stembark and fruit cotyledons used as nervine tonic, restor., stim., astrin. and to improve physical and mental state; pharmacol., transient stim. followed by depression (*Fitoterapia*, 1982, **53**, 147).

Cola ext. contains caffeine and theobromine (*Farm Obz*, 1967, **36**, 549; *CA*, 1969, **70**, 105260h); caffeine spectrophotom. detn. in nuts; and theobromine in bark, bean, leaves and pods (*J Food Sci*, 1974, **38**, 911; 1976, **41**, 458). Introduced into India.

COLCHICUM (*Colchicaceae*)

C. luteum Baker

Several alks.; colchamine, its derivs.; colchicine, its derivs.; and 2 new alks.; str. detn. (*Khim Prir Soedin*, 1970, **6**, 82; 275; *CA*, **73**, 45635j; 45536k); collutine, its str. (*ibid*, 1975, 758; *CA*, 1976, **84**, 150804p). Str. of luteidine, luteicine & luteine (*ibid*, 1976, 354; 359; 801; *CA*, 1977, **87**, 43863b; 42864c; 190283r).

Alk. distribution in Indian plant (*Indian J Pharm*, 1977, **39**, 115).

COLEBROOKEA (*Lamiaceae*)

C. oppositifolia Smith

Leaves contain rare flavones; 5,6,7-tri- & 5,6,7,4"-tetra-MeO- flavones (*Indian J Chem*, 1974, **12**, 1327). Aerial parts, 2 new flavones and a known one (*ibid*, 1981, **20B**, 627).

COLEUS (*Lamiaceae*)

C. amboinicus Lour. syn. *C. aromaticus* Benth.

In Samoa, weed used for cold (*Econ Bot*, 1974, **28**, 15); herb against fractures (*Sri Lanka For*, 1980, **14**, 145); leaves applied as poultice in centipede or scorpion sting, and headache; internally in asthma and broncht. (Hocking, 56).

Leaves, exalacetic acid (large amt.) (*Naturwissenschaften*, 1963, **50**, 667); cirsimaritin and β-sitosterol glucd. (*Indian Chem Soc*, 1976, **53**, 1064); several triterp. acids (*Arch Pharm Wein*, 1977, **310**, 910; *CA*, 1978, **88**, 101548g). Leaves of S. American plant; flavones, salvigenin, 6-OMe-genkwanin, quercetin, chrysoeriol, luteolin and apigenin; flavanone, eriodyctol; and flavanol, taxifolin (*Planta Med*,

1977, **31**, 308). Med. properties and antibact. activity against *Pneumococcus* and *Staphylococcus* 209 P, may be attributed to codeine, carvacrol, flavones, arom. acids, tannin, etc. [*Duoc Hoc*, 1979, (5), 15; *CA*, 1980, **93**, 53857m].

Essent. oil from herb, characteristics and chem. compn. (*Perfum Essent Oil Rec*, 1967, **58**, 622); chem. exam.; thymol, 41.30% and carvacrol, 13.25% (*J Indian Chem Soc*, 1981, **58**, 103).

*C. forskohlii Briq. syn. *C. barbatus* Benth.

Herb, arom. (Wlth India, II, 308). EtOH(50%) ext. of aerial parts, spasmol. (*Indian J Exp Biol*, 1971, **9**, 91); that of roots, hypoten. and spasmol. (*ibid*, 1974, **12**, 512). Roots given to children in constip. (*Bull Med Ethno Bot Res*, 1980, **1**, 1).

Leaves, a diterp. methylenequinone, coleon E (*Helv Chim Acta*, 1972, **55**, 1994); coleon F (*ibid*, 1973, **56**, 1129); str. of diterp. barbatusin and cyclobutatusin (*J Am Chem Soc*, 1973, **95**, 598; 1974, **96**, 580); diterps., barbatusin and cyclobutatusin; former inhibitory against Lewis lung carcinoma and lymphocytic leukemia P 388 in mice (*Tetrahedron*, 1977, **33**, 1457).

Roots, a new diterp. with hypoten. and spasmol. activity, isolation procedure (Indian Pat, 1976, 140419; *CA*, 1980, **92**, 146993x); substance useful for heart and cardiovascular ailments, isolation procedure (Ger. Offen. 1977, 2557784; *CA*, **87**, 106735ę); str. of 5 diterps. including coleonol; diterps., B.P. lowering, and cardioactive (*Tetrahedron Lett*, 1977, 1669); coleonol, hypoten. and spasmol. (*Indian J Chem*, 1977, **15B**, 880);diterps.; deoxycoleonol, coleonol B & C; also E & F; and new diterp. coleosol (*ibid*, 1978, **16B**, 341; 1055; 1979, **18B**, 214); str. of coleonol D, coleol and coleonone isolated from roots (*ibid*, 1979, **17B**, 321).

Roots naphthopyrone; compd. decreased B.P. in cats (Indian Pat., 1979, 145926; *CA*, 1980, **92**, 99564w); also crocetin dialdehyde (*Helv Chim Acta*,

1979, **62**, 2706). Process for preparation of pharmacol. active substance of root; activity in benzene, EtOAc fractions, yield diterp. with mol. formula $C_{22}H_{34}O_7$ (Can. Pat., 1980, 1083589; *CA*, **93**, 245443y).

Coleforsin—extn. procedure of pharmacol. active substance from roots (Belg. Pat., 1977, 8532644; *CA*, 1978, **89**, 30750z); it caused decrease in B.P. in cats (Indian Pat., 1979, 147030; *CA*, 1980, **92**, 203575 p); antihyperten., vasodilatory and inotropic activity (Brit. Pat., 1981, 1589326; *CA*, **95**, 103308 x).

Forskolin—yield, 0.05% dry wt from whole plant and 0.1% from roots; a potent cardioactive and hypoten. diterp. (*Planta Med*, 1980, **39**, 183); assay by GLC (*J Pharm Sci*, 1980, **69**, 1449); a potent adenylatecyclase activator [*Arzneim Forsch*, 1981, **31**(II), 1248]; forskolin, mp 230- 32° identical with coleonol (*Indian J Chem*, 1985, **24B**, 583); pharmacol. of coleonol, a hypoten. diterp. (*J Enthnopharmacol*, 1981, **3**, 1).

Phytochem. studies of *Coleus* genus; chem. compn., med. uses and biol. activity of *C. forskohlii* [*Herba Hung*, 1981, **20** (1-2), 213].

Commonly found on dry barren hills.

C. scutellarioides Benth. syn. *C. blumei* Benth.

Leaves ext., antibiot. and antitumour (*Philipp J Sci*, 1973, **102**, 1). In Samoa, herb used in elephantiasis (*Econ Bot*, 1974, **28**, 15).

Leaves, hydrocarbons, β-sitosterol & stigmasterol; and triterp.(*Philipp J Sci*, 1973, **102**, 1; 1978, **107**, 95). Phytochem. studies of *Coleus* genus, chem., med. uses, and biol. activity of *C. blumei* (*Herba Hung*, 1981, **20**, 213).

Rosmarinic acid (caffeol ester, yield 15%) in cell culture (*Naturwissenschaften*, 1977, **64**, 585; *Planta*, 1977, 137; *in* Beal & Reinhard, 475-76).

COLOCASIA (*Araceae*)

C. esculenta (Linn.) Schott syn. *C. antiquorum* Schott

Tuber—chewing fresh tuber irritates mouth and throat (*Acta Phytother*, 1979, **16**, 121). Sick persons suffering from localized scleoderma nourish exclusively on cooked tuber, this eases pain and decreases T.B. ulcers. Sap of raw pulverised rhizomes or pulp as poultice used to treat ulcers; sap also applied for crippled extremities and for fungal abscesses of animals; anthelm.; causes dermatitis (*Econ Bot*, 1969, **23**, 104; 1974, **28**, 4).

EtOH(50%) ext. of rhizome, hypoten. (*Indian J Exp Biol*, 1973, **11** , 43).

Culm—in Brazil, juice of crushed corm used as effective abortif. Raw grated corms mixed with sugarcane juice, in pulmonary congestion; in Hawaii, corm, as laxt. (*Econ Bot*, 1969, **23**, 104; 1972, **25**, 245).

Leaves—juice (also of roots) used in tumours ulcerated polyp, cancer of nose and warts (*Lloydia*, 1967, **30**, 414); in Hawaii, in styptics and poultices. Leaves cause severe irritation of mouth, and may cause leprosy, toxicity greatest in dry season (*Econ Bot*, 1969, **23**, 104). In Samoa, and in New Guinea, to treat boils (*Econ Bot*, 1974, **28**, 4; *Q J Crude Drug Res*, 1980, **18**, 33). Ext., antifung. (*Geobios*, 1978, **5**, 49).

Plant—said to cause glomeruletubular nephritis and degeneration of adrenals; various plant parts used in atrophy, emaciation or cachexy, wounds, consumption, dry cough and broncht., and anthrax (*Econ Bot*, 1969, **23**, 104; 1970, **24**, 241).

Tubers, trypsin inhibitor (*Indian J Biochem Biophys*, 1975, **12**, 383); also 2α-amylase inhibitors sterols (*J Agric Food Chem*, 1980, **31**, 981; 1977, **25**, 1222); chem. compn. of cultivars of Bangladesh (*Sci Hortic*, 1979, **10**, 127).

Nigerian plant, HCN and oxalic acid (*Indian J Nutr Diet*, 1970, **7**, 119). Leaves sterols, hypocholesterolemic in mice (*Bangladesh J Biol Sci*, 1979, **8**, 17; *CA*, 1980, **93**, 237544 p).

Content and compn. of seed mucilage from Egyptian plant (*Planta Med*, 1980, **38**, 73).

*C. fornicata Kunth

B.–*Biskachu*.

EtOH(50%) ext. of rhizome, anti-amphetaminic (*Indian J Exp Biol*, 1973, **11**, 43).

Plant sterols and flavons. (*Phytochemistry*, 1972, **11**, 2621).

Hoogli, W. Bengal.

C. macrorrhiza Schott; see **Alocasia macrorrhiza**

*C. nymphaefolia Kunth

EtOH(50%) ext. of leaves, spermic. (*Indian J Exp Biol*, 1980, **18**, 594).

Burdwan, W. Bengal.

C. virosa Kunth; see **Studnera virosa**

COLOPHOSPERMUM (*Caesalpinaceae*)

*C. mopane Kirk ex Leon. syn. *Copaifera mopane* Kirk ex Benth.

Root infusion used against tapeworm. In N. Zimbabwe, stem decoct. given in epilepsy. Wood ext. applied to inflam. eyes. Young leaves purg. to bovines (White, 121; Uphof, 150; Allen & Allen, 176; Watt & Breyer Brandwijk, 577).

Heartwood contains (+)-mopanol & its 4-epimer and other flavons.; also mopanin and fisetin (*J Chem Soc C*, 1966, 1644; 1967, 1407).

Grown in Rajasthan.

COLQUHOUNIA (*Lamiaceae*)

*C. coccinia Wall.

EtOH(50%) ext. of aerial parts, spasmol. (*Indian J Exp Biol*, 1973, **11**, 43).

Found in Uttar Pradesh.

COLUBRINA (*Rhamnaceae*)

*C. asiatica Brongn.

In Samoa, leaves used to treat bone fracture (*Econ Bot*, 1974, **28**, 23).

Essent. oil (1.2%) from ripe fruit, hypoten. in dogs and depress. effect on frog heart; antagonised spasmodic effect of Ac-choline on smooth muscles (*Planta Med*, 1970, **18**, 222); antibact. (*ibid*, 1974, **26**, 196; *Qual Plant Mater Veg*, 1970- 71, **20**, 231). Antimicrob. activity of essent. oil from seeds [*Indian Drugs Pharmac Ind*, 1977, **12**(2), 15].

Bark contains OMe-dauricine as major alk. (*Phytochemistry*, 1970, **9**, 1683).

Coastal forests of S. India and Andamans.

COLUTEA (*Fabaceae*)

C. nepalensis Sims syn. *C. arborescens* Linn. var. *nepalensis* Baker

Poisonous plants, rev. on taxonomy, morphology, active principles and their toxic effects and treatment, use and biol. (*PTA Prakt Pharm*, 1979, **8**, 172; *CA*, 1980, **92**, 160469n).

COMBRETUM (*Combretaceae*)

*C. dasystachyum Kurz

EtOH(50%) ext. of aerial parts, CNS depress., hypoten. and diur. (*Indian J Exp Biol*, 1974, **12**, 512).

Found in Assam.

C. nanum Buch.- Ham. ex D. Don

Various plant parts used in enlarged spleen, stomach complaints, colic, cholera and dysen. (*Econ Bot*, 1970, **24**, 241).

*C. ovalifolium Roxb.

EtOH(50%) ext. of aerial parts, CNS depress. and diur. (*Indian J Exp Biol*, 1974, **12**, 512).

Found in Gujarat.

*C. ovalifolium Roxb. var. **cooperi** Haines

EtOH(50%) ext. of aerial parts, hypoten. and spasmol. (*Indian J Exp Biol*, 1973, **11**, 43).

Reported to occur in Orissa.

C. roxburghii Spreng. syn. *C. decandrum* Roxb.

Seed oil used against eczema (*Econ Bot*, 1965, **19**, 241). Plant, in burns (*ibid*, 1970, **24**, 241). Raw leaves eaten in diar. and

gastric troubles (*Bull Bot Sur India*, 1980, **22**, 161).

COMMELINA (*Commelinaceae*)

C. benghalensis Linn.

Various plant parts used in otitis media suppurativa, sores and snake-bite (*Econ Bot*, 1970, **24**, 241).

Plant contains alkanols and sterols [*J Res Indian Med*, 1975, **10**(1), 79].

C. diffusa Burm. f. syn. *C. nudiflora* auct. non Linn.

In Samoa, leaves used as emetic and laxt. (*Econ Bot*, 1974, **28**, 4). In Hawaii, plant as blood purifier (*ibid*, 1971, **25**, 245).

C. paludosa Blume syn. *C. obliqua* Buch.-Ham.

EtOH(50%) ext. of plant, hypoten., CNS depress. and diur. (*Indian J Exp Biol*, 1974, **12**, 512).

C. suffruticosa Blume

Plant used in menor. (*Econ Bot*, 1970, **24**, 241).

*C. undulata R. Br.

-EtOH(50%) ext. of plant, anticancer (*Indian J Exp Biol*, 1974, **12**, 512).

Maharashtra.

COMMIPHORA (*Burseraceae*)

*C. caudata Engl.

Eng.–*Hill mango*; Kan.–*Kondamavu*; Tel.–*Kiluvai*.

Bark and leaves yield a gum-resin used in medicine (Santapau & Henry, 43).

EtOH(50%) ext. of stem, spasmol. and antivir. (*Indian J Exp Biol*, 1968, **6**, 232).

Found in Tamil Nadu.

C. wightii Bhandari syn. *C. mukul* Engl.; *Balsamodendron mukul* Hook. ex Stocks

Gum-resin—called *guggul(u)*, one of the constituents of several indigenous drugs, extensively investigated w.r.t. pharmacol. & clin. Highly rated in Ayurvedic medicine for treatment of rheumatoid arthritis, obesity and several other disorders. Pharmacol. studies of crude drug as well as its fractions and pure constituents revealed significant antiinflam., antirheum. and hypocholesterimic activity, lending credence to ancient claims. Active constituents, guggulsterol-I, -II & - III(*in* Wagner & Wolff, 223). Clin. trials; in rheum., rheumatoid arthritis, osteoarthritis, frozen shoulder and sciatica; also rev. on drugs used on rheum. [*Rheumatism*, 1976-77, **12**, 32; 1977- 78, **13**, 1; 10; 1978-79, **14**, 118; 153; 53; 1980-81, **16**, 54; *J Res Indian Med*, 1978, 13(3), 14]. Major component of *Navakagaggulu*, its efficacy in rheum.; effective drug (*Rheumatism*, 1980-81, **16**, 106; 118; 159). Effect of *guggulu* on estrogen-induced hyperlipidemia in chicks [*J Res Indian Med*, 1974, 9(2), 4]. Clin. trials: in obese subjects effective, safe and cheap drug [*ibid*, 1973, 8(4), 1; 1976, **11**(2), 132; 1979, 14(2), 11]; long-term clin. studies on hypolipidaemic effective gum resin (*Indian J Med Res*, 1977, **65**, 390); also with a fraction of *guggulu* (*J Assoc Physns India*, 1978, **26**, 376). Hypocho-lesteremic and hypolipidaemic action of *guggulu* in patients of coronary heart disease [*J Res Indian Med*, 1976, **11**(2), 1]; inhibition of platelet aggregation (*Planta Med*, 1979, **37**, 367); increased serum fibrinolytic activity and decreased platelet adhesive index in human (*Indian J Med Res*, 1979, **70**, 992); gum dependable agent for hemiplegia and other atherosclerotic disorder like coronary insufficiency, clin. observations (*Rheumatism*, 1979-80, **15**, 107); increased fibrinolytic activity in ischaemic heart disease patients; more effective hypolipidaemic agent than garlic, clin. study (*Rajasthan Med J*, 1980, **19**, 84; 1981, **20**, 73).

Indigenous compn. '*Gugullipid*' useful in heart diseases, spondilitis and gout [*East Pharm*, 1979, **22**(258), 69]; clin, trials; also effect in animals, on coagulation and fibrinolysis (*Indian J Pharmacol*, 1981, **13**, 59; 89).

Resin, in indolent ulcers and as gargle in pyrrhoea alveolaris, chr. tonsilitis and pharyngitis. Inhalation of fumes from burning gum is recommended in hay fever, chr. broncht., nasal catarrh, laringitis and phthisis (*J Agric Trop Bot Appl*, 1966, **13**, 281).

Major constituent of indigenous drug, '*Septilin*' prescribed in rhinosinal infection; also used in exodontia (*J Indian Med Assoc*, 1965, **45**, 38; *Probe*, 1979-80, **19**, 124). Also one of the constituents of Chinese med. used in extradural haematomas (*Chin Med J*, 1981, **94**, 221).

Constituent of indigenous drug '*Biliarin*' useful in infective hepatitis (*Indian Pract*, 1978, **31**, 683); also of '*Arogya-wardhini*' used in acute viral hepatitis (*Indian J Med Res*, 1980, **72**, 588).

One of the constituents of Ayurvedic drug '*Myostal*' useful in puerperal patients, clin. trials (*Maharashtra Med J*, 1979, **26**, 433).

Oleoresin caused reduction in wt. of rat uterus, may be useful as antifert. agent (*Indian J Exp Biol*, 1978, **16**, 1021).

Chem. and biol. standardization of gum; w.r.t. antiinflam. activity [*J Res Indian Med*, 1972, 7(2), 6; *ibid*, 1973, 8(1), 20]. Source of *guggul* in Indian med., rev. (*Econ Bot*, 1975, **29**, 209); med. properties [*Nagarjun*, 1975-76, **19**(12), 20]; standardisation [*ibid*, 1976-77, **20**(2), 24]. *Guggul* gum, rev., 57 refs. (*Indian Drugs*, 1980-81, **18**, 417). Resin smoke, mosquito-repellent (*J Econ Tax Bot*, 1981, **2**, 175).

Str. of gum (*Indian J Chem*, 1966, **4**, 87). Guggul contains myricyl alc. and β-sitosterol (*Pak J Sci Ind Res*, 1967, **10**, 21; *CA*, 1968, **68**, 47009d).

Guggul(u)sterols—antiinflam. (*Indian J Exp Biol*, 1971, **9**, 403; *Indian J Med Res*, 1972, **60**, 929); anal. of gum and identn. of its steroidal constituents (*Tetrahedron*, 1972, **28**, 2341). Effect of ketosteroid from plant on induced hypercholesteremic & hyperlipidaemic in chick; regression by active steroid fraction; on thyroid glands in animals [*Indian J Exp Biol*, 1975, **13**, 15; *J Res Indian Med*, 1975, **10**(2), 11; *Q J Surg Sci*, 1974, **10**, 158; *CA*, 1975, **83**, 188662h]. Str. of guggulusterols-I,-II,-III, -IV & -V and sterones Z & E (*Indian J Chem*, 1976, **14B**, 802). Pharmacol. active principle for use as blood lipid lowering agent, isolation from oleogum resin of golden yellow var. (Indian Pat., 1976, 138525; *CA*, 1980, **92**, 11215x). Stereochem. of guggulsterol-1 (*Tetrahedron Lett*, 1981, **22**, 4623).

Indian gum resin, diterps. α-comphorene and cembrene (*Arch Pharm Wein*, 1972, **305**, 486; *CA*, **77**, 11154 t); str. of cembrene A and cembrane alc., mukulol (allylcembrol) (*Tetrahedron*, 1973, **29**, 341; 1976, **32**, 1437; *Khim Prir Soedin*, 1976, 108; *CA*, **85**, 59570u). Long-chain aliphatic tetrols (*Tetrahedron*, 1973, **29**, 1595).

Chem. of Indian essent. oil, rev. (*Perfum Essent Oil Res*, 1967, **58**, 622); antibact. (*Reichst Aromen Kosmet*, 1977, **27**, 303; *CA*, 1978, **88**, 99656v).

Flowers, flavons. (*Fitoterapia*, 1981, **52**, 221).

CONIUM (*Apiaceae*)

C. maculatum Linn.

Eng.–*Hemlock.*

Plant, causes poisoning in sheep (*Rev Zooteh Med Vet*, 1969, **19**, 74; *CA*, 1970, **73**, 12674t). In Europe, used as sed., anodyne, spasmod., in epilepsy, acute mania and whooping cough (*Acta Phytother*, 1971, **18**, 21). Plant ext., a constituent of med. preparation for treating obstruction of lymphatic system (Ger. Offen., 1971, 1963706; *CA*, **75**, 91299s). Mother tincture of hemlock of different homeopathic potencies beneficial in prevention of immature cataract (*Hahnemannian Gleanings*, 1979, **46**, 70).

Fruits, GLC estn. of volat. alks., coniine, N-Me-coniine and γ-coniceine; their pharmacol. (*Planta Med*, 1963, **11**, 92; *J Pharm Pharmacol*, 1963, **15**, 1). Exp. confirmation of teratogenic properties of plant

(*Lloydia*, 1975, **38**, 56). Tetratogenic effects in cattle, of plant and conium alks. α-analogues (*Clin Toxicol*, 1978, **12**, 49). Pharmacognosy of fruits (*Planta Med*, 1980, **39**, 88; 216).

Ripe seeds yield coumarins, bergapten and xanthotoxin (*An Quim*, 1969, **65**, 1165; *CA*, 1970, **72**, 129379w).

All organs contain alk. (1.77%), highest in aerial parts and lowest in stems; plant also contains coumarins (0.17%) (*Izv Akad Nauk Tadzh SSSR Otd Biol Nauk*, 1976, 81; *CA*, 1977, **86**, 86115b).

CONNARUS (*Connaraceae*)

C. monocarpus Linn.

Plant used in fractures (*Sri Lanka For*, 1980, **14**, 145).

Roots contain rapanone, bergenin and (–)-leucopelargonidin (*Phytochemistry*, 1964, **3**, 335). Fruits, rapanone, hentriacontane, lycopene, leucopelargonidin, and β-sitosterol (*Indian J Chem*, 1976, **14B**, 475).

***C. paniculatus** Roxb.

EtOH(50%) ext. of aerial parts, diur. and hypoten. (*Indian J Exp Biol*, **12**, 512).

Assam.

***C. wightii** Hook. f.

Mar.–*Fatfati.*

EtOH(50%) ext. of aerial parts, antivir., CNS depress. and hypoten. (*Indian J Exp Biol*, 1973, **11**, 43).

Ratnagiri, Maharashtra.

CONSOLIDA (*Ranunculaceae*)

C. ambigua (Linn.) Baill. & Heywood syn. *Delphinium ajacis* auct. non Linn.

Seeds, diterp. alks. (0.4%): ajaconine, delcoside & Ac-delcoside, and a related unknown alk.; mass spectrum of ajaconine (*Chem Ind Lond*, 1967, 320; 1972, 381). Diterp. alks. as plant growth regulator (*Nature Lond*, 1969, **222**, 576). As source of raw material for producing med. alks. (*Rastit Resur*, 1970, **6**, 243; *CA*, 1971, **74**, 10387y); identn. of delsoline (*Phytochemistry*, 1971, **10**, 1961). Mass spectra of delsoline, delcosine & OAcdelosine (*Proc Okla Acad Sci*, 1973, **53**, 92; *CA*, **79**, 137325k); alk., detn., highest in seeds; ajacine 10% of total alk. (*Bull Fac Pharm Cairo Univ*, 1974, **13**, 217); new alks. ajacusine and adadine; ambiguine and dihydroajaconine; several new and known alks. (*Heterocycles*, 1978, **9**, 463; 1241; *CA*, **89**, 39376q; 215615c; *J Natl Prod*, 1980, **43**, 395).

Flowers, anthocyanin and flavonol glycds. (*Phytochemistry*, 1975, **14**, 2677). Plant, new alks., [*Recent Dev Mass Spectrom Biochem Med Proc Int Symp*, 4th, 1977, (Pub., 1978), 1; 429; *CA*, 1978, **89**, 176315h].

C. regalis S.F. Gray syn. *Delphinium consolida* Linn.

Plant insectic. due to alks., esp. veratrine (*Epidemiol Mikrob Infektsiozni Bolesti*, 1964, **1**, 23; *CA*, 1965, **62**, 16628p). Flower, alks. (*Acta Pol Pharm*, 1965, **22**, 453; *Diss Pharm*, 1965, **17**, 497; 1968, **20**, 635; *CA*, 1966, **64**, 14482f; 18001g; 1969, **70**, 84937s); plant alks. (*Bull Acad Sci Ser Sci Chim*, 1965, **13**, 213; *CA*, **63**, 11976b). Variation in alk. content with growth (*Ukr Bot Zh*, 1969, **26**, 60).

Flavons. in different plant parts; kaempferol and quercetin in all parts. Presence of 10 free and bound aglycones established (*ibid*, 1971, **28**, 525). Petal anthocyanins (*Farm Glas*, 1966, **22**, 493; *CA*, 1967, **66**, 52834g).

CONVALLARIA (*Liliaceae*)

C. majalis Linn.

Eng.–*Lily-of-the-valley*.

Flowers—glycds. strengthen and regulate heart action; in dropsy they assist urine secretion; cause less secondary reactions (nausea, diar.) than leaves in med. doses.

Entire plant, very poisonous (Med. Plants, 36). Hypoglyc. (*in* Med Bot, 219).

Cardenolides—10 cardiac glycds.: convalloside, convallatoxol, convallatoxin, etc. (*Acta Pol Pharm*, 1963, **20**, 329; *CA*, 1964, **61**, 15931 de). Comparison of activities of cardiac glycds. from various plants, in mice and rats (*Arch Int Pharmacodyn*, 1965, **155**, 165; *CA*, **63**, 12171g). Clin. pharmacol. of drugs, rev., 125 refs. on *Convallaria* glycds. [*Farm Zh Kiev*, 1977, (2), 56; *CA*, **87**, 47812c].

'Corglycon' (total glycds.), technol. of production [*Khim Farm Zh*, 1975, **9**(8), 25; *CA*, 1976, **84**, 35237u]; extn., new glycds., etc. [*Khim Prir Soedin*, 1977, 537; *CA*, **87**, 197261m; *Herba Hung*, 1977, **16**, 1; 62; *CA*, 1978, **88**, 71452b; *Herba Pol*, 1978, **24**, 27; *Farmatsiya Sof*, 1979, **29**(2), 30; **29**(3), 36; *CA*, **91**, 137155c; 1980, **92**, 72670r; *Planta Med*, 1980, **40**, 1; *Sci Pharm*, 1981, **49**, 265].

Convallatoxol—chem., pharmacol., and clin., rev. (*Pharm Zentralhalle*, 1965, **104**, 377; *Dtsch Gesundheitswes*, 1965, **20**, 1435; *CA*, **63**, 9741g; 13909a); extn. (East Ger. Pat., 1970, 72348; *CA*, **73**, 123505h).

Convallatoxin—extremely effective diur. in rats (*Arch Exp Pathol Pharmacol*, 1963, **241**, 553; *CA*, 1965, **62**, 5765c); cytotoxic against Eagle KB strain of human epidermoid carcinoma (*J Med Chem*, 1965, **8**, 547). Alteration in lung blood supply under its effect (*Fiziol Zh Kiev*, 1968, **14**, 244; *CA*, **69**, 9609n); effective in impairment of coronary circulation in cats (*Farmakol Toksikol Moscow*, 1968, **31**, 421); detn. in leaves [*Khim Farm Zh*, 1969, **3**(6), 42; *CA*, **71**, 98960b].

Herb, flavons. (*Acta Pol Pharm*, 1972, **29**, 351; 1976, **33**, 767; *CA*, **77**, 149649r; 1977, **87**, 180762c). Extn. of flavons. having cholagogic action (USSR Pat., 1973, 378245; *CA*, **79**, 70209e).

Flavon. fraction, slightly diur. and spasmol. (*Herba Pol*, 1976, **22**, 163; *CA*, 1977, **86**, 50752t). Aerial parts, 6 flavons. (*Planta Med*, 1978, **33**, 412).

Lily-of-the-valley flower oil and others, rev., 20 refs. [*Perfum Flav*, 1980, **5**(6), 1].

CONVOLVULUS (*Convolvulaceae*)

C. arvensis Linn.

Plant—ext., hypoten. in cats, raises coronary circulation rate. Alks., hypoten. without vasodilation (*Farmakol Toksikol*

Moscow, 1966, **29**, 70; *CA*, **64**, 14811d); soaked in water, used as cooling drink (*J Agric Trop Bot Appl*, 1966, **13**, 262). EtOH ext., anticonvuls. in rats (*Izv Inst Fiziol Bulg Akad Nauk*, 1969, **12**, 205; *CA*, 1970, **72**, 98942t); aq. ext. mascarinic and nicotinic activity (*Indian J Pharm*, 1977, **39**, 89).

All parts of plant contain β-Me-esculetin (*Rev Med, Targu-Mures*, 1967, **13**, 354; *CA*, 1968, **68**, 102555f). Aerial parts, *n*-alkanes, *n*-alkanols, α-amyrin and sterols (*J Pharm Sci*, 1973, **62**, 678).

Roots, cuscohygrine (*Phytochemistry*, 1974, **13**, 519). Coumarins in Saudi Arabian plant (*Pharmazie*, 1981, **36**, 569; *CA*, **95**, 200551d).

C. auricomus Bhandari syn. *C. glomeratus* Choisy ex DC.

Roots and shoots, 2-C-Me-*D*-erythritol; its configuration (*Acta Chem Scand*, 1976, **30B**, 91; 903).

C. cuneatus Willd.; see **Argyreia cuneata**

C. microphyllus Sieb. ex Spreng. syn. *C. pluricaulis* Choisy
H.–*Shankhpushpi.*

Leaves and flowers—comparative study of hypoten. and potentiation of barbiturate hypnosis of different plant parts; max. activity in leaves and flowers [*J Res Indian Med*, 1972, **7**(4), 74; 1974, **9**(2), 19]; max. activity in leaves and flowers (*Planta Med*, 1975, **28**, 62); effective in anxiety neurosis; as sed., etc.; w.-insol. portion, most active [*J Res Indian Med*, 1977, **12**(3), 18; 42; 48; 58; 1977, **12**(4), 108; 1979, **14**(3-4), 7; 132; 136].

Clin. antianxiety effects and improved mental function (*Probe*, 1980-81, **20**, 201); plant effective in thyrotoxicosis (*Ancient Sci Life*, 1981-82, **1**, 46).

Leaves and flowers, antifung; pet. ext., antifung., probably due to some flavons. [*J Res Indian Med*, 1974, **9**(2), 69; *Geobias*, 1981, **8**, 66].

Plant ext., ceryl alc., 6-OMe-OH-coumarin and β- sitosterol (*J Indian Chem Soc*, 1969, **46**, 759). Fatty acids and waxy constituents of wildly growing Indian plant (*J Am Oil Chem Soc*, 1975, **52**, 318); hydrocarbons, aliphatic alcs., and sterols (*Z Naturforsch*, 1978, **33B**, 249). Alc. ext. of plant yield kaempferol, its glucd., di-OH-cinnamic acid and β-sitosterol glucd. (*Planta Med*, 1978, **34**, 222). Coumarins of plant grown in Saudi Arabia (*Pharmazie*, 1981, **36**, 569).

Essent. oil from plant, characteristics (*Perfum Essent Oil Rec*, 1967, **58**, 622). Str. of microphyllic acid, main glycd. acid, from plant resin (*Phytochemistry*, 1977, **16**, 715).

CONYZA (*Asteraceae*)

*C. stricta willd.

EtOH(50%) ext. of plant, antiamphetaminic, hypoten. and CNS depress. (*Indian J Exp Biol*, 1969, **7**, 250).

Plant contains diterp. resin acid, conyzic acid; diterp., strictic acid; str. of conyzic acid, identical with strictic acid and secconidoresedaic acid (*Indian J Chem*, 1975, **13**, 504; 1979, **18**, 494; 1981, **20**, 850). Flavons. (*ibid*, 1976, **14B**, 849); and 2 flavones including conyzatin (*Phytochemistry*, 1977, **16**, 1455).

Roots gave +ve test for alk. (*Lloydia*, 1972, **35**, 288).

Dehra Dun, U.P.

*C. viscidula Wall.

EtOH(50%) ext. of plant, antivir. (*Indian J Exp Biol*, 1971, **9**, 91).

Himachal Pradesh.

COPAIFERA (*Caesalpinaceae*)

C. mopane Kirk ex Benth.; see **Colophospermum mopane**

COPERNICIA (*Arecaceae*)

C. cerifera Mart.

Wax contains triterp., carnaubiol (*Aust J Chem*, 1965, **18**, 1411).

COPTIS (*Ranunculaceae*)

C. teeta Wall.

Local uses, distribution and cultivation. In Dibang valley rhizomes used in fever and in backache (*Bull Bot Sur India*, 1980, **22**, 179). In Siang (Arunachal Pradesh), used in dysen., cuts and wounds (*Bull Med Ethno Bot Res*, 1980, **1**, 440).

Rhizomes, 8-9% berberine (Hocking, 59); the drug, due to berberine & its related alks. promotes reticuloendothelium to increase phagocytosis of leucocytes in dog blood, both *in vitro* and *in vivo* (*in* Beal & Reinhard, 382). For other uses of berberine, see *Berberis*.

CORBICHONIA (*Aizoaceae*)

*C. decumbens Exell syn. *Orygia decumbens* Forsk.

P.–*Tambreswari*.

Roots infusion taken for biliousness and as emetic; leaves eaten in scarcity (Wlth India, VII, 110),

From drier regions of India.

CORCHORUS (*Tiliaceae*)

C. aestuans Linn. syn. *C. acutangulus* Lamk

EtOH(50%) ext. of plant, anticancer (*Indian J Exp Biol*, 1969, **7**, 250). Alc. ext. and glycd. of seeds, cardiotonic (*Acta Pharm Sin*, 1980, **15**, 193).

Plant, quercetin (*Indian J Chem*, 1963, **1**, 502). Seeds, erysimoside and olitoriside; fat, β-sitosterol and ceryl alc. (*ibid*, 1969, **7**, 1276; 1974, **12**, 780); oligosaccharides (*Indian J Pharm*, 1970, **32**, 17).

C. capsularis Linn.

Eng.–*Jute plant*.

Seed cardiac glycds., colorim. detn. (*Uzb Khim Zh*, 1965, **9**, 18; *CA*, **63**, 3315f); extn. on enzymic treatment; glycd. very effective in acute and chr. cardiac insufficiency, peroxystic tachycardia, tachyarythmia in oral dosing (Belg. Pat., 1968, 701544; *CA*, 1969, **70**, 38053c); helveticoside (*Tetrahedron Lett*, 1969, 789); oligosaccharides (*Indian J Pharm*, 1970,

32, 17); erysimoside and a polar glucd.; its str. (*ibid*, 1971, **33**, 58; *Indian J Chem*, 1972, **10**, 479); str. of corchoroside B (*Helv Chim Acta*, 1971, **54**, 1960). New bitter glycd., corchoside C along with strophanthidin, glycd. A and corchoside B (*Bangladesh J Sci Ind Res*, 1978, **13**, 127; *CA*, 1979, **90**, 148453d).

Leaves contain 3 bitter principles; corchoral, capsularol and capsularone, β-sitosterol & its glucd. (*Sci Res Dacca*, 1965, **2**, 152; *CA*, 1966, **65**, 10964c); a new triterp. glucd. (*J Bangladesh Acad Sci*, 1980, **4**, 155; *CA*, 1981, **95**, 43408t); ext. antifeedant against *Myllocerus discolor* (*Boh J Entomol Res*, 1980, **4**, 148).

Roots contain a triterp. corosin and β-sitosterol (*Pak J Sci Ind Res*, 1970, **13**, 363; 1971, **14**, 49; *CA*, 1971, **75**, 1339c; 106046h). Str. of corosin; oxo- corosin, corosilic and ursolic acids from fresh undried roots (*Z Naturforsch*, 1974, **29C**, 209; 1979, **34B**, 1320).

Bark exam. (*Bangladesh J Biol Agric Sci*, 1972, **1**, 64; *CA*, 1973, **78**, 26523h). Phytochem. of tissue culture (*Planta Med*, 1975, **27**, 77).

C. depressus (Linn.) Stocks syn. *C. antichorus* Rausch.

Infusion of leaves, demulc., laxt., carmin., stim., appetizer and bitter tonic useful in dysen., dyspep., and liver disorders. Decoct. of ripe fruit, in diar. Dried plant with goats milk, in sexual impotency (*J Agric Trop Bot Appl*, 1966, **13**, 285).

A tri-OH-dicarboxylic acid from plant; its tri-OAc, antipyr. and analg. in mice (*Indian J Pharm Sci*, 1979, **41**, 249; *J Ethnopharmacol*, 1981, **4**, 223). Distribution of coumarins, in plant grown in Saudi Arabia (*Pharmazie*, 1981, **36**, 569).

C. fascicularis Lamk

Plant, betulinic acid and β-sitosterol (*Indian J Appl Chem*, 1971, **34**, 237). Glycd. from plant, spasmol. (*Indian J Exp Biol*, 1973, **11**, 248).

Autofermented defatted seeds yield cardenolides including trilocularin (*Indian J Pharm*, 1976, **38**, 157).

C. olitorius Linn.

Eng.–*Jew's mallow.*

Seeds, ecbolic in mice; cardenolides, pharmacol, w.r.t. its cardiovascular activity (*Qual Plant Mater Veg*, 1968-69, **17**, 153; 305).

Olitoriside—a cardiac glycd., from seeds [*Izuch i Ispol's Lekarstv Rastit Resur SSSR (Leningrad : Med) Sb*, 1964, 200; *CA*, 1965, **63**, 2048h]. In patients, with chr. cardiac insufficiency, olitoriside equivalent to strophanthin (*Nauch Konf Vop Morfol Patol Serdechno-Sesudistoi Sist Yaroslavak Med Inst*, 1965, 44; *CA*, 1967, **67**, 31504e). Clin. efficacy of olitoriside A, k-strophanthin and KCl combination in heart diseases (*Ref Zh Otd Vyp Farmakol Khimioter Sredstva Toksikol*, 1967, No.7, 54, 358; *BA*, 1968, **49**, 13037). Isolation method of olitoriside from seeds (*Khim Prir Soedin*, 1969, **5**, 327; 1970, **6**, 702; 1972, **8**, 81; *CA*, 1970, **72**, 82921z; 1971, **74**, 84004t; 77, 85668m); coroloside along with olitoriside and erysimoside (*Khim Prir Soedin*, 1975, **11**, 525; *CA*, **83**, 203758q); raffinose and corchoroside A as by-products of olitoriside preparation (*ibid*, 1977, 285; *CA*, **87**, 86621j).

Seeds, helveticoside (*Tetrahedron Lett*, 1969, 789); corchoroside A, on reduction gave strophinthidol boirinoside (*Arch Pharm Wein*, 1969, **302**, 184; *CA*, **71**, 57533w); evonoside (*Khim Prir Soedin*, 1971, **7**, 378; *CA*, **75**, 115866c); also corchoroside A, strophanthidol, strophanthidin & its trioside; helveticoside and olitorin (*Indian J Pharm*, 1972, **34**, 168; *Curr Sci*, 1973, **42**, 731); preparation of strophanthidin-OAc (*Deposited Doc*, 1975, VINITI, 745; *CA*, 1977, **87**, 44175m). Cardiotonic action of corchoroside A, ouabin and strophanthin-K on heart-lung preparation of guinea- pig and cat (*Acta Pharm Sin*, 1979, **14**, 257).

Roots, a triterp. corosin and β-sitosterol (*Pak J Sci Ind Res*, 1971, **14**, 49; *CA*, **75**, 106046h).

Distribution of glycds. in Egyptian plant (*Egypt J Chem*, 1976, **19**, 153).

C. trilocularis Linn.

Autofermented seeds yield glycds., trilocularin and corchoroside B (*Phytochemistry*, 1975, **14**, 533).

CORDIA (*Ehretiaceae*)

C. dichotoma Forst.

EtOH(50%) of leaves of stems, antimicrob. (*Fitoterapia*, 1980, **51**, 231). Leaf decoct. used in cough and cold (*Bull Med Ethno Bot Res*, 1980, **1**, 318).

C. gharaf Ehrenb. ex Aschers syn. *C. angustitolia* Roxb.; *C. rothii* Roem. & Schult.

Fruits useful in constip., stomach worms, piles and toothache (*J Agric Trop Bot Appl*, 1966, **13**, 265). EtOH(50%) ext. of aerial parts, CNS depress. (*Indian J Exp Biol*, 1973, **11**, 43).

Stem, sitosterol (*Indian J Chem*, 1976, **14B**, 473). Unsap. matter of fruits, *n*-hentriacontane, β-amyrin and β-sitosterol (*J Indian Chem Soc*, 1978, **55**, 419). Compn. of leaf wax (*Acta Ciencia Indica*, 1980, **6**, 226).

C. macleodii Hook. f. & Thoms.

Plant used in gravel and dysen. (*Econ Bot*, 1970, **24**, 241).

C. myxa Roxb. non Linn. syn. *C. obliqua* Willd.

Various plant parts used in dropsy, anasarca, urticaria, cholera and dysen. (*Econ Bot*, 1970, **24**, 241). EtOH(50%) ext. of aerial parts, hypothermic and diur. (*Indian J Exp Biol*, 1974, **12**, 512; 1977, **15**, 208).

Fruit mucilage, a valuable anticapping agent for amidopyrine tablets (*J Drug Res*, 1969, **2**, 117; *CA*, 1971, **74**, 91137s); Mono- & polysaccharides (*Pak J Sci Ind Res*, 1976, **19**, 64; *CA*, 1978, **88**, 60115t).

Seed oil, β-sitosterol (*Planta Med*, 1967, **15**, 241). Seeds, flavonol glycd., taxifolin 3-rhamnoside (*Indian Drugs*, 1978-79, **16**, 105); also 3,5-dirhamnoside (*Phytochemistry*, 1979, **18**, 2058); and distylin 3-xyloside (*Indian J Pharm Sci*, 1980, **42**, 95).

Stem bark, allantoin, β-sitosterol and a flavanone rhamnopyranoside (*Planta Med*, 1979, **36**, 191).

Roots, β-sitosterol (*Vijnana Parishad Anusandhan Patrica*, 1977, **20**, 153); flavon. glycd. (*Indian J Chem*, 1977, **15B**, 760); hesperetin 7-rhamnoside; also maltoside (*Phytochemistry*, 1978, **17**, 334; 1005).

CORDYLINE (*Agavaceae*)

C. fruticosa Goeppert syn. *C. terminalis* Kunth

In Hawaii, flowers used against growth in nostrils, asthma, dry fever and run-down condition; in Tonga, leaves squeezed in water and liquid used to cure eye infections. Leaves crushed with Tongan oil and applied to abscesses of gums (*Econ Bot*, 1971, **25**, 245; 440). In Samoa, leaf juice with coconut oil used to treat inflam. in aching limbs, fever and earache. Pounded bark or root juice given in illness (*ibid*, 1974, **28**, 5).

COREOPSIS (*Asteraceae*)

*C. grandiflora Hogg ex Sweet

EtOH(50%) ext. of plant, hypoten. (*Indian J Exp Biol*, 1973, **11**, 43).

5-Ph-Et-thiophene-2-aldehyde (*Chem Ber*, 1967, **100**, 2518). Flavon. chem. of *C. grandiflora* vars. (*Brittonia*, 1980, **32**, 154).

Reported from Uttar Pradesh.

CORIANDRUM (*Apiaceae*)

C. sativum Linn.
Eng.–*Coriander*.

Fruit—also referred to as seeds. Used to prevent gripping; decoct. in sore throat, catar.; also to wash eyes in conjuctivitis. Leaves useful as carmin. and antibil. [*Indian Fmrs Dig*, 1978, **11**(6 & 7), 74].

Seed ext., antimicrob. (*Khim Farm Zh*, 1968, **2**, 40; *CA*, **69**, 944k); ext. beneficial as antibact. and sed., used in lotions and shampoos (*Maslo-Zhir Promst*, 1969, **35**, 25; *CA*, **71**, 42162a); with caster oil useful in rheum. [*J Res Indian Med*, 1978, **12**(4), 53]. Roasted, useful in dyspep. As poultice, they are applied in chr. ulcers and carbuncles [*Indian Frms Dig*, 1978, **11**(6 & 7), 74]. EtOH(50%) ext. fungitoxic against *Helminthosporium oryzae* (*Nat Acad Sci Lett*, 1978, **1**, 287).

Essent. oil from fruit, antimicrob. (*Indian Drugs*, 1976- 77, **14**, 62; *Herba Pol*, 1980, **26**, 245).

Various plant parts used in spleen complaint, sores, veneral sores and syphilis (*Econ Bot*, 1970, **24**, 241). Leaves useful as carmin. and antibil. [*Indian Frms Dig*, 1978, **11**(6 & 7), 74].

Fruits, umbelliferone and scopoletin (*Khim Prir Soedin*, 1974, **10**, 94; *CA*, **81**, 60810w); seeds, quercetin 3-O- caffeyl glucd. and kaempferol 3-glucd. (*Z Lebensm Unters Forsch*, 1977, **164**, 194; *CA*, **87**, 166146 y). Samples of coriander contains aflatoxins B_1 & B_2 (*Can Inst Food Sci Technol J*, 1975, **8**, 124; *CA*, **83**, 145901t); gave +ve test for alk. (*Lloydia*, 1972, **35**, 117).

Essent. oil, from seeds, chem. constituents; some promising selections [*Indian Perfum*, 1977, **21**, 86; 1976, **20**(IA), 14]; from fruits grown around Mysore, high geranyl content [*Indian Spices*, 1979, **16**(1), 7]; of Vietnamese origin (*Tap Chi Hoa Hoc*, 1980, **18**, 30; *CA*, 1981, **94**, 52670p); recent advances in chem. (*Perfum Flav*, 1980, **5**, 6; 55).

Seed fat, small amts. of $\Delta^{5,6}$-octadecenoic acid (*Chem Ind Lond*, 1970, 831). Extn. of 6-octadecenoic acid from Taiwan coriander [*Hua Hsueh*, 1973, (2), 52; *CA*, 1974, **80**, 45638g]. Seeds, β-sitosterol (*Indian J Chem*, 1974, **12**, 226).

Plant, chlorogenic and caffeic acids, 7 coumarins, quercetin, and rutin (*Khim Prir Soedin*, 1974, **10**, 94; *CA*, **81**, 60810w).

Volat. flavour compds. of leaves (*J Sci Food Agric*, 1976, **27**, 721).

Coriander, various aspects (Parry, 108-11; 193-94; *in* Purseglove *et al*, II, 736-91).

CORIARIA (*Coriariaceae*)

C. nepalensis Wall.

Seed oil contains (*R*)-13-OH-*cis*-9, *trans*-11- octadecadienoic acid as principal fatty acid (*Tetrahedron Lett*, 1966, 4329).

CORNUS (*Cornaceae*)

See **BENTHAMIDIA**

CORONOPUS (*Brassicaceae*)

*C. didymus Smith

Seeds, cooling, used in headache (*J Econ Tax Bot*, 1980, **1**, 138).

Leaves gave +ve test for alk. and flavon. (*Lloydia*, 1972, **35**, 288).

Found in Rajasthan.

CORTADERIA (*Poaceae*)

*C. selloana (Schult.) Aschers & Graeb.

Grass contains phytotoxic substance (*J Chem Ecol*, 1975, **1**, 183).

Native of S. America; introduced into India as an ornamental.

CORYDALIS (*Fumariaceae*)

*C. cornuta Royle

EtOH(50%) ext. of plant, hypoten. (*Indian J Exp Biol*, 1980, **18**, 594).

Leaves and stems contain alks., (-)-stylopine, protopine and (-)- coreximine (*Indian J Chem*, 1977, **15B**, 389).

Temperate Himalayas: from Kumaun to Kashmir, at 4,000 m.

C. govaniana Wall.

Plant—decoct. in chr. fever and liver complaints [*J Res Indian Med*, 1973, **8**(1), 76]; juice useful in eye diseases; contains alks. protoine, choline, corlumine, biculline and isocorydine (*Khadi Gramodyog*,

1976-77, **23**, 115); EtOH(50%) ext., hypoten. and spasmol. (*Annu Rep RRL Jammu*, 1970-71, 24; *Indian J Exp Biol*, 1977, **15**, 208).

Str. of govanine; also of 3 alks., corygovanine, govadine & govanine and base, biscuculline from leaves and stems (*Indian J Chem*, 1976, **14B**, 58; 216; 844).

*C. meiofolia Wall.

Ladakh—*Stogzil*.

Herb used as hepato-tonic and stomch. (*in* Atal & Kapur, Med. Plants, 519).

Root, stems and leaves contain alk. (*Lloydia*, 1971, **34**, 94).

Occurs in Ladakh.

CORYLUS (*Corylaceae*)

C. avellana Linn.

Leaves contain taraxerol,β-sitosterol and stigmast- 5-en-3 α, 7 α-22 α- triol (*Z Naturforsch*, 1966, **21B**, 78).

C. jacquemontii Decne. syn. *C. colurna* auct. non Linn.

EtOH(50%) ext. of aerial parts, hypoten. (*Indian J Exp Biol*, 1971, **9**, 91).

COSCINIUM (*Menispermaceae*)

C. fenestratum Colebr.

Eng.–*Vine*; H.–*Thar-ki-Haldi*.

Roots resemble turmeric, considered bitter tonic and stomch. (Uphof, 154).

Plant used against fractures (*Sri Lanka For*, 1980, **14**, 145).

Stem and root yield same pattern of alks., berberine and jatrarrhizine (major); berbarrubine and N,N-di-Me-lindacarpine (appreciable amt.) and thalifendine and palmitine (small amts.) (*Planta Med*, 1980, **38**, 24).

COSMOS (*Asteraceae*)

*C. bipinnatus Cav.

Seed ext, antifung. [*Environ India*, 1981, **4**(I & II), 83]. Astringency of leaves due to poor extractibility of tannins (*Phytochemistry*, 1980, **19**, 982).

Seeds yield β-sitosterol glucd. (*Indian J Appl Chem*, 1963, **26**, 174).

Flowers, flavon. cosmosin [*Nagoya Shiritse Daigaku Yakugakubu Kenkyu Nempo*, 1968, (16), 29; *CA*, 1669, **70**, 93947x]; distribution of flavons. in various plant parts; contains trifolin and luteolin glucuronide (*Z Pflanzenphysiol*, 1974, **71**, 80). Flowers, 7-glucuronides of chrysoeriol and luteolin (*Planta Med*, 1976, **30**, 349). Identn. of flavones in plant (*Agric Biol Chem*, 1978, **42**, 475).

Physicochem. characteristics of essent. oil from flowers (*Indian Oil Soap J*, 1969-70, **35**, 136).

Cultivated in Indian gardens.

COSMOSTIGMA (*Asclepiadaceae*)

C. racemosum Wight

Juice of leaves used against neck inflam. of bullocks (*J Econ Tax Bot*, 1981, **2**, 187).

COSTUS (*Costaceae*)

C. speciosus Smith

Rhizomes—*chutney* made from burnt tuber, sugar and tamarind taken for dysen. and other digestive troubles (*Econ Bot*, 1965, **19**, 245). Powd. in indign. (*Bull Bot Surv India*, 1973, **15**, 20); paste taken internally when urine contains blood (*Bull Med Ethno Bot Res*, 1980, **1**, 8).

Carbontetrachloride ext. of rhizome, strong. stim. on uterine musculature in animals and human; rhizomes and saponin mixt., spasmodic [*J Res Indian Med*, 1972, **7**(2), 14; 1974, **9**(1), 164]; antifung. [*ibid*, 1976, **11**(1), 105].

Plant—various plant parts, in fever, ardor, dropsy, anasarca, gravel, cholera, phthisis, and bronch. asthma (*Econ Bot*, 1970, **24**, 241). EtOH(50%) ext., antivir. (*Indian J Exp Biol*, 1973, **11**, 43). One of the constituents of indigenous drug '*Amber mezhugu*', useful in rheum. (*Rheumatism*, 1976-77, **12**, 38). Juice of stem bark taken in burning sensation on urination (*Q J Crude Drug Res*, 1979, **17**, 66); juice of

boiled plant used in earache (*Bull Med Ethno Bot Res*, 1980, **1**, 8).

Rhizome essent. oil, physicochem. characteristics (*Perfum Essent Oil Rec*, 1967, **58**, 622); antimicrob. [*Indian Perfum*, 1971, **15**(Pt.2), 89]; roots, aliphatic OH-ketone; also 5α-stimast-9(11)-en-3β-ol (*Phytochemistry*, 1981, **20**, 2557).

Rhizomes yield diosgenin (2.12%) and tigogenin, saponins & genins cause spasmodic uterine contraction (*Experientia*, 1970, **26**, 475); saponins showed estrogen-like activity in albino rats similar to stilbestrol (*Indian J Med Res*, 1972, **60**, 287); estrogenic activity of 1600 μg diosgenin equivalent to 150 μg neoclinestrol; abortif. in rats; caused abortion and early parturation in rabbits [*Indian J Pharm*, 1973, **35**, 35; 114; *Med Surg*, 1972, **12**(1), 177]. Saponin mixt., antiinflam.; rhizomes also contain β-sitosterol glucd. (*Indian J Pharm*, 1972, **34**, 116).

Diosgenin—rhizome, as potential source, various aspects such as cultivation, extn., etc. (Asolkar & Chadha, 47-51; 65; 89). Optimum conditions for max. yield; effect of rhizome diameter: thinnest contained max. (*Indian Drugs*, 1976-77, **14**, 101; 1977-78, **15**, 14). Method of high production (*Indian J Pharm Sci*, 1981, **43**, 184). Variation of content in rhizomes with locality (*Indian Drugs*, 1979-80, **17**, 3).

Diosgenin and tigogenin from stem and rhizome callus (*Lloydia*, 1978, **41**, 640); steroidal constituents of callus cultures (*Planta Med*, 1979, **35**, 289). NMR of dioscin and gracillin from rhizome (*Indian J Chem*, 1980, **19B**, 817).

Seeds, diosgenin as major genin (*Q J Crude Drug Res*, 1979, **17**, 113); as additional source of diosgenin (2.4% dry wt) (*Planta Med*, 1980, **38**, 185); saponin, potent hypoten. and bradycardiac in dogs (*Indian Drugs*, 1980-81, **18**, 121).

*C. speciosus Smith var. argyrophyllus Wall.

EtOH(50%) ext. of plant, hypoten. and CNS depress. (*Indian J Exp Biol*, 1974, **12**, 512).

Found in Goalpara, Assam.

COTINUS (Anacardiaceae)

C. coggygria Scop. syn. *Rhus cotinus* Linn.
H.–*Tunga.*
Leaf and seed decoct. used in cancer (*Lloydia*, 1967, **30**, 100). Leaves, astrin., vesic. and diur.; given in colic and dysen. (*Indian Drugs*, 1976-77, **14**, 47).
EtOH(50%) ext. of aerial parts, antiprot., antivir. and CNS depress. (*Indian J Exp Biol*, 1968, **6**, 232); ext., antifung. (*Labdev*, 1971, **9B**, 136).
Leaf tannin useful for production of gallic acid (*Kem Ind*, 1965, **14**, 147; *CA*, 1966, **64**, 927g); polyphenols [*Fenol' nye Soedin lkh Biol Funkts Mater Vses Simp* 1966 (Pub. 1968), 78; *CA*, 1969, **71**, 10255s]; anthocyanins (*Phytochemistry*, 1969, **8**, 2367); total flavons., antiphl. in mice (*Farmakol Toksikol Moscow*, 1969, **32**, 596). Seasonal variation of tannin, flavon. glycds. and gallic acid in leaves (*Rastit Resur*, 1972, **8**, 237; *CA*, **77**, 39094y); str. of gallotannin (*Khim Prir Soedin*, 1973, 789; *CA*, 1975, **82**, 28556c); selective extn. for tannin [*Khim Farm Zh*, 1981, **15**(12), 68].

COTONEASTER (Rosaceae)

*****C. acuminatus** Lindl.
EtOH(50%) ext. of aerial parts, CNS depress. (*Indian J Exp Biol*, 1973, **11**, 43).
Chamoli, U.P.

C. bacillaris Wall. ex. Lindl. syn. *C. affinis* Lindl. var. *bacillaris* (Lindl.) Schneid.
New leaves and shoots poisonous to livestock [*Indian Livestk*, 1963, **1**(2), 28]. EtOH(50%) ext. of aerial parts, antivir. and diur. (*Indian J Exp Biol*, 1973, **11**, 43).
Twigs, leaves and fruits contain flavon. (*Lloydia*, 1971, **34**, 100).

*****C. integrifolius** (Roxb.) Klotz.
EtOH(50%) ext. of plant, semen coagulant (*Indian J Exp Biol*, 1980, **18**, 594).
Chamoli. in U.P., and Khasi hills of Meghalaya.

*****C. marginatus** Schldl.
EtOH(50%) ext. of aerial parts, spasmol. and anticancer (*Indian J Exp Biol*, 1969, **7**, 250).
Shimla, H.P.

COTULA (Asteraceae)

*****C. hemisphaerica** (Roxb.) Wall. ex Benth. & Hook. f.
EtOH(50%) ext. of plant, spermic. (*Indian J Exp Biol*, 1980, **18**, 594).
Kheri, U.P.

COTYLEDON (Crassulaceae)

C. laciniata Roxb.; see **Kalanchoe laciniata**

CRASSOCEPHALUM (Asteraceae)

*****C. aurantiaca** DC.
Eng.–*Velvet plant.*
Leaves used for ringworm in Java (Wlth India, IV, 281).
Grown in Indian gardens.

*****C. crepidioides** (Benth.) S. Moore syn. *Gynura crepidioides* Benth.
Meghalaya–*Jali.*
Leaf decoct. used as a lotion for headache and mild stomch. (Wlth India, IV, 280); juice taken to treat constip. and other stomach disorders (*Econ Bot*, 1981, **35**, 4).
Native of Tropical Africa, found in Tamil Nadu, Orissa, W. Bengal, Assam and elsewhere.

CRATAEGUS (Rosaceae)

*****C. crenulata** Roxb.
Fruit—med. used as fruits of *C. songarica* (*Indian Drugs*, 1976- 77, **14**, 47).
Himalayas from Sutlej and Bhutan.

C. songarica Koch syn. *C. oxyacantha* auct. non Linn.
Eng.–*Hawthorn.*
Berries eaten fresh as heart tonic; tea of dried ones equally effective (*Acta Phytother*, 1963, **10**, 1). Plant ext., ingredient of a compn. for behaviour

disturbances and insomnia in infants (*Clin Term*, 1969, **51**, 15; *CA*, 1970, **72**, 99037p); propylene glycol ext. in cosmetic preparation for skin improvement (Fr. Pat., 1970, 1588770; *CA*, 1971, **75**, 67391v).

Leaves contain leucocyanidins (*Bull Acad Pol Sci Ser Sci Biol*, 1965, **13**, 121); flavons.; principal, vitexin-4- rhamnoside (*Arzneim Forsch*, 1966, **16**, 80; 1965, **15**, 1417; *CA*, 1966, **64**, 18023d; 20193e); vitexin glycds.; oligomeric leucoanthocyanidin; and polymeric flavons. (*Rocz Chem*, 1966, **40**, 445; 2025; 1970, **44**, 1733; *CA*, **65**, 5730h; 1967, **67**, 8713p; 1971, **74**, 108111d); oligomeric procyanidins decreased B.P. in cats and affected CNS (*Arzneim Forsch*, 1971, **21**, 886; *CA*, **75**, 13926f); estn. of flavons. and preparation of flavon.- enriched exts. (*Acta Pharm Jugosl*, 1977, **27**, 75); catechins and oligomeric proanthocyanidins in callus and suspension culture (*Planta Med*, 1977, **32**, 297). Hyperoside and vitexin glycds. main flavons. in plant (*Acta Pharm Hung*, 1977, **47**, 11; *CA*, **87**, 28903s). Cardiotonic activity due to *l*-epicatechin present in leaves and fruits; flavones vitexin and hyperoside potentiate activity (*Indian Drugs*, 1980-81, **18**, 302).

Str. units of condensed tannins (polymer proanthocyanidins); also comparison of strs. of tannins from leaves and fruits (*J Sci Food Agric*, 1981, **32**, 711).

CRATEVA (*Capparaceae*)

C. nurvala Buch.- Ham. syn. *C. religiosa* Hook. f.& Thoms. non Forst.f.

Bark—Contracep.; juice of bark given to women after childbirth (*Econ Bot*, 1965, **19**, 239; 1980, **34**, 264); oxytocic (*Annu Rep, ICMR*, 1967-68, 64); bitter and poisonous (*Q J Crude Drug Res*, 1972, **12**, 1922). W.- sol. fraction of alc. ext., spasmol. on animal and human uterii and cholinergic on smooth muscles of animals; pet. ether ext., antiinflam. against different types of inflam. [*J Res Indian Med*, 1966, **1**, 120; 1974, **9**(3), 9]. Ingredient in indigenous drug for polycythaemia [*ibid*, 1976, **11**(1), 117].

Various plant parts used in baldness, sores and epidydimitis and hydrocele (*Econ Bot*, 1970, **24**, 241). Plant inhibited phosphatic stone formation in rats [*J Sci Res Plants Med*, 1980, **1**(3-4), 9]. Plant used in fractures (*Sri Lanka For*, 1980, **14**, 145).

Root ext., antibact. against Gram +ve and Gram –ve bacteria [*Med Surg*, 1965, **5**(2), 11]. Alc. ext. of stem, antibact. against *E. coli* [*J Res Indian Med*, 1974, **9**(2), 66].

Bark yields ceryl alc., friedelin, lupeol, betulinic acid and diosgenin; fruits, glucocapparin, β-sitosterol, triacontane, triacontanol, cetyl and ceryl alcs. (*Planta Med*, 1978, **34**, 223). Bark and stem gave +ve test for alk. (*Lloydia*, 1972, **35**, 1).

Leaves, *l*-stachydrine (*Phytochemistry*, 1973, **12**, 2893). Rootbark, rutin, quercetin and β-sitosterol (*J Indian Chem Soc*, 1974, **51**, 1058); lupen-3-one, lupeol; 3-epilupeol, its-OAc, and ψ-taraxasterol; a new triterp. (*Curr Sci*, 1975, **44**, 227; *Planta Med*, 1975, **27**, 254; 1977, **32**, 214).

CREPIS (*Asteraceae*)

C. fleuosa (DC.) Benth.

Ladakh–*Samboo*.

Milky latex of palnt used in constip. (*in* Atal & Kapur, Med. Plants, 519).

Found in Ladakh.

CRESCENTIA (*Bignoniaceae*)

C. cujete Linn.

Used to treat mangy dogs (*Econ Bot*, 1970, **24**, 344).

EtOH(50%) ext. of aerial parts, antiprot. (*Indian J Exp Biol*, 1980, **18**, 594).

CRESSA (*Convolvulaceae*)

C. cretica Linn.

Plant contains quercetin glycd. [*J Res Indian Med*, 1974, **9**(3), 109]; also a coumarin (*Pharmazie*, 1981, **36**, 569).

CRINUM (*Amaryllidaceae*)

C. asiaticum Linn.

In Samoa, bulb used as emetic and antid. (*Econ Bot*, 1974, **28**, 4).

Fruit of var. *japonicum* yields alk. hamayne (*Bull Chem Soc Jpn*, 1976, **49**, 3369); bark, sterols and triterp. (*Yakugaku Zasshi*, 1977, **97**, 1155).

C. defixum Ker.–Gawl.

Anti-T.B. activity of lycorine (*Indian J Pharm*, 1967, **29**, 157).

*****C. defixum** Ker.- Gawl. var. **defixum**

EtOH(50%) ext. of plant, CNS depress., diur. and antiinflam. (*Indian J Exp Biol*, 1977, **15**, 208).

Bastar, M. P.

C. latifolium Linn. syn. *C. zeylanicum* Linn.

Plant used in tubercular fistula (*Econ Bot*, 1970, **24**, 241).

C. powellii Hort. var. **album** Hort.

Plant alks., crinosine, crinidine and powelline (*Pharmazie*, 1965, **20**, 586; *CA*, **63**, 18649g); also cherylline (*J Org Chem*, 1970, **35**, 1100).

CROCUS (*Iridaceae*)

C. sativus Linn.

Saffron—bot., chem. and med. details, rev., 37 refs. (*Econ Bot*, 1966, **20**, 377). Different preparations have been used in various kinds of cancers (*Lloydia*, 1969, **32**, 252). In Europe, used as carmin., diaphor., emmen.; in amenor.; dysmen. and hysteria (*Acta Phytother*, 1971, **18**, 21). Med. uses (*J Sci Ind Res*, 1975, **34**, 644). Used as aphrodis. (*Nagarjun*, 1979-80, **23**, 170). In Unani med., used as exhilarant, helps absorption of cardiotonics and strengthens inner part of the body [*East Pharm*, 1980, **23**(272), 39].

Constituent of pharm. preparations for preventing premature ejaculation (Ger. Offen., 1975, 2405115; *CA*, **83**, 197817q). In indigenous drug 'Amber Mezhugu', useful in rheum. [*Rheumatism*, 1976-77, **12**(2), 38]; in Unani drug 'Jawarish Jalinoos', useful in gastro-intestinal disorders [*J Res Indian Med*, 1979, **14**(3-4), 34]. Minor constituent of indigenous drug Geriforte' useful as antifatigue drug and also in senile pruritus (*Indian Drugs*, 1980-81, **18**, 346; *Rajasthan Med J*, 1980, **19**, 23).

Plant ext., uterine stim.; effect myogenic and neurogenic (*Yao Hsueh Hsueh Pao*, 1964, **11**, 94; *CA*, **61**, 2348b). Alc. ext. of stigma, antifung. (*Geobios*, 1978, **5**, 49).

Saffron chem., rev., 51 refs. [*East Pharm*, 1969, **12**(141), 52]; evaluation of purity of saffron (*Res Ind*, 1971, **16**, 294). Isolation of picrocrocin (*Helv Chim Acta*, 1973, **56**, 1121). Stigmas of flowers minor carotenoid (*Indian J Chem*, 1975, **13**, 339). Characteristics of essent. oil from petals (*Perfum Essent Oil Rec*, 1967, **58**, 622). Volat. constituents of plant (*Lebensm Wiss Technol*, 1971, **4**, 43; *CA*, **75**, 87198r; *Phytochemistry*, 1971, **10**, 2755).

CROTALARIA (*Fabaceae*)

C. spp. source of hepatotoxic pyrrolizidine alks. (*J Natl Prod*, 1981, **44**, 129-52).

*****C. agatiflora** Schw.

Eng.–*Canary-bird bush.*

Alc. ext. of plant, hypoten., spasmol. and smooth muscle relaxant in animals (*Indian J Exp Biol*, 1967, **5**, 149).

Contains alk. madurensine (*Tetrahedron Lett*, 1966, 537).

Cultivated at RRL, Jammu.

*****C. alata** Buch.- Ham. ex Roxb.

Plant pounded and applied as paste on boils and abscesses (*Nagarjun*, 1980-81, **24**, 1).

Seeds contain alk. usaramine (*Indian J Pharm*, 1976, **38**, 156).

Kumaun, Assam and Khasi hills and parts of Tamil Nadu up to 2,500m.

C. albida Heyne ex Roth

Pyrrolizidine alk., croalbidine (*Indian J Chem*, 1973, **11**, 88). Stereochem. of croalbinecine (*Aust J Chem*, 1974, **27**, 1805).

C. anagyroides H.B. & K.

Seeds, alk. *l*-methylenepyrrolizidine and senecionine (*Planta Med*, 1964, **12**, 173); anacrotine (*Tetrahedron Lett*, 1966, 537); flavon., isovitexin (*Curr Sci*, 1967, **36**, 403); flavons. (*Phytochemistry*, 1970, **9**, 2581); trachelenthamidine (small amts.) (*Indian J Pharm*, 1976, **38**, 156);β-amyrin and β-sitosterol (*Indian J Chem*, 1978, **16B**, 78).

*C. assamica Benth.

Seeds, antitumour effect and toxicity in mice of alk. isolated; source for pyrrolizidine alk., monocrotaline, antitumour (*Chung Hua I Hsueh Tsa Chih*, 1973, 472; *Chih Wu Hsueh Pao*, 1974, **16**, 380; *CA*, 1974, **82**, 11176f; **83**, 25052v); see *C. spectabilis*.

Found in Assam.

*C. brevifolia Linn.

Seeds, β-sitosterol (*Indian J Pharm*, 1966, **28**, 274); alks. usaramine and integerrimine (*Indian J Chem*, 1967, **5**, 655); usaramine, hypoten., relaxant and spasmol.; pharmacol. properties of integerrimine (*Indian J Exp Biol*, 1969, **7**, 144; 1971, **9**, 177).

Cultivated at RRL, Jammu.

*C. brownei Bert. ex DC.

EtOH(50%) ext., pharmacol. (*Indian J Exp Biol*, 1971, **9**, 91).

Baripada, Orissa.

C. burhia Buch.-Ham. ex Benth.

Plant useful in gout, hydrophobia and swellings (*J Agric Trop Bot Appl*, 1966, **13**, 268). EtOH(50%) ext. of roots, anticancer (*Indian J Exp Biol*, 1980, **18**, 594).

Leaves and branches, hentriacontane and β- sitosterol (*Pak J Sci Ind Res*, 1967, **10**, 80; *CA*, **68**, 57385n). Plant, alk. crotalarine (*ibid*, 1973, **16**, 227; *CA*, 1974, **81**, 120836w); and croburhine (*Indian J Chem*, 1975, **13**, 835).

Rotenoids in tissue culture (*Planta Med*, 1979, **36**, 181). Isolation of antimicrob. principle from tissue culture (*Indian J Pharm Sci*, 1980, **42**, 113).

*C. calycina Schrank

Plant parts used in pain, convuls., wounds, venereal sores, syphilis, carbuncle, haemat., cholera, dysen. and spider-lick (*Econ Bot*, 1970, **24**, 241).

Found in Hassan district of Karnataka.

*C. fulva Roxb.

Plant, cause for outbreak of cirrhosis of liver in Jamaica (*in* Plant and Fungal Toxins, 649, 660); toxic [*Int Symp Hepatotoxic*, 1973 (Pub. 1974), 142; *CA*, 1975, **83**, 1555k]. EtOH(50%) ext. of aerial parts, diur. (*Indian J Exp Biol*, 1974, **12**, 512).

Tirupati, A.P.

C. juncea Linn.

Leaves, emmen. and abortif. (*Q J Crude Drug Res*, 1972, **12**, 1922). Ext. of leaves and seeds antifert. in albino rats (*Indian J Med Res*, 1979, **70**, 517). Seed ext.,hepatotoxic in mice (*Nagpur Vet Coll Mag*, 1976-79, **7**, 13). Plant known to cause hepatic veno-occlusive disease originating in Ecuador (*Gastroenterology*, 1976, **70**, 105).

Seed, phytoagglutinin (*Biochim Biophys Acta*, 1973, **310**, 446). Quercetin from tissue cultures (*Indian J Exp Biol*, 1974, **12**, 466); alk. production from tissue culture (*ibid*, 1977, **15**, 807).

C. laburnifolia Linn.

EtOH(50%) ext. of aerial parts, CNS depress. (*Indian J Exp Biol*, 1974, **12**, 512).

Seeds, alk.; its pharmacol. (*Indian J Pharm*, 1964, **26**, 322); alk., anacrotine (*Indian J Chem*, 1967, **5**, 655); alk. crotalaburnine and β-sitosterol (*Indian J Pharm*, 1966, **28**, 277); anacrotine identical with crotalaburanine (*J Indian Chem Soc*, 1971, **48**, 887). Major alks.; and flavons., orientin & isoorientin (*Curr Sci*, 1967, **36**, 363; 364). Pharmacol. of crotalaburnine (*Indian J Med Res*, 1968, **56**, 1386); crotalaburnine extn., its pharmacol.; flowers, hyperoside (*Planta Med*, 1968, **16**, 432).

Whole plant, alk. nadurensine (*Indian J Chem*, 1969, **7**, 308; *Tetrahedron Lett*, 1966, 537).

C. medicaginea Lamk

EtOH(50%) ext. of plant, CNS depress. (*Indian J Exp Biol*, 1971, **9**, 91).

Chem. examination of whole plant ext. (*Curr Sci*, 1966, **35**, 460). Seeds, 2 pyrrolizidine alks., Me-ethers of supnidine & heliotridine (*J Indian Chem Soc*, 1970, **47**, 741).

*C. medicaginea Lamk var. luxuriona Baker

EtOH(50%) ext. of plant, spasmol. (*Indian J Exp Biol*, 1977, **15**, 208).

Plant yields rotenone, elliptone and tephrosin (*J Natl Prod*, 1979, **42**, 689).

Rajasthan.

*C. nana Burm f.

Ultra-str. of liver in veno-occlusive diseases due to grain (*Indian J Med Res*, 1978, **68**, 790).

Western Peninsula ascending to 2,500 m.

C. pallida Ait. syn. *C. mucronata* Desv.; *C. striata* DC.

EtOH(50%) ext. of plant, hypoton. (*Indian J Exp Biol*, 1973, **11**, 43).

Seeds, alks. mucronatine (*Yao Hsueh Hsueh Pao*, 1964, **11**, 246; *CA* **61**, 8129c); usaramine (*Indian J Chem*, 1967, **5**, 655); nilgirine; str. of nilgiric acid obtained from alk. nilgirine (*Tetrahedron Lett*, 1968, 5605; *Planta Med*, 1972, **21**, 435); mucronatinine (*Tetrahedron*, 1968, **24**, 6319); crotastriatine (*Curr Sci*, 1968, **37**, 285; *Indian J Chem*, 1975, **13**, 989). Total alks., antitumour against Walker 256 and sarcoma 180 rat tumours (*Peiching I Hsueh Yuan Hsueh Pao*, 1981, **13**, 81; *CA*, **95**, 138474a).

Seed agglutinins to human antigen A (*Izv Akad Nauk SSSR Ser Biol*, 1968, 59); flavons. (*Curr Sci*, 1969, **38**, 65). Leaves and stembark, flavons. (*Phytochemistry*, 1970, **9**, 2581).

C. retusa Linn.

EtOH(50%) ext. of aerial parts, spasmol. and CNS depress. (*Indian J Exp Biol*, 1977, **15**, 208). Effect of seed feeding on broiler chickens and growing pigs (*J Agric Sci*, 1977, **89**, Pt.1, 95; 101; *CA*, **87**, 162495p; 162496q). Outbreak of hepatic disease in horses, pigs and poultry due to plant (*in* Plant and Fungal Toxins, 647-48).

Seed, as high as 10% pyrrolizidine alks.; toxic species typically contain 0.2-3.0% alks., also flavons. (*Curr Sci*, 1966, **35**, 549; 1969, **38**, 65); alks. monocrotaline, retusine and spectabiline; monocrotaline, antitumour agent (*Peiching I Hsueh Yuan Hsueh Pao*, 1981, **13**, 15; 9; *CA*, **94**, 162632a).

Monocrotaline—from seeds, used in preparation of pharmacodynamic compd. (*Indian J Pharm*, 1972, **34**, 123). Pulmonary vascular occlusions initiated by endotheliosis in monocrotaline-intoxicated rats (*Exp Mol Pathol*, 1970, **13**, 59). *C. sessiliflora* containing monocrotaline as active principle, used for treatment of skin cancer (*in* Beal & Reinhard, 369); the alk., cytotoxic and carcinogenic in certain dose levels (*in* Plant and Fungal Toxins, 657-58); str. (*Sci Sin*, 1981, **24**, 497).

C. spectabilis Roth syn. *C. sericea* Retz.

Plant—known to cause outbreak of hepatic disease in horses, cattle, pig and poultry (*in* Plant and Fungal Toxins, 647-48). Twig ext. given to children suffering from intestinal worms (*Econ Bot*, 1965, **19**, 241). EtOH(50%) ext. of plant, spasmol. (*Indian J Exp Biol*, 1969, **7**, 250). Clin. signs and pathological changes in plant-intoxicated rats (*Am J Vet Res*, 1970, **31**, 1059); pulmonary arterial changes in rats fed on plant (*Am J Pathol*, 1979, **94**, 37). Fresh plant toxic to sheep, goat and cow (*Bull Bot Surv India*, 1980, **22**, 96).

Seeds—rats fed on seeds developed pulmonary hypertension (*Experientia*, 1968, **24**, 1149); toxicity in rats (*Am J Parhol*, 1970, **60**, 75); in turkeys (*Liver Proc Int Gstaad Symp*, 1975, 448; *CA*, 1978, **89**, 210083t).

C. verrucosa Linn.

EtOH(50%) ext. of plant, CNS depress. and diur. (*Indian J Exp Biol*, 1977, **15**, 208).

Seeds contain 4 alks. including crotalaburnine, flavons., and β-sitosterol (*Indian J Pharm*, 1967, **29**, 311); alks. isosenkirkine & OAc-isosenkirkine (*ibid*, 1972, **34**, 168); crotaverrine & OAc-crotaverrine (*Phytochemistry*, 1976, **15**, 1061).

Leaves, tropane alk. (*Indian J Pharm Sci*, 1979, **41**, 252).

CROTON (*Euphorbiaceae*)

Cocarcinogenic diterps. of tigliane (phorbol esters) present in plants; ingestion of plants or plant products or extensive contact of these plant parts with skin should be avoided (*J Cancer Res Clin Oncol*, 1981, **99**, 103-24).

C. bonplandianum Baill. *C. sparsiflorus* Morong

EtOH(50%) ext. of plant, hypoten. and spasmol. (*Indian J Exp Biol*, 1969, **7**, 250). Latex used to heal cuts and wounds (*J Econ Tax Bot*, 1980, **1**, 144).

Plant and/or leaves alks.; sparsiflorine, antibact. action (*J Indian Med Assoc*, 1964, **43**, 592); str. (*Tetrahedron Lett*, 1965, 1539); isoquinoline dienone alk. crotoflorine, str. (*J Indian Chem Soc*, 1968, **45**, 1087); proaporphine alk.; crotsparinine (*Experientia*, 1968, **24**, 10; 1969, **25**, 354); alks.; their biosynth.; and their absolute configuration (*Phytochemistry*, 1970, **9**, 2573; 1974, **13**, 2767; *Tetrahedron*, 1972, **28**, 4579); pharmacol. of alks. (*Annu Rep CDRI Lucknow*, 1970, 64); N-Me-crotsparine, significant hypoten. in cats given 5-15 mg iv dose lowered B.P. by 50-70% for 1-3hrs; hypoten. activity appears to be mainly due to α-adrenergic blockade associated with a negative inotropic effect and direct supraspinal vasomotor loci (*Indian J Pharmacol*, 1969, **1**, 23; 1971, **3**, 18). Str. of isocrotsparinine, its N-Me deriv. and (+)-

tetrahydroglazievine from aerial parts (*J Chem Soc Perkin Trans I*, 1975, 1659).

Leaves, rutin in significant amts.; leaves and stems, β-sitosterol and taraxerol; vomifoliol and ursolic acid (*Phytochemistry*, 1971, **10**, 2548; 2247; 1972, **11**, 2888).

Seeds, phorbol diesters, phorbol triesters (known as new 'cryptic irrit.'), cocarcinogen (*ibid*, 1976, **15**, 1070; *Lloydia*, 1978, **41**, 193); alks., 3-OMe-4,6-di-OH-morphinandien-7-one and norsinoacutine (*Phytochemistry*, 1981, **20**, 863).

C. caudatus Geisel.

EtOH(50%) ext. of aerial parts, hypoten. (*Indian J Exp Biol*, 1969, **7**, 250); of fruit, hypoten., CNS depress. and diur. (*ibid*, 1977, **15**, 108). Root decoct. used against malaria (*Bull Bot Surv India*, 1980, **22**, 161).

Stem bark, dotriacotanol, β-amyrin and β-sitosterol (*J Indian Chem Soc*, 1969, **46**, 323); diterps. teucvidin (major), crotocaudin (minor); and 3 triterps. (*Tetrahedron*, 1977, **33**, 2407); isocrotocaudin (*Phytochemistry*, 1978, **17**, 1777).

C. oblongifolius Roxb.

Plant—various plant parts used in headache, fever, spleen trouble, madness, epilepsy, convuls., icterus, scabies, venereal sores, syphilis, ulcer, hydrocele, foul breath, cholera, neuralgia, pleur., pneum., etc. (*Econ Bot*, 1971, **24**, 241). EtOH(50%) ext., hypoten. (*Indian J Exp Biol*, 1971, **9**, 91).

Root—paste against constip.; rootbark decoct. with black pepper given in diar. and dysen., also in inflam. and fever (*Bull Bot Surv India*, 1976, **18**, 247; 1980, **22**, 59).

Bark, β-sitosterol and a diterp. alc., oblongifoliol (*Tetrahedron Lett*, 1968, 4685); deoxyoblongifoliol, their strs.; minor compds. (*Indian J Chem*, 1969, **7**, 838; 1971, **9**, 1055; 613; 1028); oblongifolic acid (*Tetrahedron*, 1970, **26**, 5275).

C. polyandrus Roxb.; see **Baliospermum montanum**

*C. scabiosus Bedd.

EtOH(50%) ext. of aerial parts, hypoten. (*Indian J Exp Biol*, 1974, **12**, 512).

Reported from Courtallam, T.N.

C. tiglium Linn.

Plant—causes haemat., diur. and swelling of lymph glands in animals [*Indian Farming*, 1966-67, **16**(9), 43]. Chem., pharmacol. and therapeutic uses, rev. (*Pharm Tijdsche Belg*, 1970, **47**, 218; *CA*, 1971, **74**, 79519k). An ingredient of indigenous drug '*Amber Mezhugu*' useful in rheum. (*Rheumatism*, 1976-77, **12**, 38).

Seed—ext., 2 active cocarcinogenic compds. (*Cancer Res*, 1965, **25**, 1871; 1966, **26**, 1729); fish poison (*J Bombay Natl Hist Soc*, 1968, **65**, 236). See plant also. Ext., inhibitory against P-388 lymphocytic leukemia in mice (*Science*, 1976, **191**, 571); increases intestinal motility and produces intestinal relaxant action in albino rat (*Bull Chiang Mai Assoc Med Sci*, 1979, **12**, 125). Clin. use of seed and its alk. in alopecia aerata (*Indian J Pharmacol*, 1981, **13**, 62).

Seed oil—inflam. and cocarcinogenic compds. (*Z Anal Chem*, 1966, **221**, 424); oil and resin, insectic. but their highly vesic. properties represented a distinct limitation; active constituents have resemblance to those from commercial plant insecticides sabadilla and ryania (*in* Jacobson & Crosby, 222, 224-25).

Phorbol-12,13-diesters — a series of toxic, irritating cocarcinogenic diesters of tigliane type of diterp. polyol, phorbol with simple acids such as acetic, 2-Me-butyric, tiglic, myristic (tetradecanoic), etc. from seed oil; 14 such diesters of which 3 being hydrolysis products of naturally occurring triesters, called 'cryptic irrit. or cocarcinogens' studied for tumour-promoting activity; most potent cocarcinogen, 12-O- tetradecanoyl-phorbol-13-OAc; str.-activity; etc. (*in* Plant and Fungal Toxins, 262-67). Str. & stereochem. of phorbol,

parent of cocarcinogen from seed oil (*Tetrahedron Lett*, 1967, 3165; *J Chem Soc C*, 1968, 1347). From seed oil, rev., 44 refs.; mode of action; tumour-promoting activities (*Cancer Res*, 1968, **28**, 2338; 2349; 1969, **29**, 624).

Phorbol esters, rev., 185 refs. (*Fortschr Chem Org Naturst*, 1974, **31**, 377-467). Phorbol 12 tiglate 13-decanoate from oil which is tumour-promoting at certain dose levels, is antileukemic in. mice at lower dose range (*Science*, 1976, **191**, 571). Tigliane (phorbol esters), daphnane and ingenane diterps., their chem., distribution and biol., activities, rev., 277 refs. (*Lloydia*, 1978, **41**, 193). Phorbol myrystate OAc, from oil activates nitroblue tetrazolium reduction in human polymorphs (*Experientia*, 1979, **35**, 830). As possible human risk factor (*J Cancer Res Clin Oncol*, 1981, **99**, 103).

Seeds, β-sitosterol (*Indian J Appl Chem*, 1969, **32**, 211); also haemolytic protein, crotin-I (*Taiwan Yao Hsueh Tsa Chih*, 1977, **28**, 104; *CA*, 1978, **88**, 33458a); purification and properties of seed lectin (*Arch Biochem Biophys*, 1981, **212**, 740).

CRYPTOCARYA (*Lauraceae*)

*C. amygdalina Nees

EtOH(50%) ext. of stem bark, hypoten., CNS depress., spasmol. and diur. (*Indian J Exp Biol*, 1974, **12**, 512).

Stem bark contains reticuline and di-2-*n*-Pr-pentyl phthalate; reticuline showed spasmol. activity in guinea pig intestine (*Indian J Chem*, 1979, **17B**, 411); also 2 olefinic acids, cryptocaryic acid and amygdalinic acid and alks. orientaline and laudanidine (*Phytochemistry*, 1981, **20**, 501).

From Eastern Himalayas, Khasi hills and Andamans.

*C. bourdilloni Gamble

Roots, lactone cryptocaryalactone (*Tetrahedron Lett*, 1971, 340). Cryptocaryalactone, moderate antifung. *in vitro*, against *Candida albicans*, slight sed. in mice and prolonged hypoten. in dog (*in* Wagner & Wolff, 216-17); another lactone; and β-sitosterol (*Indian J Chem*, 1972, **10**, 149; 1971, **9**, 611); a chalcone, cryptocaryone; its str. (*Tetrahedron Lett*, 1972, 3419; *Tetrahedron*, 1973, **29**, 3091).

Reported to occur in India.

CRYPTOLEPIS (*Asclepiadaceae*)

C. buchanani Roem. & Schult.

Plant—various plant parts used in sores, ascites, dropsy, anasarca, cholera, dysen., bodyache and snakebite (*Econ Bot*, 1970, **24**, 241); *C. sinensis* with active principles Na-OAc and protocatechuic acid showed a marked protective action to snake toxin in mice (*in* Beal & Reinhard, 386). Plant, as blood purifier (*Khadi Gramodyog*, 1972-73, **19**, 269). Used in fractures (*Sri Lanka For*, 1980, **14**, 145).

Roots—EtOH(50%) ext. of roots and stem, hypoten., CNS depress., and antiamphetaminic (*Indian J Exp Biol*, 1969, **7**, 250). Paste given internally in abdominal pain (*Bull Med Ethno Bot Res*, 1980, **1**, 8); pounded roots given to women to increase milk secretion (*Nagarjun*, 1980-81, **24**, 1). Rootbark used in rheum. (*Bull Bot Surv India*, 1980, **22**, 59).

Plant, alk. buchanamine; stem, a new nicotinoyl glucd. alk. (*Phytochemistry*, 1978, **17**, 2047; 1980, **19**, 1278); sold in market under the name Sariva, rev., 21 refs., also chem. studies [*J Res Indian Med*, 1979, **14**(2), 69; 126]. Stem constituents, alks., triterp., etc; leaf constituents, α- & β-amyrin (*Proc Indian Sci Congr*, 1980, Pt III, 72; 1981, Pt III, 106).

*C. elegans Wall.

EtOH(50%) ext. of aerial parts, diur. (*Indian J Exp Biol*, 1977, **15**, 208).

Found in Assam.

CRYPTOMERIA (*Taxodiaceae*)

*C. japonica (Linn. f.) D. Don

EtOH(50%) ext. of aerial parts, CNS depress., antivir. and spasmol. (*Indian J Exp Biol*, 1969, **7**, 250).

Essent. oil from heartwood, constituents (*Bull Chem Soc Jpn*, 1964, **37**, 886; 1029); anal. (*Koen Yoshishu-Koryo Terupen Oyobi Seiyu Kagaku Ni Kansuru Toronkai*, 1979, 187; *CA*, 1980, **92**, 194429q). Extn. (*Indian For*, 1981, **107**, 107). Monoterps. and sesquiterps. (*Agric Biol Chem*, 1981, **45**, 1493).

Heartwood, phenolic compds., their str. (*Nippon Mokuzai Gakkaishi*, 1963, **9**, 139; 1965, **11**, 23; *Mokuzai Gakkaishi*, 1968, **14**, 425; 430; *CA*, 1964, **60**, 1626c; 1965, **62**, 16553g; 1969, **70**, 114956a-57t). Wood of Yaku var. yields bisabolane sesquiterp. cryptomerone (*Tetrahedron Lett*, 1969, 3185).

Leaf, constituents; indication of chemovars. (*Phytochemistry*, 1966, **5**, 391; 1970, **9**, 591; 1968, **7**, 135).

Plant releases terp. (*Kyoto-fu Eisci Kogai Kenkyusho Nempo*, 1977, **22**, 111; *CA*, 1979, **90**, 51392v).

Native of Japan and China; introduced into hills of India.

CRYPTOSTEGIA (*Asclepiadaceae*)

C. grandiflora (Roxb.) R. Br. ex Lindl.

Young regrowth after burning, when eaten by cattle caused mortality due to cardiac arrest (*Queensl J Agric Anim Sci*, 1969, **26**, 9).

Latex, proteolytic (*Curr Sci*, 1966, **35**, 42). EtOH ext. of aerial parts, hypoglyc. in rabbits (*Indian J Med Res*, 1967, **55**, 1277). EtOH(50%) ext. of aerial parts, CNS depress. and barbiturate potentiating (*Indian J Exp Biol*, 1977, **15**, 208). Stem ext. in MeOH, promising molluscicide against snails (*Planta Med*, 1980, **39**, 57).

EtOH ext. of aerial parts, cytostatic against KB cell culture (human nasopharynx carcinoma);contains 5 cardenolides, oleanodrigenin, its derivs. 3-rhamnoside (rhodexin B), 16- propionyl-and 16-anhydrogitoxigenin and gitoxigenin; rhodexin B responsible for activity (*J Pharm Sci*, 1972, **61**, 570).

CUBEBA (*Lauraceae*)

C. officinalis Miq.; see Litsea cubeba

CUCUBALUS (*Caryophyllaceae*)

C. baccifer Linn.

Various plant parts, haemolytic; roots have highest haemolytic index.

Flavons. (*Sb Nauchn Tr Ryazan Med Inst*, 1975, 50, 22; *CA*, 1976, 84, 56522y). Anal. of various plant parts; roots contain a mixt. of saponosides, aglycone, gypsogenin & its glucuronoside (*Herba Pol*, 1979, 25, 277).

CUCUMIS (*Cucurbitaceae*)

C. callosus Cogn. syn. *C. pseudo-colocynthis* Royle; *C. trigonus* Roxb.; *Bryonia callosa* Rottl.

Fruit—EtOH ext. stimulates isolated uterus of guinea pigs (*Indian J Pharm*, 1962, 24, 218); ext., analg. and antiinflam. (*Pharmacology*, 1980, 20, 52). Fruit ext., diur. in albino rats (*J Ethnopharmacol*, 1981, 3, 15).

Fruit, proteolytic enzyme (*Bull RRL Hyderabad*, 1962-63, 1, 198); steroid and triterp. compds. (*Planta Med*, 1976, 30, 144); cucurbitacin B (*Indian J Chem*, 1979, 17B, 417).

C. melo Linn.

Eng.–*Muskmelon, sweetmelon.*

Fruit—pulp and juice, demulc., useful in tan freckles. Med. plants, rev. (*Hamdard*, 1981, 24, 102).

Seeds—NaHCO₃ and HCl exts., anticancer against Ehrlich ascites tumour cells (*Philipp J Sci*, 1964, 93, 57). Ext., diur. (*Indian J Med Res*, 1970, 58, 505). Seed oil useful in urinary infections. Root emetic and purg. [*Indian Fmrs Dig*, 1978, 11(6 & 7), 74]. Alongwith other plant products used as antifert. drug (*Econ Bot*, 1980, 34, 274).

Fruits, ferulic, caffeic and chlorogenic acids detn. (*Z Lebensm Untersuch Forsch*, 1966, 132, 193; *CA*, 1967, 66, 45594a). Korean plant β-sitosterol, 70% of total sterols (*Yakhak Hoeji*, 1969, 13, 144; *CA*,

1971, 75, 40312h). Fruit oil, volat. constituents (*Phytochemistry*, 1971, 10, 1925; *J Food Sci*, 1977, 42, 32). Characterisation of cucurbitin (*Eur J Biochem*, 1980, 103, 577); fruit stalk with active principles cucurbitacin B & E, lowers elevated SGPT levels in carbon tetrachloride-intoxicated rat (*in* Beal & Reinhard, 375).

C. prophetarum Linn.

Roots used in indign. and fever (*J Agric Trop Bot Appl*, 1966, 13, 265).

Fruits, cucurbitacin C (*Curr Sci*, 1968, 37, 361); also cucurbitacin Q1, which is antitumour agent (*Phytochemistry*, 1973, 12, 2741); propheterosterol and cucurbitacin Q1 (*Pak J Sci Ind Res*, 1976, 18, 12; *CA*, 85, 51656f).

C. sativus Linn.

Eng.–*Cucumber.*

Fruit—juice of cucumber, major constituent of anti-acne lotion (US Pat., 1981, 4255418; *CA*, 94, 180703d). Pink eyes, sunburn and eyestrain relieved by application of cooling and refreshing slices to closed eyes (Herbal Med., 150).

Plant—used in headache (*Econ· Bot*, 1970, 24, 241). Evaluation of allelopathic cucumbers as an aid to weed control (*Weed Sci*, 1979, 27, 54). Med. plants, rev. covering chem. and pharmacol., alongwith other plants [*Hamdard*, 1981, 24(1), 102].

Cucumber, rutin (*Kaseigaku Zasshi*, 1965, 16, 193; *CA*, 63, 15449e). Seeds, glucds. including cucurbitaside (*Khim Prir Soedin*, 1972, 306; *CA*, 1973, 78, 2008t). Fruits, volat. compds. (*J Agric Food Chem*, 1974, 22, 717). Characteristics of cucurbitin (*Eur J Biochem*, 1980, 103, 577).

Leaves, free cucurbitasides B & C; ferredoxin (*Khim Prir Seedin*, 1972, 306; *CA*, 1973, 78, 2008t; *Biokhimiya*, 1972, 35, 1012); stigmast-7-en-3β-ol and α-spinosterol (*Chem Pharm Bull*, 1970, 18, 213). Free and bound sterols in seedlings (*Phytochemistry*, 1974, 13, 2235; 1975, 14, 296); sterols from different organs (*Khim Prir Seedin*, 1975, 660; *CA*, 1976, 84, 102281u).

Male and female flowers, sterols (*Planta*, 1977, **134**, 115).

*C. sativus Linn. var. **hardwickii** Royle

Fruit pieces, in hot fomentation used on chest in pneum. (*Econ Bot*, 1971, **25**, 418). Occurs in Kumaun.

CUCURBITA (*Cucurbitaceae*)

C. maxima Duch. ex Lamk

Eng.–*Pumpkin.*

Seed—ext., anthelm., *in vivo* and *in vitro* (*Indian J Med Res*, 1967, **55**, 629; *Labdev*, 1967, **5**, 64); inotropic on frog heart (*Indian J Pharmacol*, 1978, **10**, 315). Seed oil used in migraine and neuralgia.

Fruit—pulp, sed., emol. and refrig. Useful in haemoptysis and pulmonary haemor.

Plant, in curing *kapha*, gonor. and urinary diseases (*Planta Med*, 1973, **23**, 381).

Seed oil, sterols (*J Am Oil Chem Soc*, 1977, **54**, 525); sterols and triterps. (*Planta Med*, 1979, **37**, 264).

Fruits, vit. A [*Dacca Univ Stud*, 1973, **21** (2,Pt.B), 65; *CA*, 1974, **81**, 90294y].

Korean plant ext., saponin (*Hanguk Yongyang Hakhoe Chi*, 1977, **10**, 22; *CA*, **87**, 66777m).

Pollen, vits.(*Nippon Nogei Kagaku Kaishi*, 1967, **41**, 184; *CA*, **67**, 88308y). Pollens and stigmas of male and female flowers, flavons. (*Experientia*, 1979, **35**, 13).

*C. moschata Duch.

Used in headache, phthisis, bronch. and asthma (*Econ Bot*, 1970, **24**, 241). Seedlings, fungistatic principle (*Curr Sci*, 1975, **44**, 279).

Seeds—inhibit growth of young worms of *Sehistosoma japonica* (*in* Beal & Reinhard, 380); anthelm. against tapeworm, diur., in gonor. and urinary diseases.

Fruit—pulp poultice for boils, and ulcers. Dried pulp, in haemptysis and haemor. from pulmonary organs [*Indian Frms Dig*, 1978, **11**(6 & 7), 73]. Peduncle and thalamus of mature fruit, as antid. to scorpion sting (*J Econ Tax Bot*, 1980, **1**, 141).

Pollens and stigmas of male and female flowers contain flavons. (*Experientia*, 1979, **35**, 13).

Cultivated in India.

C. pepo Linn.

Eng.–*Hungarian pumpkin.*

Seed—seed coat, anthelm. (*Bull Soc Pharm Bordeaux*, 1966, **105**, 189; *CA*, 1967, **67**, 29843w); ext. fungitoxic against *Helminthosporium oryzae* (*Nat Acad Sci Lett*, 1978, **1**, 287); minor insectic. (*in* Jacobson & Crosby, 226).

Seeds contain cucurrbitine, an anthelm., active principle, rev., 22 refs. (*Med Parazitol Parazit Belezai*, 1966, **35**, 487; *CA*, **65**, 18425d); seeds, +ve test for alk. (*Lloydia*, 1974, **37**, 506); stigmasta-7, 24(28)-dien-3β-ol (*Tetrahedron Lett*, 1968, 2443); sterols (*Z Anal Chem*, 1966, **217**, 268; *Phytochemistry*, 1976, **15**, 1533; *J Am Oil Chem Soc*, 1977, **54**, 525).

Plant organs contain light-dependent Ac-choline (*Experientia*, 1974, **30**, 1387). Leaves and stems, alk. (*Q J Crude Drug Res*, 1980, **18**, 105). Detn. of ulcer-preventing vit. U [*Gig Sanit*, 1981, (6), 85].

Pollens and stigmas of male and female flowers, flavons. (*Experientia*, 1979, **35**, 13). Flowers, flavonol glycds. (*Phytochemistry*, 1981, **20**, 2421).

CUMINUM (*Apiaceae*)

C. cyminum Linn.

Eng.–*Cumin.*

Fruits—EtOH(50%) ext., spasmol. and hypoten. (*Indian J Exp Biol*, 1968, **6**, 232). Alc. or aq. ext. (or seed) showed significant antiimplantation activity in albino rats (*Indian J Med Res*, 1976, **64**, 1133). Along with leaves of *Ficus arnottiana*, taken as sterilizer (*Econ Bot*, 1980, **34**, 273). Ext. inhibits *Clostridum botulinum* (*J Food Prot*, 1980, **43**, 195); inhibits toxin production by *Aspergillus* (*Appl Environ Microbiol*, 1980, **39**, 818).

Essent. oil—from fruit, larvicidal (*Nippon Suisan Gakkaishi*, 1974, **40**, 1241; *CA*, 1975, **82**, 84722r); antibact. against pathogenic microorganism (*Pak J Sci Res*, 1974, **26**, 25; *CA*, 1977, **86**, 84191z); from seed, antifung. [*Indian Drugs Pharmac Ind*, 1980, **15**(6), 7]; antimicrob. activity (*Herba Pol*, 1980, **26**, 245; *Fitoterapia*, 1980, **51**, 201).

Fruit, cuminin (*J Pharm Sci UAR*, 1963, **4**, 35; *CA*, 1965, **63**, 11921b); volat. oil (2.5-4.5%), fixed oil (*c*.10%), protein, etc. (Parry, 194). Flavons. (*Phytochemistry*, 1972, **11**, 1741); glucopyranosides of luteolin and apigenin (*Egypt J Pharm Sci*, 1977, **18**, 245; *Pharmazie*, 1978, **33**, 296; *CA*, **89**, 103738p).

Essent. oil, physicochem. characteristics (*Perfum Essent Oil Rec*, 1967, **58**, 622); chief constituent, cumaldehyde (*p*- isoPr-benzaldehyde, *p*-cuminicaldehyde) (Parry, 194); from seed (fruit), volat. components (*J Agric Food Chem*, 1970, **18**, 234; 239); chem. constituents (*Indian Perfum*, 1978, **22**, 164; 1979, **23**, 34; *Proc Indian Sci Congr*, 1980, Pt.III, 94); cuminal & cuminol; oil, antimicrob. (*J Sci Res Bhopal*, 1980, **2**, 83). Progress in essent. oils, rev., 46 refs. [*Perfum Flav*, 1981, 5(7), 49].

Seed fat, anal. for content of volat. acids; $\Delta^{5,6}$-octadecenoic acid (*Chem Ind Lond*, 1969, 1869; 1970, 831).

CUPRESSUS (*Cupressaceae*)

C. spp. commonly known as Cypress. Bioflavones of *Cupressaceae* plants as taxonomic markers (*Phytochemistry*, 1970, **9**, 575).

*C. funebris Endl.

EtOH(50%) ext. of aerial parts, semen coagulant (*Indian J Exp Biol*, 1977, **15**, 208).

Leaf essent. oil contains tricyclic sesquiterp. hydrocarbon (*Indian J Chem*, 1973, **11**, 508).

Vishakhapatnam, A.P.

C. sempervirens Linn.

Essent. oil of leaves, antimicrob. (*Herba Pol*, 1980, **26**, 245).

Undried cones contain communic acid (*Bull Soc Chim Fr*, 1964, 348); terp. from cones; identified as cupressic acid (*Trav Soc Pharm Montpellier*, 1973, **33**, 373, 367; *CA*, 1974, **80**, 130497e; 143047h); also neocupressic acid II and isocupressic acid (*ibid*, 1976, **36**, 219; *CA*, 1977, **86**, 27662e).

Oleoresin acid fraction yields communic acid, cupressic acid & its iso deriv. as major constituents; tolarol, one of the 2 minor constituents. Several diterps. including sempervirol (*Tetrahedron Lett*, 1964, 2643; 1967, 673); 2 terp. ketones (*Gazz Chim Ital*, 1966, **96**, 206).

Leaves, Me-*muco*-inositol; constituents of leaf wax and heartwood; also wood sesquiterps. (*Phytochemistry*, 1972, **11**, 245; 1981, **20**, 1135; 1299).

Essent. oil from fruits, characteristics and constituents (*Perfum Essent Oil Rec*, 1967, **58**, 622); constituents (*Helv Chim Acta*, 1975, **58**, 1184).

*C. torulosa D. Don

EtOH(50%) ext. of aerial parts, antivir., şpasmol., CNS depress. and diur. (*Indian J Exp Biol*, 1974, **12**, 512).

Essent. oil from leaves, constituent, *d*-limonene antibact., from fruit, less effective (*Indian Oil Soap J*, 1972, **37**, 230).

Heartwood, constituents (*Acta Chem Scand*, 1961, **15**, 1313). Stembark, 5 closely related diterp. acids, β- sitosterol & its glucd. (*Indian J Chem*, 1973, **11**, 87); diterps. of leaves and stembark (*ibid*, 1977, **15B**, 397).

Essent. oil from leaves, constituents and physicochem. characteristics (*Perfum Essent Oil Rec*, 1967, **58**, 622); from fruits; its chem. characteristics and antimicrob. action [*Indian Perfum*, 1971, **15**(Pt.1), 11; 1973, **17**(Pt. 2), 31].

Ootacamund, T.N. and Kumaun, U.P.

CURCULIGO (*Amaryllidaceae*)

C. orchioides Gaertn. syn. *Hypoxis orchioides* Kurz

Rhizomes—pounded and applied on cuts and wounds; pounded with *ajwain* and its decoct. given to unconscious children (*Econ Bot*, 1965, **19**, 245). Powd. used externally to heal wounds (*Bull Bot Surv India*, 1973, **15**, 21); with milk taken as tonic for impotency (*J Econ Tax Bot*, 1980, **1**, 144).

Leaves used in whitlows (*Lloydia*, 1967, **30**, 391). EtOH(50%) ext. of plant, hypoglyc. and anticancer (*Indian J Exp Biol*, 1968, **6**, 232).

Rhizomes, glycd. (*Planta Med*, 1976, **29**, 291); also yuccagenin and alk. lycorine (*Indian J Pharm Sci*, 1978, **40**, 104). Roots afforded a new aliphatic MeO-ketone, 3-MeO, 5-Ac,31-tritriacontene (*Acta Ciencia Indica*, 1981, **7C**, 174).

Plant contains flavone glycd., a powerful uterine stim. in guineapig, rats and rabbits [*J Res Indian Med*, 1975, **10**(3), 104].

CURCUMA (*Zingiberaceae*)

C. aromatica Salisb.

Rhizome—EtOH(50%) ext., spasmol. (*Indian J Exp Biol*, 1969, **7**, 250). Powd. used as anthelm. (*Econ Bot*, 1981, **35**, 4).

Essent. oil—from rhizomes, anthelm., antifung., antimicrob. [*Indian J Hosp Pharm*, 1971, **8**, 150; *Econ Bot*, 1972, **26**, 255; *Indian J Pharm*, 1976, **38**, 53; *East Pharm*, 1978, **21**(244), 183; *Indian Perfum*, 1978, **22**, 69]. Oil, commercially available; inhibitory effect on sarcoma 180 in mice; used for treatment of early stage of cervix cancer; active constituents, curcumol and curdione (*in* Beal & Reinhard, 370).

Essent. oil from rhizome, characteristics and constituents (*Perfum Essent Oil Rec*, 1967, **58**, 622; *Flavour Ind*, 1974, **5**, 234); detn. of curcumol (*Acta Pharm Sin*, 1979, **14**, 356; 1980, **15**, 251).

C. longa Linn. syn. *C. domestica* Valeton

Rhizome—in Hawaii, used against growth in nostrils, for cleaning blood and gargle; green rhizome given for whooping and other coughs (*Econ Bot*, 1971, **25**, 245; 420); cough and dysponoea management by rhizome; in Unani med., powd. used as antifert. agent [*J Res Indian Med*, 1979, **14**(2), 110; 1978, **13**(1), 107]. Used in a compn. for migraine (*Q J Crude Drug Res*, 1979, **17**, 62). Minor ingredient of Ayurvedic drug for malarial fever (*Indian J Med Res*, 1976, **64**, 1451); also of indigenous antifatigue drug 'Geriforte'; effective in senile pruritis (*Indian Drugs*, 1980-81, **18**, 346; *Rajasthan Med J*, 1980, **19**, 23). Ingredient of Unani drug '*Majnoon-E-Falsfa*' useful in gastro-intestinal complaints [*Nagarjun*, 1977-78, **21**(11), 23]; of drug 'Vitafix' prescribed in premature ejaculation [*Indian Pract*, 1980, **33**(2), 81].

Ext. effective as insect repellent against houseflies (*Bull RRL Jammu*, 1963, **1**, 169); insectic.; and antifung. effect (*Labdev*, 1965, **3**, 212; 1971, **9B**, 136). Effect of turmeric ext. on cholesterol level in rats; fractions on intestinal and pathogenic bacteria *in vitro* (*Indian J Exp Biol*, 1964, **2**, 104; 1979, **17**, 1363). Inhibition of *Clostridium botulinum* by ext. (*J Food Prot*, 1980, **43**, 195). Inhibitor effect of curcuma on growth and toxin production of toxigenic fungi (*Appl Environ Microbiol*, 1980, **39**, 818). Exts., antiinflam.; comparison of activity of various exts. (*Indian J Med Res*, 1971, **59**, 1289; 1976, **64**, 601). In Tonga, decoct. in conjunctivitis and rhizome mixt. with coconut oil as vulnerary; powd., to heal umbilicus of new born child; with coconut oil for inflam.; asthma, broncht., fever and as emetic (*Econ Bot*, 1971, **25**, 447; 1974, **28**, 7). Effect on growth of some intestinal and pathogenic bacteria (*J Food Sci Technol*, 1978, **15**, 152; *Indian J Exp Biol*, 1979, **17**, 1363).

EtOH(50%) ext., spasmol., antiprot. and CNS depress.; hypoten.; antifert. in albino rats; toxicity of rhizome in rats, guinea pigs and monkey (*Indian J Exp Biol*, 1968, **6**, 232; 1969, **7**, 250; 1978, **16**, 1077; 1980, **18**, 73).

Various plant parts—used in hazy vision and blindness, sores, spleen consumption, pain, rheum., lock-jaw, icterus, indistinct speech, scabies, syphilis, atrophy, indign., *prolapsus ani, fistula ani,* cholera, slow lactation, anthrax, etc. (*Econ Bot*, 1970, **24**, 241). In Samoa, plant used against inflam., gall stones, jaundice, sores and jaws; also as diur. Leaves, ingredient for stomachache (*ibid*, 1974, **28**, 7). In skeletal fracture (*Sri Lanka For*, 1980, **14**, 145).

Essent. oil—from rhizomes, fungitoxicity (*Shoyakugaku Zasshi*, 1971, **25**, 11; *CA*, 1972, **76**, 21838p). Antiinflam. and antiarthritic activity (*Indian J Med Res*, 1972, **60**, 138). Effect of alc. ext., essent. oil and active ingredient, curcumin on bacteria and fungi (*Planta Med*, 1974, **26**, 9). Antibact. and antifung. action [*Herba Pol*, 1980, **26**, 245; *J Res Indian Med*, 1977, **12**(1), 89; 1978, **13**(2), 63].

De-bittering of turmeric (US Pat., 1967, 3340250; *CA*, **67**, 107522g).

Turmeric, chem. and uses, rev. [*Indian Spices*, 1974, **10**(3), 7]; chem., technology and quality, rev., 185 refs. (*CRC Crit Rev Food Sci Nutr*, 1980, **12**, 199; *CA*, **93**, 148154x). Studies of *haridra*, rev., 13 refs. covering med. uses, pharmacol. and chem. (*J Nat Integ Med Assoc*, 1980, **22**, 79).

Oleoresin extn. (*J Food Sci Technol*, 1981, **18**, 101). Essent. oil, extn. (Ger. Offen., 1981, 2924345; *CA*, **94**, 109341d).

An unsymmetrical diaryl heptanoid yielding on oxidation curcumin, of biogenetic significance; ether ext. of rhizome highly cytotoxic; toxicity higher than those from known curcuminoids, may be due to highly active minor curcuminoids (*Phytochemistry*, 1980, **19**, 2031; 2643).

Curcumin—from rhizomes (Parry, 211; *J Indian Chem Soc*, 1967, **44**, 985); 1,7-bis(4-OH-3-MeO-Ph)-1, 6-heptadiene-3,5-dione from rhizome (turmeric) (Dictionary Org Compds., II, 1321). Cur-

cumin, its alkali salts and oil on induced gastric ulcers in guineapigs; curcumin, effective [*Indian J Exp Biol*, 1964, **2**, 158; *Nagarjun*, 1975-76, **19**(6), 11]. Pharmacol. of diferuloyl methane (curcumin); more effective and less toxic than Ph-butazone as antiinflam. agent (*J Pharm Pharmacol*, 1973, **25**, 447); synth. (*Heterocycles*, 1977, **7**, 241). Cytotoxicity (*Phytochemistry*, 1980, **19**, 2643). Antirheum., clin. trials; mech. of curcumin-induced gastric ulcer in rats (*Indian J Med Res*, 1980, **71**, 632; 806); metabolism (*Xenobiotica*, 1978, **8**, 761; *Acta Pharmacol Toxicol*, 1978, **43**, 86); no effect on liver, but it apparently gets cleaved in liver to a choleretic cinnamic acid deriv. (*in* Beal & Reinhard, 221); *in vitro* absorption in rats intestine (*Toxicology*, 1981, **20**, 251).

Extn. and detn. of curcumin content in rhizomes (*Res Ind*, 1970, **15**, 258). Effect of extn. conditions on content of active constituents (*Herba Pol*, 1971, **17**, 40; *CA*, **75**, 143947y). HPLC detn. (*Yakugaku Zasshi*, 1981, **101**, 374); simple method for curcumin detn. in turmeric [*Indian Spices*, 1981, **18**(2-4), 21].

C. zedoaria Rosc.

Rhizome—decoct. of fresh rhizome used for blood purification (*Bull Bot Surv India*, 1973, **15**, 20). Med. uses in indigenous systems, rev. (*J Sci Ind Res*, 1975, **34**, 644). Antifung. evaluation, clin. study [*J Res Indian Med*, 1977, **12**(1), 25; 1978, **13**(2), 63]. An ingredient in Chinese medicine for extradural haematomas (*Chin Med J*, 1981, **94**, 241). One of the six ingredients of Ayurvedic recipe for antifert. [*J Sci Res Plants Med*, 1981, **2**(1 & 2), 1].

Essent. oil—from rhizome efficacy on pathogenic fungi (*Flavour Ind*, 1972, **3**, 368); antimicrob. (*Indian J Med Res*, 1970, **58**, 627; *Indian Perfum* 1978, **22**, 214).

Antifung. activity of various parts (*Econ Bot*, 1972, **26**, 255).

Rhizomes, sesquiterps. curcumol; curdione; curcolone; procurcumenol; isocurcumenol; furanodiene & its iso-deriv.; curcumadiol; dehydrocurdione; zederone; str. (*Chem Pharm Bull*, 1965, **13**, 1484; 1967, **15**, 1390; 1968, **16**, 827; 1605; 1969, **17**, 959; 1970, **18**, 752; 1971, **19**, 93; 1972, **20**, 987; 1966, **14**, 550; *J Chem Soc C*, 1971, 688). Antifung. compd., Et- *p*-Me-cinnamate (*Lloydia*, 1976, **39**, 218). Cytotoxic components, curcuminoids (*Phytochemistry*, 1980, **19**, 2643).

Essent. oil, from rhizomes characteristics and compds. (*Perfum Essent Oil Res*, 1967, **58**, 622). Sesquiterp. zedoarone; str. of sesquiterp. curzerenone, main constituent of essent. oil; isolation of curcuminoids (*Yakugaku Zasshi*, 1968, **88**, 792; 1970, **90**, 863; 1467).

CUSCUTA (*Cuscutaceae*)

*C. capitata Roxb.

Plant used in anginal and renal pain (*in* Atal & Kapur, Med. Plants, 519).

Found in Ladakh.

C. chinensis Lamk

Plant—various parts used in dropsy, anasarca, cancer, rinderpest, trouble during pregnancy and bone fracture (*Econ Bot*, 1970, **24**, 241). In Chile, as diur. (*Planta Med*, 1974, **25**, 183). Pharmacognosy of drug in natural and powd. form (*Bull Med Ethano Bot Res*, 1980, **1**, 494).

C. reflexa Roxb.

Seeds—purg. (*Bull Bot Surv India*, 1973, **15**, 19). In Unani med., germinative and anodyne [*East Pharm*, 1980, **23**(272), 39]; powd. used as antifert. drug (*Ancient Sci Life*, 1981-82, **1**, 64).

Plant—w.-sol. portion of fresh alc. ext., relaxant and spasmol. on guinea pig and rabbits ileum; also has a Ac-choline like action (*Indian J Med Res*, 1965, **53**, 465). EtOH(50%) ext. of aerial parts, antivir. (*Indian J Exp Biol*, 1969, 7, 250). Juice of stem and leaves, to kill lice (*Econ Bot*, 1971, **25**, 418); ext. antifert. in albino rats (*Indian J Med Res*, 1979, **70**, 517). One of the constituents of Unani drug '*Itrifal Ustakhudus*' used for purging viscid matters from brain and stomach (*Nagarjun*,

1978-79, **22**, 237). Application of *Cuscuta* in folk med. throughout the world, chem. constituents and clin. studies, rev. [*Ethnomedicine*, 1978-79, 5(1/2), 47]; paste used to cure dislocated joints (*ibid*, 1980, **6**, 139); to check falling of hair; also in treatment of swellings of testicles and in headache (*Bull Med Ethno Bot Res*, 1980, **1**, 1; 318; 494). Juice useful in hookworm and in diphtheria; pharmacognostic studies to help identify the drug in natural and powd. form.

Parasitic plant grown on *Mangifera indica*, contains mangiferine (*Indian J Chem*, 1966, **4**, 335).

CYAMOPSIS (*Fabaceae*)

C. tetragonolobus Taub.

Eng.–*Guar*.

Bean—addn. of guar in meal of normal subjects reduced blood glucose and plasma insulin and in diabetics caused decrease in max. postprandial plasma GIP and decrease in blood glucose (*Diabetologia*, 1979, **17**, 85). Oral administration of flour produced fall in serum cholesterol, total lipids and uric acid in male subjects (*Indian J Nutr Diet*, 1980, **17**, 297). Aq. ext. of fruits and seeds, hypoglyc. in rabbits (*Indian J Med Res*, 1980, **72**, 128).

Seed—ext., constituent of a cream for treating hair and skin (Fr. Demande, 1978, 2437829; *CA*, 1980, **93**, 245268s).

Gum—versatile, rev. with patents (*Res Ind*, 1965, **10**, 101); appetite suppressor or depressor in human diet (*Pharm J*, 1971, **207**, 65; *Dtsch Apoth*, 1973, **25**, 614; *CA*, 1974, **80**, 58732h); decrease in postprandial insulin and glucose levels by gum and pectin in human subjects (*Ann Intern Med*, 1977, **86**, 20); uses [*Indian Farming*, 1980-81, **30**(9), 19]; useful in diabetes, clin. trials (*Lancet*, 1979, **1**, 612, 434, 271, 435); mixt. of guar gum and pectin also useful (*Isr J Med Sci*, 1980, **16**, 1). Reduction of glycosuria during gum supplimentation in non-insulin-dependent diabetics (*Dan Med Bull*, 1981, **28**, 41). Lowered serum total cholesterol and low-density lipoprotein cholesterol in volunteers (*Am J Chem Nutr*, 1981, **34**, 2446).

Hypocholesteremic and hyperglyc. in albino rats (*Proc Soc Exp Biol Med*, 1967, **124**, 749; *Indian J Pharm Sci*, 1981, **43**, 166).

CYANOTIS (*Commelinaceae*)

*C. fasciculata Schult.
EtOH(50%) ext. of plant, anticancer and diur. (*Indian J Exp Biol*, 1974, **12**, 512).
Amboli, Maharashtra.

CYATHEA (*Cyatheaceae*)

*C. gigantea Holtt.
EtOH(50%) ext. of aerial parts, antiinflam. (*Indian J Exp Biol*, 1977, **15**, 208).
Mahabaleshwar, Maharashtra.

*C. nilgirensis Holtt.
EtOH(50%) ext. of aerial parts, hypoten., spasmol., CNS depress. (*Indian J Exp Biol*, 1977, **15**, 208).
Coorg, Karnataka.

CYATHOCLINE (*Asteraceae*)

C. purpurea Kuntze syn. *C. lyrata* Cass.
Roots given in stomach pain (*Bull RRL Jammu*, 1962-63, **1**, 126). EtOH(50%) ext. of plant, spasmol. (*Indian J Exp Biol*, 1969, **7**, 250).

Essent. oil—from plant, antimicrob. activity (*Indian J Pharm*, 1975, **37**, 129; *Indian Perfum*, 1980, **24**, 219); anthelm. against nodularworms (*Sci Cult*, 1981, **47**, 39); also against tapeworms and hookworms; better than piperazine phosphate or hexylresorcinol; hypoten. in cat, cardiac depress. on isolated auricle of guineapig; also spasmol. and oxytocic (*Indian J Pharm Sci*, 1979, **41**, 228; 249).

Essent. oil from plant, chem. constituents (*Curr Sci*, 1967, **36**, 205); terp., lyratol, str. (*Tetrahedron*, 1969, **25**, 3217); lyratic acid (*Indian J Chem*, 1971, **9**, 186). Plant, 2 new sesquiterp. lactones, an eudesmanolide called isoivangustin and a

guaianolide (*Phytochemistry*, 1981, **20**, 2034).

CYATHULA (*Amaranthaceae*)

C. prostrata Blume
Plant, ecdysterone (*Yakugaku Zasshi*, 1968, **88**, 1293).

*C. tomentosa Moq.
EtOH(50%) ext. of plant, spasmol. (*Indian J Exp Biol*, 1969, **7**, 250).
Temperate Himalayas up to 2,500 m.

CYCAS (*Cycadaceae*)

C. circinalis Linn.
Eng.–*Cycads*.
Clin., pathological and biochem. results of toxicity of seeds to rhesus monkeys [*Fed Proc Fed Am Soc Exp Biol*, 1964, **23**(Pt.1), 1368]; seed contains alk. (*Lloydia*, 1973, **36**, 231). Population using cycads as food, cognizant of toxic properties; processes of fermentation, heating, water extn. or sundrying detoxified final product, flour; processed material exp., nontoxic and non-carcinogenic (*in* Liener, 350-53).

Fresh nuts—cycads produce gastrointestinal irrit., vomiting, abdominal cramps and bloody diar. (*Acta Phytother*, 1969, **16**, 41). Oncogenicity of cycads and its implications, rev. (*Adv Mod Toxicol*, 1977, **3**, 209; *CA*, **87**, 162248k).

Plant—neurological disorder involving irreversible paralysis in cattle in addition to hepatotoxic and carcinogenic effect (*Fed Proc Fed Am Soc Exp Biol*, 1966, **25**, 533; *in* Liener, 439-40). Cycad poisoning (*in* Plant and Fungal Toxins, 462-71).

Cycasin—from nut ext., toxic; it is Me-azoxy-MeO-glucd. toxic constituent, Me-azoxymethanol, aglycone of cycasin (which is hydrolysed by β-glucosidases) (*Arch Biochem Biophys*, 1963, **101**, 299; 1965, **110**, 373). Cycasin, carcinogenic in rats (*J Natl Cancer Inst*, 1963, **31**, 919). Azoxyglycds. macroamin and cycasin from green outer shells (*Agric Biol Chem*, 1964, **28**, 575). Effect of cycasin or endosperm on liver nucleic acids and lipids in rats; both produce liver and kidney tumours (*Proc Soc Exp Biol Med*, 1965, **118**, 1).

Me-azoxy methanol, neurotoxin, carcinogen and teratogen. Freshly removed kernels of Indian plant contain 0.96 and dried nuts 0.55% of cycasin; effect of boiling and storage on cycasin content (*Nature Lond*, 1965, **206**, 1363; 1966, **210**, 841). Cycads, rev. on toxic principle, 25 refs. (*Toxic Const Plant Foodst*, 1969, 159; *CA*, 1970, **72**, 20130g). Cycasin induced severe ataxia in mice (*Fed Proc Fed Am Soc Exp Biol*, 1972, **31**, 1517).

Plant contains α-amino-β-Meaminopropionic acid markedly neurotoxic in chicks and rats; its str. and physiol. effects, amino acid similar to those amino acids causing lathyrism (*Biochem J*, 1968, **106**, 15p).

C. revoluta Thunb.

Untreated raw, untreated cycad nuts used in small toy dolls contain considerable amts. of cycasin and hence carcinogenic risk to humans coming in contact with them (*Fed Proc Fed Am Soc Exp Biol*, 1972, **31**, 1476). Intestinal tumour induction by cycads exts. (*Kagoshima Daigaku Igaku Zasshi*, 1977, **29**, 71; *CA*, 1978, **88**, 147141x). Biflavones from leaves (*Phytochemistry*, 1971, **10**, 1936; *Indian J Chem*, 1973, **11**, 1209).

C. rumphii Miq.

Large scale extn. of cycasin from seeds [*Kagoshima Daigaku Nogakubu Gakujustsu Hokoku*, 1971, No. 21, (3), 120; *CA*, 1972, **76**, 86091y]. Seeds, β-glycosidase, purification and properties (*Mem Fac Agric Kogoshima Univ*, 1977, **13**, 109).

Biflavones of leaves (*Indian J Chem*, 1973, **11**, 1209).

CYCLAMEN (*Primulaceae*)

C. europaeum Linn.

Fresh tubers, a saponin cyclamine which on hydrolysis gave cyclamiretine A, B, C & D (*Ann Chem*, 1964, **680**, 107; *CA*,

1965, **62**, 16309b). Cyclamin, barrier to fungal infection (*in* Plant & Fungal Toxins, 753). Corms, cyclamigenins (*Tetrahedron Lett*, 1963, 2223).

C. persicum Mill.

Alc. ext. of tubers, inhibitory, *in vitro* against cells derived from human carcinoma of nasopharynx (KB), saponin fraction inhibitor of Walker 256 tumour in rats (*J Pharm Sci*, 1967, **56**, 603).

CYCLEA (*Menispermaceae*)

C. barbata Miers syn. *C. peltata* Hook. f. & Thoms.; *C. burmanii* Hook. & Thoms.

Crushed root ext. taken as remedy against small pox (*Bull Bot Surv India*, 1980, **22**, 161). Plant used in bone fractures (*Sri Lanka For*, 1980, **14**, 145).

Roots contain alks., *d*-tetrandrine (main); *dl*- tetrandrine, isotetrandrine, limacine, berbamine and bomoarmoline (*Planta Med*, 1972, **22**, 402; 1974, **25**, 315); 5 bisbenzylisoquinoline alks., cycleapeltine, cycleadrine, cycleacurine, cycleanorine and cycleahomine chloride (*J Org Chem*, 1973, **38**, 1846).

Tetrandrine—bisbenzylisoquinoline alk. from roots, irrit. on mucous membranes; produced hyperglyc. in rats, and emesis in pigeons; also cardiac depress. Destroys polymorpho nuclear cells and lymphocytes in rabbits (*Q J Crude Drug Res*, 1971, **11**, 1665); both *d* & *dl* forms, antileukemic; crystal str. (*J Org Chem*, 1973, **38**, 1846; *J Am Chem Soc*, 1976, **98**, 1947); affects CNS, respiratory and skeletal muscles (*Pharmacology*, 1974, **12**, 97); i.v. injection of *d* form, hypoten. and bradycardiac in anaesthetized rhesus monkey, and in high doses, toxic (*Cancer Chemother Rep*, 1974, **58**, 637); compd. in phase II studies at M.D. Anderson Hospital, Houstan, Texas (*in* Wagner & Wolff), 63). Biosynth. (*Phytochemistry*, 1980, **19**, 2347).

CYCLOPHORUS (*Polypodiaceae*)

See **PYRROSIA**

CYCLOSORUS (Thelypteridaceae)

C. dentatus Ching syn. *Dryopteris dentata* C. Chr.

Aq. ext. (autoclaved) of the pinnae of fern, antibact. (Wlth India, III, 115).

Occurs wild throughout India in plains and also on hills up to 3,000 m.

CYDONIA (Rosaceae)

C. oblonga Mill. syn. *C. vulgaris* Pers.; *Pyrus cydonia* Linn.

Eng.–*Quince.*

In Europe, seed mucilage applied to inflammed skin as soothing and protective; useful in soreness of mucous membrane (*Acta Phytother*, 1971, **18**, 21).

Fruit skin flavonols, hyperin, isoquercitrin and quercetin (*Soobshch Acad Nauk Gruz SSR*, 1972, **65**, 701; *BA*, 1973, **55**, 9760); terp. lactones (*Agric Biol Chem*, 1980, **44**, 957).

CYLISTA (Fabaceae)

See **PARACALYX**

CYMBIDIUM (Orchidaceae)

*C. giganteum Wall.

EtOH(50%) ext. of plant, spasmol. (*Indian J Exp Biol*, 1980, **18**, 594).

Triterp. glucd., cymbidoside (*Phytochemistry*, 1978, **17**, 1975). Isolation and str. of compds., rev. [*Chem Commun Univ Stockholm*, 1978, (3), 29; *CA*, 1979, **90**, 200209v].

Chamoli, U.P.

C. stimulans Rolfe syn. *C. aloifolium* Swartz

Tuberous roots, a constituent of salep (*Q J Crude Drug Res*, 1971, **11**, 1742).

CYMBOPOGON (Poaceae)

*C. caesius Stapf

Bangalore–*Kachi grass.*

EtOH(50%) ext. of plant, spasmol. (*Indian J Exp Biol*, 1968, **6**, 232). Essent. oil, antibact. (*ibid*, 1977, **15**, 339).

Essent. oil, characteristics and constituents (*Perfum Essent Oil Rec*, 1967, **58**, 622).

Abundant in neighbourhood of Bangalore.

C. citratus(DC.) Stapf syn. *Andropogon citratus* DC.

Eng.–*Lemon grass.*

Leaves—in Samoa, chewed for sore gums; also used in elephantiasis; juice applied in headache (*Econ Bot*, 1974, **28**, 5); in Panama, carmin, diaphor., expect., depurative and in indign. (*Q J Crude Drug Res*, 1979, **17**, 115).

Essent. oil—antimicrob. (*Sci Cult*, 1971, **37**, 195; *Indian Drugs*, 1977-78, **15**, 30); CNS depress., analg. and antipyr. (*Indian J Exp Biol*, 1976, **14**, 370); fungitoxic (*Econ Bot*, 1980, **34**, 186); oil and plant, insect repellent (*Nagarjun*, 1979-80, **23**, 177).

Leaves, essent. oil and rhizomes, alk. (*Garcia de Orta*, 1960, **8**, 626; *CA*, 1964, **61**, 12325g); constituents of essent. oil; also antimicrob. activity (*Bull Med Ethno Bot Res*, 1980, **1**, 401); 78- 82% citral (*Indian Perfum*, 1979, **23**, 178); citral, insectic., fumigant and repellent properties [*Pesticides*, 1980, **14**(12), 6].

Leaf wax, triterps., cymbopogonol; cymbopogone; their strs. (*Phytochemistry*, 1976, **15**, 1074; *Tetrahedron Lett*, 1975, 3099; 1981, **21**, 3701).

Nigerian plant, β-sitosterol, hexacosanol, triacontanol, alk., and saponin glucd., used against fever (*Planta Med*, 1975, **28**, 186). Yield trial and tissue culture of Thai lemon grass (*Shoyakugaku Zasshi*, 1981, **36**, 128).

*C. distans Wats.

Essent. oil, antibact. (*Indian J Exp Biol*, 1977, **15**, 339); chem. constituents (*Proc Indian Sci Congr*, 1981, Pt.III, 83); terps. (*Phytochemistry*, 1981, **20**, 2770).

Found in N-W India.

C. flexuosus Wats. syn. *Andropogon nardus* Linn. var. *flexuosus* Hack.

Plant—EtOH(50%) ext. spasmol. (*Indian J Exp Biol*, 1977, **15**, 208); plant and its essent. oil, insect repellent (*Nagarjun*, 1979-80, **23**, 177).

Essent. oil—from leaves, antibact. activity (*Indian Perfum*, 1978, **22**, 118; 1979, **23**, 205); and antifung. [*Indian Drugs Pharmac Ind*, 1979, **14**(4), 29].

Essent. oil known as East Indian Lemongrass oil, constituents (*Indian Perfum*, 1978, **22**, 278); sesquiterp. alc., isointermedeol; its str. (*Phytochemistry*, 1979, **18**, 671; 1980, **19**, 2468); new trace constituents [*Pafai J*, 1981, **3**, 22; *Perfum Flav*, 1981, **6**(2), 29].

Leaves, triacontane, triacontanol, β-sitosterol and triterp., arundoin (*Indian J Chem*, 1975, **13**, 1108). Essent. oil from var. *sikkimensis*, its constituents (*Indian Drugs*, 1976-77, **14**, 195).

C. jwarancusa Schult. syn. *Andropogon jwarancusa* Jones

Essent. oil, antimicrob. [*Indian J Exp Biol*, 1977, **15**, 339; *J Res Indian Med*, 1978, **13**(3), 122].

Essent. oil, characteristics and constituents of Indian spp., rev. (*Perfum Essent Oil Rec*, 1967, **58**, 662); constituents (*Indian Perfum*, 1979, **23**, 14); variation in compn. (*Planta Med*, 1981, **41**, 386).

C. martinii (Roxb.) Wats. syn. *Andropogon martinii* Roxb.

EtOH(50%) ext. of plant, CNS depress. (*Indian J Exp Biol*, 1977, **15**, 208).

Essent. oil from leaves — in rheum. (*Bull Bot Surv India*, 1973, **15**, 21); antimicrob. (*Acta Ciencia Indica*, 1978, **4**, 248; *Indian Drugs*, 1977-78, **15**, 30); antimicrob. and antifung. [*Indian Drugs Pharmac Ind*, 1979, **14**(5), 11; **14**(1), 3]; fungitoxic (*Econ Bot*, 1980, **34**, 186); used in mosquito repellent ointments (*Nagarjun*, 1979-80, **23**, 177).

Two vars., *sofia* and *motia*, former yielding 'Gingergrass oil'. Constituents of essent. oil from *C. martinii* var. *motia* known as 'Palmrosa oil'(*Perfum Essent Oil Rec*, 1965, **56**, 435; *R A K Riechst Aromen Kosmet*, 1980, **30**, 20; *CA*, **92**, 160599e); terps. (*Indian Perfum*, 1980, **24**, 115); detection of trace constituents (*Pafai J*, 1981, **3**, 11).

C. nardus Rendle syn. *Andropogon nardus* Linn.

Essent. oil, *in vivo*, antimicrob. (*Flavour Ind*, 1970, **1**, 725; *Sci Cult*, 1971, **37**, 195); sed. (*Indian J Exp Biol*, 1971, **9**, 515); antimicrob. activity test for essent. oil, insect-repellent (*Nagarjun*, 1979-80, **23**, 177).

Constituents of essent. oil of *C. nardus* var. *stracheyi* (*J Indian Chem Soc*, 1978, **55**, 621).

*C. pendulus Wats.

Essent. oil, superior source of citral [*Indian J Pharm*, 1976, **38**, 61; *Indian Perfum*, 1976, **20**(Pt.1A), 29]. Essent. oil, antibact. and antifung. [*ibid*, 1978, **22**(2), 76; *J Res Indian Med*, 1978, **13**(4), 111].

N-E India.

*C. winterianus Jowitt

Essent. oil, *in vitro*, antimicrob. (*Indian Drugs*, 1977-78, **15**, 30); plant and its essent. oil, insect repellent (*Nagarjun*, 1979-80, **23**, 177).

Constituents of essent. oil (*Indian Perfum*, 1979, **23**, 167).

Cultivated for its valuable cintronella oil in many parts of the world.

CYNANCHUM (*Asclepiadaceae*)

*C. heydei Hook.f.

EtOH(50%) ext. of aerial parts, cardiac stim. (*Annu Rep RRL Jammu*, 1970-71, 24).

Cultivated at RRL, Jammu.

C. vincetoxicum Pers.; see **Vincetoxicum officinale**

CYNARA (*Asteraceae*)

C. scolymus Linn.
Eng.–*Artichoke*.

Herb—preparation of ext. for use in liver diseases (Rom. Pat., 1968, 51326; *CA*, 1969, **70**, 90724n); w.-sol. ext. for treating hepatic ailments, hypercholesteremic and renal incapacity; also magnesia exts. from baldo and artichoke plants having cholagogic and choleretic action; and herb ext. a constituent of antitoxic, diur. and laxt. compn. (Fr. M. 1969, 6613; 6880; *CA*, 1971, **74**, 45602s; 57291c; Fr. Demande, 1977, 2336922; *CA*, 1978, **88**, 94850u). Ext. in antimeteoristic preparation (Ger. Offen, 1972, 2040425; *CA*, **76**, 158338v).

Plant, fresh herb, cyanoroside (luteolin 7-glucd.) & scolynoside (luleolin 7β-rutinoside) (*Med Promst SSSR*, 1964, **18**, 23; *CA*, **61**, 11010b). Therapeutically active in jaundice; activity relationship with constituents (*Corr Farm*, 1967, **22**, 59; *CA*, **67**, 89667b). Phenolic carboxylic acids (*Rastit Resur*, 1967, **3**, 250; *CA*, 1968, **68**, 910a).

Sesquiterp. lactone, cynarolide (*Diss Pharm Pharmacol*, 1968, **20**, 217; *CA*, **69**, 52330b). Italian plant, sesquiterp. lactones, cynaropicrin and grosheimin; Polish plant, cynaropicrin & its dehydro deriv. (*Tetrahedron Lett*, 1971, 4775); stereochem. of guaianolides (*J Chem Soc Chem Commun*, 1972, 386). Cynaropicrin, cytotoxic properties in tissue cultures of human and animal malignant cells (*Immunol Ther Exp*, 1975, **23**, 845; *in* Wagner & Wolff; 162). Volat. aroma constituents of cooked herb (*J Agric Food Chem*, 1978, **28**, 791). A new guaianolide, cynaratriol from leaves (*Helv Chim Acta*, 1979, **62**, 1288).

Leaves, polyphenolic cynarin (*Med Promst SSSR*, 1965, **19**, 13; *CA*, **63**, 6786b); flavone complex from leaves in diur. compn. (Fr. M., 1968, 6074; *CA*, 1970, **72**, 6237r); choleretic compds. from leaves (Jpn Kokai, 1976, 76118814; *CA*, 1977, **86**, 78665r).

Cynarin—active principle, present as 1,3-dicaffeoylquinic acid which gets trans esterified to 1,5-dicaffeoyl isomer during extraction and hydrolysed in gastrointestinal tract to caffeic acid which may be true active substance possessing hepatotropic and choleretic activity (*in* Beal & Reinhard, 220-21); various polyphenolic constituents from leaves; and detn. (*Khim Prir Soedin Akad Nauk Uz SSR*, 1966, **2**, 16; *CA*, **65**, 3947f; *Pharmazie*, 1967, **22**, 176; *CA*, **67**, 51052j; *Plant Med Phytother*, 1970, **4**, 56; 1971, **5**, 39; *CA*, **73**, 84642d; **75**, 15879r).

Flower, receptacles constituents (*Egypt Pharm Bull*, 1962, **44**, 19; *CA*, 1965, **62**, 8116a). Fruits gave +ve test for alk. (*Lloydia*, 1972, **35**, 8).

CYNODON (*Poaceae*)

C. dactylon (Linn.) Pers.

Rhizome useful in genito-urinary disorders (*J Agric Trop Bot Appl*, 1966, **13**, 272). Pollen ext. beneficial in rhinitis and asthma, clin. study (*Philipp J Sci*, 1972, **101**, 15). In Mexico, leaves wetted with morning dew rubbed on warts to cure them; various plant parts used in headache, convuls., cramps, sores, carbuncle, wounds and snakebite (*Econ Bot*, 1977, **31**, 347; 1970, **24**, 241).

Plant—used in inflammed tumours, whitlows and fleshy excrescences of nails (*Lloydia*, 1969, **32**, 192). EtOH(50%) ext., antivir. (*Indian J Exp Biol*, 1968, **6**, 232). Ext., antifung. (*Labdev*, 1971, **9B**, 136); hypoglyc. (*Acta Phytother*, 1972, **19**, 141); juice applied to stop nose-bleeding and skin diseases [*J Res Indian Med*, 1977, **12**(4), 53]; produces dermatitis (*Indian J Med Res*, 1978, **68**, 650). Pharmacol. (*Philipp J Sci*, 1978, **107**, 71; *Indian J Pharm*, 1967, **29**, 347). Ext., more diur. than theophylline solution (*An Inst Bot A J Cavanilles*, 1977, **34**, 703; *BA*, 1980, **69**, 18954); antilithic (*Proc Indian Sci Congr*, 1981, Pt III, 156).

CYNOGLOSSUM (*Boraginaceae*)

Genus contains hepatotoxic pyrrolizidine alks. (*J Natl Prod*, 1981, **44**, 129-52).

*C. denticulatum DC. var. zeylanica C.B. Clarke

Root paste given in vomiting and diar. (*Bull Med Ethno Bot Res*, 1980, **1**, 8).

Found in Dang forest of Gujarat.

C. glochidiatum Wall. ex Benth. syn. *C. wallichi* G. Don

Alc. ext. of plant contains alk. amabiline (*Indian J Pharm*, 1975, **37**, 69); pyrrolizidine alks., major cynaustraline (*Indian J Pharm Sci*, 1978, **40**, 225).

C. lanceolatum Forsk. syn. *C. micranthum* Desf.

EtOH(50%) ext. of plant, anti-Accholine activity (*Indian J Exp Biol*, 1969, **7**, 250).

Plant, alk. cynaustraline and cynaustine (*Indian J Pharm*, 1975, **37**, 69).

CYPERUS (*Cyperaceae*)

C. articulatus Linn.

In Hawaii, bud, leaves, roots used in aches (*Econ Bot*, 1971, **25**, 245).

Essent. oil from roots, sesquiterp. ketone cyperone (*Tetrahedron*, 1968, **24**, 3891).

C. brevifolius Hassk.; see **Kyllinga brevifolia**

*C. compactus Retz. syn. *Mariscus microcephalus* Presl

EtOH(50%) ext. of aerial parts, antiinflam., diur. and anticancer (*Indian J Exp Biol*, 1980, **18**, 594).

Found in Madhya Pradesh and Uttar Pradesh.

C. esculentus Linn.

Plant, uterine stim. (*Qual Plant Mater Veg*, 1968-69, **17**, 153). Tuberous rootstocks, purg. (*Nagarjun*, 1979-80, **23**, 217).

Tuber oil, unsap. matter constituents (*Riv Ital Sostanze Grasse*, 1970, **47**, 252; *CA*, **73**, 108455y).

C. iria Linn.

Rhizomes, hentriacontanol (*Curr Sci*, 1973, **42**, 622). Essent. oil of roots, constituents (*Nippon Nogei Kagaku Kaishi*, 1978, **52**, 379; *CA*, 1979, **90**, 192372a).

*C. laevigatus Linn.

In Hawaii, plant used in urine trouble (*Econ Bot*, 1971, **25**, 245).

Found in Madhya Pradesh.

*C. niveus Retz.

EtOH(50%) ext. of plant, antivir. and spasmol. (*Indian J Exp Biol*, 1968, **6**, 232).

Reported from Madhya Pradesh.

C. rotundus Linn.

Tubers—aq.-alc. exts., hypoten. in cats and cause systolic heart arrest in frogs (*Azerb Med Zh*, 1966, **43**, 12). Ext. potential antiinflam., also antipyr. and analg.; active constituent, a triterp. (*Indian J Med Res*, 1971, **59**, 76); used in dysen. EtOH(50%) ext., diur. (*Indian J Exp Biol*, 1980, **18**, 594).

Root paste applied for healing wounds, sores, etc. (*Bull Bot Surv India*, 1973, **15**, 21; *Econ Bot*, 1974, **28**, 4); used in intestinal diseases; contain essent. oil of antibiot. nature (*Indian Drugs*, 1977-78, **15**, 145). Aq. ext. from MeOH ext., useful in conjunctivitis, clin. trials (*J Res Ayur Sidha*, 1980, **1**, 115); ingredient in herbal drug for giardiasis, clin. trials (*Sachitra Ayurveda*, 1981-82, **34**, 401).

Plant—minor ingredient of Unani drug *Jawarish Jalinoos'* used in diseases of stomach, intestine and urinary bladder (*Planta Med*, 1971, **20**, 60). In Bahama Island, tea taken in cold (*Econ Bot*, 1975, **29**, 307); to cure jaundice [*J Res Indian Med*, 1978, **12**(4), 92].

Essent. oil—pharmacol. (*Indian J Med Res*, 1970, **58**, 103); anti-insect and juvenile hormone mimicking activity (*Indian J Pharm Sci*, 1979, **41**, 250); antimicrob. and anthelm. (*Indian J Hosp Pharm*, 1980, **17**, 102).

Diur. effect of drug from galenicals; chem. constituents [*Izv Akad Nauk Az SSR Ser Biol Nauk*, 1964, (4), 98; *CA*, 1967, **66**, 64135t]. Tubers, oleanolic acid & its glycd. (*Phytochemistry*, 1980, **19**, 2056);β-sitosterol (*Planta Med*, 1980, **39**, 157).

Essent. oil, Indian, sesquiterps. (*Tetrahedron Lett*, 1967, 4661); characteristics, rev. on oil from Indian spp. (*Perfum Essent Oil Rec*, 1967, **58**, 522). Characteristics and constituents of essent.

oil from tubers (*J Res Ludhiana*, 1969, **6**, 383).

Essent. oil from other countries, monoterp., and sesquiterp. compds. including patchoulenone (*Collect Czech Chem Commun*, 1964, **29**, 1675; *CA*, **61**, 5697h). Identn. of sesquiterp. ketone cypernone (*Tetrahedron*, 1968, **24**, 3891). Tubers, sesquiterp., α- & β- retunol; their str. (*Tetrahedron Lett*, 1969, 2741; *Tetrahedron*, 1971, **27**, 4831). Str. of cyperotundone from tubers. Norsesquiterps., kobusone & isokobusone (*Chem Pharm Bull*, 1966, **14**, 890; 1969, **17**, 1390); sesquiterps. (*Phytochemistry*, 1976, **15**, 1265; *Zasso Kenkyu*, 1977, **22**, 14; *CA*, 1978, **88**, 86013h).

C. scariosus R. Br.

Essent. oil—from tuber, hypoten. and CNS stim. (*Annu Rep RRL Jammu*, 1970-71, 24); antiinflam. (*Indian J Exp Biol*, 1972, **10**, 41); antimicrob. [*Indian Drugs*, 1978- 79, **16**, 150; *Indian Drugs Pharmac Ind*, 1979, **14**(4), 25].

Essent. oil, from tuber, sesquiterp., cyperenone, its identn. (*J Pharm Sci*, 1965, **54**, 1823; *Tetrahedron*, 1968, **24**, 3891). Cyperenol and patchoulenol.; also isopatchoulenone (*Tetrahedron Lett*, 1967, 2447; 1965, 4053); str. of sesquiterp. enedione (*Sci Cult*, 1969, **35**, 110); (-)-β-selinene and isopatchoula-3,5-diene (*Indian J Chem*, 1978, **16B**, 148); tricyclic sesquiterp., retundene & rotundenol; their str. (*ibid*, 1970, **8**, 854; *Tetrahedron Lett*, 1977, 2121).

Leaves, new glycd. of leptosidin (*Phytochemistry*, 1981, **20**, 2605).

C. stoloniferus Retz. syn. *C. juncifolius* Klein

Essent. oil from tubers, hypoten. and CNS stim. (*Annu Rep RRL Jammu*, 1970-71, 24).

*C. tegetum Roxb.

Plant used in atrophy, emaciation, cachexy and snakebite (*Econ Bot*, 1970, **24**, 241).

Found throughout India.

C. triceps (Rettb.) Endl.; see **Kyllinga tenuifolia**

CYRTOPHYLLUM (*Loganiaceae*)

C. peregrinum Reinw. ex Blume; see **Fagraea cochinchinensis**

CYTISUS (*Fabaceae*)

C. scoparius Link syn. *Sarothamnus scoparius* Koch

EtOH(50%) ext. of aerial parts, hypoten., spasmol. and diur. (*Indian J Exp Biol*, 1969, **7**, 250).

Seed agglutinin aggregated blood platelets (*Biochem Biophys Res Commun*, 1977, **75**, 200).

Plant, alk., sparteine, *l*-α-isosparteine, lupanine and OH-lupanine (*Diss Pharm*, 1964, **16**, 261; *CA*, 1965, **62**, 6800e). Antimicrob. substance from plant tissue culture ext. (*Lloydia*, 1968, **31**, 180). Synth. of Vit. B6 by cultured callus (*Agric Biol Chem*, 1980, **44**, 2683). Glycd. sarothamnoside (*Tetrahedron Lett*, 1981, **22**, 1223).

Leaves, extn. of alk. oxysparteine, lupanine and genisteine, all minor alks. (*Acta Pol Pharm*, 1967, **24**, 619; *CA*, 1968, **68**, 66331u); genitoside, scoparoside and 5 other flavones (*Lloydia*, 1977, **40**, 591).

Flowers, essent. oil constituents (*Yakugaku Zasshi*, 1980, **100**, 1054). Flower and fruits gave +ve test for alk. (*Lloydia*, 1972, **35**, 17).

Seeds, DOPA (*Herba Pol*, 1975, **21**, 366; *CA*, **85**, 83147g); tocopherol estn. (*Plant Med Phytother*, 1979, **13**, 278; *CA*, **92**, 194479f).

Sparteine—also called lupinidine, is an quinolizidine alk.; present in all parts of plant including seeds; it is a cardiac and respiratory stim. and an oxytocic but not altogether safe (Sim, 83-87). Natural drying of herb yields higher amts. (*Farm Pol*, 1966, **22**, 537; *CA*, 1967, **67**, 76234h).

DACTYLICAPNOS (*Fumariaceae*)

D. macrocapnos Hutchins.; see **Dicentra scandens**

DACTYLIS (*Poaceae*)

*D. glomerata Linn.

Eng.–*Cocks-foot-grass.*

Plant—estrogenic activity equivalent to 17.4μg of di-Et-stilbestrol/kg (*Agric Louvain*, 1962, **10**, 353;*CA*, 1964, **60**, 4463b); boiled with lard and bread used against tumours (*Lloydia*, 1969, **32**, 192). EtOH(50%) ext., preliminary pharmacol. (*Indian J Exp Biol*, 1980, **18**, 594).

Pollen, antigenic properties and their allergenic ext. studied (*Byull Eksp Biol Med*, 1964, **58**, 80; *Allerg Asthma*, 1965, **11**, 301; *CA*, 1968, **68**, 20482r). Commercial extn. of sterols from pollen (*Acta Chem Scand*, 1968, **22**, 2161).

Estn. of estrogenic substance present in undetectable quant. (*Mie Daigaku Nogakubu Gakujutsu Hokoku*, 1963, **27**, 7; *CA*, 1964, **61**, 6045h). Aerial parts, chelidonic acid (*Aust J Biol Sci*, 1965, **18**, 437). Plant, cholecalciferol, isolation (*FEBS Lett*, 1968, **1**, 59); γ- *l*-glutamyl-*l*-glutamine (*Bull Acad Pol Sci Ser Sci Biol*, 1971, **19**, 95).

N-W Himalayas, and also grown on hill farms.

DACTYLOCTENIUM (*Poaceae*)

D. aegyptium Willd. syn. *Eleusine aegyptica* Desf.

Grass—fish poison (SEPASAT, 165).

Grass contains oxalic acid (total, 0.5; w.-sol.,0.06%); oxalate- level not likely to cause any deleterious effect in animals on feeding (*Indian J Anim Sci*, 1973, **43**, 476). Grains taken with husk cause stomach troubles. Presence of cynogenic glycd. reported (*Bull Bot Soc Bengal*, 1978, **32**, 48).

*D. scindicum Boiss. syn. *Eleusine scindica* Duthie

Grains when consumed cause internal disorders (*Econ Bot*, 1974, **28**, 76).

Found in hotter parts of the Middle East, extending into N-W India.

DACTYLORHIZA (*Orchidaceae*)

D. hatagirea (D. Don) Soo syn. *Orchis latifolia* auct. non Linn.

Tubers used to relieve hoarseness, as nervine tonic and aphrodis. Mucilageous root useful in diar., dysen. and chr. fevers; decoct. or salep given to sick person (Wlth India, VII, 104). Tubers alongwith leaves of *Urtica dioica* and leaf and bark of *piyoss* made into paste and applied to fractures (*Bull Med Ethno Bot Res*, 1980, **1**, 440).

DAEDALACANTHUS (*Acanthaceae*)

See **ERANTHEMUM**

DAEMIA (*Asclepiadaceae*)

See **PERGULARIA**

DAEMONOROPS (*Aracaceae*)

D. draco Blume syn. *Calamus draco* Willd.

Resin as powd. or in pills used against cancer and malignant tumour (*Lloydia*, 1970, **33**, 316).

Resin, flavonols, chalcones, quinone methides, nordracorhodin and nordracorubin; and secobiflavonoid (*J Chem Soc C*, 1971, 3967; *J Chem Soc Perkin Trans I*, 1976, 1570); diterp. acids; and triterps. (*Phytochemistry*, 1974, **13**, 2231; 1981, **20**, 514).

DALBERGIA (*Fabaceae*)

*D. cultrata Grah. ex Benth.

EtOH(50%) ext. of aerial parts, spasmog. (*Indian J Exp Biol*, 1974, **12**, 512). Seed ext., antibact. (*J Exp Med*, 1980, **50**, 263).

Found in Darjeeling, W. B.

D. lanceolaria Linn.f.

Leaves, ether, EtOH and aq. exts. slightly antiarthritic in albino rats (*Indian J Med Res*, 1965, **53**, 71; 1966, **57**, 363). Clin. trials of drug (leaves and tender branch) for rheum., inflam. and osteroarthritis; as antiinflam. drug better than Ph- butazone (*Rheumatism*, 1978-79, **14**, 53; 118; 153).

ψ-Baptigenin from leaves and flowers, possessed properties to treat arthritic ailments of human and animal patients (*Curr Sci*, 1967, **36**, 484).

Root bark, isoflavone glycd., lanceolarin; its str. (*Tetrahedron Lett*, 1965, 3191; *Tetrahedron*, 1967, **23**, 405).

D. latifolia Roxb.

Bark—pounded with *D. paniculata* in water, given to relieve body pain (*Econ Bot*, 1965, **19**, 236). EtOH(50%) ext., spasmog., and anthelm. against *Ascaridia galli* (*Indian J Exp Biol*, 1968, **6**, 232).

Bark contains hentriacontane, latifolin, β- sitosterol, sucrose and tannins (*Bull Nat Inst Sci India*, 1965, No. 31, 165); and triacontane, dalbergichromene, lupeol, Ac-oleanolic acid, γ-sitosterol, (*R*)-latifolin, (*R*)-4-OMe-dalbergione, Me-dalbergin & dalbergin;last 6 compds. also found in sapwood (*Phytochemistry*, 1971, **10**, 2551).

Seeds, 4-Ph-coumarin, sisofolin [*Proc Nat Acad Sci India*, 1970, **40A**(Pt.2), 165]; and a new rotenoid, dalbin & a new OH-rotenoid, dalbinol (*Phytochemistry*, 1979, **18**, 188; 1978, **17**, 1442).

Heartwood, (*R*)-dalbergione, 2,4,6-tri-OMe-acetophenone, β-sitosterol, dalbergin, and latifolin; its str. (*Tetrahedron Lett*, 1965, 4451; 1966, 3761); latifolin, liquiritigenin and dalbergenone (*Indian J Chem*, 1965, **3**, 422).

Quinones of heartwoods of *Dalbergia* spp., rev., 13 refs (*Bull Nat Inst Sci India*, 1965, No.28, 1). A phenanthrene-1, 4-quinone, latinone (*Phytochemistry*, 1981, **20**, 1089).

*D. paniculata Roxb.

EtOH(50%) ext. of aerial parts, antiprot. against *Entamoeba histolytica* strain, and spasmog. (*Indian J Exp Biol*, 1980, **18**, 594).

Plant contains a rotenoid, dalpanol (*J Chem Soc D*, 1971, 29).

Flowers, apigenin, luteolin, caviunim, dalpanin, *d*- pinitol, and an aliphatic alc. (*Phytochemistry*, 1973, **12**, 2543; *Proc Indian Acad Sci*, 1975, **81A**, 23); leaves, luteolin and apigenin; heartwood, biochanin-A-7-O-glucd. and paniculatin (*Indian J Chem*, 1973, **11**, 969; 89).

Seeds, caniunin (*Curr Sci*, 1971, **40**, 602); dalpanitin, dalpatin, and dalpanin (*Tetrahedron*, 1972, **28**, 5377); dalpatien and dalpanol-O-glucd. (*Phytochemistry*, 1973, **12**, 3003); 6a, 12a- dehydrodalpanol, and milldurone (*Indian J Chem*, 1975, **13**, 425).

Bark,β-sitosterol, paniculatin, biochanin A (*Phytochemistry*, 1976, **15**, 1025); and isocaviunin-7-O- glucd. (*Indian J Chem*, 1980, **19B**, 429).

Root, triacontane, *d*-panitol, caviunin & its -7-O-glucd.; also -7-O-rhamnoglucd. (*J Indian Chem Soc*, 1979, **56**, 81; *Phytochemistry*, 1980, **19**, 1563).

Found almost throughout India.

D. sissoo Roxb. ex DC.

Leaf mucilage mixed with sweet oil applied in excoriations (Wlth India, III, 11).

Leaves, isoflavone, sissotrin (*Indian J Chem*, 1966, **4**, 70). Flowers, 7,4′-di-Me-tectorigenin (*Curr Sci*, 1966, **34**, 431).

Pods, green, *meso*-inositol, 7-Me-tectorigenin & its 4′-rhamnoglucd. (*Indian J Chem*, 1965, **3**, 474); mature pods isocaviunin, tectorigenin, dalbergin, biochanin A and 7-OH-4-Me-coumarin; also 7-O-glucds. of tectorigenin and caviunin (*ibid*, 1979, **18B**, 472; 1980, **19B**, 237); and 7- getiobiosides of caviunin; & isocaviunin (*Phytochemistry*, 1979, **18**, 1253; 1980, **19**, 715).

Stem bark, dalbergenone, dalbergin, Me-dalbergin and a 4-Ph- chromene, dalbergichromene (*Tetrahedron*, 1971, **27**,

799); and fresh bark, isotectorigenin (*Indian J Chem*, 1974, **12**, 1118).

Heartwood, dalbergin, OMe-dalbergin and dalbergenone (*Curr Sci*, 1963, **32**, 455); hydroxy- & OMe-dalbergenones (*Bull Nat Inst Sci India*, 1965, No. 28, 1); dalbergichromene, nordalbergin and isodalbergin (*Tetrahedron*, 1971, **27**, 799); and allylphenol of latifolin, dalbergiphenol (*Indian J Chem*, 1974, **12**, 10); and 3,5-di-OH-*trans*-stilbene; and biochanin A (*J Indian Acad Wood Sci*, 1975, **6**, 57; 59).

Found almost throughout India.

D. spinosa Roxb. syn. *Drepanocarpus spinosus* Kurz

EtOH(50%) ext. of aerial parts, diur. and spasmog. (*Indian J Exp Biol*, 1977, **15**, 208).

D. sympathetica Nimmo ex Grah. syn. *D. multiflora* Heyne ex Wall.

EtOH(50%) ext. of aerial parts, spasmog. (*Indian J Exp Biol*, 1977, **15**, 208).

D. volubilis Roxb.

EtOH(50%) ext. of aerial parts, diur. (*Indian J Exp Biol*, 1971, **9**, 91).

Flowers, β-sitosterol, stigmasterol, biochanin A and glycds., volubilin; volubilinin (*Phytochemistry*, 1974, **13**, 2301; 1976, **15**, 235); rhamnoside, isovolubilin (*Indian J Chem*, 1975, **13**, 444).

Glycd. from leaves, significant antiinflam. and antiarthritic in rats, low level toxic (*Indian J Med Res*, 1975, **63**, 93); flavon, glycd., chrysoẹriol-7-O- β-D-glucopyranosidyl-(2→1) - D - apiofuranoside, possessing antiinflam.and antiarthritic properties; leaves also contain triacontane, myricyl alc., β-sitosterol, biochanin A, formononetin, tectoregenin and 7-OH-4-Me-coumarin (*Indian J Chem*, 1977, **15B**, 395; 492).

Wood, friedelin (*An Assoc Bras Quim*, 1962, **21**, 33; *CA*, 1965, **63**, 4655b); bark dalbergin, tectorigenin, tectoridin, cearoin, *d*-medicarpin and 8-OMe-tectorigenin; & its glycds. (*Indian J Chem*, 1978,**16B**,

76;641); also tectc rigenin-7-gentiobioside (*Phytochemistry*, ⸱J78, **17**, 596).

DAPHNE (*Thymelaeaceae*)

D. oleoides Schreb. syn. *D. mezereum* Linn.

Plant—as vesic. and counter irrit. In Baluchistan, crushed leaves with wheat flour and oil, for poulticing boils (*Wlth India*, III, 13); for treatment of cancer (*Lloydia*, 1971, **32**, 204).

Plant growing in Moscow, daphnin (major compd.), 8- β-glucd. of 8-OH-coumarin, daphneretin, a phenoglucd. daphnoside, β-sitosterol, an unidentified tri-OH-flavone, sucrose and mezerein resin [*Tr Vses S'ezda Farm*, 1967, (Pub. 1970), 245; *CA*, 1971, **75**, 126577k]. All parts of plant, umbelliferone, daphnetin and daphnin. In addn. fruits, leaves and roots, also daphnoretin, branch barks and root rinds, a flavon. [*Farmatsiya Moscow*, 1970, **19**(5), 36; *CA*, 1971, **74**, 10324a].

Bark yields poisonous daphnetoxin (0.02%), its str. (*J Am Chem Soc*, 1970, **92**, 1070).

Leaves, β-sitosterol and luteolin-7-glucd. (*Curr Sci*, 1966, **35**, 178); α-amyrin, lupeol and a fatty alc. (*J Indian Chem Soc*, 1979, **56**, 437); leaves and stems, daphnetin, tectochrysin and lignans, sesamin and pinoresinol (*Indian J Chem*, 1981, **20B**, 937).

Seeds, a coumarin glycd. daphnoside, β-sitosterol sucrose (*Farmatsiya Moscow*, 1968, **17**, 40; *BA*, 1969, **50**, 89448).

Mezerein—An antiinflam. and anticarcinogenic constituent from seeds; its NMR (*Chem Ztg Chem Appar*, 1970, **94**, 347; 849; *CA*, **73**, 64459w; 1971, **74**, 136353c). Isolation, str., daphnane ester (0.1%), and dephnetoxin (0.02%) from seeds (*Tetrahedron Lett*, 1970, 4261). EtOH ext. significantly active against P-388 lymphocytic leukemia and L-1210 leukemia, due to mezerein, which is active at a dose of 50 μg/kg body wt. of mice (*Science*, 1975, **187**, 652); mech. of antileukemic action (*Z Naturforsch*, 1977, **32C**, 678);

tumour-promoting activity on mouse skin (*in* Plant and Fungal toxins, 270).

Roots contain 14 constituents of which 3 are coumarins including daphnin (*Nauchn Tr Aspir Ordinatorov Pervogo Mosk Med Inst*, 1967, 138; *CA*, 1969, **71**, 105149z).

D. papyracea Wall. ex Steud.

Plant—used for curing insanity (*Curr Sci*, 1962, **31**, 463). EtOH(50%) ext. of aerial parts exhibits potent activity against P-388 lymphocytic leukemia in mice and antagonism of amphetamine hyperactivity (*Indian J Exp Biol*, 1973, **11**, 43).

Roots—roots, as also leaves poisonous, purg., used against skin diseases and gonor. (*Indian Drugs*, 1976-77, **14**, 47). In Sikkim, used for internal trouble (*Econ Bot*, 1979, **33**, 52). EtOH ext., cardiac depress. (*Annu Rep RRL Jammu*, 1970-71, 25).

Unsap. fraction of plant ext. yields sterol (mp 131- 32°); alc. ext. contains 3 glucds., G$_1$(mp 195- 97°), G$_2$(mp 175-77°) and G$_3$. Detanned alc. ext. of plant, and glycd. G$_3$, hypoten., tranquillizing and B.P. depress.; fatal in higher doses (*Curr Sci*, 1962, **31**, 463). Aerial parts, taraxerol & its - OAc, taraxerone, taraxeric acid, genkwanin, dephnetin and β-sitosterol. glucd. (*Indian J Chem*, 1979, **18B**, 189).

Roots, coumarin glycd., daphnin (*Indian J Chem*, 1964, **2**, 509); and daphnetin & its 8-β-glucd. (*J Pharm Sci*, 1973, **62**, 1358).

DAPHNIPHYLLUM (*Daphniphyllaceae*)

Alks. (*in* Manske, XV, 41-82).

*D. neilgherrense Rosenth. syn. *D. glaucescens* Blume

Kan.–*Nirijappe*; Tam.–*Collavan*; Tel.–*Putike*.

EtOH(50%) ext. of aerial parts, spasmog. (*Indian J Exp Biol*, 1974, **12**, 512).

Bark contains alks., calycine, glaucescine, and glaucescenine; leaves, calcycine (*Phytochemistry*, 1965, **4**, 627).

Found in Shola forests of Nilgiris, Anamalais, Pulney and other S. Indian mountain ranges, up to 1,200 m.

DATISCA (*Datiscaceae*)

D. cannabina Linn.

Plant—used in fevers, and gastric and scrofulous complaints (Wlth India, III, 14); having compd. with insulin-like activity, useful against diseases of fat metabolism (Ger. Offen. 1973, 2159923; *CA*, **79**, 57679p).

EtOH(50%) ext. of seeds and flowers, marked sed., highly antiinflam. and mild analg., antipyr. and diur. in rats [*J Res Indian Med*, 1979, **14**(2), 53].

Aerial parts yield same flavons. as root (*Khim Farm Zh*, 1978, **12**, 81; *CA*, 1979, **90**, 3155y), also rutin and Mg salt of datiscetin (*Khim Prir Soedin*, 1980, 125). Plant, hentriacontane, α-amyrin, oleanolic acid, erythrodiol, β-sitosterol & its glucd. (*Indian J Pharm Sci*, 1980, **42**, 24).

Root contains flavons., datiscin and datiscetin [*Vestn Mosk Univ Khim*, 1962, **17**(6), 64; *CA*, 1964, **60**, 4447d]; datiscetin, galangin-3-rutinosides (*Phytochemistry*, 1968, **7**, 51); datiscoside and an enzyme (*C R Acad Sci Ser D*, 1969, **268**, 2495); also galangin, cannabin, isalpinin and a chalcone (mp 350°) (*Khim Prir Soedin*, 1969, **5**, 179; *CA*, **71**, 98962d); datin, datinoside and datinate-CM (M=Ca and Mg) (*ibid*, 1974, 788; *CA*, 1975, **82**, 135689q);and galanginoside (*Rastit Resur*, 1976, **12**, 237; *CA*, **85**, 59588f).

DATURA (*Solanaceae*)

D. arborea auct. non Linn.; see **Brugmansia candida**

D. innoxia Mill. syn. *D. metel* auct. non Linn.

Seeds—smoked like tobacco for curing gum troubles such as pyorrhoea (*Econ Bot*, 1971, **25**, 414). EtOH ext., antimicrob. (*Indian Drugs*, 1976-77, **14**, 160); ext., depress. properties, increased by Δ^9-tetrahydrocannabinol (*Indian J Pharm*, 1978, **40**, 1).

EtOH(50%) ext. of plant, spasmol. (*Indian J Exp Biol*, 1969, **7**, 250).

All parts of plant including seeds, alks., hyoscine (scopolamine) and hyoscyamine. Roots, also tropine, ψ-tropine and meteloidine; sap, nortropine (*J Pharm Pharmacol*, 1965, **17**, 115; 1964, **16**, 337); oncogenetic changes in alk. content (*Pharmazie*, 1966, **21**, 48); accumulates more scopolamine than hyoscyamine (Sim, 37); levels of atropine and scopolamine during growth (*Diss Pharm Pharmacol*, 1972, **24**, 307; *CA*, **77**, 85746k). Roots, a new tropane deriv. (*Phytochemistry*, 1974, **13**, 1249).

A saponin-like compd. in green parts of plant (*Zesz Nauk Akad Econ Poznaniu Ser I*, 1975, **62**, 37; *CA*, 1976, **85**, 59613k).

Scopolamine isolation from aerial parts during fruit ripening [*Farmatsiya Sof*, 1967, **17**(4), 37; *CA*, 1968, **68**, 6129g].

From cell suspension culture, *p*-OH-benzoic acid glucose ester in comparatively high yield; glucosylation reaction having biochemical potential (*Phytochemistry*, 1976, **15**, 1225; *Planta*, 1972, **105**, 342).

Scopolamine (Hyoscine)—extn., from seed economic method (*Farmacia Buc*, 1973, **21**, 403; *CA*, 1974, **80**, 100142t); extn., with small amts. of *l*-hyoscyamine, 2 unknown alks. (*Bull Fac Sci Riyadh Univ*, 1973, **5**, 1; *CA*, 1974, **81**, 101848h). Cultivation studies for tropane alk. production (*Indian Drugs*, 1976-77, **14**, 39; *Indian J Pharm*, 1978, **40**, 14). Sepn. from hyoscyamine from aq. ext. (Hung. Teljes, 1979, 17040; *CA*, 1980, **92**, 82421z); extn. (Rom Pat., 1978, 64869; 1980, **92**, 64774c). In India, leaves used for extn. of hyoscine (Wlth India, IA, 485-86); see also *D. stramonium*.

D. metel Linn. syn. *D. alba* Nees; *D. fastuosa* Linn.var. *alba* C.B. Clarke

Plant—various parts used in headache, otitis media suppurative, sores, mumps, pain, dropsy, anasarca, madness, rheum., rigid thigh muscles, hemiplegia, epilepsy, convuls., cramps, delirium febris, pimples, smallpox, venereal sores, syphilis, orchitis, epidydimitis, and hydrocele (*Econ Bot*,

1970, **24**, 241). EtOH(50%) ext., anthelm., anticancer, and also of fruits, spasmog. and B.P. depress. (*Indian J Exp Biol*, 1968, **6**, 232). Aq. ext., strong nematicidal (*Indian J Entomol*, 1979, **41**, 326).

Leaves—smoked to cure cough (*Econ Bot*, 1978, **32**, 278). EtOH ext., so also aq. ext. of fruits, anticholinergic [*An Acad Bras Cienc*, 1970, **42**(Suppl.), 245]; ext., antivir. (*Indian Phytopathol*, 1981, **34**, 452).

Seeds used in asthma, hydrophobia, malaria and making liquor more intoxicating; roots used to cure toothache and for brushing teeth (*J Agric Trop Bot Appl*, 1966, **13**, 247).

Plant accumulates more hyoscine than hyoscyamine (Sim, 37); hyoscine content of dried leaves and flowering tops between 0.02-0.55% (Markets Selected Med. Plants, 104).

Leaves, alk. content 0.55 and stem, 0.4% (*Planta Med*, 1970, **18**, 266); nicotianamine (*Phytochemistry*, 1976, **15**, 1701); scopolamine, hyoscyamine and 2 unidentified alk. in leaves from Thailand (*J Nat Res Counc Thailand*, 1978, **10**, 7).

Seeds, alks., 0.19 (in pericarps, 0.8%); mainly hyoscine (scopolamine) and hyoscyamine (*Indian J Pharm*, 1964, **26**, 140); other alks. (*Sci Res Dacca*, 1965, **2**, 147; 1966, **3**, 212; *CA*, 1966, **65**, 12246h; 1968, **68**, 29909t); scopolamine extn. from seeds and pods, 90% recovery (*Khim Farm Zh*, 1970, **4**, 42; *CA*, 1971, **74**, 34568j).

Seeds, daturaolone and fastusic acid (*Pak J Sci Ind Res*, 1967, **10**, 85; *Sci Res Dacca*, 1968, **5**, 66; *Indian J Chem*, 1976, **14B**, 1007); seed oil, α-Me-sterols (*Phytochemistry*, 1978, **17**, 971).

Fruit pericarp, alks. and β-sitosterol (*Bangladesh J Sci Ind Res*, 1974, **9**, 79); triterp., daturaolone and daturadiol (*Indian J Pharm*, 1977, **39**, 119).

Roots, alk.; content (at flowering of plant), 0.77% (*Lloydia*, 1965, **28**, 71; *Planta Med*, 1970, **18**, 266); tropane deriv. (*Bull Fac Pharm Cairo Univ*, 1967, **6**, 9; *CA*, 1970, **73**, 77448s).

*D. quercifolia H.B. & K.

Tam.–*Vellum-matti.*

EtOH(50%) ext. of whole plant and fruit, spasmog., and B.P. depress.; hypoglyc.; plant ext., also hypoglyc.; fruit ext., anthelm. (*Indian J Exp Biol*, 1968, **6**, 232).

Plant organs, scopolamine, atropine and 5 other alks. (*Diss Pharm Pharmacol*, 1967, **19**, 371; *CA*, **67**, 102710g).

Leaves contain withanolides, daturalactone; its oxo-deriv., daturalactone-3 & -4 (*Phytochemistry*, 1973, **12**, 476; 1976, **15**, 339; 1979, **18**, 283; 1756); daturalactone, effective interceptive; weak estrogenic (*Indian J Exp Biol*, 1978, **16**, 419; 648).

Found in Coimbatore and Madras, T. N.

*D. sanguinea Ruiz & Pav.

Roots and aerial parts, tropane alks.; scopolamine, major; roots, possible commercial source. Leaves, new tropane deriv. (*Planta Med*, 1965, **13**, 353; 1975, **28**, 105); alks. from various plant parts; seed alks. (*J Chem Soc C*, 1968, 1621; 2775). Aerial parts, tropanol (*Phytochemistry*, 1978, **17**, 171).

D. stramonium Linn. syn. *D. tatula* Linn.

Eng.–*Jimson weed, thorn apple.*

Plant—an analg. compn. containing minor amts. of stramonium powd. with other ingredients (US, 1972, 3865933; *CA*, 1976, **84**, 35344b); ext., insectic. (*Indian J Agric Sci*, 1979, **49**, 295).

Seeds—ext. agglutinated human red cells, non-specific to any blood group (*J Chem UAR*, 1963, **6**, 191); seed lectin, non-specific in human electrolyte ABO system (*Biochem Biophys Acta*, 1978, **532**, 92).

Species accumulates more hyoscyamine than scopolamine (Sim, 47); most suitable for scopolamine extn. (*Farmatsiya Sof*, 1968, **18**, 50; *CA*, **68**, 109846f); atropine, scopolamine in leaves, roots and stem, cuscohygrine in roots (*Diss Pharm Pharmacol*, 1970, **22**, 35; *CA*, **73**, 939v); leaves of Iranian wild plant yield alks. hyoscyamine as major (*Pazhoohandeh Tehran*, 1977, **16**, 118; *CA*, 1978, **88**,

71501s); cultivated in S. Europe and the Far East; hyoscyamine (major alk.) extracted (Markets Selected Med. Plants, 11).

Whole plant alk., 0.26% (Seeds, 0.98; and stem, 0.08%); hyoscyamine, 44.1-67.1%; hyoscine, 13.2-25.3%; and atropine, 0.01-0.1% of total alks. (*Dokl Akad Nauk Tadzh SSR*, 1978, **21**, 34; *CA*, 1979, **90**, 51420c).

Hyoscyamine N-oxide from all parts [*J Pharm Pharmacol*, 1973, **25** (Suppl), 116p; *Phytochemistry*, 1975, **14**, 999]. Aerial parts of plants from two places, different pattern of alks. (*Khim Prir Soedin*, 1977, 126; *CA*, **87**, 50201h).3 Coumarins from aerial parts (*Rastit Resur*, 1972, **8**, 373; *CA*, **77**, 111527m); tropane deriv. from leaves (USSR Pat., 1978, 634747; *CA*, 1979, **90**, 99687x); new withanolide, withastramonolide (*Khim Prir Soedin*, 1978, 91; *CA*, **89**, 43962v); daturalactone & its keto deriv. (*Tezisy Dokl Sav Indiiskii Simp Khim Prir Soedin 5th*, 1978, 53; *CA*, 1980, **93**, 146292p).

Seeds, scopolamine and hyoscyamine (*Aptech Delo*, 1962, **11**, 29; *CA*, 1964, **60**, 13093h); total alks., 0.35%, atropine, 0.17% (*Diss Pharm*, 1963, **15**, 313; *CA*, 1964, **61**, 2903g); alk. in seeds, 0.03-0.23% (in leaves, 0.06-0.26%) [*Farmatsiya Sof*, 1965, **15**(2), 96; *CA*, **63**, 13699h]; alk. detn., amperometric (*Yao Hsueh Hsueh Pao*, 1965, **12**, 388; *CA*, 1966, **65**, 15159h).

Hyoscine (scopolamine)—extn. from seed (USSR Pat., 1963, 158281; *CA*, 1964, **60**, 10485e); more than 10% increase in hyoscyamine and scopolamine by the application of trace elements (*Tartu Riikliku Ulikooli Toim*, 1971, No. 270, 3; *CA*, 1972, **76**, 33212t); atropine and scopolamine, colorim. detn. (*Ann Acad Med Lodz*, 1971, **12**, 403; *CA*, 1973, **79**, 35195a); alk. detn., accurate method (*Arch Pharm Berl*, 1972, **305**, 273; *CA*, **77**, 39316x); hyoscine and hyoscyamine from callus cultures (*in* Beal & Reinhard, 82). Extn., simple method, hyoscyamine as byproduct (*Res Ind*, 1973, **18**, 160); pure isolation (Indian Pat., 1976,

130397; *CA*, 1979, **91**, 181445w). Scopolamine in aerial part,≥ 70.5% of total alks.; hyoscyamine in roots, 66.5% (*Rev Med Hanoi*, 1977, 118; *CA*, 1979, **91**, 207479n); hyoscine 5 times as active as atropine in producing mydriasis but its main use is as antimotion sickness drug; minor use in combination as a sed. Salts of its esters in antiperspirant preparations (Markets Selected Med. Plants, 11).

D. suaveolens Humb. & Bonpl. ex Willd.; see **Brugmansia suaveolens**

DAUCUS (*Apiaceae*)

D. carota Linn. var. **sativa** DC.

Eng.–*Carrot.*

Root (Carrot)—EtOH(50%) ext. effective on isolated coronary vessels of rats, flavons., sugars and a quaternary base present; preliminary pharmacol. (*Biul Inst Rosl Leczn*, 1964, **10**, 113; *CA*, 1965, **63**, 6197f; *Indian J Exp Biol*, 1971, **9**, 91); a coronary vasodilator (0.5%) (Pol. Pat., 1969, 57079; *CA*, 1970, **72**, 24596m); antimicrob. (*Fitoterapia*, 1980, **51**, 303).

Used in leprosy, piles, tumours, etc., considered blood purifier, antisep., etc. Carrot decoct. beneficial in biliousness and jaundice. An ointment with lard useful in burns and scalds; used with leaves as poultice for oozing sores and ulcers (*Planta Med*, 1973, **23**, 381); ext. exhibits thiamine inactivation, uneffected by cooking or gastric juice (*Int Z Vitaminforsch*, 1963, **34**, 135; *CA*, 1964, **61**, 6277a).

Seeds—chitinase and Ac-glucosaminidase activity (*Comp Biochem Physiol*, 1965, **14**, 127); aq. ext., antisp. and cardiotonic, contains compd. with papavarine-like action; choline and a cholinergic active quaternary base (*Indian J Med Res*, 1966, **54**, 178; 1053). EtOH(50%) ext., diur. (*Indian J Exp Biol*, 1974, **12**, 512). Also antifert. activity; 60% inhibition of implantation and 80% of ovulation [*Indian J Med Res*, 1974, **62**, 1225; *Indian J Exp Biol*, 1976, **14**, 506; 1981, **19**, 1058; *Nagarjun*, 1977-78, **21**(4),

8; *J Karnatak Univ*, 1977, **12**, 167; *Probe*, 1977-78, **17**, 315; *J Res Indian Med*, 1979, **14**(1), 128].

Essent.oil from seeds, anthelm. against earthworm, comparable to piperazine citrate (*Indian J Hosp Pharm*, 1971, **8**, 150); antimicrob. [*Indian Drugs Pharmac Ind*, 1978, **13**(1), 39]; and antifert. (*Chung Ts'ao Yao*, 1981, **12**, 13; *CA*, **95**, 1032g).

Carrot, tertiary base with papavarine-like activity (*Indian J Physiol Pharmacol*, 1979, **23**, 225); and also toxin, *trans*-2-nonenal which killed carrot fly larvae (100% in 24hrs) (*Experientia*, 1980, **36**, 1387).

Toxicant, carotatoxin (*J Chem Soc D*, 1967, 439; *Tetrahedron*, 1967, **23**, 465). Toxicants anal., myristicin, 17.4 and falcarinol, 36.6ppm (*J Agric Food Chem*, 1978, **26**, 1390); myristicin, 12 related ethers, an acetylenic alc. and falcarinol (*J Chromatogr*, 1978, **161**, 271).

Carrot volat. components a survey (*Chem Ind Lond*, 1971, 1212); α-humulene, β-farnesene, α-bergamotene, γ-munrolene and γ-bisabolene; no β-bisabolene (*J Agric Food Chem*, 1978, **26**, 181); volat. constituents, detn. (*ibid*, 1980, **28**, 594).

Wild carrot, essent. oil constituents (*Rastit Resur*, 1965, *1*, 227; *CA*, **63**, 9737g; *Int Pharm Abstr*, 1966, **3**, 402e; *J Agric Food Chem*, 1968, **16**, 1009; 1975, **23**, 229; 1979, **27**, 1; 1980, **28**, 549).

β-Carotene (Hung. Teljes, 1971, 2461; *CA*, **75**, 132992h); *L*(+)- lactic acid, isolation (Ger. Offen, 1972, 2001874; *CA*, **77**, 4044e); iodine, 12.8±0.3μg/100g (*Vopr Pitan*, 1972, **31**, 77); pyruvate kinase (*Biochem Biophys Acta*, 1973, **329**, 128); steryl glucd. acyltransferase (*FEBS Lett*, 1975, **52**, 153); dauic acid from mature carrot (*J Chem Soc Perkin Trans I*, 1975, 2069); 7 flavons. from leaves (*Z Lebensm Unters Forsch*, 1977, **165**, 147; *CA*, 1978, **88**, 34565v); cholesterol detn. in carrots (*Egypt J Hortic*, 1978, **5**, 83; *CA*, 1979, **90**, 102159j); carrot, 5 aglycones, 4 glycds., and leaves, 2 glucds. (*Planta Med*, 1980,

40, 382); also alkane, *n*-hexacosanol, cholesterol, β- sitosterol & stigmasterol (*J Indian Chem Soc*, 1980, **57**, 1044); ulcer-preventing vit.U (*Gig Sanit*, 1981, 85).

Seeds, *n*-alkanes, β-sitosterol, glucose, and amino acids (*Indian J Chem*, 1975, **13**, 639); lipid glycerides and higher hydrocarbons (*Phytochemistry*, 1975, **14**, 2726).

Essent. oil from seeds, constituents (*J Sci Food Agric*, 1968, **19**, 383); and also from seeds of red, black, yellow and wild carrots from Pakistan (*Pak J Sci Ind Res*, 1977, **20**, 103; 1979, **22**, 258).

Lycopersene (*C R Acad Sci*, 1965, **260**, 1013); and also ferulic, caffeic and chlorogenic acids (*Z Lebensm Unters Forsch*, 1966, **132**, 193; *CA*, 1967, **66**, 45594a); mutalochrome and flavochrome; an enzyme (*Phytochemistry*, 1967, **6**, 1037; 109); a phosphodiesterase (*Biochemistry*, 1967, **6**, 3689); and bergapten (*Bergyogy Venerol Sz*, 1969, **45**, 118; *CA*, 1969, **71**, 110986z).

Lipoxygenase content and antioxidant activity (*J Food Sci*, 1971, **36**, 571); coumarins in roots, leaves and stalk (*Tr Bot Inst Akad Nauk SSSR*, 1971, **17**, 136; *CA*, 1973, **78**, 26472r);linuron extn. (*Pr Inst Przem Org*, 1971, 245; *CA*, 1973, **79**, 14285q).

Potentially useful biotransformation reactions in plant cell cultures of *D. carota* (cardiac glycd.-free) when digitoxigenin was supplied (*Lloydia*, 1978, **41**, 476).

D. visnaga Linn.; see **Ammi visnaga**

DAVALLIA (*Davalliaceae*)

See **SPHENOMERIS**

DECALEPIS (*Asclepiadaceae*)

D. hamiltonii Wight & Arn.

Roots—used as substitute of Ayurvedic drug, *Sariva* (*Hemidesmus indicus*). Pharmacognacy (*Indian J Pharm*, 1977, **39**, 167); identified as source of Ayurvedic drug '*Shweta Sariva*' [*J Res Indian Med*, 1978, **13**(4), 75].

DECASCHISTIA (*Malvaceae*)

*****D. crotonifolia** Wight & Arn.

EtOH(50%) ext. of plant, hypoglyc. and diur. (*Indian J Exp Biol*, 1977, **15**, 208).

Yellow flowers contain gossypitrin, quercimeritrin and gossypin (*J Indian Chem Soc*, 1981, **58**, 101).

Peninsular India and Upper Gangetic Plain.

DECASPERMUM (*Myrtaceae*)

*****D. fruticosum** Forst. syn. *D. paniculatum* Kurz

Ass.–*Diengauro-la-pyrno*, *dieng-la-phynia*.

Berries, as a remedy for stomach pains. Leaves and terminal shoots, astrin. Former chewed with betel in dysen. (Wlth India, III, 24).

Occurs in Sikkim, and Khasi hills.

DEERINGIA (*Amaranthaceae*)

D. amaranthoides Merrill syn. *D. celosioides* R. Br.

Leaves, anticancer against inflam. tumours (*Lloydia*, 1967, **30**, 379). EtOH(50%) ext. of aerial parts, diur.; and spermic. in rats but not against human spermatozoa (*Indian J Exp Biol*, 1974, **12**, 512; 1977, **15**, 231).

DELONIX (*Caesalpiniaceae*)

D. elata Gamble syn. *Poinciana elata* Linn.

EtOH(50%) ext. of plant excluding roots, spasmog. (*Indian J Exp Biol*, 1969, **7**, 250).

Trunk bark contains *d*-asparagine and aspartic acid; sucrose, β-amyrin, β-sitosterol & its glucd. (*Curr Sci*, 1966, **35**, 437; 1969, **38**, 460); bark, γ-methylene glutamine as major amino acid (*Indian J Pharm*, 1968, **30**, 212).

Seeds, uncommon amino acids (*Phytochemistry*, 1978, **17**, 1127).

*D. regia Rafin. syn. *Poinciana regia* Boj. ex Hook.

Bark—aq. ext., emetic and CNS depress.; EtOH ext. yields erythritol and a long chain hexahydroxy alc. (*Herba Pol*, 1972, **18**,160; *CA*, 1973, **78**, 13768s). Ext. inhibits potato virus X (*Technology Sindri*, 1972, **9**, 415). Alc. ext., molluscacidal (20% mortality) (*Planta Med*, 1980, **39**, 57).

Flowers—aq. and alc. ext. active against roundworm (*Haemonchus contortas*) (*Indian J Pharm*, 1971, **33**, 74).

Bark,leucocyanidin (*Curr Sci*, 1966, **35**, 437); bark, as also leaves, tannin (*Qual Plant Mater Veg*, 1967, **14**, 28; 1971, **20**, 285); lupeol and β-sitosterol (*J Indian Chem Soc*, 1968, **45**, 464); and free OH-proline as major amino acid (*Indian J Pharm*, 1968, **30**, 212).

Flower anthers rich source of zeaxanthin (*Biochem J*, 1966, **101**, 250). Chem. compn. of yellow and red flowers (*Curr Sci*, 1967, **36**, 376). Hentriacontane, hentriacontanol, quercetin, protocatechuic acid, β-sitosterol & its glucd. (*Indian J Pharm*, 1971, **33**, 74). Buds and floral parts, compn.; flowers, glycds. of cyanidin, quercetin and naringenin (*Phytochemistry*, 1975, **14**, 1915;1976, **15**, 835).

Seeds, saponin, (*Sci Cult*,1971,**37**, 351); galactomannan; and uncommon amino acids (*Phytochemistry*, 1972, **11**, 1129; 1978, **17**, 1127).

Planted as avenue tree in gardens and also on roadsides throughout India.

DELPHINIUM (*Ranunculaceae*)

Alks. (*in* Manske & Holmes, IV, 275; *in* Manske, VII, 473-504; XII, 2-135; 136-206).

D. ajacis Linn.; see **Consolida ambigua**

D. cashmerianum Royle

Alk., (all *d*-forms) cashmiradelphine, anthranoyllycoctonine, lycaconitine, avadhridine, lappaconitine & its N-de-OAc deriv. from plant; arrhythmogenic and heart rate effect of alks. in isolated guinea-pig atria (*J Natl Prod*, 1979, **42**, 615).

D. consolida Linn.; see **Consolida regalis**

D. denudatum Wall. ex Hook. f. & Thoms. syn. *D. pauciflorum* Royle

Aq. ext. of roots had a protective effect against hepatocellular damage in rats (*Indian J Pharm Sci*, 1981, **43**, 120).

Root alks. (*Tetrahedron Lett*, 1966, 4217); β-sitosterol & its glycd., an unsaturated hydrocarbon and an alc. (*Pak J Sci Ind Res*, 1965, **8**, 173); alks. condelphine and isotalatizidine (*J Am Chem Soc*, 1967, **89**, 4146); str. of alk. denudatine; and X-ray crystallogr. of delnudine (*Tetrahedron Lett*, 1969, 4369; 5245); standardisation of drug., chem. anal.; EtOH(50%) ext., anticonvuls. (*Nagarjun*, 1979-80, **23**, 188; 208); stigmasterol, sitosterol, cholesterol Δ^5- avenasterol and plant, fatty acids (*Fette Seifen Anstrichm*, 1981, **83**, 323; *CA*, **95**, 129413c).

Seeds contain delnuline (*Tetrahedron Lett*, 1969, 5335).

D. elatum Linn.

Seeds used in itch and other skin eruptions. Flowers, astrin. and used in eye troubles (Wlth India, III, 32).

Commercial extn. of alk., elatine (*Planta Med*, 1965, **13**, 200). Alk. mixt. from root, identn. of Me-lycaconine; and magnoflorine (*Diss Pharm Pharmacol*, 1967, **19**, 85; 81; *CA*, **67**, 41011f; 36360q). Eldeline and Me-cycaconitine, extn. from roots (*ibid*, 1968, **20**, 325; *CA*, 1969, **70**, 29152g).

D. vestitum Wall. ex Royle

Plant, cardiac and respiratory depress. (Wlth India, III, 31-32). In Tibet, roots used as chief ingredient in preparation of drugs for dysen. and diar. Root powd., to heal cattle wounds. Powd. flower mixed with mustard oil, to kill lice (*Nagarjun*, 1978-79, **22**, 190).

Alks., A & B; alk. A, on saponification converted to lycoctonine (*Pak J Sci Ind Res*, 1970, **13**, 51).

DENDROBIUM (*Orchidaceae*)

D. densiflorum Lindl. ex Wall. syn. *D. thyrsiflorum* Reichb. f.

A glycd. densifloroside (2-β-D-glucopyranosyloxy)- 4,5-di-OMe-*trans*-cinnamic acid & its *cis* isomer (*Acta Chem Scand Ser B*, 1975, **29**, 627).

*D. herbaceum Lindl.

Whole plant ext., antiprot. against *Entamoeba histolytica* strain (*Indian J Exp Biol*, 1980, **18**, 594).

Bihar and in Western Peninsula from Konkan to Coorg.

D. macraei Lindl.; see **Ephemerantha macraei**

*D. moschatum Wall.

Leaf juice used as ear drops for ear pain (*Econ Bot*, 1981, **35**, 4).

Khasi and Garo hills of Meghalaya.

D. ovatum (Willd.) Kranzl.

Leaves contain alks. (traces) [*J Res Indian Med*, 1974, **9**(1), 56].

DENDROCNIDE (*Urticaceae*)

D. sinuata (Blume) Chaw. syn. *Laportea crenulata* Gaud.

Plant hairs caused dermatitis with acute burning pain in body. Effect lasts several days, aggravated by water. Max. effect during flowering season causing violent sneezing, sleeplessness and fever. Roots and leaves applied to swellings and blind abscesses. Seed, also med. (Wlth India, VI, 34).

DENDROPHTHOE (*Loranthaceae*)

D. falcata (Linn.f.) Etting. syn. *Loranthus falcatus* Linn. f.; *L. longiflorus* Desr.

Plant—when growing as parasite on *Calotropis gigantea*, considered useful in increasing brain power and when growing on *Tamarindus indica*, valuable for treating impotency (*Econ Bot*, 1965, **19**, 236). EtOH(50%) ext. (plant without roots), hypoten. and antivir. (*Indian J Exp Biol*, 1969, **7**, 250; 1971, **9**, 91); diur. [*J Res Indian Med*, 1974, **9**(3), 33].

Leaves—aq. ext. produces rise in B.P. of anaesthetised cat, myocordial effect on frog heart, dose-related contraction in guineapig and contractile response on rat uterus (*Indian Drugs*, 1980-81, **18**, 183).

Young shoots contain 10% tannin (*Pak J For*, 1965, **15**, 250). Leaves, flavons. (*Lloydia*, 1975, **38**, 346); hexokinase activity (*Phytochemistry*, 1976, **15**, 1859).

Stems contain β-amyrin-OAc, oleanolic acid & its Me-ester acetate, β-sitosterol & stigmasterol (*Curr Sci*, 1977, **46**, 850).

D. pentandra (Linn.) Miq. syn. *Loranthus pentandrus* Linn.

Aq. ext. of leaves, toxic, hypoten., ether ext., papavarine-like spasmol. activity; leaves contain quercetrin (large amt.), hydrocarbons and fats (*Shoyakugaku Zasshi*, 1974, **28**, 7; *CA*, 1975, **83**, 90793b).

DERRIS (*Fabaceae*)

D. elliptica Benth.

Leaves contain 2 amino acids of pipecolic acid (*Phytochemistry*, 1976, **15**, 183); tubaic (0.01%) & β-tubaic (0.05%) acids, both antimicrob. (*Agric Biol Chem*, 1976, **40**, 1245); imino alc., 2,5-dihydroxy Me-3, 4-di-OH-pyrrolidine (*Phytochemistry*, 1976, **15**, 747).

Rotenoid—production by tissue culture (Jpn Kokai, 1977, 77108090; *CA*, 1978, **88**, 11904r); rotenone from this genus, carcinogenic (*Cancer Treat Rep*, 1976, **60**, 1171; *in* Plant and Fungal Toxins, 259). Rotenone insecticides vis-a-vis synthetic ones; may play important role because of low toxicity and rapid degradation to nontoxic substances (*in* Crosby & Jacobsen, 71-97).

Root, *d*- & *l*-maackiain (*Meijo Daigaku Nogakubu Gakujutsu Hokoku*, 1981, **17**, 40; *CA*, **95**, 200536c).

D. indica (Lamk) Bennet. syn. *Pongamia glabra* Vent.; *P. pinnata* (Linn.) Pierre H.–*Karanja*.

Differences in *Pongamia glabra* and *P. pinnata* (*Curr Sci*, 1964, **33**, 644).

Seed oil—stim. and antisep., destroys parasites; antibact. *in vitro* (*Indian J Med Res*, 1962, **50**, 218); useful in treatment of sarcoptic mange in goats (*Indian Vet J*, 1969, **46**, 622); used in leucoderma [*J Res Indian Med*, 1977, **12**(3), 76].

Seeds—powd. used as expect. in broncht. and whooping cough (*Bull Bot Soc Bengal*, 1975, **29**, 97). In Unani med., powd. considered as febge. and tonic in asthmatic and debilitating conditions, also used in broncht. and whooping cough; paste used in leprous sores, skin diseases and painful rheum. joints. Decoct. with decoct. of seeds of *Azadirachta indica*, *Terminalia belerica* and *Trichosanthes cucumerina* cures wounds when washed externally [*J Res Indian Med*, 1978, **13**(4), 92]. Seeds applied on eczema; juice of bark and root also used (*J Res Ayur Siddha*, 1981, **2**, 109).

Leaves—essent. oil, antifung. (*Indian Drugs*, 1977-78, **15**, 41); ext., antibact. (*Indian J Hosp Pharm*, 1978, **15**, 166); paste useful in paromychia (whitlow), clin trials (*Sachitra Ayurveda*, 1981-82, **34**, 295).

Plant—used in leprosy; roots as piscic. (*Econ Bot*, 1970, **24**, 241; 134). Uses and constituents, rev., 54 refs. (*J Sci Ind Res*, 1976, **35**, 608). Used in fractures (*Sri Lanka For*, 1980, **14**, 145).

Seed oil contains di-Me-chromenoflavanone, isolonchocarpin and de-MeO-kanugin; oil from immature seeds yields new OH- furanoflavone, pongol (*Indian J Chem*, 1973, **11**, 1097; 1979, **18B**, 525).

Seeds, new β-diketone, karanjin (bitter principle effective in skin diseases), pongapin, lanceolatin-B, kanjone and isoponga flavone (*Indian J Chem*, 1977, **15B**, 1138); seed shells, flavones and furanoflavones: pongamol, karanjin, de-OMe- kanugin, kanugin, pongapin, kanjone and pinnatin (*Curr Sci*, 1977, **46**, 743).

Leaves, furanoflavone, 3'-OMe-pongapin, karanjin, kanjone & its 2 isomers (*Indian J Chem*, 1976, **14B**, 229; 1977, **15B**, 536); 4'-MeO-furone- (2",3":7,8) flavone and known ones (*Planta Med*, 1979, **37**, 73).

Stem bark, chromenoflavone, pongachromene (*Tetrahedron*, 1969, **25**, 1063); tetra-OMe-fisetin(also in root bark) (*Indian J Chem*, 1969, **7**, 1275); glabrin (*Tetrahedron Lett*, 1971, 4451); glabra-I, glabra-II, karanjin, pongapin, and other known flavones (*Indian J Chem*, 1978, **16B**, 658). Stem bark compds. pongapin, kanugin & de-MeO-kanugin, toxicity and pharmacol. tests; last two compds., toxic [*East Pharm*, 1980. **23**(265), 113].

Heartwood, pongachalcone, glabrachromen, β- sitosterol, de-MeO-kanugin, kanugin, pongaglabrone and pongachromene (*Curr Sci*, 1973, **42**, 128); pongaflavone from stems (Indian Pat., 1976, 140321; *CA*, 1980, **92**, 91185c).

Flowers, new OH-furanoflavone, pongaglabol, aurantiamide-OAc, 4 known furano flavones and β-sitosterol (*Phytochemistry*, 1980, **19**, 1199).

*D. robusta Benth.

Seeds—alc. ext. showed significant, *in vitro*, activity against some human and plant pathogenic bacteria; compared with acromycin and streptomycin, other exts. showed varying degree of activity (*Indian Drugs*. 1979-80, **17**, 41); antifung, against keratiophilic fungi and related dermatophytes (*Bull Bot Soc Univ Sagar*, 1980, **27**, 24).

Seed shell contains chalcone rubone; isoflavone derrugenin; rubustigenin; its 5-Me ether; derrusnin, Me ethers of robustone and robustin, alpinum, isoflavone di-Me-ether, β-sitosterol & its glucd. (*Phytochemistry*, 1979, **18**, 2056; 1583; 1082; *Indian J Chem*, 1979, **17B**, 649; 471); 5-OH-7- OMe-isoflavone (*Planta Med*, 1979, **36**, 379); derrone; its Me-ether (*Phytochemistry*, 1980, **19**, 1857; *Curr Sci*, 1981, **50**, 818).

Roots, 4 isoflavones, derrustone, derrubone, robustone & its Me ether, and 5 coumarins, derrusnin, robustic acid & their Me esters (*J Chem Soc C*, 1969, 365).

In Himalayas from Kumaun eastwards, Assam and Western Peninsula.

D. scandens (Roxb.) Benth.

EtOH(50%) ext. of aerial parts, antibact. and spasmog. (*Indian J Exp Biol*, 1977, **15**, 208). Lupeol, taraxerol, β-sitosterol and a saturated compd. (*J Indian Chem Soc*, 1971, **48**, 95).

Roots, scandenin and lonchocarpic acid; also osajin, scardenone and scandinone (*J Chem Soc C*, 1966, 192; 701); Indian roots, isoflavones warangalone (scandenone), chandalone, and coumarins, lonchocarpic acid, scandenin, and lonchocarpenin (*ibid*, 1969, 374). New oxygen heterocyclics of *D. scandens* and *Mundulea suberosa*, rev., 34 refs. (*J Indian Chem Soc*, 1974, **51**, 83).

D. trifoliata Lour. syn. *D. uliginosa* Benth.

Plant, stim., antisp. and counter-irrit. An oil preparation used as an embrocation (Wlth India, III, 39). In Samoa, leaves used to treat indign. (*Econ Bot*, 1974, **28**, 1).

Roots, dehydrorotenone, lupeol and a ketone (*Indian J Chem*, 1976, **14B**, 1012).

DESCURAINIA (*Brassicaceae*)

D. sophia (Linn.). Webb ex Prantl syn. *Sisymbrium sophia* Linn.

Seeds, cardiotonic and diur. (*in* Beal & Reinhard, 371).

Plant, as mosquito repellent in Ladakh (*Bull Med Ethno Bot Res*, 1980, **1**, 301).

Seeds yield mustard oil (0.025%) with isothiocyanates of benzyl, 60; allyl, 7.5; and propenyl, 5%; and also allyl disulphide, 2.5% (*Perfum Essent Oil Rec*, 1967, **58**, 782); cardiac glycds. strophanthidin, evomonoside, helveticoside, evobioside and erysimoside (*Yao Hsueh Hsueh Pao*, 1981, **16**, 62).

Plant, isorhamnetin, helioscopiol and β-sitosterol (*Pak J Sci Ind Res*, 1970, **12**, 505). Stem, leaves, flowers and seed ext. gave +ve test for alk. (*Lloydia*, 1972, **35**, 10).

DESMODIUM (*Fabaceae*)

D. caudatum DC.; see **Catenaria caudata**

D. elegans DC. syn. *D. tiliaefolium* G. Don
EtOH(50%) ext. of plant excluding roots, spasmog. (*Indian J Exp Biol*, 1969, **7**, 250).

Plant, tyramine, hordenine, salsoline, salsolidine, tryptamine, abrine, hypaphorine, 4 quaternary β-Ph-Et amines, etc. and root, choline and betaine (*Phytochemistry*, 1973, **12**, 193).

Leaves, wax ester (major hexacosanyl eicosanoate) alcs., *n*-aliphatic and wax acids (*ibid*, 1972, **11**, 3546).

D. gangeticum DC. syn. *Hedysarum gangeticum* Linn.
Plant used for hazy vision and dysen. (*Econ Bot*, 1970, **24**, 241).

Aerial parts contain 5 tryptamine derivs., Nb-Me-tetrahydroharman and 6-OMe-2-Me-β-carbolinium cation. Root alk., N,N- di-Me tryptamine & its N-oxide, N-Me-tyramine, hypaphorine, hordenine, candicine, and a β-Ph-Et-amine base (*Aust J Chem*, 1969, **22**, 275, 2029). Total alks. from aerial parts show hypoten. and other pharmacol. activities; seeds contain β-carboline alk. [*Biochem Physiol Alkaloide Int Symp 4th*, 1969, (Pub. 1972), 107; *CA*, 1972, **77**, 118146v]; indole -3-alkylamine and carbolines; roots, several carboxylated and decarboxylated tryptamines and β-alkylamine derivs.; aerial alks., anticholinesterase activity, smooth muscle and CNS stim., and cardiac depress.; root alks., less active (*Planta Med*, 1972, **22**, 434).

Roots, a pterocarpan (*J Chem Soc C*, 1971, 2420); pterocarpanoids, gangetinin and desmodin (*Phytochemistry*, 1975, **14**, 1129); gangetin, method of isolation (Indian Pat., 1976, 140367; *CA*, 1980, **92**, 125293d).

D. heterocarpum DC. syn. *D. polycarpum* DC.; *Hedysarum purpureum* Roxb.
EtOH(50%) ext. of plant excluding roots, spasmog. (*Indian J Exp Biol*, 1974, **12**, 512).

*D. laxiflorum DC.

EtOH(50%) ext. of plant, antiinflam., diur. and spasmog. (*Indian J Exp Biol*, 1973, **11**, 43).

Found in Himalayas from Garhwal to Assam up to 1,300 m.

*D. motorium Merrill syn. *D. gyrans* DC.

Eng.–*Telegraph plant, semaphone plant*; H.–*Sarivan*; Tam.–*Pulladi*.

Roots—in Indian system of medicine, pounded and used in fever (*Nagarjun*, 1980-81, **24**, 1). Also used as emol., laxt., antidysen. and in cough and asthma (*Phytochemistry*, 1972, **11**, 1863).

Leaves—tonic, diur., febge. and aphrodis., applied to wounds; fruits for same use (*Bull RRL Jammu*, 1962-63, **1**, 126).

EtOH(50%) ext. of plant, weak hypoglyc. (*Indian J Exp Biol*, 1980, **18**, 594).

Root alk./bases (0.33%), N,N-di- Me-tryptamine, its Nb-oxide, choline, hypaphorine, and unidentified indole-3-alkylamines and β-Ph-Et-amines; leaves, alks./bases (0.036%), β-Ph-Et-amine, bufotenine, choline, etc. (*Phytochemistry*, 1972, **11**, 1863).

Assam hills and Peninsular India.

D. pulchellum (Linn.) Benth.

EtOH(50%) ext. of plant, hypoten. and spasmog. (*Indian J Exp Biol*, 1971, **9**, 91).

β-Carbolines, 15 indole-3-alkylamines, and several quaternary derivs. from individual plant parts; alks./bases pharmacol. active (*Planta Med*, 1972, **21**, 398).

Whole plant, alk. (0.3%), bufotenin & its Me ether (0.2-0.25%), N,N-di-Me-tryptamine & its oxide; 2 tryptamine derivs. and gramine (*Chem Ind Lond*, 1964, 1800; 1965, 793); 7 indole- 3- alkylamine bases of tryptophan (*J Org Chem*, 1966, **31**, 2284).

Seed galactomannan; 1-glucosyl rhamnoside of physcion (*Phytochemistry*, 1970, **9**, 1881; 1971, **10**, 1921).

Roots, betulin, α-amyrin and β-sitosterol (*Indian J Chem*, 1975, **13**, 869).

*D. triangulare Merrill var. **congestum** Santapau syn. *D. cephalotes* Wall. ex Wight & Arn.

Plant used in cataract, blindness, stomach pain and diar. (*Econ Bot*, 1970, **24**, 241). Preliminary pharmacol. (*Indian J Exp Biol*, 1973, **11**, 43).

Alks. (0.011%) of stem roots contain β-Ph-Et-amine, salsolidine, hordenine, tyramine, candicine, etc.; leaves, β-Ph-Et-amine (major), tyramine, salsolidine; curative properties probably due to alks. (*Phytochemistry*, 1974, **13**, 1628).

Eastern Himalayas up to 1,200 m.

D. triflorum DC. syn. *Hedysarum triflorum* Linn.

Plant used in blindness, eye diseases, sores, whitlow, spleen complaints, pain, stomach trouble, colic diar., menor., or flooding and breast pain (*Econ Bot*, 1970, **24**, 241). Roots for cough, asthma, and applied to wounds and abscesses (*Phytochemistry*, 1971, **10**, 3312). EtOH (50%) ext. of plant, diur., affects CNS in mice and potentiates barbiturate (*Indian J Exp Biol*, 1980, **18**, 594).

Leaf alks. (0.01-0.15%) β-Ph-amine (major), indole- 3-acetic acid, tyramine, trigonelline, hypaphorine, its Me ester and N,N-di- Me- tryptophan Me-ester; root alks. (0.01-0.02%) hypaphorine (major) and other leaf alks. Base HCl possesses nicotine-like activity (*Phytochemistry*, 1971, **10**, 3312). In addn., leaves contain S-*l*-stachydrine and root, 3,4- di-OH-Ph-Et-tri-Me ammonium cation; on drying alk./base content decreases. Chloroform-sol. root alks. show antisp., sympathomimetic, CNS stim. and curarimimetic effects (*Planta Med*, 1973, **23**, 321).

D. triquetrum (Linn.) DC.

EtOH(50%) ext. of plant (excluding roots), antivir. (*Indian J Exp Biol*, 1973, **11**, 43).

D. velutinum (Willd.) DC. syn. *D. lasiocarpum* DC.; *D. latifolium* DC.
EtOH(50%) ext. of plant (excluding roots), anticancer (*Indian J Exp Biol*, 1980, **18**, 594).

DESMOTRICHUM (*Orchidaceae*)

See **EPHEMERANTHA**

DIANELLA (*Liliaceae*)

*D. ensifolia DC.
Roots used in poultices and cosmetics. Ash of leaves and roots, as ingredient of an ointment for herpis (Wlth India, III, 52).
Tropical Himalayas up to 600-1,500 m and also in Khasi hills and Manipur.

DIANTHUS (*Caryophyllaceae*)

*D. barbatus Linn.
Eng.–*Sweet william.*
Aerial parts, saponins, barbatoside A & B; aglycone, quillaic acid; saponins, analg. and antiinflam.; astragalin, kaempferol-3-sophoroside, *d*-pinitol and *l*-leucine also isolated (*Lloydia*, 1977, **40**, 361).
Grown in Indian gardens.

D. caryophyllus Linn.
Juice of plant, potent· antivir. (*Indian J Microbiol*, 1979, **19**, 198).
Leaves contain glucoproteins, dianthin 30 & 32; dianthins mixed with tobacco mosaic virus strongly decreased the number of local lesions on leaves of *Nicotiana glutinosa* (*Biochem J*, 1981, **195**, 399).

DICENTRA (*Fumariaceae*)

*D. canadensis Walp.
Eng.–*Squirrel corn.*
Dried tubers, tonic and diur. Plant contains alk. bulbocapnine; alk. used for the relief of paralysis agitans and as pre-anaesthetic (Wlth India,III, 54); novel dimeric benzylisoquinoline alk., cancentrine; & its dehydro deriv.; their str. (*J Am Chem Soc*, 1970, **92**, 4998; *Can J Chem*, 1972, **50**, 853; 862).
Cultivated in Indian gardens.

*D. scandens Hook.f. & Thoms. non Walp. syn. *Dactylicapnos macrocapnos* Hutchins.
EtOH(50%) ext. of plant, spasmog. (*Indian J Exp Biol*, 1980, **18**, 594).
Plant contains alk. allocryptopine, protopine and β-, *l*- & *dl*-stylopine (Wlth India, III, 53); leaves and stems, β-stylopine and protopine (*Indian J Chem*, 1977, **15B**, 399).
From Kumaun Himalayas to Khasi hills.

DICHANTHIUM (*Poaceae*)

*D. annulatum Stapf var. **annulatum**
Grass, diur., used in kidney complaints (SEPASAT, 165).
Found throughout India.

*D. glabrum Jain & Deshpande syn. *Bothriochloa intermedia* (R.Br.) A. Camus; *Andropogon intermedius* R.Br.
Extn. of grass rich in sesquiterp. acorenone B, showed limited antitumour activity (*J Natl Prod*, 1980, **43**, 598).
Constitution of *neo*-intermediol obtained from essent. oil from plant (*Chem Ind Lond*, 1964, 194); configuration of acorenone B (*J Chem Soc Chem Commun*, 1968, 1135). Leaf oil constants [*Indian Perfum*, 1967, **11**(Pt.I), 53].
Occurs throughout India.

*D. pertusum Clyton syn. *Bothriochloa pertusa* A. Camus; *Andropogon pertusus* Willd.
Plant—used against tumour (*Lloydia*, 1970, **33**, 288). EtOH(50%) ext., diur. (*Indian J Exp Biol*, 1977, **15**, 208). Grass, weak estrogenic (*Indian Vet J*, 1974, **51**, 610).
Essent. oil., antimicrob. activity (*Acta Ciencia Indica*, 1978, **4**, 248; *Indian Drugs*, 1978-79, **16**, 122).
Cultivated in Indian gardens.

DICHROA (*Saxifragaceae*)

D. febrifuga Lour.
Febrifugine & isofebrifugine—febrifugine, dichrone B, β-dichroine and γ-dichroine are one and the same alk.;

isofebrifugine is its cyclic hemiketal tautomer (Dictionary Org. Compds., III, 2604); former, antimal.; 50 times as active as quinine in rats (*Yao Hsueh Hsueh Pao*, 1964, **11**, 437; *CA*, 1965, **62**, 946b); colorim. estn. (*Hua Hsueh Hsueh Pao*, 1965, **31**, 482; *CA*, **64**, 14028 e). Total alks. (including others) during Sept.- Oct.; in roots, 0.02-0.05%; in leaves, 0.5-0.7% with febrifugine, 0.15-0.19%; & isofebrifugine, 0.1% (*Tr Vses Nauchno Issled Inst Lek Aromat Rast*, 1969, **15**, 356; *CA*, 1971, **75**, 20733t). Both alks. have high antimoth activity but very toxic (*Lekarstv Rast*, 1969, 356; *CA*, 1972, **76**, 32240p); see also antimalarials (*in* Manske & Holmes, V, 156-57). α- Dichroine, 98-152 times as strong as quinine-HCl (*in* Beal & Reinhard, 358).

DICHROCEPHALA (*Asteraceae*)

*D. integrifolia Kuntze syn. *D. latifolia* DC.

Herb, as diur. (Santapau & Henry, 54).

Himalayas, Khasi hills and Western Ghats.

DICHROSTACHYS (*Mimosaceae*)

D. cinerea Wight & Arn.; see **Cailliea cinerea**

DICOMA (*Asteraceae*)

D. tomentosa Cass.

Herb, as tooth cleaners (SEPASAT, 116).

DICRANOPTERIS (*Gleicheniaceae*)

D. linearis (Burm.f.) Underwood syn. *Gleichenia dicotoma* Willd.; *G. linearis* Bedd.

Young fronds—ground with cow's milk, used for 7 days continuously to remove sterility in women (*J Sci Res BHU*, 1969- 70, **20**, 227); used as poultice and decoct.; useful in fever.

Plant—reported to be antiasthmatic and anthelm. (*Indian Drugs*, 1976-77, **14**, 136);

anticancer activity (*Annu Rep CDRI Lucknow*, 1970, 73).

Plant, β-sitosterol (*Indian J Appl Chem*, 1969, **32**, 401). Roots and rhizomes gave +ve test for flavon. (*Lloydia*, 1972, **35**, 288).

DICTAMNUS (*Rutaceae*)

D. albus Linn. syn. *D. hispanicus* Web.

Roots, a lactone mixt., 0.30% and alk. dictamnine, 0.1% (*Tr Nauchnoizsled Inst Farm*, 1961, **3**, 86; *CA*, 1964, **61**, 8130a); a lactone, fraxinellone (*Monatsch Chem*, 1965, **96**, 1324); alk., γ-fagarine (*Pharmazie*, 1966, **21**, 77; *CA*, 1967, **66**,108194t); preskimmianine, a biogenetic precursor of skimmianine (*Tetrahedron Lett*, 1972, 2199); alks., isodictamnine and isomaculosidine (*Herba Hung*, 1973, **10**, 123; *CA*, **79**, 2768m), and also isopteleine and β-sitosterol (*Khim Prir Soedin*, 1978, 472; *CA*, **89**, 176371y).

Leaves and inflorescence contain a rutinoside (0.1% in leaves), diosmin and isoquercitrin (*Diss Pharm*, 1964, **16**, 177; *Int Pharm Abstr*, 1965, **2**, 752a).

Plant, coumarins, bergapten (*Experientia*, 1964, **20**, 615); aurapten (*Planta Med*, 1967, **15**, 320); and psoralen and xanthotoxin (*Pharmazie*, 1968, **23**, 76; *CA*, **68**, 112185z).

DIDYMOCARPUS (*Gesneriaceae*)

D. pedicellatus R. Br.

Plant—lithotriptic (*Q J Crude Drug Res*, 1972, **12**, 1881). Drug 'Cystone' containing 65 mg plant/223 mg of drug for urolithisis; very effective for urinary tract infection (*Probe*, 1979-80, **19**, 270).

Essent. oil from plant, weak antimicrob. [*J Res Indian Med*, 1978, **13**(4), 111]; contains 70% humulene (*Indian Perfum*, 1978, **22**, 16).

Plant, didymocarpin A (*Chem Ind Lond*, 1979, 348). Didymoflavonone, 2'-OH-4',5',6'- tri-OMe chalcone, both new compds. and a tetra-OMe flavanone (*Planta Med*, 1981, **43**, 86).

Leaves, pedicinin, pedicin, pedicellin, methylated quinones, pedicellic and stearic acids (*J Indian Chem Soc*, 1965, **42**, 343); pashanone and Me-pedicin (*Indian J Chem*, 1973, **11**, 404); a new flavone, didymocarpin (*Phytochemistry*, 1978, **17**, 587; *Indian J Chem*, 1978, **17B**, 176; 394); isodidymocarpin (*J Indian Chem Soc*, 1978, **55**, 1198); 2 new flavones and a known one (*Phytochemistry*, 1981, **20**, 1755). Study of antifung. and antibact, properties of leaf chalcones and flavanones (*Experientia*, 1981, **37**, 393).

Roots yield pedicin, pedicellin, pashanone and β- sitosterol (*Indian J Chem*, 1973, **11**, 9).

DIEFFENBACHIA (*Araceae*)

D. seguine (Linn.) Schott

Plant—juice used against cancer, warts and corns, in Cuba (*Lloydia*,1967, **30**, 379); as oral contracep. (*Planta Med*, 1973, **23**, 167). Juice, highly poisonous; stem when chewed, renders the person speechless (Santapau & Henry, 55). Extremely caustic causing severe burning of skin and mucous membranes.

Leaves—withered by heat used by Caribs of West Indies to wrap around dropsical, scarred or varicose legs to draw out the water, and to treat yaws, or use an ointment made by boiling juice in hog's lard. Decoct. used in gargling for angina and in lotions for inflam. oedemas. In Cuba, juice, aphrodis. (*Econ Bot*, 1969, **23**, 106).

Infusion of cane used in dysmen., and cane used to poison rats and cockroaches. A tincture of root juice used as lotion to cure genital prurigo. Toxicity due to a proteolytic enzyme (*Econ Bot*, 1969, **23**, 106; 1972, **26**, 364).

DIGERA (*Amaranthaceae*)

D. alternifolia Asch. syn. *D. muricata* Mart.; *D. arvensis* Forsk.

Flowers and seeds useful in urinary discharges; plant laxt. in high doses [*J Res Indian Med*, 1973, **8**(2), 81]; EtOH(50%) ext. of plant, diur. (*Indian J Exp Biol*, 1980, **18**, 594).

Plant, α- & β-spinasterol (*Plant Biochem J*, 1977, **4**, 14).

DIGITALIS (*Scrophulariaceae*)

D. lanata Ehrh.

Eng.–*Woolly foxglove.*

Tinctures lost 16% activity in one year (*Acta Pol Pharm*, 1961, **18**, 423;*CA*, 1964, **60**, 15684d); study of phytochem. at different growth stages and pharmacol. of ext. (*Boll Chim Pharm*, 1963, **102**, 801; *CA*, 1964, **60**, 12367d); semipurified ext. of tissue culture evoked pronounced vasodilation and bradycardia in animals resulting in their death (*J Pharm Pharmacol*, 1967, **19**, 760); estrogen-like activity of ext. in mature female rats; ext. accelerates sexual maturation and no. of ovarium follicles in sexually immature female rats (*Dokl Bolg Akad Nauk*, 1980, **33**, 1565; 1981, **34**, 145; *CA*, 1981, **94**, 16793x; **95**, 1036q).

Cardenolide distribution in various parts (*Farm Glas*, 1963, **19**, 353; *CA*, 1965, **63**, 3309h); all plant parts contain cardenolides; glycd. content unaffected by climatic conditions (*Planta Med*, 1981, **41**, 161; 1966, **14**, 302). Plant, in vegetative state had more glycd. content than in generative state; 1st-year leaf tissue much richer than 2nd-year leaf (*Rec Med Tirgu-Mures*, 1967, **13**, 79; *CA*, **67**, 84795g); variation in compn. during first vegetation period (*Dtsch Apoth Ztg*, 1978, 794; *CA*, **89**, 204065x).

Leaves yield 5 primary glycds. (with terminal glucose intact; in extn. glucose gets hydrolysed) digilanidobiosides of digitoxigenin, gitoxigenin, etc. (*Ann Chem*, 1964, 137; *CA*, 1965, **63**, 10054g); from fermented leaves, cardenolide pattern, digitoxigenin allomethyloside among others (*Experientia*, 1965, **21**, 575); digoxin, digoxoside, neodigoxoside and digitoxose (Ac-γ-digoxin); digoxoside on hydrolysis gave digoxin, digoxoside-mono- & bisdigitoxoside and digoxigenin;

digitoxigenin- β- glucd. (*Naturwissenschaften*, 1963, **50**, 668; 1965, **52**, 108). 2 bisdesmosidic 22-OH-furostanol, lanatigoside and lanagitoside; purpureagitoside (*Chem Ber*, 1972, **105**, 3397; 1974, **107**, 2828).

Cardiac glycds.—digitalis and allied cardiac glycds., pharmacol. basis to therapeutics (*in* Goodman & Gilman, 665-98). Preliminary pharmacol. of mixt. used to prepare 'Carlanoid', results compared with lanatoside (*Farmatsiya Sof*, 1967, **17**, 49; *CA*, 1968, **68**, 1869f). Cardiac glycds. (*in* Miller, I, 351-75); extn., improved method from *D. lanata* and *D. purpurea* leaves (East Ger Pat., 1965, 41820; 1974, 106369; *CA*, 1966, **64**, 14036a; 1975, **82**, 70392w); with water and centrifugation, recovery from *D. lanata*, 96.36%; from *D. purpurea*, 98.91% (*Herba Pol*, 1978, **24**, 27); detn. (*Farmatsiya Sof*, 1970, **20**, 41; *CA*, **73**, 112893f); flourim. (*Planta Med*, 1972, **21**, 5); quick method for anal. (*Herba Pol*, 1971, **71**, 68; *CA*, 1972, **76**, 1527h); detn. by chromatogr.-colorim. (*Tr Nauchnoizsled Khim Farm Inst*, 1972, 7; 211; *CA*, 1973, **78**, 15165c); sepn. (Rom. Pat., 1974, 57006; 56948; *CA*, 1975, **82**, 121990z- 91a). Use of 2-dimensional TLC for extn. (*J Chromatogr*, 1979, **168**, 541); occurrence, chem. and recovery, rev., 10 refs. (*Pharmazie*, 1979, **34**, 477; *CA*, 1980, **92**, 99478w); extn., 15 kg leaves, 15g glycds. (Rom. Pat., 1978, 65413; *CA*, 1980, **92**, 28558n); extn. from fermented leaves with dil. alc. and water (*Hem Ind*, 1981, **35**, 128; *CA*, **95**, 67845j); glycd. content of leaves from Tamil Nadu, max. in June (0.35%) and min. in Dec.-Jan. (0.29%) (*J Agric Sci*, 1981, **96**, 255).

Digoxin & digitoxin—used in med. Cardiac glycds. of digoxigenin and digitoxigenin; those of former restricted to genus *Digitalis* and mainly occur in *D. lanata* (*in* Miller, I, 360). TLC detn. of *D. lanata* and *D. purpurea* glycds.; recovery of digitoxin, digoxin and lanatoside A, B & C, 94.9-97.8% (*Yau Hsueh Hsueh Pao*, 1966, **13**, 273; *CA*, **65**, 4267b); digoxin and Ac-digitoxin; sepn. of digoxin, gitoxin, digitoxin (Hung. Pat., 1962, 149778; 1972, 4706; *CA*, 1964, **60**, 7878b; 1973, **78**, 30163h). Digitoxin and gitoxin, spectrophotom. detn. (*Khim Farm Zh*, 1971, **5**, 51; *CA*, 1972, **76**, 27966a). Biosynth. of digoxigenin glycds. in fresh leaves, increase in yield of digoxin 30% and lanatoside C 25% (Czech Pat., 1974, 154113; *CA*, 1975, **82**, 54445k); extn. by alkaline hydrolysis (Rom. Pat., 1978, 63683; *CA*, 1980, **92**, 64741a).

Acute toxicity to cats (i.v.) LD_{50}(mg/kg) of digitoxin, 0.43; of digitoxigenin, 0.58 (*Arzneim Forsch*, 1978, **28**, 1365); TLC Rfs in given solvent systems for digitoxin & its genin. Prototype and mostly widely used glycd. digoxin (36 h biol. half- life); extracted from leaves of *D.lanata* and *D. purpurea*; digitoxin is obtained from the latter sp., less used because of prolonged action time (5 to 7 days biol. half- life) and more toxic side effects; toxic dose close to therapeutic dose. Digoxin holds its own as 3 million cardiac sufferers in US routinely use it, a tremendous mendate for success of herbal med. (*in* Plant and Fungal Toxins, 69-70; 787-88).

Digoxin due to superior pharmacokinetic properties, most in demand, whereas digitoxin is generally regarded highly toxic by- product of isolation procedure; basic goal of biotransformation here is to convert digitoxin into digoxin by 12 β-hydroxylation. Since digoxin-rich plant in cell culture showed strain heterogeneity in cell products and for exclusive 12 β-hydroxylation, strain selection is absolutely necessary in development of biotechnol. processes; a process for commercial application discussed (*in* Beal & Reinhard, 489- 99); radioimmunoassay to select strain with high digoxin content; digoxin sepn.; effect of growth regulators and age on leaf and root culture, older the culture greater the glycd. yield, gibberellic acid or mofluidide increases yield (*Planta Med*, 1979, **35**, 316; 1980, **40**, 320; 1981, **41**, 90; **42**, 250).

Lanatosides—detn. of lanatoside C (*Farmatsiya Sof*, 1964, **14**, 12; *CA*, 1967, **66**, 49273t); max., when leaves dried at 40° (*Herba Pol*, 1966, **12**, 178; *CA*, 1967, **67**, 847788g). Extn. (USSR Pat., 1967, 205228; *CA*, 1968, **69**, 5205e; *Acta Pharm Jugosl*, 1972, **22**, 145; *CA*, 1973, **78**, 75814n); content increases on keeping leaf at ≤60° in wet air for 1 - 30 days (Hung Teljes, 1971, 3118; *CA*, 1972, **76**, 117503b); of A & C when leaves kept at relative humidity of 45- 55%; rapid quant. detn. for A & C, digitoxin & its genin (*Planta Med*, 1971, **20**, 253; 1976, **29**, 393); chromatogr. sepn. from pure concentrations and crude ext. of plant (Czech. Pat, 1971, 142413; *CA*, 1972, **77**, 52312m).

Ac-digoxin & Ac-digitoxin—sepn. of Ac-digitoxin from glycd. mixt.; recovery alongwith Ac-gitoxin after lanatoside sepn. by counter current method (Pol. Pat., 1966, 51184; 1968, 54579; *CA*, 1967, **67**, 14834v; **69**, 109821n); sepn. (*J Pharm Sci*, 1972, **61**, 1320; Rom. Pat., 1974, 57799; *CA*, 1976, **85**, 17399q); manufacture by partial hydrolysis of lanatoside A & C (Ger.Offen., 1975, 2344710; *CA*, **83**, 55796h); preparative method (Brit. Pat., 1976, 1429690; *CA*, **85**, 51736g).

Content of glycd. in seeds and cotyledons; cotyledons contain no lanatoside C (*Sci Pharm*, 1972, **40**, 242; *CA*, 1973, **78**, 94870u).

Flavons. (*C R Acad Sci Ser D*, 1969, **269**, 1675; *Planta Med*, 1977, **32**, 24; 1978, **34**, 225; 443); in leaves and flowers w.r.t. growth of plant (*Sci Pharm*, 1979, **47**, 173; *CA*, 1980, **92**, 37854g). Anthraquinones from callus culture (*Phytochemistry*, 1972, **11**, 1073).

D. purpurea Linn.

Leaves—stability of liq. ext. 'Corditon' and 'Digipan' decreased by 10% in 3 months at 20° (*Herba Pol*, 1966, **12**, 243; *CA*, 1967, **67**, 93945h); method of production of 'Kordigit' (USSR Pat., 1973, 366862; *CA*, **78**, 164081p).

Cardenolides and spirostanol in 1st- and 2nd-year plants at various development stages: digitoxigenin main cardenolide and gitogenin main spirostanol (*Phytochemistry*, 1972, **11**, 2971).

Leaves, saponins, degalactotigonin, F-gitonin, and cardiac glycds. (*Chem Pharm Bull*, 1964, **12**, 1311; *CA*, 1965, **62**, 9391g); F-gitonin, str. (*Tetrahedron*, 1965, **21**, 299).

Cardiac glycds. — extn. of secondary glycd. with water (*Arch Farm*, 1972, **22**, 201; *CA*, 1973, **79**, 149304r); extn., sepn., and quant. detn. by fluorim. (*Planta Med*, 1973, **23**, 176). Glycds. of Dutch and cultivated English strains of *D. purpurea* and *D. lanata* leaves [*J Pharm Pharmacol*, 1973, **25** (Suppl.),145]; fluorim. detn.; also micro method (*Planta Med*, 1974, **25**, 267; 350).

Digitoxin & digoxin—preparation of digitoxin from *D. purpurea* leaves after gitalin sepn.; extn. and purification; sepn. and isolation of pure digitoxin (*Acta Pol Pharm*, 1964, **21**, 257; *Herba Pol*, 1965, **11**, 201; 1966, **12**, 260; *CA*, 1965, **63**, 432b; 1967, **66**, 79523s; **67**, 111376e); production of digitoxin by aq. autofermentation of leaves; of digoxin, 10kg of leaves on autofermentation yield 7.5g digoxin (*Khim Pharm Zh*, 1972, **6**, 31; 1973, **7**, 33; *CA*, 1973, **78**, 33852t; 1974, **80**, 19462a); extn. of both, high yield (*Hem Ind*, 1977, **31**, 683; *CA*, 1978, **88**, 177079a); extn. of both, as also gitoxin and diginatin (East Ger Pat., 1979, 134644; **91**, 96620e); digitoxin extn. by enzymic hydrolysis (USSR Pat., 1981, 833251; *CA*, **95**, 138616y); see also *D. lanata*.

Seeds, saponin mixt. of deglucodigitonin, digalonin, deglucotigonin and gitonin (*Chem Pharm Bull*, 1964, **12**, 1250; *CA*, 1965, **62**, 2818f).

Digitonin—extn. from seed; extn.; improved method (East Ger. Pat., 1964, 32625; Ger. Offen, 1973, 2141410; Brit. Pat., 1973, 1317838; *CA*, 1965, **63**, 5457c; **78**, 133640r; **79**, 57663d); max. yield during milky ripeness of seeds. 4.3-9.1%; 14.52-17.84 kg/ha when seeds harvested at waxy ripening stage; quant. detn., 3.67%;

(*Herba Pol*, 1980, **26**, 111; 1975, **21**, 377; *CA*, 1976, **86**, 68337a).

Seed and seedlings, sterol mixt., cholesterol and usual sterols, plant grown in dark contain more sterol; in 25-days-old seedlings, β-sitosterol (major); in older plant, stigmasterol (major) (*Arch Biochem Biophys*, 1968, **127**, 655); sterols, spectrophotom. detn. in leaves and seeds (*Planta Med*, 1971, **19**, 249); distribution in plant; seed oil, Me-sterols; herb steryl esters (*J Pharm Pharmacol*, 1971, **23**, Suppl., 232 S; 1972, **24**, 227; 1973, **25**, 156).

Flower polyphenols (*Ann Pharm Fr*, 1966, **24**, 245; *CA*, **65**, 18986g). Leaf flavons. (*J Chem Soc C*, 1971, 2007; *Planta Med*, 1977, **32**, 347); anthraquinones, etc.; growing tips, cyclohexanone (*Phytochemistry*, 1968, **7**, 1423; 1973, **12**, 2287).

DILLENIA (*Dilleniaceae*)

D. indica Linn.

H.–*Aggai*.

Plant used in chest trouble, sores of Hg poisoning, sores and carbuncle, and cholera (*Econ Bot*, 1970, **24**, 241). EtOH(50%) ext. of leaves, antiamphetamine activity (*Indian J Exp Biol*, 1969,**7**, 250).

Seed ext., antimicrob. (*Chem Petrochem J*, 1979, **10**, 21); fatty oil (23%), active antifung. agent and its unsap. matter,antibact. [*J Sci Food Agric*, 1972, **23**, 53; *Indian Drugs Pharmac Ind*, 1980, **15**(3), 35].

Leaves, cycloartenone, *n*-hentriacontanol, betulinic acid and β-sitosterol (*J Indian Chem Soc*, 1981, **58**, 97); flavone content in leaves (*Phytochemistry*, 1971, **10**, 1055).

Flavons. distribution in bark, timber, fruit and pericarp (*ibid*, 1975, **14**, 1127); betulinic acid content, in bark 1.3; timber 0.25; and pericarp 1.9% (*ibid*, 1974, **13**, 2002). Fruits, an arabinogalactan (2%) (*Indian J Chem*, 1978, **16B**, 662); β-sitosterol in wood, betulin in fruit, betulinic acid in

both; their contents alongwith lupeol content in Indian spp. (*J Indian Chem Soc*, 1976, **53**, 638; 1980, **57**, 760).

Stem bark, betulinaldehyde, betulin, lupeol, β- sitosterol, myricetin, and a new hydroxylactone (*Phytochemistry*, 1975, **14**, 1447); also dihydroisorhamnetin and dillentin (*J Chem Soc Perkin Trans I*, 1975, 612); glucds. (*Planta Med*, 1979, **35**, 188).

*D. pentagyna Roxb.

Plant used in T.B. fistula, sores, carbuncle, neuralgia, pleur. and pneum. (*Econ Bot*, 1970, **24**, 241). Roots, preliminary pharmacol. (*Indian J Exp Biol*, 1971, **9**, 91).

Stem,α - L - rhamnopyranosyl - 3 - OH-lup-20(29)-en-28-oic acid (*Phytochemistry*, 1980, **19**, 980); and a flavonone glycd. (*Chem Scr*, 1979, **13**, 191); bark, lupeol, betulin, betulinic and morolic acids (*J Indian Chem Soc*, 1981, **58**, 817).

Found in subtropical Himalayas.

*D. scabrella Roxb.

Used for sores (*Econ Bot*, 1970, **24**, 241).

Occurs in Assam, and Khasi hills, up to 1,000 m.

DIMERIA (*Poaceae*)

*D. gracilis Nees ex Steud.

EtOH(50%) ext., diur. (*Indian J Exp Biol*, 1974, **12**, 512); spermic., *in vitro*, in rat and human spermatozoa (*ibid*, 1977, **15**, 231).

Found in Tamil Nadu and Karnataka.

DIMOCARPUS (*Sapindaceae*)

D. longan Lamk syn. *Euphoria longan* Steud.; *E. longan* Lamk; *Nephelium longan* Camb.

EtOH(50%) ext. of aerial parts, preliminary pharmacol. (*Indian J Exp Biol*, 1973, **11**, 43).

DIOCLEA (*Fabaceae*)

*D. javanica Benth. syn. *D. reflexa* Hook.f.

Seeds to kill lice. In Africa, seeds alongwith those of *Aframomum* spp., used as tonic and stim. (Wlth India, III, 67).

W. Bengal and Assam.

DIOSCOREA (*Dioscoreaceae*)

D. alata Linn. syn. *D. atropurpurea* Roxb.; *D. globosa* Roxb.; *D. purpurea* Roxb.; *D. rubella* Roxb.

Tuber—in Hawaii, used in fever, leaves in rash and itch; plant in constip. (*Econ Bot*, 1971, **25**, 245). EtOH(50%) ext.,diur. (*Indian J Exp Biol*, 1974, **12**, 512).

Tubers of a purple-fleshed cultivar contain anthocyanins; red ones, acylated anthocyanins with ferulic acid (*Experientia*, 1967, **23**, 611; 1968, **24**, 445); cholesterol, compesterol, β-sitosterol & stigmasterol (*J Agric Food Chem*, 1977, **25**, 1222); *trans*-crotonic and palmitic acids (*Pharmazie*, 1978, **33**, 766); effect of X-ray irradiation on contents of sapogenin, alk. and starch; increase in diosgenin content (*Indian J Exp Biol*, 1979, **17**, 144).

D. bulbifera Linn. syn. *D. crispata* Roxb.; *D. pullchella* Roxb.; *D. sativa* Thunb. non Linn.; *D. versicolor* Buch.-Ham. ex Wall.

Santals use plant against madness (*Econ Bot*, 1970, **24**, 241); rhizomes, anorexiant (*Indian J Med Res*, 1969, **57**, 1075); EtOH(50%) ext. of aerial parts, diur. (*Indian J Exp Biol*, 1977, **15**, 208).

Tubers, of *D. bulbifera*, *D. spontanea* (a wild type of *D. bulbifera*) yield furanoid norditerps., see diosbulbines from different varieties with varying bitterness, either in cooked or uncooked; all contained some of the bitter and non-bitter terps. (*J Agric Food Chem*, 1974, **22**, 332); norditerp. glucds., diosbulbinoside D & F (*Chem Pharm Bull*, 1978, **26**, 435). Mutant, increase in diosgenin content and a new steroid sapogenin in 3 generations (*Proc Indian Nat Sci Acad*, 1976, **42B**, 156). A new dihydrophenanthrene, a known phenanthrene, *d*-sorbitol, diosbulbin B & D (*Indian J Chem*, 1978, **16B**, 643).

Diosbulbin(e)s — a diterp. lactone, str. (*Indian J Chem*, 1969, **7**, 452); furanoid norditerps., diosbulbins, A, B & C, all having bitter taste (*Chem Pharm Bull*, 1968, **16**, 2430); str. of D, E, F, G & H; hunger-suppressing properties of tuber due to diosbulbin, showed no biol. properties (*Justus Liebigs Ann Chem*, 1978, 818; 1973, 978).

Bulbils, diosgenin, 0.22% (*Indian J Pharm Sci*, 1978, **40**, 228).

*D. composita Hemsl. syn. *D. macrostachya* Benth.

Of the various spp. tried for introduction; successful cultivation of *D. floribunda* and *D. composita* reported from different parts of the country from 1973 onwards, and are established sources of diosgenin.

Various aspects of cultivation for tubers; see also *D. deltoidea* and *D. floribunda* (Asolkar & Chadha, 11-59).

Diosgenin—extn. from tubers by aq. HCl (US Pat., 1970, 3510400; *CA*, **73**, 38530t); detn. spectrophotom.-TLC (*Analyst Lond*, 1972, **97**, 973); content increases with maturation of tubers (*Q J Crude Drug Res*, 1977, **15**, 67); comparison of content of old and new world spp. with special reference to chromosomal race (*Indian J Exp Biol*, 1977, **15**, 1109); synth. in shoot cultures (*Planta Med*, 1980, Suppl, 120).

Introduced and cultivated at Bangalore, Jammu, Jorhat, Darjeeling and in Goa and Anaimalai hills.

D. deltoidea Wall. ex Kunth

India depended entirely on *D. deltoidea* rhizomes for its diosgenin; a steroid drug precursor in the 60s. Large scale collection resulting in depletion of forest resources and in some areas complete eradication of wild plant. Natural regeneration requires 7 years, hence it was necessary to bring it under cultivation and also to introduce exotic *Dioscorea* spp. for regular and assured supplies of tubers.

D. deltoidea, much valued in India for its purest possible source of diosgenin, has been reported to be brought under cultivation.

Rhizomes— in trade called tubers, commercial source of purest diosgenin. Sources of diosgenin from wild spp., viz. *D. deltoidea* and *D. prazeri*, their cultivation and of two introduced spp., viz. *D. composita* and *D. floribunda*; genetics, breeding and plant improvement; tissue culture (Asolkar & Chadha, 11-59).

Diosgenin—see details under *D.floribunda*.Diosgenin glucopyranoside (*Indian J Chem*, 1976, **14B**, 735). Preliminary fermentation of rhizomes resulted in increase of diosgenin yield by 17-35% (*Prikl Biokhim Microbiol*, 1975, **9**, 583). Diosgenin obtained by cultivation of pretreated isolated tissues (USSR Pat., 1974, 440404; *CA*, 1975, **82**, 83265g); extn. from tubers of Uttar Pradesh hills, 2.5-6.3% (*Indian Drugs*, 1977-78, **15**, 103).

Change in haemolytic index of total saponins in relation to extn. method (*Rastit Resur*, 1972, **7**, 574; *CA*,1973, **78**, 75813m); rhizomes also contain stigmasterol, β- sitosterol, and campesterol (*Planta Med*, 1975, **28**, 101). Sepn. of w.-sol. and insol. saponins; new saponins from rhizome, deltonin and deltoside, isolation and their fungitoxic properties (*Prikl Biokhim Microbiol*, 1974, **10**, 467; 1975, **11**, 94; 1977, **13**, 172).

Seed ext., antimicrob. (*Lloydia*, 1968, **31**, 180). Plant, 4-OH-isoleucine (*Phytochemistry*, 1976, **15**, 325). Leaves, new steroid deltofolin; its str.; fresh leaves, bound diosgenin (*c*. 0.4- 0.6%); increase on slow-drying (*Dokl Akad Nauk SSSR*, 1979, **249**, 241; 1981, **256**, 741; *Prikl Biokhim Microbiol*, 1980, **16**, 755; 1975, **11**, 784).

*D. floribunda Mart. & Gal.

Successful cultivation since 1973; see *D. composita*; of all the *Dioscorea* spp.,

this is the one which is mainly cultivated for extn. of diosgenin.

Tubers—commercial source of diosgenin, a steroid drug precursor; various aspects of cultivation of species for tubers (Asolkar & Chadha, 11-59). Diosgenin greater in tuber-propagated tubers (2.68% on dry wt) than in seed and vegetatively propagated ones; same is the case with tuber wt., etc. [*Indian Drugs Pharmac Ind*, 1975, **10**(1), 9]. Cultivation of diosgenin-rich plant (*Indian J Pharm*, 1976, **38**, 144); diosgenin extn. from tubers by aq. HCl (US Pat., 1970, 3510400; *CA*, **73**, 38530t); tubers suitable for diosgenin extn. (*Indian Drugs*, 1978-79, **16**, 182).

Saponins including 5 spirostanol glucd. and 2 furostanol glucd. (*Phytochemistry*, 1975, **14**, 539); 4 new steroid saponins, floribunda saponins C,D,E & F; str. of A & B from yams (*Indian J Chem*, 1978, **16B**, 350; *Phytochemistry* 1981, **20**, 1943).

Diosgenin—a steroid sapogenin, not itself very active principle, but best example of molecular manipulations for manufacture of highly effective pharmaceutics, and successful integration of higher plant for the purpose (*in* Wagner & Wolff, 267-68). Extn. in India from tubers of *D. composita*, *D.deltoidea*, *D. floribunda* and *D. prazeri*; before 1976, *D. deltoidea* wild rhizomes ruled supreme; later on, *D. floribunda* cultivated tubers are the mainstay of Indian steroid industry. Extn. and assay procedures; extn. methods, isolation, identn.; various assay procedures with their merits and demerits. Diosgenin conversion to steroid drugs; corticosteroids, contraceptive pills and sex hormones with uses and other relevant details (Asolkar & Chadha, 60-111). GLC anal. (*Chih Wu Hsueh Pao*, 1980, **22**, 204; *CA*, 1981, **94**, 170363d); detn. of diosgenin and other saponins by HPLC (*J Natl Prod*, 1981, **44**, 750; *J Chromatogr*, 1981, **206**, 169).

Introduced and commercially cultivated mainly at Bangalore and Goa, and experimentally, at Lucknow and New Delhi.

D. hispida Dennst. syn. *D. daemona* Roxb.; *D. hirsuta* Dennst.; *D. triphylla* auct: non Linn.

Plant parts used in whitlow, sores, boils, bite of rabid jackal or dog (*Econ Bot*, 1970, **24**, 241).

Tubers used for ulcer, to kill worms in wounds, and as fish poison [*J Res Indian Med*, 1976, **11**(3), 54].

Tubers contain alk. dioscorine & 4-epidioscorine; latter a neuromuscular blocking agent (*Indian J Pharm Sci*, 1978, **40**, 235); biosynth. of dioscorine (*J Chem Soc D*, 1971, 1499; *Phytochemistry*, 1972, **11**, 3219).

D. oppositifolia Linn.

Plant used in sores, orchitis, epidydimitis or hydrocele and dysen. (*Econ Bot*, 1970, **24**, 241). Preliminary pharmacol. of EtOH(50%) ext. of plant (excluding roots) and of its var. *dekhunensis* (*Indian J Exp Biol*, 1977, **15**, 208).

D. pentaphylla Linn. syn. *D. jacquemontii* Hook.f.

Plant, used in dropsy and anasarca (*Econ Bot*, 1970, **24**, 241); decoct. of tubers in rheum. (*Bull Bot Surv India*, 1973, **15**, 13); EtOH(50%) ext., antiinflam. (*Indian J Exp Biol*, 1980, **18**, 594).

Tubers, alk. dioscorine (*Indian J Chem*, 1966, **4**, 457).

D. prazeri Prain & Burkill syn. *D. clarkei* Prain & Burkill; *D. deltoidea* Wall. var. *sikkimensis* Prain; *D. sikkimensis* Prain & Burkill.

Rhizomes, source of diosgenin; various aspects (Asolkar & Chadha, 11-59); see also *D. deltoidea* and *D. floribunda*; 2 diosgenin and a prazerigenin glucopyranosides (*Q J Crude Drug Res*, 1977, **15**, 67). Studies with short-term fertilisation (N, potash and bact. fertilizers). Synth. of diosgenin favoured in plant undergoing defruiting operation (*Indian J Exp Biol*, 1979, **17**, 1418).

Rhizomes, 3 new steroidal sapogenins, prazerigenin A, B & C, str. (*J Chem Soc Perkin Trans I*, 1975, 1460); 2 new, 9, 10-hydrophenanthrenes, str. (*Indian J Chem*, 1975, **13**, 1137).

DIOSPYROS (*Ebenaceae*)

D. candolleana Wight

Stem and bark contain betulin, betulinic acid and lupeol; leaves taraxerol (*Indian J Chem*, 1970, **8**, 851; 1973, **11**, 840).

*D. chloroxylon Roxb.

Eng.–*Green ebony persimmon*; Mar.–*Ninai*; Oriya–*Ondodi*; Tam.–*Kamvakkunai*; Tel.–*Illinda*.

EtOH(50%) ext. of plant excluding root, antivir. (*Indian J Exp Biol*, 1973, **11**, 43).

Stem and bark yield 7-Me-juglone, diospryrin, its isomer, xylospyrin, β-sitosterol; 2 new naphthalenes (*Tetrahedron Lett*, 1967, 2905; 1970, 1739).

Maharashtra, Orissa and in S. India.

D. ebenum Koenig syn. *D. hebecarpa* A. Cunn. ex Benth.

Heartwood contains 2β-naphthaldehydes (*J Chem Soc*, 1965, 4292); 2 naphthoic acid derivs. (*Phytochemistry*, 1969, **8**, 789); ceryl alc., betulin, α-amyrin, ursolic acid (free & as -OAc), baurenol and stigmasterol; leaves, ursolic acid, lupeol, and a triterp alc. (*Indian J Pharm*, 1967, **29**, 289; 1968, **30**, 93).

D. exsculpta Buch.-Ham. syn. *D. tomentosa* Roxb.

Plant—various parts in bleeding of gums, fever, atrophy, tumours, emaciation or cachexy, sores, T.B., fistula, syphilis, carbuncle, dysuria, gravel, stomach trouble, *prolapsus ani*, *fistula ani*, blood and mucus in bowel excretion, dry cough, broncht., neuralgia, pleur., pneum., rinderpest, etc. (*Econ Bot*, 1970, **24**, 241). Preliminary pharmacol. (*Indian J Exp Biol* 1971, **9**, 91).

Unsap. matter of seeds produced fall in B.P. and increase in respiration rate; also showed anorexia, CNS depress. and antibact. activities (*Indian J Hosp Pharm*, 1980, **17**, 73).

Leaves and stems, β-sitosterol, lupeol, betulin, betulinic and oleanolic acids & their -OAc (*Phytochemistry*, 1971, **10**, 2829).

*D. insignis Thw.

Tam.–*Pottuvarai.*

EtOH(50%) ext. of plant excluding roots, antifert. activity (*Indian J Exp Biol*, 1977, **15**, 208).

Evergreen forest of Kerala and Anaimalai, at low altitudes.

D. kaki Linn.f.

Carotenoid detn. (*C R Acad Agr Fr*, 1961, **47**, 336; *CA*, 1965, **62**, 8113b); betulic, oleanolic and ursolic acids (*Yakugaku Zasshi*, 1971, **91**, 905). Astragalin and a pyranoside; astragalin and isoquercitrin, hypoten. principles from leaves (*Chem Pharm Bull*, 1978, **26**, 1936; 1979, **27**, 2865).

Tannins—capable of detoxifying snake venoms and bacterial toxins; activity much stronger than tannic acid (*Toxicon*, 1979, **17**, 524); simple method for purification (*Agric Biol Chem*, 1981, **45**, 1885).

Roots, 7-Me-juglone, mamegakinone, plumbagin, diospyrin, etc. (*Chem Pharm Bull*, 1972, **20**, 2029).

Calyx constituents (*Yakugaku Zasshi*, 1977, **97**, 452); callus growth inhibitors (*Agric Biol Chem*, 1977, **41**, 2495).

D. lotus Linn.

Plant, antivir. (*Lloydia*, 1978, **41**, 463).

Roots yield 7-Me-juglone, mamegakinone, isodiospyrin & its dimer (*Tetrahedron Lett*, 1970, 7); also tetralone deriv., shinanolone and common triterps. (*Chem Pharm Bull*, 1971, **19**, 2314).

Leaves, hentriacontanol, betulinic acid, oxy-allobetulin, taraxerol and β-sitosterol (*Phytochemistry*, 1971, **10**, 2829). Bark triterps. (*Khim Prir Soedin*, 1975, **11**, 103; *CA*, **83**, 75369z).

D. melanoxylon Roxb.

Eng.–*Ebony.*

Unsap. matter of seed oil, antibact. (*Indian Drugs*, 1978- 79, **16**, 261).

Bark, sapwood and ebony (heartwood) contain betulin, lupeol and tannin; ebony ext., naphthaquinones (*Indian J Appl Chem*, 1963, **26**, 29); bark, also betulinic acid and β- sitosterol (*Indian J Chem*, 1964, **2**, 467).

Heartwood, a naphthaquinone, diomelquinone A (*Ann Chem Warsaw*, 1966, **691**, 172; *CA*, **64**, 14142g); 5 naphthaquinones and 4 naphthol derivs.; a binaphthaquinone (*Indian J Chem*, 1968, **6**, 681; 1973, **11**, 507); a naphthaldehyde; pentacyclic quinones, diosindigo A & B, and biramentaceone (*Phytochemistry*, 1971, **10**, 458; 1981, **20**, 1093).

Leaves, ceryl alc., sequoyitol; bauerenol, and ursolic and oleanolic acids; a flavone (*Proc Indian Acad Sci*, 1964, **60A**, 36; *Indian J Chem*, 1969, **7**, 204; 1973, **11**, 840).

*D. mollis Griff.

Fruit—exts. of fresh ones widely used in Thailand as anthelm. against hookworm (*in* Wagner & Wolff, 222); ext. very active against hookworm, less against tapworm (*Proc Pac Sci Congr Pac Sci Assoc*, 1957, **5**, 52; *CA*, 1964, **60**, 12371a).

Berries contain diospyrol, dinaphthol and 3-Me-naphthalone-1,8- diol (*J Chem Soc*, 1965, 1533); constituents of fruit, bark and roots (*Chem Pharm Bull*, 1971, **19**, 2261; *CA*, 1972, **76**, 45990h). Plant yields 2 *n*-alkanes, lupeol, α-amyrin and β-sitosterol (*Planta Med*, 1972, **21**, 61).

Diospyrol—anthelm. principle from berries; LD_{50}, 3000 mg/kg in exp. animals; its str.; its new diglucd. (*Tetrahedron Lett*, 1967, 4857; 1976, 105); in hamsters infected with human hookworm, *Necator americanas.* Sound basis for use of fresh juice against parasitic infections (*Proc Life Sci*, 1977, 222; *Arzneim Forsch*, 1974, **24**, 2000; *CA*, 1975, **82**, 149297c).

Introduced and cultivated at Coonoor in Tamil Nadu.

*D. montana Roxb. var. cordifolia Hiern syn. *D. cordifolia* Roxb.

Plant—various parts, in fever, dysuria, gravel, neuralgia, pleur., pneum., menor. and flooding, puerperal fever, diar. and spider-bite poison (*Econ Bot*, 1970, **24**, 241).

Bark—ext., significant antiinflam., antipyr. and analg. [*J Res Indian Med*, 1973, **8**(2), 15]; alc. ext. inhibits Ehrlich ascites carcinoma in mice (*J Indian Chem Soc*, 1981, **58**, 627).

Leaves and seeds, non eq. ext. antibact. (*Indian J Pharm*, 1973, **35**, 93).

Stems yield lupeol (*Indian J Chem*, 1970, **8**, 851); diospyrin & its cyclo deriv. from Indian wood; diospyrin derivs. & related compds. from bark (*J Chem Soc Perkin Trans I*, 1976, 2155); tetrahydrodiospyrin from bark (*Phytochemistry*, 1979, **18**, 684).

Leaves, triterp. constituent (*Phytochemistry*, 1972, **11**, 1180); β-dihydrodiospyrin (*Tetrahedron Lett*, 1972, 4201); diospyrin, lupeol and betulic acid (*Curr Sci*, 1978, **47**, 345).

Fruit pulp, triterps. and also esters of α-amyrin, ursolic, oleanolic and betulinic acids; seeds, betulinic acid (*Phytochemistry*, 1972, **11**, 1508).

Throughout the greater part of India.

D. peregrina Gurke syn. *D. embryopteris* Pers.

Fruit—unripe, pounded and its ext. used in diar.; chewing of fruit cured blisters in mouth (*Econ Bot*, 1965, **19**, 236).

Plant or plant parts used in gravel, cholera; menor. or flooding and rinderpest (*ibid*, 1970, **24**, 241). EtOH(50%) ext. of stem bark, antiprot., antivir. and hypoglyc.; that of plant excluding roots, diur. and anticancer (*Indian J Exp Biol*, 1968, **6**, 232; 1980, **18**, 594).

Fruit pulp, alkanes and triterps.; seeds, betulinic acid (*Phytochemistry*, 1971, **10**, 904); seeds yield fatty oil (32%); unsap. matter, β-amyrin (*Proc Nat Acad Sci India*, 1974, **44A**, 319).

Leaf triterps. (*Indian J Chem*, 1964, **2**, 129). Bark, myricyl alc., triterps. and saponin (*Proc Nat Acad Sci India*, 1964, **34A**, 180).

Stem, β-sitosterol and a leucoanthocyanin (*J Indian Chem Soc*, 1978, **55**, 1068). Plant, nonadecan-7-ol-2-one (*Phytochemistry*, 1980, **19**, 2637).

Str. of new glycds. from roots (*Planta Med*, 1979, **35**, 373; *Indian J Chem*, 1982, **21B**, 167).

*D. viriginiana Linn.

Tannin—from plant produced tumour in rats (*J Nat Cancer Inst*, 1976, **57**, 207). Fruit tannin has strong detoxifying action against snake venoms and bacterial toxins, 8-32 times stronger than tannic acid (*Sankyo Kenkyusho Nampo*, 1978, **30**, 104; *CA*, 1979, **90**, 181233e); controls plant virus (Jpn Kokai Tokkyo Koho, 1979, 7914515; *CA*, **90**, 18158v).

Fruit pectin, cholesterol-lowering (*Nutr Res Inst*, 1979, **20**, 519; *CA*, 1980, **92**, 40333s).

Bark and seed, isodiospyrin (*J Chem Soc C*, 1968, 2279); wood, 7-Me-juglone (*J Agric Food Chem*, 1978, **26**, 869).

Introduced and cultivated at Coonoor in Tamil Nadu.

DIPLOCLISIA (*Menispermaceae*)

D. glaucescens (Blume) Diels syn. *Cocculus macrocarpus* Wight & Arn.

Roots contain alk. stepharine (*Chem Ind Lond*, 1964, 282). Plant, ginnol, β- & γ-sitosterol, trilobine, and a neutral substance (mp, 226-28°) and probably sesquoyitol (*Indian J Chem*, 1974, **12**, 226).

DIPLOCYCLOS (*Cucurbitaceae*)

D. palmatus Jeff. syn. *Bryonopsis laciniosa* (Linn.) Naud.; *Bryonia lanciniosa* Linn.

Seeds—Powd. given to help conception in women; roots for same purpose (*Bull RRL Jammu*, 1963, **1**, 126; *Econ Bot*, 1965, **19**, 242; 1971, **25**, 422). Seeds and plant serve as tonic and aphrodis. (*Khadi Gramodyog*, 1972-73, **19**, 271).

Plant—various organs used in headache, ague, enlarged spleen, paralysis of tongue, colic pain, delirium and convuls., foaming at mouth, sores, adenitis scrofulosa colli, syphilis, carbuncle, stomach swelling or tumour, constip., phthisis; and snakebite; EtOH(50%) ext. of aerial parts, spasmol. (*Econ Bot*, 1970, **24**, 241; 1971, **25**, 422); *Indian J Exp Biol*, 1974, **12**, 512).

Seed oil, source of punicic acid (38.2%) (*Lipids*, 1981, **16**, 558).

DIPLOKNEMA (*Sapotaceae*)

D. butyracea Lamk; see **Aisandra butyracea**

DIPSACUS (*Dipsacaceae*)

*D. fullonum Linn.

Decoct. in wine used against inflammed tumours. A liniment preparation of juice used against warts, wens, felon and whitlow. Aq. ext. of leaves used against warts in fundament (*Lloydia*, 1969, **32**, 104).

Cultivated in India.

DIPTERACANTHUS (*Acanthaceae*)

*D. longifolius Stocks syn. *Ruellia longifolia* T. Anders.

M.P. – *Surata.*

Used as powd. or in *ghee* to cure abdominal tumours (*Lloydia*, 1967, **30**, 387).

Found jn Madhya Pradesh.

D. prostratus (Poir.) Nees syn. *Ruellia prostrata* Poir.

EtOH(50%) ext. of plant, mild hypoglyc., and anticancer against human epidermoid carcinoma of nasopharynx, in tissue culture (*Indian J Exp Biol*, 1980, **18**, 594).

Flowers and buds, luteolin, its 7-glucd. and apigenin, its 7- glucd. & 7-glucuronide (*J Indian Chem Soc*, 1972, **49**, 825).

D. suffruticosus Voigt syn. *Ruellia suffruticosa* Roxb.

Used in fever, atrophy, emaciation and cachexy, cough and broncht., dropsy, puerperal fever, and as diur. by Santals (*Econ Bot*, 1970, **24**, 241).

DIPTEROCARPUS (*Dipterocarpaceae*)

D. alatus Roxb. syn. *D. incanus* Roxb.

Essent. oil, 2 sesquiterps. of eudesmane series (*Tetrahedron Lett*, 1970, 279).

D. indicus Bedd. syn. *D. turbinatus* Dyer

EtOH(50%) ext. of plant excluding roots, diur. and spasmog. (*Indian J Exp Biol*, 1977, **15**, 208).

Oleoresin and its essent oil; β-caryophyllene, humulene, à hydrocarbon and a sesquiterp. alc. (*Indian Soap J*, 1961, **26**, 97; *J Indian Chem Soc*, 1952, **29**, 590). Bark, bergenin (*Indian J Chem*, 1967, **5**, 523).

D. pilosus Roxb.

Sesquiterp., γ-gurjunene (*Tetrahedron*, 1969, **25**, 1785). Oleoresin, a mixt. of tetra and pentacyclic sesquiterps. (18%) containing caryophyllene, its oxide, humulene, etc.; and triterps. fraction (≈ 80%) with dipterocarpol and several related compds., asiatic acid & its 2- Ac derivs., and 2-α-OH-ursolic acid (*ibid*, 1971, **27**, 635; 823).

DISPORUM (*Liliaceae*)

*D. pullum Salisb.

Stem eaten raw or cooked in rheum. (*in* Jain, 124).

Khasi and Jaintia hills of Meghalaya.

DODONAEA (*Dodonaeaceae*)

D. viscosa (Linn.) Jacq.

Plant—aq. and alc. exts., cardioinhibitory and coronary constricting and also spasmol., sed., hypoten., anthelm. and antibact. (*J Sci Ind Res*, 1962, **21C**, 349).

Leaves contain hautriwaic acid (*Phytochemistry*, 1971, **10**, 2813); leaves and pods, 3-O-rutinosides of isorhamnetin and quercetin & 3-O-galactoside of latter (*Indian J Chem*, 1975, **13**, 639).

Bark, a new isomer of 5,7,3′,4′-tetra-OH-flavan, shikimic and chlorogenic acids and glucose (*Leath Sci*, 1966, **13**, 174). Yellow flowers, 2 kaempferol-Me ethers (*Rev Latinoam Quim*, 1978, **9**, 97;*CA*, **89**, 143352q).

DOLICHANDRONE (*Bignoniaceae*)

*D. arcuata C.B. Clarke

EtOH(50%) of plant excluding roots, diur. (*Indian J Exp Biol*, 1974, **12**, 512). Coimbatore and Ootacamund, T.N.

D. falcata Seem.

Leaves yield luteolin, chrysin & its 7-rutinoside and glucd. (*Phytochemistry*, 1972, **11**, 438).

D. stipulata Benth. syn. *Markhamia stipulata* Seem.

Stem heartwood yield lapachol, dehydro-α-lapachone, β-lapachone, β-sitosterol, tectol, paulownin and palmitone; bark, first 4 compds., dehydrotectal and tectoquinone (*Planta Med*, 1978, **34**, 219; *Pharmazie*, 1980, **35**, 701).

DOLICHOS (*Fabaceae*)

D. lablab Linn. var. typicus; see Lablab purpureus

D. uniflorus Lamk syn. *D. biflorus* auct. non Linn.

Plant—used in tumours, adenitis, sores, burns, measles, smallpox, dysuria, *prolapsus ani, fistula ani*, dysen., neuralgia, pleur., pneum., leprosy, and rinderpest (*Econ Bot*, 1970, **24**, 241). Ext., as radio-label reagent in ABO-blood grouping of human hair (*Vox Sang*, 1973, **25**, 420).

Seeds—EtOH(50%) ext. of spasmol. and affected respiration (*Indian J Exp Biol*, 1968, **6**, 232).

Seed lectins—in detn. of subgroups of blood groups A and AB (*Probl Gematol Perveliv Krovi*, 1967, **12**, 13; *CA*, **66**, 114144t); ext. (also of root and stem) agglutinated human leukocytes and erythrocytes (*Nature Lond*, 1968, **217**, 654). Extn. (*Biochemistry*, 1970, **9**, 869; *Izv Akad Nauk SSSR Ser Biol*, 1968, 59); isolation of anti-A phytoagglutinin (*Biochem Biophys Acta*, 1971, **243**, 434); non-toxic in mice and rats, while that of *Lablab purpureus* (*D. lablab*), toxic (*Toxicon*, 1972, **10**, 89).

Seeds, 4 active glycosidases (*Biochimie*, 1973, **55**, 5); an unusual allantoinase (*Phytochemistry*, 1978, **17**, 397).

Globulin fraction showed hypolipidaemic effects in rats (*Atherosclerosis*, 1973, **18**, 369). A lectin-like glycoprotein from stems and leaves, possesses carbohydrate-binding activity (*Biochem Biophys Res Commun*, 1980, **96**, 92); also in leaves and stems, coumesterol and psoralidin (*Z Naturforsch*, 1980, **35C**, 923); pterocarpans from bacteria-treated leaves (*Phytochemistry*, 1981, **20**, 807).

DOLOMIAEA (*Asteraceae*)

D. macrocephala DC.; see Jurinea dolomiaea

DOREMA (*Apiaceae*)

D. ammoniacum D. Don

Str. of gum resin (*Ann Chim Paris*, 1970, **60**, 3; 17).

DORONICUM (*Asteraceae*)

D. hookeri Hook.f.

'Mufarreh' of plant used as exhilarant and cardiotonic, useful in melancholia; dissolves trapped gases and acts as stomch. [*East Pharm*, 1980, **23**(272), 39].

D. pardalianches Linn.

Roots and aerial parts yield new sesquiterp. alc., pardalianchol & its acetophenone deriv. (*Phytochemistry*, 1979, **18**, 668).

DRACAENA (*Dracaenaceae*)

D. angustifolia Roxb.

EtOH(50%) ext. of plant excluding roots, diur. (*Indian J Exp Biol*, 1974, **12**, 512).

D. cinnabari Balf. f.

Roots yield gum resin used in gargle water, as stim., astrin. and in toothpaste. Roots for treatment of rheum. Leaves, as carmin. (*Planta Med*, 1974, **26**, 65).

*D. fragrans Ker-Gawl. var. **lindenii** Hort.

EtOH(50%) ext. of plant excluding roots, diur. and anticancer against P388 lymphocytic leukemia in mice (*Indian J Exp Biol*, 1980, **18**, 594).

Cultivated in Indian gardens.

DRACOCEPHALUM (*Lamiaceae*)

D. moldavica Linn.

Extn. of 4 flavons. including moldavoside (*Farm Zh Kiev*, 1968, **23**, 75; *CA*, **69**, 44172m).

Triterp. compn. (*Rastit Resur*, 1980, **16**, 286; *CA*, **93**, 41546w). Essent. oil, citral a & b as major constituents (*Farmacia Buc*, 1978, **26**, 93; *CA*, 1979, **90**, 43662t).

DRACONTIUM (*Araceae*)

D. polyphyllum Linn.

Plant used as antid. for snakebite and a remedy against spasms; considered a powerful stim. (*Econ Bot*, 1969, **23**, 97).

DREGEA (*Asclepiadaceae*)

D. volubilis Benth. ex Hook.f.; see **Wattakaka volubilis**

DREPANOCARPUS (*Fabaceae*)

D. spinosus Kurz; see **Dalbergia spinosa**

DRIMIA (*Liliaceae*)

D. indica (Roxb.) Jessop syn. *Urginea indica* Kunth; *U. coromandeliana* Hook. f. Eng.–*Indian squill*.

Bulb—known as Indian squill. EtOH(50%) ext., antiprot., anticancer,

hypoglyc. (*Indian J Exp Biol*, 1968, **6**, 232). Powd. used externally to check skin diseases (*Bull Bot Surv India*, 1973, **15**, 21); fried and applied to wounds [*J Res Indian Med*, 1973, **8**(1), 85]. As drug, rev., 45 refs. [*Q J Crude Drug Res*, 1976, **14**(2), 49]. Paste applied as lep on forehead in '*sannipat*'(*Nagarjun*, 1980-81, **24**, 1). Cardiotonic potency of tincture, half that of European squill (*U. maritima*) in guineapigs (*J Pharm Pharmacol*, 1976, **28**, 81); reflex expect. action (Martindale, 693).

Cardiotonic action resembles that of digitalis, rapid and less cumulative in its effect, its use as substitute for digitalis undesirable due to irritating effect and poor absorption entailing larger dosage; use restricted to patients hypersensitive to digitalis. Squill available in Indian market is admixed with a small portion of bulbs of *Scilla hyacinthiana* (Wlth India, X, 417).

Bulbs max. content of glycds. at dormant stage; seasonal variation in content (*Curr Sci*, 1980, **49**, 276). See also cardiovascular drugs; cardiac glycds. (*in* Goodman & Gilman, 666- 68).

Diploid and triploid cytotypes, better in vitamin (B_1, B_6 and niacinamide) content than tetraploids (*Indian Drugs*, 1980- 81, **18**, 350).

Bulbs yield hentriacontanol, octacosanoic acid and sitosterol (*Phytochemistry*, 1972, **11**, 2888). Sterol content varies with age of root in diploid and tetraploid form (*Indian J Exp Biol*, 1980, **18**, 291). Bulbs of 12 cytotypes; those of di-, tri-, tetra- and hexaploid contain glycds. proscillaridin A, scillopheoside and anhydroscilliphaosidin; sterols in different cytological races of Indian squill; leaves, bulb and roots screened (*Phytochemistry*, 1981, **20**, 524; 1442).

Powd. bulb contains alc.-insol. mucilage (51%); distinguishing it from European squill which contains alc.-sol. sinistrin & related carbohydrates; mucilage consists of mannose, glucose and xylose (*Indian For*, 1971, **97**, 408).

Leaves eaten in times of scarcity; plant, cyanogenic (*Annu Rep CDRI Lucknow*, 1965-66, 69).

DROSERA (*Droseraceae*)

D. peltata Smith syn. *D. lunata* Buch.-Ham.

Resin from plant used in chr. broncht. and whooping cough [*Nagarjun*, 1974-75, **18**(1), 31]. Extn. of plumbagin by steam distillation (*Yao Hsueh Young Pao*, 1980, **15**, 3; *CA*, 1981, **95**, 49260k).

DRYMARIA (*Caryophyllaceae*)

D. cordata Willd. ex Roem. & Schult.

Plant—used in snakebite. Tribes of Meghalaya use juice in burns and skin diseases (*Econ Bot*, 1981, **35**, 4).

An antileukemic compd., cordacin ($C_{17}H_{22}O_7$) inhibitory to primary cultures of human leukemia cells, at 0.25 µg/ml; and established epithelial cells, at 10 µg/ml (*Chin J Microbiol*, 1974, **7**, 74).

*D. villosa Cham. & Schult.

Meghalaya–*Sohkha*.

Plant mashed and taken in case of food poisoning (*in* Jain, 124).

Khasi and Jaintia hills of Meghalaya.

DRYNARIA (*Polypodiaceae*)

D. quercifolia Smith

Oriya–*Garuda pakshini*.

Rhizome paste applied to forehead to relieve headache (*in* Jain, 232); as bitter tonic in bowel inflam. and in cough [*J Res Indian Med*, 1973, **8**(3), 71].

Whole plant, anthelm., pectoral, expect. and tonic. Used in treatment of chest and skin diseases, and for loss of appetite (*Indian Drugs*, 1976-77, **14**, 136).

DRYOBALANOPS (*Dipterocarpaceae*)

D. aromatica Gaertn. f. syn. *D. camphora* Colebr.

Resin contains caryophyllene, humulene, several triterp. alc. and ketones with dipterocarpol and dryobalanone as major; oxygenated deriv. of asiatic acid (*Tetrahedron Lett*,1967, 2807; 1968, 4363). Oleanoic, oleanolic, maslinic, asiatic and aliphitolic acids; hederagenin and arjunolic acid as artifacts; also non-acidic triterps., erythrodiol, dammarenediol II and ocotillol II (*J Chem Soc C*, 1968, 1047; 2686); oleanolic-OAc, dehydronic and dryobalanonoloic acids, Me-11-oxo-asiatate and dryobalanolide (*Phytochemistry*, 1972, **11**, 1771).

Wood contains essent. oil, its constituents; also triterps. OH-dammarenone II, dryobalanone, ocotillone, kapurone, and kupurol (*Nippon Mokuzai Gakkaishi*, 1967, **13**, 360; 1968, **14**, 59; *CA*, 1968, **69**, 25078u; 10582e).

DRYOPTERIS (*Dryopteridaceae*)

*D. chrysocoma (Christ) C. Chr.

Rhizome, anthelm. Phloroglucinol derivs. of crude filicin from dried rhizomes consisted of albaspidin, filixic and flavaspidic acids (*Phytochemistry*, 1976, **15**, 343).

Shillong and Khasi hills up to 1,500 m.

*D. cochleata (D. Don) C. Chr.

Eng.–*Kakolisag*; Bihar–*Netharhat*.

Leaf juice used in epilepsy (*J Sci Res BHU*, 1969- 70, **20**, 227). Pounded rhizome, as lep for rheum. swelling and pain (*Nagarjun*, 1980-81, **24**, 1); antifung. (*Econ Bot*, 1980, **34**, 284).

Ranchi district of Bihar; and Khasi hills of Meghalaya, up to 1,300 m.

D. dentata C. Chr.; see **Cyclosorus dentatus**

D. filix-mas (Linn). Schott syn. *Aspidium filix-mas* Linn.

Plant—fern ext. taeniacidal against dwarf tapeworm; activity due to flavaspidic acid and aspidinol (*J Pharm Pharmacol*, 1964, **16**, 464); ext., significant anthelm.; it is more toxic to mice and rats than filicin and aspidin (*Ann Med Exp Biol Fenn*, 1967, **45**, 341; 352; *CA*, 1968, **68**, 1936a; 1693u). Conserve, in cancerous tumours (*Llyodia*, 1970, **33**, 386).

283

Infusion, as contracep. (*Planta Med*, 1973, **23**, 167); as vermifuge (*Indian Drugs*, 1976-77, **14**, 136).

Oleoresin from rhizome, anthelm. (*Nagarjun*, 1974-75, **18**, 31).

Filicin—toxic principle, method of purification (*Farmatsiya Sof*, 1962, **12**, 34; *CA*, 1964, **61**, 15929f). Flavaspidic acid from U.S.P. sample (*Medd Nor Farm Selsk*, 1963, **25**, 191; *CA*, 1964, **60**, 7876h);spores contained 9 aliphatic alc. and 3 sterols (*Phytochemistry*, 1964, **3**, 89). TLC paper chromatogr. sepn. of phloroglucides (*Planta Med*, 1964, **12**, 112; *Pharm Acta Helv*, 1964, **39**, 327; *CA*, **61**, 4151h); and their content (*Ann Med Exp Biol Fenn*, 1967, **45**, 333; *CA*, 1968, **68**, 19515x); sunshine and moisture destroy activity of filicin (*Farmatsiya Sof*, 1967, **17**, 22; *CA*, 1968, **68**, 6148c). Flavaspidic acid, 50% and filixic acid, 25% of crude filicin from fern from Finland (*Farm Aikak*, 1968, **77**, 30; *CA*, **69**, 33514y). Chromatogr. sepn. of flavaspidic acid and filixic acid; recoveries, 72% and 84% resp. [*J Pharm Pharmacol*, 1969, **21**(Suppl.),55]. Contains alkanes and triterps. (*Phytochemistry* 1972, **11**, 2519). Extn. of filicin (*Farmatsiya Sof*, 1975, **25**, 20; *CA*, **83**, 152254n; Rom. Pat., 1977, 62961-62; *CA*, 1980, **92**, 99568a-69b). Flavaspidic acid BB, *p*-aspidin and albaspidin from rhizomes; therapeutic uses of compd. discussed (*Ankara Univ Eczacilik Fak Mecm*, 1976, **6**, 214; *CA*, 1977, **87**, 193871n). Phloroglucide ext. from plant, bactericidal at 25-80 µg/ml and bacteristatic at 2-10 µg/ml (*Rastit Resur*, 1978, **14**, 582; *CA*, 1979, **90**, 16950d). C_{17} Flavon., dryopterin from aerial part (*Z Naturforsch*, 1981, **360**, 607).

***D. marginalis** (Linn.) A. Gray

Used as taenfuge (Wlth India, III, 114).

Plant, a pteridoptal phloroglucinol deriv., margaspidin (major), flavaspidic acid, *p*-aspidin, etc. (*J Pharm Sci*, 1965, **54**, 1362). Margaspidin, significant antiinflam. in rats (*Takeda Kenkyusho Ho*, 1971, **30**, 225; *CA*, 1972, **76**, 126q).

Imported under the name 'filix-max' or 'male fern'

D. marginata (Wall.) Christ

Plant, antibiot. (*Econ Bot*, 1980, **34**, 284).

Contains several arom. compds., predominantly margaspidin (*Planta Med*, 1978, **33**, 177).

DRYPETES (*Euphorbiaceae*)

D. roxburghii Hurus. syn. *Putranjiva roxburghii* Wall.

Leaves and stones of fruits used in rheum. Crushed leaves applied to swollen throats of cattle.

Seeds yield a fatty oil; kernel, essent. oil with mustard smell; isothiocyanates produced on enzymic hydrolysis of glucoputranjivin, glucocochlearin and glucojiaputin; glucocleomin also present. Fruit pulp contains mannitol (large quant.), a saponin glucd. and an unknown alk. Stones, alk. (Wlth India, VIII, 325).

Seed coats yield triterp. saponin, putranjivoside (1.3%), β- sitosterol & its glucd. (*Planta Med*, 1968, **16**, 17); saponins, putranosides A-D; their str. (*Indian J Chem*, 1973, **11**, 830; 1974, **12**, 447); their isolation [*J Res Indian Med*, 1974, **9**(1), 70].

Leaves, β-amyrin, its palmitate & another ester, putrone, putrol, putranjivic acid, Me putranjivate, stigmasterol and hydrocarbons (*Curr Sci*, 1968, **37**, 301); str. of putranjivic acid & Me putranjivate; also str. revision of putrone and putrol (*Indian J Chem*, 1969, **7**, 1179; 1973, **11**, 525); saponins A-D; their constitution (*ibid*, 1971, **9**, 189; 1975, **13**, 447); triterp. roxburghonic acid; biflavones (*Phytochemistry*, 1971, **10**, 865; 1973, **12**, 1501).

Bark yields triterps friedelin, friedelanol, roxburgholone and putranjivadione;its str. detn. (*Tetrahedron*, 1968, **24**, 6259; 1205). Trunk bark, triterps., putranjivanol, putranjic acid, putranjivadione, etc. (*Phytochemistry*, 1968, **7**,

2053); str. of putranjic acid (*Tetrahedron Lett*, 1969, 231); str. of putranjivanonol; assigned str. of friedelanone (*Planta Med*, 1970- 71, **19**, 352; 359). Stem bark triterp. putrolic acid; its str. (*Curr Sci*, 1969, **38**, 101; *Indian J Chem*, 1970, **8**, 401).

*D. venusta Pax & Hoffim. syn. *Hemicyclia venusta* Thw.

EtOH(50%) of plant excluding roots, low CNS depress., gives +ve rotarod test and potentiates barbiturate (*Indian J Exp Biol*, 1977, **15**, 208).

Found in Western Ghats.

DUABANGA (*Sonneratiaceae*)

*D. sonneratioides Buch.-Ham.

Ass.–*Thera*; B.–*Banderhulla*; Trade–*Lampati*.

EtOH(50%) ext. of stem bark, anticancer and spasmog. (*Indian J Exp Biol*, 1971, **9**, 91).

Stem, bark contains hentriacontanol, hentriacontanone, lignoceryl ferulate, acacetin, betulinic acid, β-sitosterol, & its glucd. (*Phytochemistry*, 1971, **10**, 2247; 1972, **11**, 2621); also genkwanin-4'-galactoside, ellagic acid, its tetra-Me-ether and epioleanolic acid (*ibid*, 1974, **13**, 527).

Eastern Himalayas, Assam and Andamans, up to 1,000 m.

DUBOISIA (*Solanaceae*)

*D. myoporoides R. Br.

Leaves, source of tropane alks. used in medicine due to their mydriatic, anticholinergic and spasmodic actions (*CSIR News*, 1980, **30**, 108); see *Atropa, Datura* and *Hyoscyamus*.

Leaves contain alks. 3-4%, with hyoscine (60%) and hyoscyamine (30%).

Young leaves and stems contain alks. valtropine and scopolamine (major) and valeroidine (minor). Stems, also tropine and leaves, tropyl tiglate. Leaves rich in alks. than stems. Old leaves and stems contain valeroidine, tropine, nortropine, hyoscyamine, apohyoscine and tropyl butyrate. In old leaves, valtropine and

scopolamine as major alks., while in stems, former as major alk. (*Planta Med*, 1967, **15**, 459). Alks. of roots and their distribution in old and fresh roots and bark (*ibid*, 1968, **16**, 174).

Leaves used as antid. by New caledonian natives; contain nicotine, nornicotine, atropine (or hyoscyamine) and hyosine (*Toxicon*, 1976, **14**, 55; *CA*, **84**, 140651x; *Phytochemistry*, 1976, **15**, 818).

Introduced into India at FRI, Dehra Dun.

DURANTA (*Verbenaceae*)

D. repens Linn. syn. *D. plumieri* Jacq.

Plant ext., antifung. (*J Res Orissa Univ Agric Technol*, 1979, **9**, 147).

Leaves yield pectolinaringenin and scutellarein (*Phytochemistry*, 1972, **11**, 3095).

Fruit alk. (*Planta Med*, 1973, **23**, 173); new durantoside- 4(V) and triterps. from fruit (*Indian J Chem*, 1978, **16B**, 844).

Plant, lamiide and 3 new iridoids, durantosides (*Z Naturforsch*, 1974, **29C**, 111); tetra-OAc of durantosides I, II and IV & penta-OAc of durantoside I (*Experientia*, 1976, **32**, 968).

DURIO (*Bombacaceae*)

D. zibethinus Linn.

Fruits reduce lethality of alcohol (*Asian J Med*, 1973, **9**, 158; *CA*, **79**, 74546k). Fruit, volat. flavouring constituents; volat. constituents as well as fatty acid compn. of lipids (*Phytochemistry*, 1972, **11**, 2081; 1980, **19**, 79).

DYSOPHYLLA (*Lamiaceae*)

*D. rugosa Hook. f.

EtOH(50%) ext. of plant, diur. (*Indian J Exp Biol*, 1977, **15**, 208).

Found in Western Ghats.

*D. stellata Benth.

EtOH(50%) ext. of plant, diur. and spasmog. (*Indian J Exp Biol*, 1974, **12**, 512).

Plant yields 2 phenolic ketones, a chromone stellatin and stigmasterol (*J Chem Soc Perkin Trans I*, 1977, 433).

Found in Western Ghats, from Belgaum southwards in rice fields.

DYSOXYLUM (*Meliaceae*)

*D. binectariferum Hook. f.

Preliminary pharmacol.; EtOH(50%) ext. of fruit, antiinflam., diur. and CNS depress. (*Indian J Exp Biol*, 1973, **11**, 43; 1977, **15**, 208). Fruit, tetranortriterp. dysobinin, a potential CNS depress. and inflam. inhibitor (*Phytochemistry*, 1976, **15**, 2001).

Sikkim, Assam, W. Bengal and Western Ghats.

ECBALLIUM (*Cucurbitaceae*)

E. elaterium A. Rich.

Root—used to treat skin diseases and baldness (Belg. Pat., 1964, 648535; *CA*, 1965, **63**, 12981c); and for physiological or parasitic scalp diseases (Neth. Appl., 1965, 6405353; *CA*, 1966, **65**, 2074g); also for schirrhous, eruptions and oedematous tumours of throat; root and leaf decoct. for schirrhous tumours in hard uterus.

Plant—used for carcinomatous ulcers, myrmecia, acrochordon and cancer of genitals. A cataplasm preparation used for indurations in wounds and a plaster for indurations of viscera; juice used in the pastille preparation for condylomata of anus (*Lloydia*, 1969, **32**, 79); plant exts., less toxic (*Toxicol Eur Res*, 1978, **1**, 329; *CA*, 1980, **92**, 105200t).

Roots, leaves and fruits yield cucurbitacin mixt. containing cucurbitacin C, D, E, G, H & I, chromatogr. sepn.; leaves and roots, elasterol (*An R Soc Esp Fis Quim Ser B*, 1967, **63**, 959; 1123; *CA*, 1968, **68**, 6124u, 78485k); roots, allantoin (*Herba Hung*, 1969, **8**, 101; *CA*, 1970, **73**, 101980g).

Plant, di- & tetrahydroelasterol (*An Quim*, 1969, **65**, 1139; *CA*, 1970, **73**, 73798h); and also hydroquinone acetovanillone, 4-HOC$_6$H$_4$COMe, ligbalinol and 2-nitroquinol (*Tetrahedron*, 1974, **30**, 3309). All plant organs contain cucurbitacin B, D, E & I (*Egypt J Pharm Sci*, 1978, **19**, 253). Seasonal variations in sterol compn. of different parts (*Planta Med*, 1979, **37**, 37). Sepn. of elaterium (cath. drug) from plant juice; extn. of α-elaterin, elatericin A & B from elaterium (*Chim Acta Turc*, 1979, **7**, 57; *CA*, 1980, **92**, 185788d).

Fruit juice, cucurbitacins B, L & R, and derivs. (*J Chem Soc Perkin Trans I*, 1974, 2552). Fruit glycds. cucurbitacin B & D (*Pharmazie*, 1977, **32**, 605; *CA*, 1978, **88**, 86017n).

Pollen, kaempferol-3-O-rutinoside (major) and stigmas, rutin (*Experientia*, 1980, **36**, 1136).

ECBOLIUM (*Acanthaceae*)

E. viride (Forsk.) Alston syn. *E. linneanun* Kurz; *Justicia ecbolium* Linn.

Root and leaves used against tumours (*Lloydia*, 1967, **30**, 379). EtOH(50%) of plant, cardiovascular effects (*Indian J Exp Biol*, 1974, **12**, 512).

Leaves, flowers and roots yield, orientin, vitexin & their isoflavones (*Phytochemistry*, 1975, **14**, 1644).

ECHEVERIA (*Crassulaceae*)

*E. glauca Baker

Leaves contain a bactericidal substance; juice, isocitric, citric and succinic acids, Ca malate and Me-malic acid anhydride (Wlth India, III, 123).

Cultivated in Indian gardens.

ECHINOCHLOA (*Poaceae*)

*E. colonum Link syn. *Panicum colonum* Linn.

EtOH(50%) ext. of plant, diur. (*Indian J Exp Biol*, 1980, **18**, 594). Grains eaten in times of scarcity. Young shoots eaten (Wlth India, III, 124).

Cultivated throughout India up to 2,400m.

E. crus-galli (Linn.) Beauv. syn. *Panicum crus- galli* Linn.

Plant used against sore and carbuncle (*Econ Bot*, 1970, **24**, 241); and cancer (*Lloydia*, 1969, **32**, 153); estrogenic (*Indian Vet J*, 1974, **51**, 610).

ECHINOPS (*Asteraceae*)

E. echinatus Roxb.

EtOH(50%) ext. of plant, spasmog. (*Indian J Exp Biol*, 1969, **7**, 250).

Plant, hentriacontane, hentriacontanol, β-amyrin and lupeol (*J Indian Chem Soc*, 1968, **45**, 697); pharmacognosy (*Experientia*, 1980, **36**, 1136).

Seeds contain echinopsine (USSR Pat., 1968, 219748; *CA*, **68**, 99388s).

*E. niveus Wall.

Plant, alter., diur., nerve tonic, used in hysteria, dyspep. and ophthalmia (*Indian Drugs*, 1976-77, **14**, 47).

Garhwal Himalayas to Khasi hills up to 1,200 m.

ECHITES (*Apocynaceae*)

E. fragrans Moon; see Chonemorpha macrophylla

ECLIPTA (*Asteraceae*)

E. alba (Linn.) Hassk. syn. *E. prostrata* Roxb.

Herb—in skin diseases; leaves in boils (*J Agric Trop Bot Appl*, 1966,**13**, 247). Crude ext. of gum resin from herb, anticancerous against Ehrlich ascites carcinoma (*Annu Rep ICMR*, 1967-68, 64). EtOH(50%) ext., antivir. and spasmog. (*Indian J Exp Biol*, 1968, **6**, 232); pulp roasted in *ghee* and applied to wounds and burns; active against *E. coli* [*J Res Indian Med*, 1973, **8**(2), 67; 1974, **9**(2), 66]. Aq. ext., ovicidal against *Sitotroga cerealella* eggs and nematicidal (*Curr Sci*, 1979,**48**,1090). With black pepper and sugar taken twice daily for 15 days in body inflam. (*Bull Med Ethno Bot Res*, 1980, **1**, 318). Haemostatic (*Yakugaku Zasshi*, 1981, **101**, 501).

Useful in liver and gall-bladder ailments (*Acta Phytother*, 1970, **17**, 181); and leaf and root decoct. as liver tonic (*Bull Bot Surv India*, 1973,**15**, 13). Herb ext. protective against hepatotoxic action of carbon tetrachloride in female guineapigs (*Toxicol Appl Pharmacol*, 1978, **45**, 723). Powd. cured 100% patients suffering from infective hepatitis(*Curr Med Pract*, 1979, **23**, 237); taken with honey (50 mg/kg body wt.), completely cured children from jaundice in 1-5 weeks (*J Sci Res Plants Med*, 1981, **2**, 96). 'Tafroli', clin. trial, excellent drug for viral hepatitis (*Antiseptic*, 1980, **77**, 643).

Leaves—aq. ext. myocardial depress. and hypoten., unrelated to cholinergic and histaminergic effects [*J Res Indian Med*, 1976, **11**(3),91]. Juice used to cure shoulder pain caused by carrying heavy loads (*J Econ Tax Bot*, 1980, **1**, 137).

Chem. of *E. alba* and *Wedelia calandulacea* including pharmacol. details, rev., 16 refs. [*J Res Indian Med*, 1974, **9**(1), 9].

Leaves contain stigmasterol and α- terthienylmethanol (*Tetrahedron Lett*, 1966, 4227); small amt. of 2-formyl-terthienyl; wedelolactone, de-Me-wedelolactone & its 7-O-glucd. (*Indian J Chem*, 1970, **8**, 761; 664; 1972, **10**, 810). Aerial parts of Egyptian plant, β-amyrin, wedelolactone, luteolin-7-glucd., phytosterol A, its glucd., and glucd. of a triterp. acid (*Egypt Sci Pharm*, 1981, **49**, 262).

EDGEWORTHIA (*Thymelaeaceae*)

E. gardneri Meissn. syn. *E. tomentosa* Nakai

Stem bark, daphnoretin and a biscoumarin, edgeworthin (*Phytochemistry*, 1974, **13**, 1929).

EHRETIA (*Ehretiaceae*)

E. aspera Roxb. syn. *E. obtusifolia* Hochst. ex DC.

Leaves, new pyrrolizidine alk., ehretinine (*Phytochemistry*, 1980, **19**, 1273).

E. buxifolia Roxb.; see **Carmona retusa**

*E. laevis Roxb.

Plant used against syphilis (*Econ Bot*, 1970, **24**, 241).

Stem contains allantoin; leaves and roots, bauerenol (*Indian J Chem*, 1970, **8**, 851; 1971, **9**, 611).

Common in deciduous forests and in S. Andamans up to 900 m.

E. microphylla Lamk; see **Carmona retusa**

*E. wallichiana Hook. f. & Thoms.

Lepcha–*Kalet, non-kung*.

EtOH(50%) ext. of aerial parts, antileukemic (*Indian J Exp Biol*, 1980; **18**, 594).

Found in Eastern Himalayas and Assam hills up to 3,000 m.

EICHHORNIA (*Pontederiaceae*)

E. crassipes (Mart.) Solms-Laub.

Plant juice used internally for treatment of goitre alongwith poultice of plant pulp for three months [*Nagarjun*, 1974-75, **18**(2), 43].

Roots contain bound auxin (*Bull Bot Soc Bengal*, 1964, **18**, 87); pharmacognostic studies of root and rhizomes (*Bull Med Ethno Bot Res*, 1980, **1**, 37).

Plant releases Hg (*Org Geochem*, 1980, **2**, 99; *CA*, **92**, 194777b). Shoot ext. showed gibberellin-like activity (*Indian J Agric Sci*, 1973, **43**, 1). Leaves, chem. compn. (*Pak J Sci Res*, 1980, **32**, 115).

Pale purple flowers yield delphinidin-3-diglucd. (*Bot Mag*, 1965, **78**, 299). Flowers and rhizomes, quercetin, compesterol, β-sitosterol & stigmasterol [*J Res Indian Med*, 1976, **11**(3), 118].

ELAEAGNUS (*Elaeagnaceae*)

E. angustifolia Linn. syn. *E. hortensis* Bieb.

Aerial parts yield carboline alks. harman & tetrahydroharman (*Herba Pol*, 1967, **13**, 103; *CA*, 1968, **68**, 112163r); stem bark and roots, same alks.; polyphenols from leaves and bark (*Khim Prir Soedin*, 1970, **6**, 493; 765; *CA*, 1971, **74**, 1058q; 95420b); Extn. of alk. harman and harmol from different plant organs; root bark and aerial parts most suitable source of harman (*Gdansk Tow Nauk Rozpr Wydz*, 1971, No. 8, 137; *CA*, **75**, 126628c).

Flowers, fruits and leaves, flavons.; leaves, flavon. glycds. (*Farm Zh Kiev*, 1971, **26**, 56; *Pol J Pharmacol Pharm*, 1973, **25**, 599; *CA*, **75**, 95353c; 1974, **80**, 68408w).

E. conferta Roxb. syn. *E. latifolia* Linn.

EtOH(50%) ext.of aerial parts, spasmog. (*Indian J Exp Biol*, 1977, **15**, 208).

Stem, β-sitosterol (*Indian J Chem*, 1970, **8**, 851).

E. parvifolia Wall. ex Royle syn. *E. umbellata* auct. non Thunb.

Preliminary pharmacol. of plant ext. excluding roots (*Indian J Exp Biol*, 1971, **9**, 91); therapeutic preparation for athelete's foot containing MgO and EtOH ext. (Jpn Pat., 1977, 77117410; *CA*, 1978, **88**, 27826c).

ELAEIS (*Aracaceae*)

E. guineensis Jacq.

Oil used for tumours (*Lloydia*, 1970, **33**, 316). Fermented beverages from sap of *E. guineensis* and *Raphia*, rev., 30 refs. (*Tech Memo Niger Fed Inst Ind Res*, 1977, **29**, 13; *CA*, 1980, **92**, 109027q).

Campesterol, β-sitosterol, stigmasterol and other sterols from unsap. matter of oil from kernel and palm (*J Am Oil Chem Soc*, 1973, **50**, 122). Fatty acid compn. of fruit oil (*Oleagineux*, 1975, **30**, 401); seed oil, fatty acid and tocopherol pattern (*Fette Seifen Anstrichm*, 1976, **78**, 228; *CA*, **85**, 92378k). Soap prepared by saponification of oil with lye obtained from ashes of various woods, good antibact. (*Q J Crude Drug Res*, 1981, **19**, 183).

Pollen, lipid ext. *p*-OMe-allylbenzene in substantial amts. (*J Exp Bot*, 1975, **26**, 619); lipid and sterol compn. (*Phytochemistry*, 1975, **14**, 1023).

ELAEOCARPUS (*Elaeocarpaceae*)

E. floribundus Blume
Leaves, myricetin, myricitrin and mearnsetin (*Indian J Chem*, 1977, **15B**, 197).

E. serratus Linn. syn. *E. oblongus* Gaertn.
EtOH(50%) ext. of aerial parts, diur. and cardiovascular (*Indian J Exp Biol*, 1977, **15**, 208).
Leaves, myricetin, myricitrin, mearnsetin and ellagic acid (*Planta Med*, 1977, **32**, 197).

E. sphaericus K. Schum. syn. *E. ganitrus* Roxb.
EtOH(50%) ext. of stem bark, hypoglyc. (*Indian J Exp Biol*, 1968, **6**, 232). Aq. ext. of fruits, hypoten., sed., anticonvuls., spasmol., choleretic, bronchodialatory and cardiostim. (*Planta Med*, 1975, **28**, 174).
Leaves yield 7 isomeric alks.: *l-,d-epi-* & *d-* ψ-*epi*-isoelaeocarpiline, *d-* & *l-*elaeocarpiline,*l-*alloelaeocarpiline & *d-*epiadloelaeocarpiline (*J Chem Soc Chem Commun*, 1970, 804);elaeocarpidine, *dl-*élaeocarpine and other known alks. (*Aust J Chem*, 1971, **24**, 1679); quercetin, gallic and ellagic acids (*Planta Med*, 1977, **32**, 197); new alk., rudrakine (*Phytochemistry*, 1979, **18**, 700).

E. tuberculatus Roxb.
Leaves, quercetin, kaempferol, gallic acid & Et-gallate (*Planta Med*, 1977, **32**, 197).

ELAEODENDRON (*Celastraceae*)

See **CASSINE**

ELATOSTEMA (*Urticaceae*)

*****E. sessile** Forst.
Leaves used in abdominal disorders, in Malaysia (Wlth India, III, 142).
Assam hills and Nilgiris up to 2,400 m.

ELEOCHARIS (*Cyperaceae*)

*****E. dulcis** Trin. ex Hensch.
Eng.–*Chinese water chestnut*.

Tubers—juice, antibiot. against *Staphylococcus aureus, E. coli* and *Aerobacter aerogenes*; antibiot. principle, puchiin. Rich in starch (Wlth India, III, 142).
Found throughout India up to 900 m.

ELEPHANTOPUS (*Asteraceae*)

E. scaber Linn.
Roots—paste made into small pills given to children suffering from fever. Crushed roots, applied to cattle wounds; given to patients with heart and liver trouble (*Econ Bot*, 1965, **19**, 236; 1981, **35**, 4). Paste applied in rheum., and roots with mustard oil in amoebic dysen. (*J Econ Tax Bot*, 1980, **1**, 137). Roots also used to cure filariasis (*Bull Med Ethno Bot Res*, 1980, **1**, 318). EtOH(50%) ext. of plant, anticancer (*Indian J Exp Biol*, 1980, **18**, 594).
A germancranolide, elephantopin from *E. elatus* showed *in vivo* cytotoxicity (in Beal & Reinhard, 106, 109).

ELETTARIA (*Zingiberaceae*)

E. cardamomum Maton
Eng.–*Cardamom*.
Seeds—used in phthisis, broncht., asthma and consumption (*Econ Bot*, 1970, **24**, 241). Aq. ext. of crushed capsules given to breast-feeding mothers, children taking such milk free from ringworm; roasted seeds boiled with a piece of betel leaf,in indign. or worm trouble. Paste used as balm for headache; husk for rheum. [*Cardamom*, 1979, **11**(7), 23].
In Unani system, preparations used as antid., astrin., exhilarant, and in nausea [*East Pharm*, 1980, **23**(273), 39].
Minor constituent of 'Geriforte' (*Indian Drugs*,1980-81, **18**, 346; *Rajasthan Med J*, 1980, **19**, 23).
Essent. oil, antimicrob. [*East Pharm*, 1980, **23**(271), 113].
Essent. oil from Canada, constituents by gas chromatogr. (*J Pharm Sci*, 1965, **54**, 799); from India (*Perfum Essent Oil Rec*, 1966, **57**, 623). Production technology

(*Res Ind*, 1968, **13**, 623). Terps. their comparative distribution among varieties (*Phytochemistry*, 1971, **10**, 177); constituents of cardamom oil of wild plant from Sri Lanka, GLC detn. (*J Sci Food Agric*, 1979, **30**, 521).

Cardamom, bot. and chem. compn. (Parry, 23-26, 187-88); rev. covering all aspects (Purseglove *et al*, II, 581-643).

ELEUSINE (*Poaceae*)

E. aegyptica Desf.; see **Dactyloctenium aegyptium**

E. coracana Gaertn.

Used in measles, smallpox, pleur. and pneum. (*Econ Bot*, 1970, **24**, 241).

Seed coats of var. Co.7, constituents, of which 2 phenolic compds. inhibitory against 8 fungi, esp. *Helminthosporium oryzae* and *H. nodulosum* (*Labdev*, 1971, **9B**, 109); flavon. patterns in *ragi* and other *Eleusine* spp. (*Biochem Syst Ecol*, 1978, **6**, 247). α-Amylase inhibitors (*Indian J Biochem Biophys*, 1980, **17**, 181).

Plant, cyanogenic glucd., triglochinin (*Proc K Med Akad Wet Ser C*, 1977, **80**, 227). Ochratoxin A (*J Food Sci Technol*, 1979, **16**, 113).

E. scindica Duthie; see **Dactyloctenium scindicum**

ELYTRARIA (*Acanthaceae*)

*E. acaulis Lindau syn. *E. crenata* Vahl

Mar.–*Dasmori*.

In Africa, plant infusion used as cough remedy for infants. Leaf decoct. in V.D. (Wlth India, III, 167); also in fever. Roots used in mammary tumours and abscesses; root alongwith mother's milk in rickets, marasmus, pneum. and infantile diar. [*J Res Indian Med*, 1973, **8**(2), 67].

From Western Peninsula to Gangetic Plains.

EMBELIA (*Myrsinaceae*)

E. ribes Burm. f.

Plant—to cure pyorrhoea (*Madras Agric J*, 1960, **47**, 283); in cystic tumours; preparation in *ghee*, powd. bolmes and enemas used against abdominal tumours (*Lloydia*, 1970, **33**, 288); also more useful drug for tapeworm than male fern; EtOH ext., slightly active against *E. coli* [*J Res Indian Med*, 1974, **9**(2), 71; 65]. One of the constituents of 'Gasex', in abdominal discomforts; clin. results in post-operative gastro- intestinal symptoms (*Probe*, 1977-78, **17**, 330; 237; 1979-80, **19**, 277). Ayurvedic preparation, with equal parts of 5 drugs including *E. ribes*, anthelm. [*J Res Indian Med*, 1978, **13**(3), 130]. Aq. ext., nematicidal (*Indian J Entomol*, 1979, **41**, 326).

Constituent of a long-acting oral contracep., active principles of *E. ribes, Piper longum, Ferula asafoetida* and borax in 2:2:1:2 ratio; mixt., dose and mode of administration given; prevents conception for 1 yr without side effects (Brit. Pat., 1966, 1025372; *CA*, **64**, 19328h); also a mixt. containing dry exts. of *E. ribes*, among others (see *Abrus precatorius*) effective for 4 months (Brit. Pat., 1976, 1445599; *CA*, 1977, **86**, 21786b).

Fruit—cures dental, oral and throat trouble except ptyslism and cancer of lips (*Madras Agric J*, 1960, **47**, 283). Equal amts. of fruits of *E. ribes*, leaves of *Ficus religiosa* and borax with cow's milk, a quick aborticide (*Econ Bot*, 1980, **34**, 273).

Aq. ext. of fruit, antifert. activity [*J Res Indian Med*, 1971, **6**(2), 107]; powd. inhibits 62% fert. in female rats; powd. berries, given to male bonnet monkeys, at a rate 100 mg/day for 3 months adversely affected quant. and quality of semen; testasterone level reduced (*Indian J Exp Biol*, 1978, **16**, 1035; 1979, **17**, 935); ext. of berries, 62.5% resorptive in female albino rats at a dose of 150 mg/kg per day, +ve estrogenic effects of EtOH(50%) ext. on rat uterus at low dose of 75 mg/kg (*Probe*, 1977-78, **17**, 315; 1978-79, **18**, 178;267;

Planta Med, 1979, **35**, 370; **36**, 134; 369).
Aq. ext., hypoglyc. [*J Res Indian Med*, 1979, **14** (3 & 4), 159].

Aq. and EtOH ext. of fruit, anthelm. against earthworms [*Med Surg*, 1965, **5**(7), 6]. Drug composed of dry fruits of *E. ribes* among others, effective against hymenolepiasis (*Indian J Med Res*, 1970, **58**, 616). Fruit powd. (200 mg/kg) taken with curd on empty stomach expelled tapeworm (100%) within 6-24 hrs., also effective in giardia, clin. results (*Nagarjun*, 1979-80, **23**, 234).

Seeds—antibiot. and anti-T.B. (*Indian J Med Res*, 1961, **49**, 799); alter, stim., and anthelm. (*Q J Crude Drug Res*, 1970, **10**, 1555); 100% effective against common tapeworm of poultry, at a dose rate of 246 mg/kg (*Pak J Sci*, 1979, **31**, 218). EtOH(50%) ext., antifert. (66.6%) in a dose of 200 mg/kg body wt; spermic. and diur. (*Indian J Exp Biol*, 1976, **14**, 623; 1980, **18**, 594). Seeds alongwith *Hibiscus rosa-sinensis* flowers and *Ferula asafoetida* oleo-gum resin constituent of a herbal preparation 'Vidangadi Yoga', a very effective antifert. drug without side effects [*J Sci Res Plants Med*, 1980, 1(3-4), 41].

Roots—used as antifert. drug (*Q J Crude Drug Res*, 1972, **12**, 1922); powd. showed 100% antifert. activity in female albino rats at a dose, 100 mg/kg (*Indian J Exp Biol*, 1978, **16**, 1077).

Embelin—active principle (embelic acid, 2,5-di-OH-3-undecyl- 1, 4-benzoquinone) from berries; exhibits antiimplantation activity (83.33%) in female albino rats at doses of 60 & 120mg/kg (Dictionary Org. Compds., II, 2020; *Indian J Exp Biol*, 1975, **13**, 70); given orally, high antiovulatory effect in rabbits, nontoxic up to 3g/kg in rats; antiestrogenic in immature female rats at 120mg/kg [*J Res Indian Med*, 1976, **11**(4), 84; 1974, **11**(3), 115]; devoid of antifert. activity (*Indian J Exp Biol*, 1978, **16**, 1035); devoid of estrogenic or antiestrogenic activity; isolation from seeds

and antifert. activity at 100 mg/kg in rats (*ibid*, 1980, **18**, 638; 1359).

Disalts of embelin, anthelm. (*Indian J Exp Biol*, 1976, **14**, 356). Amino salts, greater narcotic analg. with less side effects than embelin. Di-isobutyl amino deriv. (2.5-5mg/kg i.v. or 5-10 mg/kg i.p.) lasted 3-4 hrs. in dogs and 6-10 hrs. in cats accompanied by sedation, also had antiinflam., hypoten., antipyr. and anthelm. properties (Neth. Appl., 1977, 7510536; *CA*, 1978, **88**, 55075a).

Embelin, isolation, mass spectrum and PMR (*J Chem Soc Perkin Trans I*, 1975, 327); extn. from berries with EtOH and TLC sepn. (Indian Pat., 1978, 144370; *CA*, 1980, **92**, 82417c).

E. tsjeriam-cottom DC. syn. *E. robusta* C.B. Clarke non Roxb.

Plant—used in weak pulse rate, ulcer, sores, carbuncle, gravel, cholera, neuralgia, pleur., pneum., diar., and complaints during pregnancy (*Econ Bot*, 1970, **24**, 241). EtOH(50%) ext. of aerial parts, slightly hypoten. (*Indian J Exp Biol*, 1969, **7**, 250).

Fruit—ext., anthelm. and antibact. [*J Res Indian Med*, 1979, **14**(1), 68]; powd. useful in dysen. (*Nagarjun*, 1980- 81, **24**, 1).

Stem contains embelin; see *E. ribes* (*Indian J Chem*, 1977, **15**, 291).

*E. viridiflora Scheff.

EtOH(50%) ext. of aerial parts, diur., antinflam. and semen coagulant (*Indian J Exp Biol*, 1977, **15**, 208).

Western Peninsula up to 1,500 m.

EMBLICA (*Euphorbiaceae*)

E. officinalis Gaertn. syn. *Phyllanthus emblica* Linn.

Eng.–*Indian gooseberry.*

Fruit—pronounced expect. (*J Sci Ind Res*, 1960, **19C**, 60); anticancerous properties (*Chem Pharm Bull*, 1965, **13**, 882); fruit, juice and its sediment, and residue, antioxidant due to gallic acid (*Pak J Sci Res*, 1966, **18**, 61). EtOH(50%) ext., antivir. (*Indian J Exp Biol*, 1968, **6**, 232); carmin. and stomch.(*Q J Crude Drug Res*, 1970, **10**, 1555). Juice with turmeric powd. and honey said to cure diabetes insipidus (*Acta Phytother*, 1972, **19**, 141). Aq. ext. increases cardiac glycogen level and decreases serum GOT, GPT and LDH in rats having induced myocardial necrosis(*Indian J Exp Biol*, 1977, **15**, 485). In Ayurveda, as cardiotonic, aphordis., antipyr., antidiabetic, cerebral and gastrointestinal tonic (*J Nat Integ Med Assoc*, 1978, **20**, 69); hypoglyc. [*J Res Indian Med*, 1979, **14** (3&4), 159]; aq. ext., mixed with fruits of *Terminalia chebula* and *T. bellirica* or *'Triphala'* used in constip. (*Bull Med Ethno Bot Res*, 1980, **1**, 318).

Juice in *ghee*, powd. and anemas used for abdominal and glandular tumours, and in cancer. Fruit preparation in induration of liver; in collyrium used in warts of eyes (*Lloydia*, 1969, **32**, 169); a constituent of the drug *'SG-1 Switradilepa'* used against vitiligo; and also of an Ayurvedic preparation used for polycythaemia [*J Res Indian Med*, 1976, **11**(2), 66; **11**(1), 117]; decoct. of powd. pericarp cures chr. peptic ulcer [*ibid*, 1977, **12**(4), 1]; minor ingredient of Ayurvedic drug *'Arogya Wardhani'* used in acute viral hepatitis; hypocholesteraemic, useful in ischaemic heart diseases and in preventing premature atherosclerosis, clin. trials (*Indian J Med Res*, 1980, **72**, 588; *J Res Ayur Sidha*, 1980, **1**, 121); and of an antibiot. drug 'Septilin', clin. trials, in exodontia, useful drug; against chr. suppurativa otitis media (*Probe*, 1979-80, **19**, 125, 276; 1980-81, **20**, 297). *Amlaki* and its pharmaceutical compns. (*Sachitra Ayurveda*, 1981-82, **34**, 118).

Plant—various plant parts used in toothache, fever, anaemia, epilepsy, sores, pimples, tubercular fistula, gonor., gravel, cholera, sterility in women, anthrax, rinder pest and convuls. (*Econ Bot*, 1970, **24**, 241).

Fresh roots as remedy for jaundice (*Acta Phytother*, 1972, **19**, 141). Leaf ext., antibact. (*Indian Drugs*, 1979-80, **17**, 148).

Fruits and leaves, tannins; polyphenolic compds.1,3,6- trigalloylglucose, terchebin, corialgin and ellagic acid (*Leath Sci*, 1965, **12**, 327; 1967, **14**, 16; 1968, **15**, 337); also alks., phyllantidine and phyllantine (*Indian J Exp Biol*, 1975, **13**, 82).

Leaves and stems yield lupeol and β-sitosterol (*Aust J Chem*, 1968, **21**,2137). Phyllemblin, antimicrob. substance from suspension cultures [*Bangladesh Pharm J*, 1974, 3(2), 15].

Roots, ellagic acid (*Indian J Chem*, 1977, **15B**, 291).

EMEX (*Polygonaceae*)

*****E. spinosa** Campd. syn.*Rumex spinsosus* Linn.

Rajasthan–*Khato-palak*.

Leaves—Decoct. used as a tonic and for indign.(Uphof, 198); in large doses, for intestinal troubles of cattle and horse (SEPASAT, 140).

Arid and semi-arid regions of India.

EMILIA (*Asteraceae*)

Genus yields hepatotoxic pyrrolizidine alks. (*J Natl Prod*, 1981, **44**, 129-52).

E. javanica C.B. Robinson syn. *E. flammea* Cass.; *E. sagittata* DC.

Pyrrolizidine alks.: 4 in flowers, 5 in leaves, and 7 in aerial parts & 7 in roots. All parts except leaves contain othosenine (*Diss Pharm Pharmacol*, 1969, **21**, 433; *CA*, 1970, **72**, 51772x).

Emiline— isolation of alk. from plant, and str. (*ibid*, 1971, **23**, 419; *CA*, 1972, **76**, 96972m). Alk. stimulated yeast grown in low concentration $(10^{-6}$mole/ml); antimicotic in *Allium* (*Pol J Pharmacol Pharm*, 1973, **25**, 293; *CA*, **79**, 83423v); pharmacol. (Pol Pat. 1975, 74735; *CA*, 1976, **84**, 122107v). Its keto esters from aerial parts (*Phytochemistry*, 1978, **17**, 557).

E. sonchifolia (Linn.) DC.

Plant used for otitis media suppurativa (*Econ Bot*, 1970, **24**, 241). Root juice alongwith water and common salt used to cure redness of eye and cataract (*Bull Bot Surv. India*, 1976, **18**, 247). Aq. ext. of plant, weak antimicrob.

EtOH ext. of aerial parts, triacontane, *n*-hexacosanol, ursolic acid and flavons. including rutin (*Fitoterapia*, 1980, **51**, 241).

ENGELHARDIA (*Juglandaceae*)

*E. acerifolia Blume

EtOH(50%) ext. of aerial parts, spasmog. (*Indian J Exp Biol*, 1973, **11**, 43).

Sikkim, and Khasi hills up to 1,500 m.

*E. colebrookiana Lindl.

P.–*Timarrakh*; Ass.–*Pasomasi*; Kumaun–*Goparmowa*.

EtOH(50%) ext. of stem bark, cardiovascular, and antivir. (*Indian J Exp Biol*, 1971, **9**, 91).

Throughout outer Himalayas and Assam.

ENHYDRA (*Asteraceae*)

See **ENYDRA**

ENICOSTEMMA (*Gentianaceae*)

E. hyssopifolium (Willd.) Verdoon syn. *E. littorale* Blume

H.–*Chota-chirayata*; Tam.–*Vellarai*.

Crushed plant with water taken as restor. (*J Agric Trop Bot Appl*, 1966, **13**, 247); also as carmin. [*J Indian Res Med*, 1973, **8**(2), 67]. Useful against diabetes [*ibid*, 1975, **10**(4), 141; 1979, **14**(3-4), 63]. Leaf ext., fungistatic (*Sci Cult*, 1977, **43**, 437). Plant decoct., in fever and snakebite (*J Econ Tax Bot*, 1980, **1**, 137).

EtOH ext. and essent. oil obtained by steam distillation of alc. ext., slightly antibact. (*Planta Med*, 1972, **22**, 42).

Aerial parts, chloroform. sol., 4 alks. and a sterol, and w.- sol., an alk. and a sterol; chloroform-sol. alks., active depress. and weak antimal. Plant yields lactonic enamino ketone, gentiocrucine; a

mixt. of two compds. (*Tetrahedron Lett*, 1974, 403). Isolation and phylogenetic significance of erythrocentaurine and related monoterp. alks. in plant (*J Pharm Sci*, 1974, **63**, 944); and a monoterp. alk. enicoflavine (*Chem Ind Lond*, 1975, 127).

EtOH ext. of plant yields swertiamarin and betulin (*Curr Sci*, 1966, **35**, 148). Plant contains a hypoten. glycd. swertisioside (*Indian J Pharm*, 1976, **38**, 167); apigenin, genkwanin, isovitexin, swertisin, saponarin, and 5-O-glucd. derivs. of sylswertisin and isoswertisin (*J Pharm Sci*, 1980, **69**, 53).

ENTADA (*Mimosaceae*)

E. pursaetha DC. syn. *E. phaseoloides* Merrill; *E. scandens* Benth.

Used in dropsy, anasarca, cancer, pain in loins, epilepsy, constip. and rinderpest (*Econ Bot*, 1970, **41**, 241). Seeds, raw or roasted, as oral contracep. (*Planta Med*, 1973, **23**, 167).

Entanin—antitumour seed saponin; inhibits (64-100%) Walker 256 tumours in rats without deaths (US Pat. 1972, 3641243; *CA*, **76**, 131474z); on hydrolysis, saponin yields entagenic acid (*Phytochemistry*, 1972, **11**, 171); prosapogenin A and lupeol; former hydrolyses to entagenic acid(*Indian J Pharm*, 1975, **37**, 67). Process of extn. of the triterp. glycd. from kernels (Indian Pat., 1976, 140384; *CA*, 1980, **92**, 107612c).

Kernels, oleanolic and echinocytic acids and Me-mercaptan (*J Indian Chem Soc*, 1972, **49**, 1199). Seeds, tyrosine glucd. and dopamine glucd. (*Phytochemistry*, 1973, **12**, 2243). Pericarp, β-sitosterol, α-amyrin, quercetin, cyanidin chloride and gallic acid (*Curr Sci*, 1974, **43**, 81).

ENYDRA (*Asteraceae*)

E. fluctuans Lour. syn. *Enhydra fluctuans* Lour.

Plant used in ascites, dropsy, anasarca, *phoka nagri ghao* and snakebite (*Econ Bot*, 1970, **24**, 241).

Plant yields a new germacranolide (sesquiterp. lactone) enhydrin; str. revision & chem.; confirmation by X-ray (*Curr Sci*, 1968, **37**, 94; 1969, **38**, 284; 1971, **40**, 167; *Indian J Chem*, 1972, **10**, 771; 249; *J Chem Soc Chem Commun*, 1972, 1327); also 2 sesquiterp. lactones fluctuanin and gluctuadin (*Tetrahedron*, 1972, **28**, 2285).

Plant, diterp. acids, kaurenoic; *l*-16 α-OH- kauranoic; 15 α-OH-*l*-kaur-16-en-19-oic & its isovalerate and angelate derivs.; 17-OH-α-kaur- 15-en-19-oic acid (*Curr Sci*, 1969, **38**, 284; *Indian J Chem*, 1970, **8**, 375; 569; 1971, **9**, 84; 1116; *J Indian Chem Soc*, 1974, **51**, 409).

Plant, myricyl alc., *l*-kaur-16-ol, stigmasterol and two unidentified compds.; cholesterol and sitosterol glucd. (*Phytochemistry*, 1970, **9**, 459; 1975, **14**, 1663).

Stigmasta-5,22,25-triene-3β-ol (in leaves) (*Tetrahedron Lett*, 1971, 365); 3 steroids (*J Indian Chem Soc*, 1974, **51**, 419).

Contains gibberellins A_9 & A_{13} (*Phytochemistry*, 1972, **11**, 3433).

EPALTES (*Asteraceae*)

*E. divaricata Cass.

Roots, bitter; used as astrin. tonic (Wlth India, III, 177).

Peninsular India.

EPHEDRA (*Ephedraceae*)

*E. equisetina Bunge

Twigs, aq. or MeOH ext. showed vit. P activity in male rats, equivalent to an ext. from tea leaves (*Rastit Resur*, 1966, **2**, 213; *CA*, **65**, 16789g).

Plant contains alks., 0.3-3.3% (*Bot Zh*, 1964, **49**, 1785; *CA*, 1965, **62**, 9455e). Herb (from Japan), alk. ephedroxane, an antiinflam. principle (*Phytochemistry* 1979, **18**, 697).

A compn. containing plant leucodelphinidin active against tumour growth in white mice, compd. had low toxicity and did not affect peripheral circulation (*Vopr Onkol*, 1966, **12**, 61). Extn. of leukoephdin(leucodelphinidin) and ephedin (a colorant); former had vitamin P activity (*Med Promst SSSR*, 1966, **20**, 27; *CA*, **65**, 19058c); 10 flavons. (*Khim Prir Soedin*, 1976, 543; *CA*, **85**, 189195m).

Reported to occur in India.

E. gerardiana Wall. ex Stapf syn. *E. vulgaris* Hook. f. non A. Rich.

Powd. stem used as snuff for headache (*Khadi Gramodyog*, 1972-73, **19**, 269). Plant used in broncht.; together with leaf powd. of *Rhododendron*, used in hydrocele, weakness and palpitation of heart (*Nagarjun*, 1978-79, **22**, 190).

Leaves contain glucaric acid (*Z Pflanzenphysiol*, 1970, **62**, 116). Plant, ephedroxane, an antiinflam. principle (*Phytochemistry*, 1979, **18**, 697). Tissues grown on medium containing kinetin (0.5mg/1) and Indole butyric acid (10 mg/1) yield max. ephedrine (0.3%); ephedrine production from callus cultures (*Indian J Exp Biol*, 1979, **17**, 227; *Phytochemistry*, 1979, **18**, 484).

E. intermedia Schrenk & Mey.

Shoots of wild plant from USSR contain alk. 0.83-1.35%; ephedrine, major (*Bot Zh*, 1964, **49**, 1785; *CA*, 1965, **62**, 9455e); alk. (1.34%) from dried shoots, ephedrine, 0.93% (*Rastit Resur*, 1973, **9**, 57; *CA*, **78**, 121283p). Aerial parts yield antiinflam. principle, ephedroxane and ψ-ephedrine (*Phytochemistry*, 1979, **18**, 697; *Chem Pharm Bull*, 1980, **28**, 2900).

E. major Host syn. *E. nebrodensis* Tineo

Aerial parts yield alk. (0.36%) with 1-N-Me-ephedrine and d- ψ-ephedrine (78% of total) (*Ankara Univ Eczecilik Fak Mecm*, 1978, **8**, 101; *CA*, 1981, **94**, 61710w).

Ephedrine & ψ-ephedrine—active principles of *Ephedra* spp.; alks. belonging to Ph-Et-amine group, closely related to epinephrine (adrenaline); extn., pharmacol. and uses (Sim, 163-66). Most commonly encountered pure compds. from higher plants, but totally synthesised (*in* Wagner & Wolff, 3). An antiallergic, bacteriostatic sol. for external treatment of respiratory tract contains sulphanilamide, 0.4; ephedrine-HCl, 1.0g; etc. (Fr. 1964, M2416; *CA*, **61**, 9366f). Antiinflam. compns. effective in treatment of local inflam.in ophthalmology, otorhinolaryngology, gynaecology and dermatology (Belg. Pat. 1963, 624834; *CA*, 1964, **61**, 13135h). It is analg., ED50, 31.5 μ g in mice (*Yao Hsueh Hsueh Pao*, 1965, **12**, 758; *CA*, 1966, **64**, 14555g). Relation between dose and its effect, in bronch. obstruction and others, clin. study (*Klin Med*, 1967, **45**, 34; *CA*, **67**, 31176z). Ephedrine decreases thirst and increases diuresis during repeated s.c, injections in rats; nucleus cells are saturated with antidiur., neurosecretory substance [*Fiziol Zh SSSR*, 1967, **53**, 1439; *CA*, 1968, **68**, 38022a; *Dokl Akad Nauk Usb SSR*, 1968, **25**(3), 47]; weak CNS depress. in cats (*Jpn J Pharmacol*, 1968, **18**, 48; *CA*, **68**, 94543h). Vasomotory action of ephedrines (optical isomers) produced hyperten. in rats (*Arch Int Pharmacodyn Ther*, 1968, **174**, 233; *CA*, **69**, 104879j); isomers, anoretic in mice, significantly reduced their food intake without being CNS stim.; *d*-ephedrine most active [*Life Sci*, 1968, **7**(Pt.1), 665]. Bronchodilator activity of ephedrine and its ψ-deriv. & their salts, compn. of tablets for oral use (Brit. Pat., 1968, 110397; *CA*, **69**, 5201a). Local application of 2% sol. useful in nasal congestion (*Ocolaryngol Pol*, 1968, **22**, 695; *CA*, 1969, **70**, 46119u); in exudate-induced oedema in rat paw (*C R Soc Biol*, 1970, **164**, 773; *CA*, 1971, **74**, 74991h).

***E. penducularis** Boiss. syn. *E. foliata* Boiss. & Kotschy var. *ciliata* (Mey.) Stapf

Aq. ext. of leaves, weak antifung. (*Proc Nat Acad Sci India*, 1972, **42**, 300).

Stem and tissue culture, ψ-ephedrine (*Indian J Pharm*, 1976, **38**, 140); effect of light on ephedrine content in callus tissue; max. ephedrine in tissue grown under red light (0.35%) (*Indian Drugs*, 1979-80, **17**, 392).

Plains of S. Punjab and Rajasthan.

EPHEMERANTHA (*Orchidaceae*)

E. macraei Hunt & Summerh. syn. *E. fimbriatum* auct. non Blume; *Dendrobium macraei* Lindl.; *Desmotrichum fimbriatum* Blume

In Ayurvedic system, as cure of disorders of *vata, pitta* and *kapha*; used as tonic in debility caused by seminal discharges. As an alter., astrin. to bowels, expect. and useful in asthma, broncht. and throat trouble. Pharmacognosy (*Bull Bot Surv India*, 1970, **12**, 29).

EPILOBIUM (*Onagraceae*)

E. angustifolium Linn.

Woolly pappus of seed, mixed with eagle down and catfish oil applied to wounds made when tumours are cut open (*Econ Bot*, 1973, **27**, 287).

Leaves contain oleanolic, maslinic, ursolic and 2-OH-ursolic acids (*J Chem Soc C*, 1967, 510).

Flowers, w.-sol. polymer chanerol, which inhibits growth of transplantable tumours (sarcoma 37 and adenocarcinoma 755) in mice (ip or iv up to 5-20 mg/k at 48 hrs intervals), LD50 20 mg/kg (*Antibiotiki Moscow*, 1970, **15**, 782). An antitumoral haemagglutinin from inflorescence ext. (USSR Pat., 1974, 396040; *CA*, **81**, 140866j).

E. hirsutum Linn.

Plant and sap used against warts (*Lloydia*, 1970, **33**, 288).

Aerial parts yield protocatechuic, gallic and 3-OMe-gallic acids and hyperoside; flavons. (*Khim Prir Soedin*, 1975, **11**, 281; 1976, **12**, 540; 1979, **15**, 731; *CA*, **83**, 93865n; **85**, 174269q; 1981, **94**, 80218f). Tannin, also a new acid, isovalonic acid.

Leaves and flowers, oleanolic, cratoegolic, arjunolic, tormentic, 23-OH-tormentic acids, etc. (*An Quim*, 1979, **75**, 135; *CA*, **91**, 57219m).

12 Polyphenolic compds., 3 aglycones, 3 acids, 5 glycds. and a tannin of ellagitannin type (*Khim Khim Tekhnol Alma-Atta*, 1977, **22**, 99; *CA*, 1980, **92**, 90957u).

EQUISETUM (*Equisetaceae*)

E. arvense Linn.
Eng.–*Horsetail.*

Plant—decoct. used for nasal polypus, and various cancers of breast, liver, intestines, stomach, kidneys and tongue; poultice for cancerous ulcers, and wash for tumours and plant for cancerous lesions of bones (*Lloydia*, 1969, **32**, 153); carcinogenicity of some edible plants (*Gann*, 1972, **63**, 383); in USSR, plant to treat lupus [*Farm Zh Kiev*, 1972, **27**(6), 78; *BA*, 1973, **56**, 56516].

Dried green shoots, diur. (only in diseased conditions); haemostatic for internal haemor. (doubtful), strengthening lungs (effect of silicic acid still uncertain); cicatrization of wounds slow to heal (Med. Plants, 26).

Plant polyphenol: polyphenolic acids, caffeic major; green parts, several flavons. (*Khim Prir Soedin*, 1975, 416; 424; 1974, 666; 794; 1978, 508; 807; 1980, 413; 499; *CA*, 1976, **84**, 40719g; 2236q; 1975, **82**, 108840f; 121650p; **89**, 211930d; 1979, **90**, 200280m; **93**, 164324c; 200980b). Stems, Me esters of protocatechuic and caffeic acids (*Khim Prir Soedin*, 1981, 658).

Plant lipids contain triacontanedioic (equisetolic) and octacosanedioic acids; rhodoxanthin (*J Chem Soc D*, 1969, 456; *Phytochemistry*, 1971, **10**, 1885; 1972, **11**, 2801; 1977, **16**, 612). Extn. of silicon compds. from herb (*Planta Med*, 1975, **27**, 145); and protogenkwanin-4'-glucd. and gossypitrin from sprouts (*Tetrahedron*, 1981, **37**, 377).

ERANTHEMUM (*Acanthaceae*)

*E. purpureum Wight ex Nees
EtOH(50%) ext. spasmog., diur. and spermic. (*Indian J Exp Biol*, 1980, **18**, 594).

Kheri, U.P.

E. roseum R. Br.syn. *Daedalacanthus roseus* T. Anders.
EtOH(50%) ext. of stem, preliminary pharmacol. (*Indian J Exp Biol*, 1980, **18**, 594).

ERECHTITES (*Asteraceae*)

*E. valerianaefolia DC.
B.–*Bung-fung.*

EtOH(50%) ext. of plant, spasmog. (*Indian J Exp Biol*, 1969, **7**, 250). Essent. oil from leaves and flowering heads inhibitory to *Bacillus* spp.

Essent. oil, α- & β-pinene, myrcene, limonene and caryophyllene as major constituents and humulene; leaves and flowers, yield β -sitosterol and 14 alkanes (*Ann Farm Quim Sao Paulo*, 1979, **19**, 259; 1977, **17**, 43; *CA*, 1981, **94**, 61738j; 1978, **89**, 3146a).

Found in Darjeeling, W. Bengal.

EREMURUS (*Liliaceae*)

*E. himalaicus Baker
Eng.–*Himalayan desert candle.*

Fresh roots, galact. (*Sachitra Ayurveda*, 1977-78, **30**, 937).

Roots, hordenine (*Indian J Chem*, 1976, **14B**, 475).

Found in temperate Himalayas.

ERIA (*Orchidaceae*)

*E. muscicola Lindl.
A preparation with butter used for nasal polypus (*Lloydia*, 1970, **33**, 288).

Khasi hills, in Meghalaya.

ERIGERON (*Asteraceae*)

E. asteroides Roxb.
EtOH(50%) ext. of plant, spermic. (*Indian J Exp Biol*, 1980, **18**, 594).

E. canadensis Linn.
Aq. ext. of plant powd. produces fall in B.P., depresses heart and increases respiration in animals (*Indian J Pharm*, 1973, **35**, 62). Preliminary pharmacol. (*Indian J Exp Biol*, 1977, **15**, 208).

Leaves and stems contain o-benzylbenzoic acid (Recl Trav Chim Pays-Bas, 1969, **88**, 1332). Aerial parts, an unstable cumulene (Tetrahedron Lett, 1970, 2465).

E. floribundus Sch.-Bip. syn. E. linifolius Willd.; E. sumatrensis Retz.

Essent. oil, fungitoxic (Geobios, 1978, **22**, 11); contains d-limonene, 24; thujone, 13; isoeugenol, 26; Me- isoeugenol, 8; eugenol, 6; & eugenol-OAc, 11% (Indian Perfum, 1978, **22**, 11).

Plant repellent against sea snail; active principle a lachnophyllum lactone with a median effective concentration of 0.9μg/cm^2 (Agric Biol Chem, 1978, **42**, 1491; 1979, **43**, 1603).

*E. multiradiatus Benth.

EtOH(50%) ext. of plant, spasmog. (Indian J Exp Biol, 1973, **11**, 43).

Sikkim Himalayas.

ERIOBOTRYA (Rosaceae)

E. japonica (Thunb.) Lindl.

Bark, aq. ext. mild inhibitory against stains of watermelon mosaic virus (Curr Sci, 1976, **45**, 696); leaf ext., antifung. against Ustilago tritici (Acta Bot Indica, 1979, **7**, 147).

EtOH(50%) ext. of aerial parts, preliminary pharmacol. (Indian J Exp Biol, 1977, **15**, 208).

Cotyledon and seed coat of mature seeds yield caffeic acid, chlorogenic acid, its iso- & neo-acids, d-catechin, etc. (Shizuoka Daigaku Nogakubu Kenkyu Hokoku, 1969, No. 19, 138; CA, 1971, **75**, 16138k). Seed, trans-4-OH-Me- D-proline and 4-methylene-DL-proline (Phytochemistry, 1972, **11**, 751, 745).

Plant, rutin and caffeic acid (Pak J Biochem, 1975, **8**, 9; CA, 1976, **85**, 190992a). Stems and leaves, quercetin-3-O-galactoside (Agric Biol Chem, 1979, **43**, 657). Fruit pulp, new glycd. of eucocyanin, loquatoside (Planta Med, 1980, **38**, 277). Leaves, sorbitol-6-phosphate dehydrogenase (Plant Physiol, 1981, **67**, 221).

ERIODENDRON (Bombacaceae)

See **CEIBA**

ERIOGLOSSUM (Sapindaceae)

See **LEPISANTHES**

ERIOLAENA (Sterculiaceae)

*E. hookeriana Wight & Arn.

Bihar–Bundum, ganguli; Kan.–Dandiyase; Oriya–Bonohandi; Tam.–Paruduppai; Tel.–Narubotuku.

Root poultice heals wounds [J Res Indian Med, 1973, **8**(2), 67].

Stem yields β-sitosterol, lupeol, α-amyrin & its -OAc (Indian J Pharm, 1977, **39**, 17). Leaves, kaempferol-3-O-galactoside (Indian J Chem, 1980, **19B**, 821).

Seed oil, malvalic 25.8 and sterculic acid 6.0% (Chem Phys Lipids, 1979, **25**, 29; CA, 1980, **92**, 55071d).

Almost throughout India.

E. quinquelocularis Wight

EtOH(50%) ext. of aerial parts, semen coagulant and diur. (Indian J Exp Biol, 1977, **15**, 208).

Bark contains taraxerone (Indian J Chem, 1976, **14B**, 473).

ERIOSEMA (Fabaceae)

*E. himalaicum Ohashi syn. E. chinense Baker non Vog.

Ass.–Soh-pen; Santal–Konden.

Plant used in sores and syphilitic ulcer (Econ Bot, 1970, **24**, 241). Cortex, also in med. (Wlth India, III, 189).

From Himalayas and Assam hills.

ERODIUM (Geraniaceae)

E. cicutarium L'Herit. ex Ait.

Petals yield 3-glucds. of malvidin, peonidin, cyanidin; 3,5- diglucds. of malvidin and petunidin; and cyanidin 3-rutinoside (An Asoc Quim Argent, 1978, **66**, 107; CA, 1980, **92**, 72665t).

ERUCA (*Brassicaceae*)

E. vesicaria (Linn.) Cav. syn. *E. sativa* Mill.

Seeds—powd., antibact.; oily benzene ext. of residue (fatty oil), antibact. against *Shigella dysenteriae* and *S. flexneri*, unsap. fraction of fatty oil, a phytosterol (*Bull RRL Jammu*, 1963, **1**, 197). Ext. agglutinated human red cells without specificity to any particular group (*J Chem UAR*, 1963, **6**, 191).

A compn. used in induration of liver (*Lloydia*, 1969, **32**, 79). Crude juice of plant inhibited *E. coli, S. typhi* and *B. subtlis* (*Qual Plant Mater Veg*, 1972, **22**, 29).

Seed, (4-Me-thio)-Bu-glucosinolate (glucoerucin) as K and tetra-Me-N salts (*Arch Pharm Wein*, 1970, **303**, 330; *CA*, **73**, 28824c); glucoerucin also from whole plant (*Phytochemistry*, 1976, **15**, 759).

Leaves, isorhamnetin & its 3-glucd. (*J Indian Chem Soc*, 1969, **46**, 286).

ERVATAMIA (*Apocynaceae*)

E. coronaria Stapf; see **Tabernaemontana divaricata**

E. dichotoma Blatter syn. *Tabernaemontana dichotoma* Roxb.

Root bark, voacristine OH-indolenine (*J Org Chem*, 1968, **33**, 1225).

E. heyneana T. Cooke syn. *Tabernaemontana heyneana* Wall.

EtOH(50%) ext. of aerial parts, preliminary pharmacol. Exts. from root, stem and leaves, anticancer against P 388 lymphocytic leukemia; root and stem ext. also active against L 1210 lymphocytic leukemia. MeOH ext. of leaves antitumour against B-16 melanoma in mice (*Indian J Exp Biol*, 1973, **11**, 43; 1971, **9**, 268; 1979, **17**, 212). A sub-line of P 388 leukemia, cross-resistant, *in vivo*, to crude ext. from plant (*Cancer Treat Rep*, 1978, **62**, 1535; *CA*, 1979, **90**, 162055g).

Whole plant including roots, contains alk., coronaridine (*Indian J Chem*, 1966, **4**, 332; 457); fruit, lupeol-OAc and β-amyrin-OAc (*ibid*, 1971, **9**, 611); fleshy skin, 3 alks.

including heyneanine and coronaridine (*J Inst Chem India*, 1971, **43**, 69).

Root alks. coronaridine, its 19-oxo deriv., voacangine, ψ-indoxyl voacangine, and ibogamine (*J Pharm Sci*, 1973, **62**, 1199).

Leaves, alk. isovoacristine; its HCl, anticholinergic, antihistaminic, etc. (*Indian J Chem*, 1979, **17B**, 414).

Wood and stem bark yield biogenetically active campotthecine and its 9-OMe deriv. (*J Natl Prod*, 1979, **42**, 475); 14 indole alks. and 3 triterps.; 6 alks., camptothecine, its 9-OMe deriv., coronaridine, pericalline, heyneatine and 10-OMe-eglandine-N- oxide, cytotoxic against P388 lymphocytic leukemia (*Phytochemistry*, 1980, **19**, 1213).

Coronoridine—alk. present in all parts of the plant (*Indian J Chem*, 1966 **4**, 332); as HCl, its oral administration prevented pregnancy in rats; compd., estrogenic (*Planta Med*, 1978, **33**, 345); also cytotoxic against P 388 lymphocytic leukemia (*Phytochemistry*, 1980, **19**, 1213).

Camptothecine—characterized by a peculiar indolizidinoquinoline skeleton, earlier isolated from *Camptotheca acuminata* and *Mappia foetida*; marked cytotoxic properties but highly toxic [*Chem Rev*, 1973, **73**, 385; *J Pharm Sci*, 1974, **63**, 163; *Cancer Chemother Rep*, 1974, **5**(Pt. 3), 25]. It is widely used in China in treatment of various forms of cancer. Failure of camptothecine to proceed to clin. evaluation must be reevaluated. Alternative formulation with aim of drug availability appears to be appropriate and efforts made with salts of acronycine from *Acronychia baueri* may be relevant for this alk. as well (*in* Wagner & Wolff, 67-68; 118-19); str.-activity relationship; one of the few alks. showing consistent high activity in resistant L1210 form; also great activity in inhibition of growth of solid tumours in animals; its analogues (*in* Beal & Reinhard, 125-39); synth. (*J Org Chem*, 1976, **41**, 699).

ERVUM (*Fabaceae*)

See LENS

ERYCIBE (*Convolvulaceae*)

E. paniculata Roxb.

EtOH(50%) ext. of aerial parts, diur. and hypoten. (*Indian J Exp Biol*, 1974, **12**, 512). Ripe fruit eaten in constip. Pounded root, given internally, cures fever (*Nagarjun*, 1980-81, **24**, 1).

ERYNGIUM (*Apiaceae*)

E. biebersteinianum Nevski ex Babrov. syn. *E. caeruleum* Bieb.

Leaves and flowers contain *d*-mannitol (*Khim Prir Soedin*, 1969, **5**, 590; *CA*, 1970, **73**, 73824p). Underground parts yield saponin mixt.; aglycone, barringenol R_1 and barringenol A_1 (*ibid*, 1971, **7**, 843; *CA*, 1972, **76**, 110304d).

E. foetidum Linn.

EtOH(50%) ext. of plant, diur. (*Indian J Exp Biol*, 1980, **18**, 594).

ERYSIMUM (*Brassicaceae*)

E. repandum Linn.

Seeds contain 10 glycds. (*Dokl Bolg Akad Nauk*, 1974, **27**, 1101; *CA*, 1975, **82**, 82963w); TLC of cardenolides, 12 including glucoperiplorhamnoside and periplorhamnoside (*Khim Prir Soedin*, 1977, 581; *CA*, **87**, 197265r); also strophanthidin, periplogenin, glucostrophalloside, strophalloside and 2 unknown glycd. (*ibid*, 1978, 533; *CA*, **89**, 176380a). Glycd. extn., 0.75%; mixt., 82.66% cardenolides (*Probl Farm*, 1978, **6**, 39; *CA*, **89**, 220790k).

ERYTHRINA (*Fabaceae*)

*E. arborescens Roxb.

Khasi–*Dhingsong*; Kumaun–*Mandiara*; Lepcha– *Gyesa*.

EtOH(50%) of stem, spasmog. (*Indian J Exp Biol*, 1968, **6**, 232). Leaves made into paste with ginger and applied to skin dis-

eases of pigs, esp. in falling hair (*Econ Bot*, 1981, **35**, 4).

Leaves and stalks, alks. erysodine, erysotrine & its 11-OH deriv., erythratidine, a tetrahydrobenzylisoquinoline alk., N- nororientaline, erbidine; in addn., erythrabine and erysotramidine (*Yakugaku Zasshi*, 1973, **93**, 1611; 1617).

Seeds show haemagglutinin activity against human ABO red cells (*Indian J Med Res*, 1973, **61**, 1478); purification and properties of *D*-galactose-binding lectins (*Arch Biochem Biophys*, 1981, **211**, 459).

Seed alks. including tetra-OH-benzylisoquinoline alk. erythrascine, 10 spiroamine erythrina alks., hypaphorine and erysophorinc; pods, alk. erysodinophorine; and quaternary alk. erysopinophorine; and isoerysopinophorine in seeds (*Phytochemistry*, 1972, **11**, 2101; 1979, **18**, 704; 2069; 1974, **13**, 2603; 1980, **19**, 490).

Bark yields *n*-alkanes, alkyl ferulates, stigmasterol, sitosterol, campesterol, and wax acids (*Indian J Chem*, 1976, **14B**, 388).

Himalayas from Kumaun to Sikkim up to 2,100 m and on Khasi hills.

*E. corallodendrum Linn.

Remedy for appendicitis (*Econ Bot*, 1970, **24**, 344). Petals and sepals contain 3-mono- & diglucds. of cyanidin (*Shokubutsugaku Zasshi*, 1969, **82**, 139; *CA*, **71**, 67945w). Seeds, new mitogenic *D*-galactosephilic lectin (*Can J Biochem*, 1981, **59**, 315).

Exotic, grown in Indian gardens.

E. stricta Roxb.

Flowers pounded and given as tonic. A lotion made by burning wood, used in facial inflam. (*Econ Bot*, 1980, **34**, 264).

Bark contains erysovine, erysodine hypaphorine, *n*-alkanes, *n*-alkanols, alkylferulates, fatty acids, esters, sterols and a coumarin (*J Natl Prod*, 1981, **44**, 526).

E. suberoba Roxb.

Seed fatty oil and unsap. matter, good antifung. against *Fusarium solani* and *Hel-*

minthosporium oryzae resp.; unsap. matter, slightly active against *Streptococcus pyogenes* and *Salmonella faecallis (Indian Drugs*, 1980- 81, **18**, 411).

Seeds contain erysodine, erysotrine and hypaphorine (*Experientia*, 1969, **25**, 785); and erythraline; unsap. matter, sterols (*J Pharm Sci*, 1970, **59**, 1179; *CA*, **73**, 117168j).

Bark, wax esters, alcs. and acids, alkyl ferulates and sterols (*Phytochemistry*, 1970, **9**, 1673). Leaves, alk. erysotyrine (*Lloydia*, 1972, **35**, 92). Flowers yield 3,5-diglucds. of delphinidin, cyanidin and pelargonidin (*Proc Nat Acad Sci India*, 1977, **47**, 71).

E. variegata Linn. syn.*E. indica* Lamk; *E. variegata* Linn. var. *orientalis* Merrill

Leaves—leaves and root ext. in HCl(1%), slightly anticancerous (*Philipp J Sci*, 1964, **93**, 57). EtOH (50%) ext. of leaves and stem, spasmog. (*Indian J Exp Biol*, 1968, **6**, 232). In Tonga, used in convuls. and stomach-ache; plant in paralysis, convuls., pimples, menor. or flooding and snakebite (*Econ Bot*,1971, **25**, 423; 1970, **24**, 241).

A mixt. of fresh leaves of *Ocimum basilicum* and *Leucas aspera* and seeds of this sp. used for demodectic mange in dogs (*Indian Vet J*, 1975, **52**, 494). In Australia and Philippines, leaves and bark, in fever [*South Pac Bull*, 1975, **25**(4), 32].

Bark used in syphilis (*Nagarjun*, 1979-80, **23**, 9).

Leaf alks. (0.035%); erysotrine (major), erysodine, ethyraline- HCl and hypaphorine; erythrinine, erysodine and de-N-Me- orientaline (*Phytochemistry*, 1970, **9**, 2397; *J Chem Soc D*, 1970, 1076).

Trunk bark yields alks. (0.11%): erysotrine (major), erysodine, erysovine, erysonine and hypaphorine; 8 spiroamine alks. and 3 carboxylated indole-3-alkylamines including hypaphorine, N, N-di-Me-tryptophan from various parts; bark alks., neuromuscular blocking, smooth muscle relaxant, CNS depress., hydrocholeretic and anticonvuls.

(*Phytochemistry*, 1970, **9**, 2397; *J Pharm Sci*, 1972, **61**, 1274).

Bark, also stachydrine, wax alcs. and acids, alkyl ferulates and phenolates and sterols (*Lloydia*, 1975, **38**, 97); and flavones, osajin, alpinum isoflavone, oxyresveratrol, its dihydro deriv. and erythrinins A, B & C (*Indian J Chem*, 1977, **15B**, 205).

Seed alks.(0.082%), hypaphorine (major); erysopine and erysotrine (*Phytochemistry*, 1970, **9**, 2397); erythraline and erysovine; fatty acid compn. of seed oil (*Planta Med*, 1970-71, **19**, 71). Seeds, erysodine (major); flowers, erysotrine (major), erythrartine (11-OH-erysotrine); both contain hypaphorine and choline (*Lloydia*, 1978, **41**, 342). Seed lectin, properties (*Biochem Biophys Acta*, 1980, **623**, 439).

*E. variegata Linn. var. **parcellii** Hort.

EtOH(50%) ext. of aerial parts, diur. and anticancer (*Indian J Exp Biol*, 1980, **18**, 594).

Lucknow, U.P.

ERYTHROPSIS (*Sterculiaceae*)

E. colorata (Roxb.) Burkill; see **Firmiana colorata**

ERYTHROXYLUM (*Erythroxylaceae*)

E. coca Lamk

Leaves—dried leaves, CNS stim. and also depress. (*Q J Crude Drug Res*, 1971, **11**, 1742); therapeutic value of coca in contemporary med., rev., 16 refs. (*J Ethnopharmacol*, 1981, **3**, 367).

Aerial parts contain tannin geraniin; leaf alks. from Peru, cuscohygrine & its *l*-dihydro deriv. (*Phytochemistry*, 1980, **19**, 547; 1981, **20**, 1403). *dl*-Ornithine, a precursor in biosynth. of cocaine and cuscohygrine (*J Chem Soc Chem Commun*, 1980, 1170).

Cocaine—tropane alk., local anaesthetic action; its systemic effect, CNS stim. but extremely toxic with several other side actions; also danger of habit formation (Sim,

49-53); cocaine salts, also anaesthetic (*Acta Phytother*, 1972, **19**, 83). In blood of coca chewers, its stimulating effect; phytochem. of genus, a rich source of tropane alks., rev., 41 refs.; gas chromatogr. anal. of cocaine and *cis* - & *trans*- cinnamoylcocaines in leaves; extn. procedure for alks., with EtOH, quant. extn.; alk. yield varies with leaf age, sp. and var. (*J Ethnopharmacol*, 1979, **1**, 69; 1981, **3**, 265; 293; 313). Ph-cocaine analogues, C-phenylated cocaine analogues show surprising pharmacol. diversity (*in* Beal & Reinhard, 165- 73).

E. monogynum Roxb.

Leaf decoct. for malarial fever and EtOH ext.; pharmacol. active in CNS (*Indian For*, 1981, **4**, 115).

Wood yields 6 diterps. including monogynol, OH-ogynol, devadarool and an artifact; *d*-hibaene, its epoxide and an olefinic hydrocarbon (*Tetrahedron Lett*, 1964, 1171; 1181; 2751). Trunkwood, diterps., erythroxydiols P,Q, X & Y; str. of allodevadarool and OH-devadarool (*ibid*, 1964, 1859; 1966, 2109; 3767). Diterp. hydrocarbons: *l*-pimaradiene, *d*-atisirene, isoatisirene, devedarene and *d*-hibaene (*Tetrahedron Lett*, 1965, 2929); and erythroxydiols P & W; also of X (allodevadarool), Y(devadarool) & Z (*J Chem Soc C*, 1967, 668; 1966, 268).

Root bark, 2 tropane derivs.; a tropane heterodiester (*J Pharm Pharmacol*, 1974, **26**, Suppl., 111P; 1975, **27**, Suppl., 85P); and 4 alks. (*J Chem Soc Perkin Trans I*, 1976, 1550); see also tropane alks. (*in* Manske, XVI, 92-93).

ESCHSCHOLZIA (*Papaveraceae*)

*E. californica Cham.

Eng.–*Californian poppy.*

Herb used in colic and toothache, to reduce milk, as poultice to sores and ulcers, soporific for children suffering from whooping cough, as antineuralgicum possessing hypnotic, anodyne and analg. properties and used in severe headache.

Herb contains eschscholtzione and alks., α- & β-homochelidonines (*Q J Crude Drug Res*, 1963, **3**, 413); harvested at fruit ripening stage yields: allocryptopine, protopine, berberine and koptisine; californine; californidine (*Acta Pol Pharm*, 1964, **21**, 127; 1965, **22**, 359; 443; *CA*, 1965, **62**, 13507d; 1966, **64**, 8636d; 11547b). Herb, HCN (Wlth India, III, 202); cynogenic glycd., triglochinin (*Proc K Ned Akad Wet Ser C*, 1978, **81**, 492).

Roots, alks. chelerythrine, α- & β- allocryptopine, protopine, sanguinarine and ionidine; alks., feeble narcotic (Wlth India, III, 202); besides chelerythrine, chelelutine and chelerubine; escholine (*Acta Pol Pharm*, 1964, **21**, 59; 1965, **22**, 367; *CA*, 1965, **62**, 12069e; 1966, **64**, 11547b); and eschscholtzine and lauroscholtzine (N-Melaurotetanine) (*Can J Chem*, 1965, **43**, 2180; 2183); escholinine and escholine (magnoflorine) (*Collect Czech Chem Commun*, 1973, **38**, 3514).

Seeds, protopine, and lauroscholtzine & its stereo isomer (*Pharmazie*, 1970, **25**, 203; *CA*, **73**, 95422h).

Blossoms, rutin and purple-red pigment eschscholtzxanthin (Wlth India, III, 202).

Grown in Indian gardens.

ETHULIA (*Asteraceae*)

E. conyzoides Linn.f.

Aerial parts, new coumarin derivs., ethuliacoumarin, cycloethuliacoumarin; 5-Me-coumarin glucd.; isoethuliacoumarin A, B & C; and a terp. coumarin deriv. (*Phytochemistry*, 1977, **16**, 1092; 1980, **19**, 2029; 1519; 1981, **20**, 177); also apigenin and luteolin & their 7-O-glucds., α-amyrin, lupeol and β-sitosterol (*Fitoterapia*, 1981, **52**, 75).

EUCALYPTUS (*Myrtaceae*)

Leaf wax in high concentration in certain *E.* spp. may create hydrophobic environment for fungal spores not to germinate (*in* Plant and Fungal Toxins, 744).

Essent. oils, weak tumour-promoter (*Food Cosmet Toxicol*, 1965, **3**, 311).

*E. alba Reinw. ex Blume

EtOH(50%) ext. of aerial parts, diur. (*Indian J Exp Biol*, 1977, **15**, 208).

Vishakhapatnam, A.P.

*E. camaldulensis Dehn. syn. *E. rostrata* Schlecht.

Essent. oil—potent antibact. against Gram +ve and Gram –ve bacteria [*Indian Drugs Pharmac Ind*, 1978, **13**(6), 25; *Indian Perfum*, 1979, **23**, 138].

Leaf essent. oil, constituents (*Pafai J*, 1981, **3**, 20). Leaves, flavon. glycds. (*Phytochemistry*, 1980, **19**, 2629).

Wood yields a proanthocyanidin with biflavin str.; and a proanthocyanidin with octaflavan str. (*Gazz Chim Ital*, 1966, **96**, 803; *Cellul Carta*, 1969, **20**, 13; *CA*, 1970, **73**, 32278v).

In plains and on hills up to 1,800 m.

E. citriodora Hook. syn. *E. muculata* Hook. var. *citriodora* Bail.

Essent. oil—antimicrob. [*Planta Med*, 1974, **26**, 184; *J Res Indian Med*,1977, **12**(3), 132; *Indian Drugs*, 1977-78, **15**,227; *Indian Perfum*, 1978, **22**, 118; 1979, **23**, 205; *Indian Drugs Pharmac Ind*, 1979, **14**(3), 35; 1979,**14**(4), 29; *Fitoterapia*, 1980, **51**, 204]; insect repellant and insectic. (*Nagarjun*, 1979- 80, **23**, 177); applied to muscle spasm (Herbal Med., 139).

Plant ext., nematicidal [*J Sci Res Plants Med*, 1980, **1**(2), 18]. Leaf tea added to bath water and joints soaked to relieve pain (Herbal Med., 160).

Essent. oil from leaves, yield 2.6%, with citronellol 60.4%; flower oil 1.5% with citronellol 11.9% (*West Afr Pharm*, 1966, **8**, 117; *BA*, 1967, **48**, 124293). Essent. oil from Jammu, with citronellol 50%; and others (*Indian Oil Soap J*, 1963-64, **29**, 160); from Kumaun, properties [*Indian Perfum*, 1967, **11**(Pt. 1), 13]; Jorhat sample (0.9%) with citronellal (81.2%) and other constituents (*Flavour Ind*, 1972, **3**, 416).

Leaves, eucalyptin (γ -lactone coumarin deriv.) (*Bull Fac Pharm Cairo Univ*, 1964,

3, 103; *CA*, 1966, **64**, 14160e); β-sitosterol, and betulinic and ursolic acids (*Curr Sci*, 1980, **49**, 116).

Juice 'Kino' from plant or stem contains 7-Me-aromadandrin, 7-Me- kaempferol and citriodoral [*Pharmaceutist*, 1965, **11**(4), 10].

E. globulus Labill.

Plant gum-resin, mild astrin., used in diar. and pharynx [*Nagarjun*, 1974-75, **18**(1), 31].

Essent. oil from leaves and fruit, antibact. (*Indian Oil Soap J*, 1972,**37**, 230; *Fitoterapia*, 1980, **51**, 201); mosquito and vermin repellent (*Nagarjun*, 1979-80, **23**, 177).

Essent. oil, cineole (major) and caryophyllene (*Q J Crude Drug Res*, 1978, **16**, 113).

Leaf wax contains an antioxidant, more effective than α-tocopherol and tert-Bu-4-hydroxyanisol in aq./alc. system but inactive in oil system (*Agric Biol Chem*, 1981, **45**, 735).

Leaves, polyphenolic acids; flavons.; rich in calyptoside (*Plant Med Phytother*, 1976, **10**, 24; 30; 119; *CA*, **85**, 25311v; 30675w; 1977, **86**, 50591q). Bark and wood, polyphenols (*Phytochemistry*, 1976, **15**, 1180).

Plant, a granulation-inhibiting agent, euglobal III; and 11 more acetogenin mevalonates viz., euglobals having strong granulation- inhibiting action (*Chem Pharm Bull*, 1980, **28**, 2546; *J Chromatogr*, 1981, **208**, 374).

Extn. of active substance from dry buds, antiinflam. effect of substance comparable with indomethacin (Jpn Kokai Tokkyo Koho, 1981, 8120597; *CA*, **95**, 49402h).

Essent. oil from fruits, constituents (*Indian Perfum*, 1972, **16** (Pt. 2), 5]; from those of Nainital [*Natl Appl Sci Bull*, 1977, **29**(2), 73].

*E. multiflora Poir. syn. *E. robusta* Smith; *E. rostrata* Cav.

Eng.–*Swamp mahogany.*

A hypoten. agent from plant, its nature and action (*Diss Abstr Int B*, 1969, **30**, 1823; *CA*, 1970, **72**, 109532n).

Leaves—ext. antimal. (*in* Beal & Reinhard, 380). EtOH(50%) ext. of leaves and stem bark, semen coagulant (*Indian J Exp Biol*, 1980, **18**, 594). Leaves, acylphloroglucinol deriv., robustaol A, antimal. in mice (*Acta Chim Sin*, 1981, **39**, 83).

In plains of N. India, sub-Himalayan tracts, and in Nilgiris and Coorg.

*E. paniculata Smith

Essent. oil, antimicrob. against human and plant pathogenic bacteria [*Indian Drugs Pharmac Ind*, 1979, **14**(4), 25].

Cultivated in Nilgiris up to 1,200m, and plains.

*E. umbellata Dum. syn. *E. tereticornis* Smith

EtOH(50%) ext. of stem bark, anticancer (*Indian J Exp Biol*, 1974, **12**, 512).

Grown in Nilgiris, Maharashtra, Punjab, Dehra Dun and Shimla hills.

EUCHRESTA (*Fabaceae*)

E. horsfieldii Bennet.

Leaves yield 9 alks. matrine, sophoranol & their N-oxides, anagyrine, cystisine & its N-Me- and N-formyl derivs. and a new lupin alk., *d*-5α, 9α-di-OH-matrine (*Phytochemistry*, 1979, **18**, 645).

EUGENIA (*Myrtaceae*)

E. aromatica Kuntze; see **Syzygium aromaticum**

*E. bracteata (Willd.) Roxb. ex DC.

Alc. infusion of leaves, hypoglyc.; essent. oil from leaves, constituents [*Indian Perfum*, 1970, **14**(Pt. 1), 4]; essent. oil, antimicrob. (*Flavour Ind*, 1970, **1**, 725; *Indian J Med Res*, 1970, **58**, 627).

Reported from E. and S. India.

E. caryophyllata Thunb.; see **Syzygium aromaticum**

E. caryophyllifolia Lamk; see **Syzygium cumini**

E. jambolana Lamk; see **Syzygium cumini**

E. jambos Linn.; see **Syzygium jambos**

EULALIOPSIS (*Poaceae*)

*E. binata C.E. Hubbard

H. & B.–*bhabar, sabai*; Oriya–*Bagali*.
EtOH(50%) ext. of plant, spasmog. (*Indian J Exp Biol*, 1973, **11**, 43).

Found throughout India.

EUODIA (*Rutaceae*)

E. fraxinifolia Hook. f. syn. *Evodia fraxinifolia* Hook. f.

EtOH(50%) ext. of aerial parts, diur. (*Indian J Exp Biol*, 1973, **11**, 43).

Stem bark yields isobauernol and β-sitosterol (*Tetrahedron Lett*, 1968, 5963; *J Indian Chem Soc*, 1970, **47**, 91).

E. lunu-ankenda Merrill syn. *E. roxburghiana* Benth.; *Zanthoxylum tryphyllum* Juss.

EtOH(50%) ext. of stem bark, antimicrob., spasmog. and diur. (*Indian J Exp Biol*, 1974, **12**, 512).

E. meliaefolia Benth.

Root bark contains isobaurenol, β-sitosterol, campesterol, stigmasterol, and limonoids viz., limonin & limonin diosphenol (*Pharmazie*, 1970, **33**, 372; *CA*, **89**, 143329n).

E. rutaecarpa Hook. f. & Thoms.

Fruit, ext. as hair tonics containing w. or polar organic solvent (Jpn Kokai Tokkyo Koho, 1979, 79145229; *CA*, 1980, **92**, 135137v). EtOH ext. and an essent. substance, analg. (*Taehan Yakrihak Chapchi*, 1980, **16**, 57; *CA*, **93**, 179704c).

Fruit, evodiamine, rutaecarpine, etc., 3 alks./bases including synephrine, a sympathomimetic substance (*Tetrahedron*, 1967, **23**, 1873; *Yakugaku Zasshi*, 1967,

87, 608; 1979, **33**, 30, 33); 3 alks. (*Symp Pap IUPAC Int Symp Chem Natl Prod 11th*, 1978, **2**, 36; *CA*, 1980, **92**, 59068f); rutaecarpine and dehydroevodiamine show, *in vitro*, uterotonic effect on rat uterus (*J Natl Prod*, 1980, **43**, 577).

Fruit collected in July-Aug., yielded limonin and during Sept.- Oct. rutaevin, and those collected in latter part of Aug.-Sept. gave rutaevin and evodol (*Shoyakugaku Zasshi*, 1967, **21**, 126; *CA*, 1968, **69**, 65151u). Leaf flavons. (*Diss Pharm Pharmacol*, 1967, **19**, 655; *CA*, 1968, **68**, 72232d); and a flavanone diglucd. (*Phytochemistry*, 1975, **14**, 838).

Leaves (fresh), 3 quinolone alk. (*Agric Biol Chem*, 1976, **40**, 605).

Plant alk., wuchuyine, antivir. (*Med Pharmacol Exp*, 1967, **16**, 407).

EUONYMUS (*Celastraceae*)

*E. atropurpurea Jacq.

Dried root bark known as euonymus, mild cath., increases flow of bile; used in constip. and hepatic derangements.

Root bark, dulcitol, furan-β-carboxylic acid, euonymol, euonosteryl, homoeuonosteryl, atropurol, citrullol and a mixt. of plant acids. Stem bark used as substitute for root bark; contains dulcitol, asparagine, atropurpurin and plant acids (Wlth India, III, 222).

Plant, seven digitaloids (cardiac glycds.), including euatroside (*J Am Pharm Assoc*, 1957, **46**, 15; *CA*, **51**, 5371c). Seeds contain alk. (*Lloydia*, 1974, **37**, 506).

Drug *Euonymus* reported to be imported into India from USA.

*E. echinatus Wall.

EtOH(50%) ext. of aerial parts, diur. (*Indian J Exp Biol*, 1977, **15**, 208).

Mawsyram, Assam.

*E. glabra Roxb.

EtOH(50%) ext. of aerial parts, diur. and CNS depress. (*Indian J Exp Biol*, 1977, **15**, 208).

Himalayas, Assam, W. Bengal and Bihar.

*E. pendula Wall.

EtOH(50%) ext. of aerial parts, CNS depress. (*Indian J Exp Biol*, 1974, **12**, 512).

Twigs contain isohexacosane, cerotic acid, dulcitol, friedelin, epifriedelinol and β-sitosterol (*Planta Med*, 1978, **34**, 211).

Himalayas and Assam.

E. tingens Wall. ex Roxb.

Bark used in eye diseases (*Khadi Gramodyog*, 1972-73, **19**, 269).

Bark, a naphthoquinone deriv. (*Bull Nat Inst Sci India*, 1965, No. 28, 61); and 2 triterp. quinone methides, viz. tingenone & its -OH deriv. (*J Chem Soc Perkin Trans I*, 1973, 2721).

Leaves, epifriedelinol and taraxerol (*Indian J Chem*, 1971, **9**, 611); triterps., pristimerin and tingenin A (*J Am Chem Soc*, 1973, **95**, 6473).

EUPATORIUM (*Asteraceae*)

E. cannabinum Linn.

Ancient drug with new perspectives, rev., 28 refs. (*Pharm Weekbl*, 1971, **106**, 738; *CA*, **75**, 143925q). Aerial parts, preliminary pharmacol. (*Indian J Exp Biol*, 1980, **18**, 594).

Herb, caffeic, chlorogenic and isochlorogenic acids, rutin and hyperin; leaves, sesquiterp. lactone, eupatolin, eupatoriopicrin; inflorescence, eupatoriopicrin (*Diss Pharm Pharmacol*, 1972, **24**, 475; 1971, **23**, 537; *BA*, 1973, **56**, 3975; *CA*, 1972, **76**, 56629y); alks., echinatine and supinine (*Phytochemistry*, 1975, **14**, 2086); see hepatotoxic pyrrolizidine alks. (*in* Plant and Fungal Toxins, 643, 658); dammaradienyl-OAc, and stigmasterol (*Aust J Chem*, 1974, **27**, 1137). Leaves and flowers, taraxasterol and a coumarin; roots, euparin and eupatoriopicrin (*Khim Prir Soedin*, 1981, 106; *CA*, **95**, 3377a).

Eupatoriopicrin—str. revision of eupatoriopicrin; aerial parts, eucannabinolide (*Collect Czech Chem Commun*, 1972, **37**, 1546). Cytostatic and pharmacol. activity of sesquiterp. lactone; *in vitro* studies on cytotoxic properties in tissue culture of human and animal malignant cells (*Arch Immunol Ther Exp*, 1975, **23**, 857; 845; *in* Wagner & Wolff, 160).

*E. capillifolium (Lamk) Small

EtOH ext. of plant contains sesquiterp., costic acid, inhibitory to *Bacillus subtilis (J Natl Prod*, 1981, **44**, 252).

Reported from Sagar, M.P.

E. odoratum Linn.; see **Chromolaena odorata**

EUPHORBIA (*Euphorbiaceae*)

Diterp. esters, irrit. and cocarcinogenicity (*Experientia*, 1974, **30**, 1438); comparative phytochem. study (*Bot J Linn Soc Lond*, 1977, **74**, 23); antileukemic principles from *Euphorbiaceae* (*Science*, 1976, **191**, 571). Med. importance and chem. constituents of 41 spp., rev., 82 refs. (*Herba Hung*, 1981, **20**, 53).

E. antiquorum Linn.

Plant used in deafness, whitlow, dropsy, anasarca, sores, venereal sores, syphilis, indign., dysen., phthisis, broncht., asthma and breast pain (*Econ Bot*, 1970, **24**, 241). EtOH(50%) ext. of stem, spasmog. (*Indian J Exp Biol*, 1968, **6**, 232).

Latex applied on burns (*Bull Bot Surv India*, 1976, **18**, 166). Milk, a constituent of drug '*Amber Mezugu*' used in rheum. in Tamil Nadu, clin. trials (*Rheumatism*, 1976-77, **12**, 38).

Stems, friedalan-3-α-ol & β-ol, taraxerol and taraxerone; and roots, taraxerol (*J Indian Chem Soc*, 1967, **44**, 123).

Latex, β-amyrin, cycloartenol, euphol and euphorbol (*Curr Sci*, 1967, **36**, 204; *Indian J Chem*, 1971, **9**, 20).

E. atoto Forst. f.

Leaves used in boils, sore eyes, stomach ache and headache; whole plant for treating wound or abscess (*Econ Bot*, 1974, **24**, 1).

Plant yields an alk.; its configuration (*Aust J Chem*, 1967, **20**, 561; 2291); baccatin and a glycd. mixt. of sterols

(campesterol, 6.7; sitosterol, 72.5 & stigmasterol, 20.9%) (*Taiwan Yao Hsueh Tsa Chin*, 1979, **31**, 114; *CA*, 1981, **94**, 127200m).

E. dracunculoides Lamk

Preliminary pharmacol. (*Indian J Exp Biol*, 1969, **7**, 250). Plant ext., cholinergic and stim. for different muscles.

Plant, alc., glycds. and sterols (*Indian J Med Res*, 1967, **55**, 73); euphorbol, sucrose and a glycd. (*Indian J Chem*, 1966, **4**, 420); and kaempferol (*J Indian Chem Soc*,1969, **46**, 1066).

Fruit, daphnetin, β-sitosterol, oleanolic acid, etc. (*Indian J Pharm Sci*, 1980, **42**, 138).

E. fusiformis Buch.-Ham. ex D. Don syn. *E. accaulis* Roxb.

Roots and leaves, in fever (*Econ Bot*, 1978, **32**, 278). Root stock boiled in *Lahi* oil, made into paste, applied on gout and rheum. (*Bull Med Ethno Bot Res*, 1980, **1**, 318).

*E. geniculata Orteg.

EtOH(50%) ext. of plant, spasmog. (*Indian J Exp Biol*, 1969, **7**, 250).

Plant contains kaempferol, its rutinoside, quercetin and quercitrin; β-amyrin-OAc, β- sitosterol, campesterol, stigmasterol and cholesterol (*Pharmazie*, 1977, **32**, 538; 1978, **33**, 540; *CA*, **87**, 197350q; **89**, 176366a); and geniculatin (*Phytochemistry*, 1980, **19**, 2163).

Latex, β-amyrin-OAc (*Fitoterapia*, 1980, **51**, 313).

Found in Dehra Dun, U.P. and in Gujarat.

E. granulata Forsk.

Plant used in phthisis, broncht. and asthma (*Econ Bot*, 1970, **24**, 241).

E. helioscopia Linn.

EtOH(50%) ext. of aerial parts, diur. (*Indian J Exp Biol*, 1977, **15**, 208).

EtOH ext. of plant yields β-dihydrofucosterol, helioscopiol and a triterp. (*Pak J Sci Ind Res*, 1967, **10**, 167); flavone, tithymalin (quercetin galactoside) (*Agric Biol Chem*, 1968, **32**, 121).

In China, drug used for chr. broncht.; yielded heliosin (quercetin-3-digalactoside), quercetin, hyperin, gallic and succinic acids; heliosin, antitussive effects in clin. trials (*Acta Pharm Sin*, 1979, **14**, 91).

Aerial parts, esters of 12-deoxyphorbol; detn. of their irrit. dose on female mice; 12-deoxyphorbol-13-Ph-OAc, 20-OAc, major and most toxic compd. (*Contact Dermatitis*, 1980, **6**, 204; *CA*, **93**, 144294s).

Extn. of 2 toxic substances euphoscopin A & B; both antitumour (*Tetrahedron Lett*, 1981, **22**, 5315). Med. importance, chem. and constituents of 41 *Euphorbia* spp., rev., 82 refs. [*Herba Hung*, 1981, **20**(3), 53].

Fruit latex, proteolytic enzyme (*Rastit Resur*, 1968, **4**, 356; *CA*, 1969, **70**, 17566g); glucd., galactoside, galactoside-2"- gallate of quercetin (*Planta Med*, 1975, **27**, 301).

E. hirta Linn.; see **Chamaesyce hirta**

E. hypericifolia Linn.

Plant flavons. (*Fitoterapia*, 1977, **48**, 99).

***E. maddeni** Boiss.

Whole plant, chloroform ext., anticancer; contains a polyacylated jatrophene-type diterp., euphorinin (*Phytochemistry*, 1981, **20**, 1665). Plant, hypoten.; activity due to kaempferol- 4'-O-glucd. and hyperin; lupeol & epilupeol-OAc, lupenone, euphol and euphorbol (*Indian J Pharm Sci*, 1981, **43**, 261).

Western Himalayas up to 2,700 m.

E. nivulia Buch.-Ham.

Latex, for cattle wounds (*Econ Bot*, 1965, **19**, 236); in cough and as cure for earache, with syrup, given in asthma; antid. in snakebite (*J Agric Trop Bot Appl*, 1966, **13**, 245; 1978, **32**, 278). EtOH ext. of fresh stem, local anesthetic (*Indian J Pharmacol*, 1979, **11**, 139).

Latex yields euphol and nerifloiol. Leaves and stems, friedelan - 3α-ol (also -3 β-ol in stem) and taraxerol; glut-5(10)-en-1-one (*Curr Sci*, 1965, **34**, 608; 432; *Tetrahedron*, 1973, **29**, 3909).

Bark, deoxyphorbol-OAc, euphol, euphorbol hexacosonate, *n*- hexacosanol and $\bar{2}$4-Me-enecycloartenol (*Indian J Pharm Sci*, 1980, **42**, 66); and 3,5-diglucds. of pelargonin and tulipanin.

Roots, 24-Me-enecycloartenol, cycloartenol, ingenol-tri-OAc, euphorbol, deoxyphorbol-OAc (*Indian J Chem*, 1980, **19B**, 717).

E. peplus Linn.

Plant, glucds. of kaempferol and quercitin; aerial parts, β-sitosterol (0.1%), quercetin(0.16%), hyperoside(0.23%), kaempferol monosaccharides(0.36%) (*Planta Med*, 1973, **24**, 145; 1975, **27**, 287); β- amyrin- OAc, lanosterol, hydrocarbons, etc. (*Fitoterapia*, 1980, **51**, 223).

E. pilosa Linn.

Preliminary pharmacol. (*Indian J Exp Biol*, 1968, **6**, 232). Root, purg.; root and stem in mixt. cause purging and vomiting (*Khadi Gramodyog*, 1972-73, **19**, 269).

***E. prolifera** Ham.

EtOH(50%) ext. of plant, antivir. and anticancer (*Indian J Exp Biol*, 1968, **6**, 232).

C. and Western Himalayas.

***E. pulcherrima** Willd. ex klotzsch
Eng.–*Poinsettia.*

Latex inhibits growth of mouse sarcoma 180 and adenocarcinoma 755 (*Gann*, 1964, **55**, 263; *CA*, 1965, **62**, 15321f). Leaf ext. in 1% acetic acid, anticancer (*Philipp J Sci*, 1967, **96**, 393).

Latex, stems, bracts and flowers (every part) contain β-sitosterol and ψ-taraxasterol; in addn. latex, pulcherrol; and stems, octaeicosanol (*J Pharm Sci*, 1967, **56**, 1184). Latex also contains esters of β-amyrin, germanicol (main constituents) and cycloartenol (*Planta Med*, 1977, **32**, 1).

Plant, germanicol; germanicyl-OAc, epigermanicyl-OAc, 2-Me- anthraquinone, etc. (*J Indian Chem Soc*, 1967, **44**, 159;

1977, **54**, 388). Aerial parts, cholesterol and other sterols (*Phytochemistry*, 1980, **19**, 1509).

Egyptian leaves contain germanicol-OAc (0.25%), germanicol, brein, β-sitosterol, its glucd., rutin, etc. (*Acta Pharm Jugosl*, 1980, **30**, 103).

Grown in gardens.

E. resinifera Berg.

Gum—resin, purg., used in sciatica, given internally to cause abortion [*Nagarjun*, 1974-75, **18**(1), 31].

Dried latex, glutaric acids, two inositol isomers (*Acta Chem Scand*, 1969, **23**, 3609). Latex, 3 diterp. esters, deoxyphorbol- OAc deriv.; their irrit. and cocarcinogenic activity (*Experientia*, 1974, **30**, 1438); also 2 nonirrit. diterp. esters and 3 irrit. factors, viz. RL 14, resiniferatoxin & proresiniferatoxin (*Tetrahedron Lett*, 1975, 1595).

E. royleana Boiss.

EtOH(50%) ext. of stem, antivir. and spasmog. (*Indian J Exp Biol*, 1968, **6**, 232).

Latex applied for a disease *khor* in which hair of head and eye brows fall out (*Econ Bot*, 1971, **25**, 414).

Latex yield euphol, cycloeucalenol and a triterp. alc. (*Pak J Sci Ind Res*, 1965, **8**, 80); taraxerol, sitosterol, coumarins, arom. carboxylic acids (*J Pharm Sci*, 1976, **65**, 772).

Bark, taraxerol; and flowers, ellagic acid (*Indian J Chem*, 1964, **2**, 254); plant, 2,3-di-OMe-ellagic and succinic acids (*Pak J Sci Ind Res*, 1966, **9**, 38).

Stem, taraxeryl-OAc and glut-5-en-3 β-yl-OAc (*J Indian Chem Soc*, 1965, **42**, 543); β-sitosterol, friedelan-3 α-ol, lupeol, β-amyrin and epitaraxerol (*Curr Sci*, 1974, **43**, 10).

E. thomsoniana Boiss.

Latex used in eruptions and other skin diseases. Plant, purg. (*Bull Med Ethno Bot Res*, 1981, **2**, 193).

E. thymifolia Linn. syn. *E. prostrata* Ait.

Plant—galact.; used in ophthalamia and other eye troubles, ardor, sores, atrophy,

dysen. and breast pain (*Econ Bot*, 1965, **19**, 236; 1970, **24**, 241). Efficaceous drug for bronch. asthma, clin. trials [*J Res Indian Med*, 1971, **6**(2), 118]. Blood purifier (*Nagarjun*, 1980-81, **24**, 263). An aq. ext. of plant mixed with *mishri* gives cooling effect to body and cures spermator. (*Bull Med Ethno Bot Res*, 1980, **1**, 317).

Plant insectic. oil used as spray to keep off flies and mosquitoes (*Nagarjun*, 1979-80, **23**, 177).

Plant, antimicrob. alk. (*Pak J Sci Ind Res*, 1965, **8**, 293).

Plant flavons. (*Pharmazie*, 1977, **32**, 538; *CA*, **87**, 197350q). Whole plant yields hexacosanol and 2 derivs. of deoxyphorbol-OAc; cocarcinogenic activity due to phrobol derivs. (*Indian J Chem*, 1980, **19B**, 717); esters, *n*-alkanes, sterols (*Proc Indian Sci Congr*, 1980, III, 90). Aerial parts, epitaraxerol, *n*-hexacosanol, euphorbol, 2 derivs. of deoxyphorbol-OAc, 24-methylene cycloartenol and quercetin galactoside (*Indian J Pharm Sci*, 1981, **43**, 182).

Root, taraxerol, triucallol, etc. (*Indian J Appl Chem*, 1966, **29**, 39).

E. tirucalli Linn.

EtOH(50%) ext. of aerial parts, antiprot. (*Indian J Exp Biol*, 1968, **6**, 232). Stem ext., antifung. (*Geobios*, 1978, **5**, 49).

Stems contain hentriacontane, hentriacontanol, β- sitosterol, Me- ellagic & ellagic acids and a glycd. (*Indian J Pharm*, 1967, **29**, 152); plant, taraxerone, triucallol, sitosterol and Me-ellagic acid (*Indian J Chem*, 1977, **15B**, 564).

Latex, from Madagascar yielded 5 new highly irrit. euphorbia factors (*Experientia*, 1977, **33**, 986); and from S. African plant latex, 4 highly irrit. diterps. (*Tetrahedron Lett*, 1977, 925; *Planta Med*, 1972, **22**, 241); new diester irrit. from latex as potent standard irrit.; chem. races in regard to diterp. profiles from plants grown in three different locations (*Lloydia*, 1978, **41**, 648; *J Natl Prod*, 1979, **42**, 112; *in* Plant and Fungal Toxins, 266). Fresh latex, new triterps. euphorbinol, and cycloeuphornol (*Pak J Sci Ind Res*, 22, 124; 173).

*E. wallichii Hook. f.

Plant ext., antimicrob. (*Fitoterapia*, 1980, **51**, 231).

Root contains euphol and euphorbol (*Planta Med*, 1979, **35**, 193).

Western and C. Himalayas at 3,000-4,000 m.

EUPHORIA (*Sapindaceae*)

E. longan Steud.; see **Dimocarpus longan**

EUPHRASIA (*Scrophulariaceae*)

E. officinalis Linn.

Homoeopathic mother tincture of plant, *in vitro*, antimicrob. against *Staphylococcus aureus, E. coli* and *Candida albicans*, preliminary investigation (*Indian J Exp Biol*, 1977, **15**, 338).

Aerial parts, phenol carboxylic acids, flavones and Me-flavoné derivs. of cinnamic acid (*Herba Hung*, 1973, **12**, 101; *CA*, 1975, **82**, 95342t); and diosmetin, quercetin, kaempferol and quercetin diglucd. [*Acta Pharm Hung*, 1974, 44(Suppl.), 83; *CA*, 1975, **82**, 28547a].

EURYA(*Theaceae*)

*E. acuminata DC.

Leaves and fruit, stomch. (*Bot Bull Acad Sin*, 1949, **3**, 136).

C. and Eastern Himalayas and Assam up to 900-2,400 m.

*E. japonica Thunb.

Ass.–*Saseni*; H.–*Baunra, deura*; Kan. & Tam.–*Huluni*; Mal.– *Arruttuvarai*.

In Malaysia, leaves used in skin eruptions; yield essent. oil (14%) containing β-, & γ-hexenol (Wlth India, III, 231); stem, sitosterol (*Indian J Chem*, **14B**, 473).

Occurs in Eastern Himalayas at 900-3,000 m, Khasi hills at 900- 1,800 m, and Western Ghats from Konkan southwards up to 2,100 m.

EURYALE (*Euryalaceae*)

E. ferox Salisb.

Seeds used as aphrodis. (*Q J Crude Drug Res*, 1971, **11**, 1742).

EURYCOMA (*Simaroubaceae*)

E. longifolia Jack

Bark contains β-sitosterol, campesterol and 2, 6- di-OMe-benzoquinone (*Ann Fac Sci Univ Saigon*, 1963, 43; *CA*, 1966, **65**, 14091a); a bitter principle eurcomalactone & its dihydro deriv. (*J Org Chem*, 1970, **35**, 1104); also str. (*Sci Pharm*, 1980, **48**, 110; *CA*, **93**, 235099y).

Roots yield usual sterols; and 3 saponins with haemolytic activity (*Planta Med*, 1978, **34**, 339; *Sci Pharm*, 1979, **47**, 243; *CA*, 1980, **92**, 37767f).

EVODIA (*Rutaceae*)

See **EUODIA**

EVOLVULUS (*Convulvulaceae*)

E. alsinoides Linn.

Plant—used in leucoderma (*Indian J Appl Chem*, 1959, **22**, 6); antisp., aphrodis.; plant and leaves used in insanity, epilepsy, nervine complaints, bleeding, spermator. [*J Res Indian Med*, 1973, **8**(2), 67]; leaf juice, in conjunctivitis (*Nagarjun*, 1980-81, **24**, 1); increases brain power, given in bowel complaints, promotes constip. and useful in internal haemor.

Roots, in intermittent fever in children (*Sachitra Ayurveda*, 1980-81, **33**, 201).

Aq. ext. of petal, antifung. (*Geobios*, 1981, **8**, 67).

Preliminary pharmacol. of alk. evolvine, powerful stim. on respiration and B.P., similar to lobeline, possible analeptic (*Curr Sci*, 1956, **25**, 119).

Plant contains pentatriacontane, triacontane and β- sitosterol (*Indian J Appl Chem*, 1959, **22**, 6).

*E. nummularius Linn.

Defatted ext. of plant, poor sed. (*Naturwissenschaften*, 1964, **51**, 411).

A weed of grassy lands found in some parts of India.

EXACUM (Gentianaceae)

E. bicolor Roxb.

Plant ext., antifung. against *Helminthosporium sativum* (*Indian J Med Res*, 1961, **49**, 799).

E. pedunculatum Linn.

EtOH(50%) ext. of plant, anticancer (*Indian J Exp Biol*, 1980, **18**, 594).

E. tetragonum Roxb.

Pounded plant applied as lep in rheum. and gout (*Nagarjun*, 1980- 81, **24**, 1).

EXBUCKLANDIA (Hamamelidaceae)

*E. populnea R. Br. syn. *Bucklandia populnea* R. Br. ex Griff.; *Syminngtonia populnea* Van Steenis

EtOH(50%) ext.of stem bark, spasmol. and diur. (*Indian J Exp Biol*, 1974, **12**, 512).

Eastern Himalayas and Khasi hills.

EXCOECARIA (Euphorbiaceae)

Genus contains carcinogenic diterps. (*Lloydia*, 1978, **41**, 193- 233).

E. agallocha Linn.

Latex used as caustic in obstinate ulcers (Wlth India, III, 234).

Latex, 3 alcs.; exocarol, agalocol & isoagalocol (*Sci Res Dacca*, 1964, **1**, 211; *CA*, 1965, **62**, 8015g); and β-amyrin, its 3-epimer, β-amyrenone, cycloartenol and an unknown compd. (*Phytochemistry*, 1971, **10**, 3308).

Leaves, epitaraxerol (*Aust J Chem*, 1968, **21**, 2137). A piscic. compd. from twigs and bark; compd. toxic to *Cryzias latipes* (fish) at 0.003 ppm after 24 hrs. (*Agric Biol Chem*, 1974, **38**, 1093).

*E. cochinchinensis Lour. syn. *E. bicolor* Hassk.

Latex, fish poison (Wlth India, III, 234). Grown in Indian gardens.

EXOGONIUM (Convolvulaceae)

E. purga Benth. syn. *Ipomoea purga* Hayne

Resin from dried root (commercial jalap) contains β-*D*-quinovoside of 11-OH-tetradecanoic acid (*Phytochemistry*, 1973, **12**, 1701).

FABA (Fabaceae)

F. vulgaris Moench; see **Vicia faba**

FAGONIA (Zygophyllaceae)

F. cretica Linn. syn. *F. arabica* Linn.; *F. bruguieri* DC.

Plant—employed in Ayurvedic formulation of '*Kumari Asava*', a drug with stim., laxt. and alter. properties; as antisep. and for wounds and scrofulous glands (Wlth India, IV, 1); useful in cough, fever, asthma, dysen. and skin diseases; boiled plant residue, used for abortion (*J Agric Trop Bot Appl*, 1966, **13**, 245). EtOH(50%) ext. of aerial parts, antivir., antiamphetaminic and spasmog. (*Indian J Exp Biol*, 1968, **6**, 232); plant ash given to children suffering from anaemia (*J Econ Tax Bot*, 1980, **1**, 137).

Leaves and twigs—decoct., blood purifier and given for skin lesions (boils and abscesses); claimed to cure tumour and cancer in preliminary stages (*Proc Pak Sci Conf*, 1965, Pt III, C- 24).

Stem, leaves and fruit powd., antimicrob. (*Fitoterapia*, 1980, **51**, 231).

Aerial parts contain alk., 0.07% (*Pak J Sci Ind Res*, 1963, **6**, 53). Plant, chinovic acid on acid hydrolysis of alc. ext. (*ibid*, 1966, **9**, 269); ceryl alc., β- sitosterol and *n*-triacontanol (*Vijnana Parishad Anusandhan Patrika*, 1966, **9**, 87); fagogenin, genin A and betulin (*Pak J Sci Ind Res*, 1966, **9**, 41; 1967, **10**, 140); fagonin and oleanolic acid (*Phytochemistry*, 1969, **8**, 2269). Lipid fraction, campesterol, β-sitosterol(major) & stigmasterol (*J Chem UAR*, 1969, **12**, 119). Harmine, 3 triterps., and 2 unidentified compds. (*Herba Pol*, 1975, **21**, 420; *CA*, 1976, **85**, 124189t).

FAGOPYRUM (*Polygonaceae*)

F. dibotrys (D. Don) Hara syn. *F. cymosum* Meissn.

Herb—EtOH(50%) ext., diur. (*Indian J Exp Biol*, 1977, **15**, 208). In China, used in lung infection.

Herb, tetra-OH-flavonol, β-sitosterol and an unknown compd. [*Yao Hsueh T'ung Pao*, 1980, **15**(8), 40; *CA*, 1981, **95**, 86201n].

Rhizome used in treatment of pulmonary abscess; active principle, 5,7,3′,4′-tetra-OH-flavan-3-ol (*in* Beal & Reinhard, 378).

F. esculentum Moench

Eng.–*Common buckwheat; brank.*

Seed oil, good antimicrob. against *Bacillus anthrasis, E. coli* and *Salmonella paratyphi* (*Proc Indian Sci Congr*, 1980, Pt. III, 94).

Whole plant, dried or green can cause photosensitization called fagopyrism in presence of oxygen to induce phototoxicity due to the presence of fagopyrin akin to hypericin (*in* Plant and Fungal Toxins, 354).

Root decoct., used in rheum. pains, lung diseases and typhoid, and juice in urinary disorders (*Bull Med Ethno Bot Res*, 1980, **1**, 1). In China, used in pulmonary sepsis; active principle, a flavanol(5,7, 3′, 4′-tetra-OH-flavan-3-ol dipolymer); compd. antipyr. in rabbits, antiinflam. in mice and rats, and expect. in mice (*Acta Pharm Sin*, 1981, **16**, 247).

Seed cotyledons of an Estonian var., germinated 48 hrs in dark contain flavons. orientin, vitexin, etc.; cotyledons, flavons. (*Biochim Biophys Acta*, 1967, **136**, 396; *J Chromatogr*, 1978, **156**, 359). Salicylamine, its Schiff's base and 4-OH-benzylamine; 2 amides (glutamine derivs.) (*Agric Biol Chem*, 1971, **35**, 1870; 1973, **37**, 2745); piperidine deriv., fagomine; and *o*- & *p*- glucopyranosyloxy benzylamine

(*ibid*, 1974, **38**, 1111; 1467); *L*-2-(2-furoyl) alanine (*Tetrahedron Lett*, 1973, 37); β- glucosidase & its properties (*Biochimie*, 1973, **55**, 353); a trypsin inhibitor (*Biokhimiya*, 1980, **45**, 2104).

Herb, rhamnodiastase and α-*L*-rhamnosidase, enzymes hydrolyse various flavon. glycds. (*Phytochemistry*, 1975, **14**, 1279).

Rutin—from fresh or dried leaves and flowers and its med. use; rutin (6 mg/100g), hyperin (13 mg/100g), etc. from buckwheat (seeds) (Wlth India, IV, 4-5; *Nippon Nogei Kagaku Kaishi*, 1975, **49**, 53; *CA*, **83**, 4922p); chromatospectrophotom. detn. (*Khim Farm Zh*, 1980, **14**, 60; *CA*, 1981, **95**, 53031h); its production, extn. of buckwheat with w., recrystallization from EtOH while periodically removing rutin, process improvement (USSR Pat., 1981, 681841; *CA*, **95**, 12754y).

F. tataricum (Linn.) Gaertn.

Effect of agronomic factors in rutin content in seeds and green parts (*Rastit Resur*, 1967, **3**, 40; *CA*, **67**, 29873f). Cultivation studies for rutin production from leaves (*Indian J Pharm*, 1971, **33**, 92). Seeds contain quercetin(2.5%), its 3-rutinoside-7-galactoside, rutin(0.024%), kaempferol & its 3- rutinoside (*Nippon Nogei Kagaku Kaishi*, 1980, **54**, 275; *CA*, **93**, 44264p).

FAGRAEA (*Loganiaceae*)

*F. ceilanica Thunb. syn. *F. obovata* Wall.

In Java, grated leaves used as poultice in headache and fever (Wlth India, IV, 6). Preliminary pharmacol. (*Indian J Exp Biol*, 1969, **9**, 250).

Found in Eastern Himalayas, Assam and Western Peninsula up to 1,800 m.

F. cochinchinensis A. Chev. syn. *F. fragrans* Roxb.; *Cyrtophyllum peregrinum* Reinw. ex Blume

Bark used in malaria (Wlth India, IV, 6).

Leaves and fruits, major alk. 4-(2-OH-Et)-5-vinylnicotinic acid lactone. Alk., max. in leaves at flowering (0.32%) and min. after fruiting (0.005%). Ripe fruits, 0.1% alk. (*J Pharm Pharmacol*, 1964, **16**, 484).

Gentianine—vinyl-pyrido -α-pyrone; alk. also available from several other plants; available by synth. (*J Chem Soc*, 1957, 2725; *Heterocycles*, 1975, **3**, 627); given to rats in 50 or 100mg/kg dose, analg. Antiinflam. and sed. [*Asian J Med*, 1972, **8**, 334; *Dokl Akad Nauk Uzb SSR*, 1972, **29**(3), 37; *Farmakol Alkaloidov Serdech Glikozidov*, 1971, 146; 148; *CA*, 1973, **78**, 11686q; 38001z; 79634b; 66918x]; also antipsychotic (*J Pharm Sci*, 1974, **63**, 1341). See also *Gentiana olivieri*.

F. racemosa Jack

In Malaysia, root taken as tonic after fever and for pains in loins. Leaf used in dropsy and rheum.; its decoct., for med. baths for children (Wlth India, IV, 6).

FAGUS (*Fagaceae*)

*F. sylvatica Linn.

Eng.–*European beech.*

Seeds—poisoning in human beings due to beechnuts and in animals due to cake; poisonous principle saponin-like, causes severe gastrointestinal distress (Kingsbury, 443-44).

Seeds, fatty oil (*c.* 20%), used externally in skin diseases, rheum. and gout (Hocking, 83); oil, non-toxic (Kingsbury, 444).

EtOH(50%) ext. of aerial parts, antivir. (*Indian J Exp Biol*, 1971, **9**, 91).

Seed cake, *p*-OH-benzoic, vanillic, *p*-OH-cinnamic, caffeic, ferulic and sinapic acids; leaves yield first 4 acids and chlorogenic acid (*Naturwissenschaften*, 1965, **52**, 208). Free amino acids and γ-glutamyl peptides from seeds (*Phytochemistry*, 1974, **13**, 2791).

Leaves also contain 3-glucds. of kaempferol and quercetin (*ibid*, 1967, **6**, 1291); *n*-nonacosane, β-sitosterol and unidentified compd. (*Rocz Chem*, 1968, **42**, 1493; *CA*, 1969, **70**, 35062u).

Rich in vit. C (*Arch Farm Belgrade*, 1962, **12**, 529; *CA*, 1964, **60**, 2249h).

Bark, β-sitosterol and betulin (*Rocz Chem*, 1965, **39**, 583; *CA*, **63**, 18204d). Wood, squalene, cycloartenyl- and β-amyrin-OAc, Ac-Me-betulinate, dihydrositosterol, sitosterol and stigmasterol (*Phytochemistry*, 1972, **12**, 2068).

Grown in Nilgiris.

FARADAYA (*Verbenaceae*)

*F. splendida F. Muell.

Bark, a powerful fish poison; contains active saponin (Wlth India, IV, 7).

Roots, 3-OAc-oleanolic aldehyde, 3-OAc-erythrodiol and K salt of a polyhydroxy triterp. diacid, faradoic acid (*Aust J Chem*, 1974, **27**, 2289).

Cultivated in gardens for ornament.

FARSETIA (*Brassicaceae*)

F. edgeworthii Hook. f. & Thoms. syn. F. aegyptiaca Turra

Contains glucosinolates of allyl; Bu-3-enyl; 2-Ph-Et; *sec*- Bu, 3-Me-thio-Pr; 4-Me-thio-Bu and benzyl [*Prog Flavour Res Proc Weurman Flavour Res Symp*, 1978 (Pub. 1979), 281; *CA*, 1980, **92**, 124889r]. Glucosinolates from leaves; allylglucosinolate (major) (*Phytochemistry*, 1980, **19**, 227).

F. jacquemontii Hook. f. & Thoms.

Tender twigs, raw tonic (Wlth India, IV, 7).

FEIJOA (*Myrtaceae*)

See ACCA

FERONIA (*Rutaceae*)

See **LIMONIA**

FERULA (*Apiaceae*)

F. alliacea Boiss.

Latex alongwith cow's milk and ashes of seeds of palash (*Butea monosperma*), moderate aborticide (*Econ Bot*, 1980, **34**, 273).

Fruit contains mixt. of furocoumarin, byakangelicin, isopimpinellin and ferulin (a mixt. of phellopterin and byakangelicol) (*Arch Pharm Ber Dtsch Pharm Ges*, 1962, **295**, 248; *BA*, **39**, 20579).

F. assa-foetida Linn. syn. F. foetida Regel

Asafoetida—latex from living rootstocks or taproots of several *Ferula* spp. e.g. *F. assa-foetida*, *F. alliacea*, *F. narthex* and *F. rubricaulis*; imported into India, useful in asthma, whooping cough, chr. broncht., hysteria, epilepsy and cholera; as enema, stimulates intestine, respiratory tracts and nervous system (Wlth India, IV, 20). Asafoetida & its ether extracted essent. oil, protective against fat-induced increase in plasma fibrinogen and decrease in coagulation time tested in human; active principle allyl persulphide (*Indian J Med Res*, 1975, **63**, 707). Diluted with vinegar and taken, acts as abortif. (*J Sci Res Plants Med*, 1981, **2**, 39).

Used in spleen, madness, pain, hemiplegia, epilepsy, convuls., cramps, colic and rinderpest (*Econ Bot*, 1970, **24**, 241). Aq. preparation, blood coagulant in dogs [*Med Zh Uzb*, 1967, (6), 46; *CA*, 1974, **81**, 166398h]. Constituents of essent. oil from seeds (*Pak J Sci Ind Res*, 1979, **22**, 308). Oleo-gum resin used alongwith others in herbal compn. '*Vidangadi Yoga*', very effective antifert. drug [*J Sci Res Plants Med*, 1980, **1**(3-4), 41].

F. galbaniflua Boiss. & Buhse

Gum-resin, carmin. and in the form of plaster applied to inflam. swellings.

Resin, umbelliferone, galbaresinotannol, galbaresinic and falbanic acids and 2 isomeric lactones. Essent. oil from gum-resin contained d-α-pinene, β-pinene, myrcene, cadinene, and α-cadinol (Wlth India, IV, 20).

F. jaeschkeana Vatke

Sesquiterp., jaeschkeanadiol (*Tetrahedron*, 1973, **29**, 985); and sesquiterp. ester, jaeschferin (*Khim Prir Soedin*, 1980, 127; *CA*, **93**, 71992f).

F. narthex Boiss.

Essent. oil, antibact. against several pathogenic and nonpathogenic bacteria (*Flavour Ind*, 1971, **2**, 111). Gum-resin, emmen. (*Q J Crude Drug Res*, 1972, **12**, 1922). Essent. oil from gum-resin, antifung. (*Planta Med*, 1973, **24**, 127). Properties and constituents of seed oil (*Pak J Sci Ind Res*, 1979, **22**, 87).

FESTUCA (*Poaceae*)

*F. elatior Linn.

Eng.—*Meadow fescue*.

Aq. ext. of grass, antioxidant (*Med Welt*, 1972, **28**, 430; *CA*, **77**, 163119z).

Grass contains 9 alks. including perloline (*J Chromatogr*, 1963, **12**, 423).

Found in Khasi hills of Meghalaya and Mikir hills of Assam up to 1,800 m.

FICUS (*Moraceae*)

Commonly known as fig family; fig leaves cause contact dermatitis due to psoralens (*in* Plant and Fungal Toxins, 355).

F. amplissima Smith syn. F. tsiela Roxb.

EtOH(50%) ext. of aerial parts, anticancer and diur. (*Indian J Exp Biol*, 1980, **18**, 594).

F. arnottiana Miq.

Powd. leaves mixed with *Cuminum cyminum* fruit (5g. each) in water, given to women after menses, moderate sterilizer (*Econ Bot*, 1980, **34**, 273).

F. benghalensis Linn.

Latex—used in toothache; infusion of young buds in diar. and dysen. and young tips of roots for obstinate vomiting (Wlth India, IV, 26). Juice mixed with sesamum oil applied to burns [*J Res Indian Med*, 1978, **13**(4), 92]. Latex used in genital diseases; mixed with sugar given to children in cough.

Bark—with black pepper used in serious cases of snakebite (*J Econ Tax Bot*, 1980, **1**, 137). Aq. ext. of bark and leaves, depress. on uterine and cardiac muscle and also cholinergic-blocking of smooth and skeletal muscle (*Indian J Physiol Pharmacol*, 1969, **13**, 143). Ext., antidiabetic in rabbits (*Indian J Pharm*, 1970, **32**, 68); decoct., showed strong antifert. activity in men and women [*J Res Indian Med*, 1978, **13**(2), 104].

Plant—used in ophthalmia and other eye troubles, mouth sores, fever, madness, atrophy, emaciation or cachexy, cholera and rinderpest (*Econ Bot*, 1970, **24**, 241).

Root—paste applied to scalp to grow hair long (*Q J Crude Drug Res*, 1979, **17**, 61); and for menor. (*Bull Med Ethno Bot Res*, 1980, **1**, 8).

Seed powd., progenitive (*Nagarjun*, 1979-80, **23**, 9).

Bark, a hypoglyc. glucd., bengalenoside, more active than crude ext. of bark but only half as potent as tolbutamide (*Indian J Physiol Pharmacol*, 1975, **19**, 218). Leucoanthocyanidins (2) and a leucoanthocyanin; latter's Me-ethers, hypoglyc. in rats (*ibid*, 1964, **8**, 60; *Indian J Chem*, 1977, **15B**, 762); phytosterolin, also hypoglyc. in rabbits (*Indian J Pharm*, 1966, **28**, 341); stem bark, β-sitosterol α-D-glucd., *meso*-inositol and 3 ketones (*Pol J Pharm*, 1978, **30**, 559; *CA*, 1979, **90**, 200267n).

Leaves, friedelin and β-sitosterol (*J Indian Chem Soc*, 1968, **45**, 285); also quercetin 3-galactoside and rutin; heartwood, tiglic acid ester of ψ-taraxasterol (0.4%) (*Phytochemistry*, 1970, **9**, 2583).

F. benjamina Linn. var. **benjamina** Linn.

EtOH(50%) ext. of aerial parts, diur. (*Indian J Exp Biol*, 1977, **15**, 208).

Fruit, bergapten (*J Indian Chem Soc*, 1971, **48**, 979).

*F. callosa Willd.

EtOH(50%) ext. of aerial parts, CNS depress. (*Indian J Exp Biol*, 1977, **15**, 208).

Coorg and Hassan districts of Karnataka.

F. carica Linn.

Anticancer compd., effective against Ehrlich sarcoma; extracted with w. (Jpn Pat., 1969, 6912747; *CA*, **71**, 94754q). EtOH ext. given orally, reduced exp. ulcers in rats and BuOH ext. reduced rat paw oedema (*Shoyakugaku Zasshi*, 1976, **30**, 61; *CA*, 1977, **87**, 62641a). Preliminary pharmacol. (*Indian J Exp Biol*, 1971, **9**, 91).

Fruit, laxt., useful in anaemia. Latex, anthelm., due to ficin (Wlth India, IV, 31).

Leaves, psoralen, 0.37; and bergapten, 0.59% dry wt.(*Phytochemistry*, 1964,**3**, 701);other coumarins/derivs. (*Experientia*, 1971, **27**, 758; *Khim Prir Soedin*, 1971, **7**, 521; *CA*, 1972, **76**, 44006e); coumarins, xanthotoxin, xanthotoxol and marmesin (*Fitoterapia*, 1980, **51**, 269); plant, umbelliferone and scopoletin (*Pharmazie*, 1981, **36**, 297).

Psoralen & bergapten—cause contact dermatitis in human; phototoxicity in animals; furocoumarins, psoralen and bergapten (5-MeO-psoralen)(*in* Plant and Fungal Toxins, 354-56); their isolation from leaves (*Acta Pharm Jugosl*, 1971, **21**,33;*CA*, **75**, 52716f); source, highest content (0.43- 0.54%) when harvested between 10th Sept-10th Oct. (*Uzb Biol Zh*, 1974, **18**, 36). Extn. with 40% & 60% aq. acetone (*Khim Prir Soedin*, 1975, **11**, 91; *CA*, **83**, 128638v; 189946r); with hot w. (USSR Pat., 1975, 464319; *CA*, **83**, 120822e); fermentation increases 2-fold psoralen content (*Rastit Resur*, 1975, **11**, 372; *CA*, **83**, 128701k). Fruits, Ph-CHO, inhibits tumour growth and Ehrlich carcinoma in mice and tumour regression in humans (*Agric Biol Chem*, 1978, **42**, 1449).

Leaf flavons., terps., and fiscusogenin (tri-OH steroid sapogenin), etc. (*Izv Akad Nauk Turkm SSR, Ser Biol Nauk*, 1981, 65; *J Chem Soc C*, 1966, 1140).

Root, guaiazulene (*Tottori Nogakkaiho*, 1963, **16**, 13; *CA*, 1964, **61**, 6853e).

*F. elastica Roxb.

Eng.–*Assam rubber*, *Indian rubber tree*; Ass. & B.–*Bor atlah bar*.

EtOH(50%) ext. of aerial parts, diur. (*Indian J Exp Biol*, 1980, **18**, 594).

Leaves, isoprenoid alc. mixt. (*Phytochemistry*, 1966, **5**, 969); polyprenol mixt., compn. (*Biochem J*, 1966, **102**, 325).

Assam hills up to 1,500 m.

F. exasperata Vahl syn. *F. asperrima* Roxb.

Preliminary pharmacol. (*Indian J Exp Biol*, 1977,**15**, 208).

Leaves, bergapten, bergaptol, β-amyrin and β-sitosterol (*Fitoterapia*, 1980, **51**, 269).

F. fistulosa Reinw.

EtOH(50%) ext. of aerial parts, diur. (*Indian J Exp Biol*, 1973, **11**, 43).

F. hispida Linn. f. syn. *F. oppositifolia* Willd.

Fruits, tonic and lactag. Leaves used for poulticing boils (Wlth India, IV, 36). Preliminary pharmacol. (*Indian J Exp Biol*, 1977, **15**, 208).

Plant contains 10-keto-tetracosyl arachidate (*Tetrahedron*, 1975, **31**, 229). Leaves, bergapten, psoralen, β- amyrin and β-sitosterol (*Fitoterapia*, 1980, **51**, 269); surface hydrocarbons (*Indian J Chem*, 1981, **20B**, 722).

F. microcarpa Linn. f. syn. *F. retusa* auct. non Linn.

Preliminary pharmacol. (*Indian J Exp Biol*, 1971, **9**, 91).

*F. nemoralis Wall.

EtOH(50%) ext. of aerial parts, spasmog. and anticancer (*Indian J Exp Biol*, 1980, **18**, 594).

Found in Eastern Himalayas.

F. palmata Forsk.

Latex of young twigs applied to draw out prickles or other foreign matter in body. *Raita* of boiled fruits, given in dysen. (*Econ Bot*, 1971, **25**, 414).

Leaves, β-sitosterol and bergapten (*J Indian Chem Soc*, 1976, **53**, 1162).

F. racemosa Linn. syn. *F. glomerata* Roxb.

Bark—decoct. used as wash for wounds (Wlth India, IV, 36). EtOH(50%) ext. of stem bark, antiprot. and hypoglyc. (*Indian J Exp Biol*, 1968, **6**, 232); antiinflam. (*Annu Conf Indian Pharm Sci*, 1980, F-16). Leaves and bark useful as poultice for eczema (*Ancient Sci Life*, 1981-82, **1**, 236).

Leaves—glycd. rich fraction of ext., hypoten. and cardiac depress. (*Indian J Med Res*, 1969, **57**, 1070); decoct. for broncht. (*Bull Bot Surv India*, 1973, **15**, 13).

Plant—used in smallpox, muscular pain, adenitis, scabies, spermator., orchitis, epididymitis, hydrocele, menor. or flooding, and failure of lactation (*Econ Bot*, 1970, **24**, 241).

Bark, ceryl behenate, lupeol, its -OAc, α-amyrin and 3 unidentified compds. (*Proc Nat Acad Sci India*, 1977, **47A**, 1); gluanol-OAc, β- sitosterol and a ketone; first two compds. also from heartwood(*J Indian Chem Soc*, 1973, **50**, 611; 1977, **54**, 1104); stigmasterol (*Herba Hung*, 1980, **19**, 17).

Leaves, gluanol-OAc, β-amyrin and β-sitosterol (*J Indian Chem Soc*, 1971, **48**, 1165).

Fruit, lupeol-OAc, β-sitosterol and a sterol (*Indian J Chem*, 1979, **17B**, 87); hentriacontane, gluanol- OAc, tiglic acid ester of taraxasterol and glucose (*J Indian Chem Soc*, 1979, **56**, 1269).

F. religiosa Linn.

Bark—infusion used in ulcers and skin diseases. Aq. ext., antibact.(Wlth India, IV, 39). EtOH(50%) ext., antiprot., anthelm. and antivir. (*Indian J Exp Biol*, 1968, **6**, 232). Decoct. given in gonor. (*Ancient Sci Life*, 1981-82, **1**, 178).

Leaves—with shoots, in skin diseases (Wlth India, IV, 39); estrogenic (*Indian J Physiol Allied Sci*, 1967, **20**, 6); aq. ext., antifung. (*Labdev*, 1970, **8B**, 58). Young leaves with wet wheat flour or *sindoor* applied on skin erruptions and swellings (*J Econ Tax Bot*, 1980, **1**, 137). Leaves with other ingredients, an aborticide (*Econ Bot*, 1980, **34**, 273).

Seeds—laxt. (Wlth India, IV, 39). Powd. (12g) taken for three days during menses, sterilizes women for long time (*Nagarjun*, 1979- 80, **23**, 2).

Plant—various parts used in otitis media suppurativa, mouth sores, atrophy, emaciation or cachexy, rheum., smallpox, carbuncle, mucus in urine, spermator., gravel, cholera, rinderpest, etc. (*Econ Bot*, 1970, **24**, 241).

Aq. ext. of root bark contains orally effective hypoglyc. principle (*J Pharm Pharmacol*, 1962, **14**, 254; 617). Phytosterolin, isolation from bark, powerful CNS stim. and hypoglyc. (*Indian J Pharm*, 1966, **28**, 241).

F. rumphii Blume

Trunk bark, β-sitosterol and 3-OH- 3'-Me-flavone glucd. (*Curr Sci*, 1979, **48**, 113).

F. semicordata Buch.-Ham. ex Smith syn. F. cunia Ham. ex Roxb.

EtOH(50%) ext. of fruit, spasmog. (*Indian J Exp Biol*, 1968, **6**, 232). Scorched raw stem applied on tiger-bite to avoid septic (*Khadi Gramodyog*, 1972-73, **19**, 269).

*F. subincisa Buch.-Ham. ex Smith syn. F. clavata Miq.

EtOH(50%) ext. of aerial parts, spasmog. (*Indian J Exp Biol*, 1971, **9**, 91).

Gorakhpur, U. P.

F. talbotii King

EtOH(50%) ext. of aerial parts, diur. and spasmog. (*Indian J Exp Biol*, 1977, **15**, 208).

F. virens Aiton. syn. F. infectoria Roxb.; F. lacor Buch.-Ham.

Leaf, estrogenic (*Indian J Physiol Allied Sci*, 1967, **20**, 6).

Plant used in sores and rinderpest (*Econ Bot*, 1970, **24**, 241).

FILICIUM (*Sapindaceae*)

*F. decipiens Thw.

Mal.–*Val muriccha*, *niroli*; Tam.–*Athalanghi*; *kattupurvaracu*, *ningal*.

EtOH(50%) ext. of aerial parts, spasmog. (*Indian J Exp Biol*, 1974, **12**, 512).

Found in Western Ghats up to 1,500 m.

FIMBRISTYLIS (*Cyperaceae*)

*F. ovata kem syn. F. monostachya Hassk.

Used in stomachache, adenitis, scrofulosa colli, *phoka nagri ghao*, sores, syphilis, carbuncle, gravel, indign., cholera, dysen., cough, phthisis, broncht., asthma and sterility in women (*Econ Bot*, 1970, **24**, 241).

Throughout warmer regions of India.

FIRMIANA (*Sterculiaceae*)

*F. colorata R. Br. syn. Erythropsis colorata (Roxb.) Burkill

Used in sores and cholera (*Econ Bot*, 1970, **24**, 241).

Leaves contain glucuronides of apigenin, luteolin & its 6-OH deriv., scutellarein (*Phytochemistry*, 1976, **15**, 839). Plant, 6-glucuronosyloxy luteolin and apigenin-8C-glucd. (*Indian J Pharm*, 1977, **39**, 164).

Assam, W. Bengal, Madhya Pradesh and Western Peninsula.

FLACOURTIA (*Flacourtiaceae*)

F. indica Merrill syn. F. ramontchi L'-Herit.

Bark—astrin. and diur. (Wlth India, IV, 44); applied to eczema (*Econ Bot*, 1965, **19**, 236); paste given internally only once, in mad dogbite (*Bull Med Ethno Bot Res*, 1980, **1**, 8).

Plant—used in burning sensation of chest, fever, carbuncle, stab wound, sores and cholera (*Econ Bot*, 1970, **24**, 241). Preliminary pharmacol.; EtOH(50%) ext. of aerial parts, diur. and spasmog. (*Indian J Exp Biol*, 1969, **7**, 250; 1980, **18**, 594). A mixt. of plant (6g) and *gairika* (red ochre)

6g taken on 4th day of cycle makes woman sterile [*J Sci Res Plants Med*, 1981, 2(1 & 2), 30].

Fruits, digest.; and stomch. [*Bull Bot Surv India*, 1973, **15**, 13; *J Res Indian Med*, 1973, **8**(2), 67].

F. jangomas Raeusch. syn. *F. cataphracta* Roxb.

Leaves and young shoots astrin. and stomch.; leaves and bark useful for bleeding gums and toothache; bark infusion as gargle (Wlth India, IV, 43). Preliminary pharmacol. (*Indian J Exp Biol*, 1971, **9**, 91).

*F. montana Grah.

Kan.–*Han sampige, gudda*; Mar.–*Attak, champari*.

EtOH(50%) ext. of aerial parts, diur. (*Indian J Exp Biol*, 1977, **15**, 208).

Found in forests of Konkan, N. Kanara and Western Ghats up to 900 m.

FLAGELLARIA (*Flagellariaceae*)

F. indica Linn.

In Penang, fruits used to treat pox. All plant parts, diur. (Wlth India, IV, 45).

Plant, 4 glycds. of kaempferol (*Phytochemistry*, 1971, **10**, 1059).

FLEMINGIA (*Fabaceae*)

F. chappar Ham. ex Benth.

EtOH(50%) ext. of aerial parts, anticancer (*Indian J Exp Biol*, 1969, **7**, 250). Root, pounded or powd. given orally in filaria (*Nagarjun*, 1980-81, **24**, 1).

Whole plant, 2′, 4′-di-OH- chalcone, a flavon. and β-sitosterol; chalcones, flemichapparin; flemichapparin-A (*J Indian Chem Soc*, 1969, **46**, 964; 1970, **47**, 508; 1023).

Flemichapparins—2′, 4′- di-OH-5′-MeO-chalcone (flemichapparin) and 2′,4′-di-OH-chalcone from whole plant (*Tetrahedron*, 1971, **27**, 211); flemichapparin B & C from roots (*Chem Ind Lond*, 1970, 745, 1113); their str. (*Phytochemistry*, 1973, **12**, 425). Antifung. activity of flemichapparin A; B & C (*Ex-perientia*, 1974, **30**, 1022; *Sci Cult*, 1974, **40**, 198). Synth. of flemichapparin A (*Chem Ind Lond*, 1975, 179).

Leaves and flowers yield 2 new chalcones and 2 known ones 2, 4′-di-OH-& 2′, 4′, 4-tri-OH-chalcones (*Tetrahedron Lett*, 1970, 4367). Roots, β-sitosterol and 7-OH-flavanone (*Montash Chem*, 1971, **102**, 1777; *CA*, 1972, **76**, 56554v).

*F. fruticulosa Wall. ex Benth.

Roots, used in epilepsy, hysteria, ulcers and swellings (*Indian Drugs*, 1976-77, **14**, 47).

Temperate Himalayas.

F. grahamiana Wight & Arn.

Inflorescences contain flemingins A-C, also deoxy- and homoflemingins (*Phytochemistry*, 1973, **12**, 2027).

*F. lineata Roxb. ex Ait.

Plant ash made into paste with coconut oil and applied in skin diseases (*Indian For*, 1978, **104**, 676).

Found throughout India.

F. macrophylla Kuntze ex Merrill syn. *F. congesta* Roxb.; *Moghania macrophylla* Willd.

Various plant parts used in spleen complaints, smallpox, *prolapsus ani, fistula ani*, cholera, dysen. and blindness (*Econ Bot*, 1970, **24**, 241).

EtOH(50%) ext. of aerial parts, preliminary pharmacol. (*Indian J Exp Biol*, 1973, **11**, 43).

Leaves and flowers, chromenochalcones: flemingin C-F (*Phytochemistry*, 1973, **12**, 2027). Leaves, myricitrin (*Shoyakugaku Zasshi*, 1977, **31**, 172; *CA*, 1978, **88**, 148947b).

Stem bark, lupeol, α-amyrin, mixt. of dialkyl phthalates, etc. (*Curr Sci*, 1976, **45**, 797); wood and bark, lupeol, α-amyrin, sitosterol and its glucd.' and tetra-OH-isoflavone; wood isoflavones, genistein and a new one (*Phytochemistry*, 1977, **16**, 1120; 1980, **19**, 2797).

F. strobilifera R. Br.

Pounded root given in fever (*Econ Bot*, 1965, **19**, 241); leaf decoct., tonic for sick animals (*Bull Med Ethno Bot Res*, 1980, **1**, 318).

Leaves leptosidin glucd., leptosin; also phloridizin and naringin (*Planta Med*, 1976, **27**, 98; 1976, **29**, 94).

Roots, chalcones, *n*-triacontane and β-sitosterol (*Indian J Chem*, 1975, **13**, 1105).

FLEURYA (*Urticaceae*)

See **LAPORTEA**

FLOSCOPA (*Commelinaceae*)

F. scandens Lour.

In Malaysia, plant used in treatment of fractured bones (Wlth India, IV, 48).

FLUEGGEA (*Euphorbiaceae*)

See **SECURINEGA**

FOENICULUM (*Apiaceae*)

F. vulgare Mill.

Eng.–*Fennel.*

Fruit(dried) and/or seeds—useful in chest, spleen and kidney troubles. Aq. ext. used as enema for infants for expulsions of flatus. Hot infusion to increase lacteal secretion and to stimulate sweating (Wlth India, IV, 52); fennel in very high doses, causes a form of intoxication (Med. Plants, 108). Tea made from bruised seeds help detoxify body by using it in bath or in a vaporizer to increase release of toxic wastes; as a lotion rarely used for inflammed eye (Herbal Med., 88; 141; 150). With other ingredients used in antiasthmatic drug [*Farmatsiya Sof*, 1976, **25**(4), 60; *CA*, 1977, **86**, 21820h]. Seeds, oil antimicrob. (*Indian Drugs*, 1979-80, **17**, 394). Ethnomed. uses and pharmacol., its estrogenic properties due to polymers of anethole, rev., 41 refs (*J Ethnopharmacol*, 1980, **9**, 331). Oral administration of recipe, containing seeds with other ingredients to female albino rats, exhibit antiimplantation properties with 61.1% foetal loss (*J Sci Res Plants Med*, 1981, **2**, 1).

Essent. oil from fruit, antimicrob (*Indian Drugs*, 1976-77, **14**, 62; 1979-80, **17**,

394); bruised plant applied on glandular swelling (Herbal Med., 153).

Leaves alongwith those of *Lycopersicon* spp. boiled and given in gonor. (*Econ Bot*, 1979, **33**, 29). EtOH ext. of plant, antisp. (*Planta Med*, 1980, **40**, 309).

Fennel (essent.) oil, chem. compn. (Parry, 195); from fruit of Indian origin, grown in Nigeria, yield 2.0-2.4% with anethole, 86% but no fenchole, coumarin and essent. oil contents of fruit varied from fruit to fruit (*Planta Med*, 1976, **29**, 1); xanthotoxin, bergapten, etc. among others (*Fitoterapia*, 1980, **51**, 273); also psoralen, scoparone, vanillin, etc. (*Rev Latinoam Quim*, 1981, **12**, 91; *CA*, **95**, 129383t).

Seed fat contains an octadecenoic acid (*Chem Ind Lond*, 1970, 831); and seed yields 6 arachidic esters (*Indian J Chem*, 1977, **15B**, 586). Fruit contains essent. oil (1.5-3%); and fatty oil (9- 21%) with petroselenic acid as major constituent (unsap. matter, 6-oxychroman derivs.). Fatty oil yields 50-60mg/100g tocopherol. Seed and fatty oil, constituents (*Fette Seifen Anstrichm*, 1976, **78**, 224; 1979, **81**, 105; *CA*, **85**, 141477c; **91**, 35693j).

Leaves and fruit flavons. (*Phytochemistry*, 1971, **10**, 399; *Z Lebensm Unters Forsch*, 1977, **164**, 194; *CA*, **87**, 166146y); abscisic acid (*Z Pflanzenphysiol*, 1978, **86**, 61).

Plant, appetite stim; constituents anethole, fenchone, anisalehyde, feniculin, etc. (*K'o Hsueh Nung Yeh Taipei*, 1979, **27**, 35; *CA*, **93**, 210148a).

Root, essent. oil constituents (*Pharmazie*, 1969, **24**, 782; *CA*, 1970, **73**, 11367h). Coumarins including umbelliferone and bergapten from root [*Azerb Med Zh*, 1972, **49**(7), 32; 1976, **53**(6), 34; *CA*, 1973, **78**, 33848w; 1977, **86**, 2357w].

FORRESTIA (*Commelinaceae*)

See **AMISCHOTOLYPE**

FORTUNELLA (Rutaceae)

F. japonica (Thunb.) Swingle syn. *Citrus japonica* Thunb.

Plant contains fortunellin (acacetin 7-neohesperoside) (*Chem Ber*, 1969, **102**, 2083); leaves and twigs, nobiletin, tangeretin, β-sitosterol and a flavone (*Phytochemistry*, 1975, **14**, 309).

FRAGARIA (Rosaceae)

F. vesca Linn. syn. *F. nubicola* Lindl.
Eng.–*Wild strawberry.*

Volat. constituents (*J Chromatogr*, 1965, **18**, 10); those of Finnish wild strawberry, 87 compds. including 2, 5-di-Me-4-OMe-3 (dihydro)-furanone as main component (*J Agric Food Chem*, 1979, **27**, 19).

Biflavans from leaves, on acid treatment yield catechin and cyanidin (*Nature Lond*, 1965, **208**, 151); abscisic acid (*Planta*, 1968, **78**, 308).

Flavones, detn. in different plant parts (*Tr Khim Soedin*, 1968, No. 7, 104; *CA*, 1970, **73**, 32346r).

Fruit, colouring matter (*J Food Sci*, 1968, **33**, 281); anthocyanidins and anthocyanosides in flowers and fruits (*Stud Cercet Biochem*, 1976, **19**, 113).

FRANCOEURIA (Asteraceae)

See PULICARIA

FRAXINUS (Oleaceae)

F. floribunda Wall. ex Roxb.

Leaves yield 8-OAc-7-OH-6-OMe-coumarin, 8-OMe coumarin and a acetophenone deriv.; also fraxetin and aesculetin (*Phytochemistry*, 1980, **19**, 2494).

F. hookeri Wenz. syn. *F. excelsior* auct. non Linn.
Eng.–*European ash, weeping ash.*

Ether ext. of fresh stem bark, inhibitory to *Bacillus subtilis* (*Angew Bot*, 1964, **38**, 1; *CA*, 1966, **64**, 20191g).

Leaves—ext., toxic to fungi, *Gloeosporium limetticola* and *Alternaria*

tenuis (*Ann Appl Biol*, 1966, **57**, 501); used usually dried, rarely fresh, almost always as tisane, diur. acting mainly on diseases of kidney and for dropsy; also to some extent for rheum. (Med. Plants, 116).

Scopoletin, and other constituents; leaves, flavonol glycd. (*Phytochemistry*, 1968, **7**, 575; 1972, **11**, 631).

Glycd. fraction of fresh bark yields a new coumarin, fraxidin 8- O-β-*D*-glucd., 10-OH-ligstroside and mandshurin (*Phytochemistry*, 1976, **15**, 221); isofraxidin, scopoletin; acid hydrolysis of MeOH ext. increases isofraxidin content (*Dtsch Apoth Ztg*, 1980, **120**, 1505; *CA*, **93**, 200959b).

F. ornus Linn.

Bark contains esculin, esculetin and fraxin [*Farmatsiya Sof*, 1971, **21**(6), 8; *CA*, 1972, **76**, 131549c]; bark, aesculin, 4%; and flowers, cichoriin (3%), fraxetin, etc. (*Tr Nauchnoissled Khim Farm Inst*, 1972, **8**, 147; *CA*, 1973, **78**, 156664r).

FRITILLARIA (Liliaceae)

F. imperialis Linn.
Eng.–*Snake's head.*

Alk. fraction—containing imperialine reduced B.P. and showed relaxant and antisp. effects; minor alk. fraction from corms, hypoten., B.P. depress. and antifibrillatory (*Indian J Exp Biol*, 1965, **3**, 249; 1966, **4**, 153); of bulb homogenates, hypoten. in dogs (*Therapie*, 1967, **22**, 231). Pharmacol. of alk. ext. (*J Physiol Paris*, 1969, **61**, 453; *CA*, 1970, **72**, 130888t). Neuromuscular metabolic effect (*C R Soc Biol*, 1969, **163**, 2117; *CA*, 1970, **73**, 23681u).

Corms contain alks. cevanin, cevacin; and imperialine & its str. (*Indian J Chem*, 1969, **7**, 1057; *Tetrahedron Lett*, 1976, 3161).

F. roylei Hook.

Bulb, Chinese drug 'Szechuan-Pei-Mu'; used as antipyr., expect. and lactag. (Wlth India, IV, 43); as tonic (*Khadi Gramodyog*, 1972-73, **19**, 269).

Bulb contains alk. kashmirine (*Tetrahedron Lett*, 1976, 2903).

FUCHSIA (*Onagraceae*)

*F. magellanica Lamk
EtOH(50%) ext. of aerial parts, diur. (*Indian J Exp Biol*, 1977, **15**, 208).
Reported from Darjeeling, W. Bengal.

FUCUS (*Fucaceae*)

F. vesiculosus Linn.
Eng.–*Rockweed*.
Plant ext. agglutinated human erythrocytes of group A, B, O & AB (*Z Allg Mikrobiol*, 1978, **18**, 355; *CA*, **89**, 87147n). Thallus contains iodine, 0.04%; BuOH ext. of plant yields 5-8% diiodotyrosine (*Pharmazie*, 1965, **20**, 176; *CA*, **63**, 6018h). Ripe female tips, hexane and unidentified compd. (*Tetrahedron Lett*, 1970, 5163). Plant, fucosterol (*Boll Chim Farm*, 1970, **109**, 454; *CA*, 1971, **74**, 146436w);[1] hexane and pentane derivs., alkanols, pristane, paraffins, phytane, phytol, squalene and β- sitosterol (*J Chem Soc D*, 1971, 448); 2 bromo benzyl derivs. and lanosol (*Z Pflanzenphysiol*, 1974, **74**, 272).

Plant antibiotics: phloroglucinol-tri-OAc, difucohexa-OAc, trifucol nona-OAc, 2 isomeric tetrafucol dodeca-OAc; and others (*Phytochemistry*, 1975, **14**, 1403; *Planta Med*, 1977, **32**, 33).

FUMARIA (*Fumariaceae*)

F. indica Pugsley syn. *F. parviflora* Lamk
Herb—used in fever and influenza (*Econ Bot*, 1971, **25**, 414); chem. and pharmacol. activity due to protopine (*Curr Sci*, 1971, **40**, 455). Aq. ext. used against leprosy (*J Nat Integ Med Assoc*, 1981, **23**, 43).

Herb alks., sanguinarine (*Trav Soc Pharm Montpellier*, 1968, **28**, 157; *CA*, 1969, **70**, 65217r); 7 alks., protopine, cryptopine, *d*- bicuculline, fumaridine, fumaramine, etc.; str. of last 2 (*Khim Prior Soedin*, 1968, **4**, 194; 1970, **6**, 588; *CA*, **69**,

57449g; 1971, **74**, 42528m); base parfumine (*Dokl Akad Nauk SSSR*, 1969, **189**, 1262). Alks.(total 0.74%): parfumidine, parfumine and others (*Folia Med Plovdiv*, 1974, **16**, 101; *CA*, 1976, **85**, 43724m); *d*- & *dl*-bicuculline, protopine, *dl*-tetrahydrocoptisine, fumariline, fumarilicine and narceimine (*J Inst Chem India*, 1974, **46**, 120); dehydrocheilanthifoline and coptisine (*Phytochemistry*, 1976, **15**, 545); narlumidine and narceimine (*Chem Ind Lond*, 1979, 744); 8 alks. (*Tetrahedron Lett*, 1980, **21**, 1693; 1909; 1981, **22**, 3127; *J Natl Prod*, 1981, **44**, 169; 475).

Leaves and stem contain protopine, nonacosanol and sitosterol (*Phytochemistry*, 1972, **11**, 2888); alcs., *n*-alkanes and sterols (*J Indian Chem Soc*, 1973, **50**, 230). Seeds contain protopine and *l*-tetrahydrocoptisine (*Curr Sci*, 1974, **43**, 748); *d*-8-OMe-dihydrosanguinarine, fumariline and oxysanguinarine (*Phytochemistry*, 1979, **18**, 695).

F. officinalis Linn.
Herb—ext., pharmacol. (*Ann Pharm Fr*, 1966, **24**, 68; *CA*, 1967, **66**, 64058v); diaphor. and tonic [*East Pharm*, 1980, **23**(272), 39].

Alks.—herb ext. and its main alk. protopine; pharmacol. (*Oyo Yakuri*, 1972, **6**, 501; *CA*, 1972, **78**, 66946e); total alk. ext., antiarrythmic in rabbits; activity equivalent to that of ethmozine (*Khim Farm Zh*, 1977, **11**, 56; *CA*, **87**, 48139a).

Herb alks. (*C R Akad Bulg Sci*, 1967, **20**, 557; *CA*, **67**, 117013f); other alks. including fumaritine and their strs. (*Can J Chem*, 1968, **46**, 2873; 2876; 1969, **47**, 1103; 3593; 1971, **49**, 139; 3020). Protopine (major) (*Acta Pharm Suec*, 1973, **10**, 520; *CA*, 1974, **80**, 80087y); alk. extn. (*Nauchn Tr Permsk Farm Inst*, 1973, **5**, 47; *CA*, 1974, **81**, 68425v); total yield (*Tr Permsk Gos Med Inst*, 1973, **118**, 33; *CA*, 1975, **83**, 128664a). Sanguinarine; max. amt. of alk. fumaritine at beginning of vegetative period (*Aktual Vopr Farm*, 1974, **2**, 15; 20; *CA*, 1976, **84**, 118428h; 118430c).

Fumaritine sepn., yield 1% (*Khim Farm Zh*, 1974, **8**, 32; *CA*, 1975, **82**, 83010v; *J Chem Soc Chem Commun*, 1975, 89).

Herb polyphenols (*Ann Pharm Fr*, 1971, **29**, 591; *Trav Soc Pharm Montpellier*, 1971, **31**, 233; 1972, **32**, 287; 283; *CA*, 1972, **76**, 151047r; 1973, **78**, 69240f; 68853w).

Unani practitioners import it. Also reported to occur in India.

*F. vaillantii Loisel. syn. *F. parviflora* Lamk; *F.vaillantii* Hook. f.

Herb—acrid, astrin., laxt., alter., beneficial in dyspep. and scrofulous skin affections (Wlth India, IV, 68). Ext. used in tuberculoid type of leprosy [*East Pharm*, 1966, **9**(100), 107]. Injection (i.p.) of aq.-alc. ext. in rats reduced muscular activity, produced ataxia and general loss of muscle tone (*Q J Crude Drug Res*, 1977, **15**, 25).

Herb contains pentatriacontane, β-sitosterol, choline and protopine (*Indian J Hosp Pharm*, 1967, **4**, 169); several alks./bases (*Khim Prir Soedin*, 1974, 476; 1979, 874; 1981, 602; *CA*, 1975, **82**, 28586n; 1980, **93**, 46912x; *Farmacia Buc*, 1979, **27**, 1; *CA*, **91**, 2538j).

Protopine—a protoberberine alk., hypoten. in dogs and cats (*Farmakol Alkaloidov Glikozidov*, 1967, 176; *CA*, 1969, **70**, 56095x). Alks. (0.59-1.55%), sepn. of protopine, fumaridine (*sic*) and fumaritine (*Fiziol Aktiv Soedin Rast Kirg*, 1970, 41; *CA*, 1971, **75**, 148464y); pharmacol. (*Oyo Yakuri*, 1972, **6**, 501; *CA*, 1973, **78**, 66946e).

Bicuculline—extracted from *Fumariaceae*, considered most specific antagonist for GABA-receptors; its str., comprises conformation of GABA itself; bicuculline completely antagonizes the action of muscimol obtained from *Amanita muscaria* (*in* Beal & Reinhard, 195; 267; 273-74).

Root alk., norpallidine (*Phytochemistry*, 1976, **15**, 1802).

Found in greater part of India as a weed.

FUNTUMIA (*Apocynaceae*)

*F. elastica Stapf

Eng.–*Lagos silk rubber, ire rubber.*

Bark, bitter, used for piles in Ghana (Wlth India, IV, 93).

Leaves contain alks., irehdiamines A & B (*Bull Soc Chim Fr*, 1963, 594). Seed, steroids and alks. (*C R Acad Sci*, 1969, **268C**, 2105); see also vegetable pregnane steroids (Asolkar & Chadha, 143). EtOH ext. of seeds, a new epimer of irehdiamine, conamine, conessine and N, N'-tetra-Meholarrhimine (*Planta Med*, 1979, **35**, 48).

Grown in Nilgiris and in Bangalore.

FURCRAEA (*Amaryllidaceae*)

F. foetida Haw. syn. *F. gigantea* Vent.

Eng.–*Mauritius hemp.*

In Venezuela, leaves used against tumours (*Lloydia*, 1967, **30**, 379).

Leaves contain gentrogenin, tigogenin (0.20%) and hecogenin (0.33%) (*Phytochemistry*, 1978, **17**, 1923).

GAILLARDIA (*Asteraceae*)

*G. pulchella Fouger.

Plant, cytotoxic sesquiterp. lactone, gaillardin, its str. (*J Pharm Sci*, 1965, **54**, 1703). Aerial parts, sesquiterp alk., pulchellidine (*Tetrahedron Lett*, 1969, 2073); of Arizona plant, pulchellin B, C, E & F isolated; flavone-C-glycds. (*Phytochemistry*, 1969, **8**, 661; 1972, **11**, 851); ψ-twistane, pulchellon, ψ-guianolide alks. pulchellidine & neopulchellidine; str. of ψ-twistane & pulchellon [*Chem Pharm Bull*, 1975, **23**, 2998; *Int Congr Essent Oils*, 1977 (Pub. 1979), 7, 349; *CA*, 1980, **92**, 146946j].

Cultivated in Maharashtra and elsewhere.

GALEGA (*Fabaceae*)

G. purpurea Linn.; see **Tephrosia pur-purea**

GALEOPSIS (*Lamiaceae*)

G. tetrahit Linn.

Eng.–*Hemp-nettle.*

Estrogenic and toxic effects of plant on mouse (*Can J Zool*, 1980, **58**, 1575).

Plant, aucubin-like substances (*Phytochemistry*, 1966, **5**, 1053); fresh leaves, iridoid glucd., galiridoside (*Tetrahedron Lett*, 1970, 3197; *Helv Chim Acta*, 1970, **53**, 2010); 5 iridoid glucds. (*Pharm Acta Helv*, 1975, **50**, 394; *CA*, 1976, **84**, 71444t); galiridoside, gluroside, harpagide & 6-deoxyharpagide (*Tetrahedron Lett*, 1975, 291).

GALINSOGA (*Asteraceae*)

*G. ciliata Blake

EtOH(50%) ext. of plant, CNS depress. (*Indian J Exp Biol*, 1973, **11**, 43).

Chakrata, U.P.

G. parviflora Cav.

EtOH(50%) ext. of plant, spasmol. and hypoten. (*Indian J Exp Biol*, 1969, **7**, 250).

Root, saponin (*Lloydia*, 1972, **35**, 288). Plant, stigmasterol (*Indian J Chem*, 1975, **13**, 97); luteolin and apigenin (*Khim Prir Soedin*, 1977, 862; *CA*, 1978, **88**, 121655t).

GALIUM (*Rubiaceae*)

G. aparine Linn.

Eng.–*Goose grass.*

In England, plant used in jaundice; leaf juice, to check bleeding of wounds (*Econ Bot*, 1974, **28**, 331).

Aerial parts, iridoid glycd., asperuloside (*Yakugaku Zasshi*, 1969, **89**, 287); asperuloside, a major iridoid, laxt. and hypoten. compd.; also 2 minor iridoids (*Planta Med*, 1980, **39**, 267).

Plant, luteolin (*Indian J Chem*, 1976, **14B**, 475). Content of anthraquinone deriv. (*Rev Med Tirgu-Mures*, 1979, **25**, 138; *CA*, 1980, **93**, 41516m).

G. asperifolium Wall. syn. *G. mollugo* auct. non Linn.

Polish var., polyphenols (*Diss Pharm*, 1964, **16**, 393; 1965, **17**, 369; *CA*, 1965, **62**, 8115h; 1966, **64**, 10085f); flavon. heteroside (*An Fac Farm Porto*, 1967, **27**, 141; *CA*, 1969, **70**, 4523r). Several flavons. (*Rastit Resur*, 1974, **10**, 66; *CA*, **81**, 35550d). Iridoid glucd., galioside (*Gazz Chim Ital*, 1978, **108**, 13).

Roots, furomollugin (*Justus Liebig Ann Chem*, 1976, 1772); naphthoquinone deriv. (*J Chem Soc Chem Commun*, 1981, 334).

G. elegans Wall. syn. *G. rotundifolium* auct. non Linn.

Plant used in epilepsy, hysteria, cutaneous eruptions, and as aper., diur., and antiscor. (*Indian Drugs*, 1976-77, **14**, 47).

*G. triflorum Michx.

Eng.–*Sweet-scented bedstraw.*

In British Columbia, plant used in chest pain (*Econ Bot*, 1973, **27**, 291).

Temperate Himalayas from Kashmir to Bhutan at 1,800-3,000 m.

G. verum Linn.

Eng.–*Lady's bedstraw.*

Dried flowering plant—infusion as diur. for dropsy and complaints of bladder and kidneys; externally as application to wounds and to cutaneous eruptions (action doubtful).

Salicilic acid (large amt.). Its high organic acid content causes curdling of milk (Med. Plant, 149); polyphenols (*Khim Prir Soedin*, 1971, 7, 529; *CA*, **75**, 148542x). Leaves and flowers, 5 flavone glycds. (*C R Acad Sci Ser D*, 1972, **274**, 1746).

GARCINIA (*Clusiaceae*)

Garcinia spp. impart good dental health probably due to their possession of antibiots. such as morellin, α- & β-guttiferins (*in* Plant and Fungal Toxins, 789); med. value, biol. activity, chem. compn., etc., rev., 51 refs. [*Herba Hung*, 1980, **19**(2), 81].

G. cambogia (Gaertn.) Desr.

Plant used in skeletal fractures (*Sri Lanka For*, 1980, **14**, 145).

Latex, benzophenone derivs., camboginol & cambogin; latter's str. (*Tetrahedron Lett*, 1980, **21**, 1975; *Indian J Chem*, 1981, **20B**, 915).

G. cowa Roxb.

Gum resin, drastic cath., may produce nausea and vomiting [*Nagarjun*, 1974-75, **18**(1), 31]. Fruit, in headache; powd., given in dysen. (*Econ Bot*, 1979, **33**, 52; 1981, **35**, 4). Med. value, biol. activity, chem. compn., etc. of *Garcinia* plants, rev., 51 refs. [*Herba Hung*, 1980, **19**(2), 81].

Stems, xanthone (*Phytochemistry*, 1977, **16**, 2038).

G. dulcis (Roxb.) Kurz

Leaves, biflavans. and a flavanone - chromone (*J Chem Soc Perkin Trans I*, 1976, 1458).

G. indica Choisy syn. *G. purpurea* Roxb.

EtOH(50%) ext. of aerial parts, semen coagulant and CNS depress. (*Indian J Exp Biol*, 1977, **15**, 208).

Heartwood, phenolic compds. (*Phytochemistry*, 1977, **16**, 148). Fruit rind, camboginol, benzophenone derivs., garcinol & isogarcinol; their strs. (*Indian J Chem*, 1981, **20B**, 983; *Tetrahedron Lett*, 1981, **22**, 793).

*G. livingstonei T. Anders.

EtOH(50%) ext. of aerial parts, spasmol., antiprot. and CNS depress. (*Indian J Exp Biol*, 1980, **18**, 594).

Seeds, flavon. eriodictyol (*Curr Sci*, 1966, **35**, 290). Heartwood, bark and leaves, biflavonyls (*Tetrahedron*, 1971, **27**, 1625).

Introduced from tropical E. Africa and grown in Bhagalpur Garden, Bihar.

G. mangostana Linn.

Eng.–*Mangosteen.*

Bark, fruit hulls and dried latex, xanthones mangostin & β- mangostin; fruit hulls, γ- mangostin (normangostin)(*Aust J Chem*, 1970, **23**, 2539). Fruits, xanthones, gartanin, its 8-deoxy deriv., and norman-

gostin; hulls, 3 minor xanthones; garcinones A, B & C (*Tetrahedron*, 1971, **27**, 3919; *Indian J Chem*, 1971, **9**, 505; 1980, **19B**, 1008); a new xanthone; and 2 minor trioxyxanthones; heartwood phenolics (*Phytochemistry*, 1980, **19**, 2223; 1981, **20**, 183; 1975, **14**, 2517).

Mangostins & derivs.—γ-mangostin [1,3,6,7- tetra-OH-2,8-bis(3- Me-2-butenyl)-9H-xanthen-9-one, 9Cl. Normangostin]; mangostin or α-mangostin (7-OMe deriv.) & β-mangostin (3,7-di-OMe deriv.) from fruit rind (Dictionary Org. Compds., IV, 3628). Xanthone deriv., NMR (*Planta Med*, 1973, **24**, 297); protective in liver injury in albino rats (*Mediscope*, 1979, **22**, 65). Mangostin & its derivs., CNS depress., antiinflam. and antiulcer (*Arch Int Pharmacodyn Ther*, 1979, **239**, 257); mangostin-3,6-di-O-glucd., CNS depress. (at 100mg/kg i.p., or above) and raises B.P. (at 25mg/kg iv) (*J Natl Prod*, 1979, **42**, 361). Mangostin, also cardiotonic, antimicrob. and antihepatotoxic; xanthone significantly inhibited primary and secondary responses of adjuvant-induced arthritis in rats; probable mode of action discussed (*Indian J Exp Biol*, 1980, **18**, 843).

G. morella Desr.

Latex, morellic & isomorellic acids, but no gambogic acid present; heartwood, morelloflavone (*Tetrahedron Lett*, 1966, 687; 3195).

Morellin & derivs.—obtained from seedcoat, morellin & isomorellin and their neo derivs., antibact. and antiprot. Of these compds., isomorellin & isoneomorellin, more active; methods.for estn. of morellin (*Indian J Exp Biol*, 1966, **4**, 27; 1967, **5**, 106). Str. of morellin (*Tetrahedron Lett*, 1974, 1259); of neomorellin, isomorellin & isoneomorellin (*Proc Indian Acad Sci*, 1978, **87A**, 75). Good dental health due to antibiots. morellin, α- & β- guttiferins (*in* Plant and Fungal Toxins, 789).

Seedcoat and gamboge, cath. principles.

Guttiferins—β-guttiferin & guttiferin; α- and γ-guttiferins & their derivs., antimicrob. activity and toxicity (*Indian J Exp Biol*, 1968, **6**, 158; 1969, **7**, 34). Seedcoat, isolation of antibact. principles, X-guttiferin and neomorellin (*Indian J Chem*, 1969, **7**, 680).

G. pedunculata Roxb.

EtOH(50%) ext. of aerial parts, CNS depress. (*Indian J Exp Biol*, 1977, **15**, 208). Infusion of dry pericarp of fruit, in constip. and other stomach disorders (*Econ Bot*, 1978, **34**, 264).

Heartwood, a benzophenone and a xanthone (*Phytochemistry*, 1974, **13**, 1241).

*G. talbotii Raizada ex Santapau syn. G. malabarica Talbot

EtOH(50%) ext. of aerial parts, hypoten. and antivir. (*Indian J Exp Biol*, 1971, **9**, 91).

Talbotaflavone & morelloflavone [*Herba Hung*, 1980, **19**(2), 81].

Found in the Western Ghats of India.

G. xanthochymus Hook. f. ex T. Anders. syn. G. tinctoria Wight

Fruit—anthelm., cardiotonic, improves appetite (*Bull Bot Surv India*, 1980, **22**, 59).

Xanthochymol & isoxanthochymol—from fruit; str. (*Tetrahedron Lett*, 1973, 4977; 1976, 2921). Str. of isoxanthochymol and its relation to cambogin (*Chem Ind Lond*, 1978, 166; 1979, 92); their isolation (*Indian J Chem*, 1980, **19B**, 627); xanthochymol, antibact. against *Streptococcus faecallis* and *Klebsiella pneumoniae*, action better than tetracycline (*Curr Sci*, 1980, **49**, 472).

Fruits, flavones and xanthones (*Curr Sci*, 1979, **48**, 814); biflavones and xanthones (*Acta Ciencia Indica*, 1981, **7C**, 31).

GARDENIA (*Rubiaceae*)

G. floribunda Roxb.; see Xeromphis spinosa

G. gummifera Linn.f.

EtOH(50%) ext. of aerial parts, CNS-depress. (*Indian J Exp Biol*, 1973, **11**, 43).

Gum, isolation of 5 flavons. including gardenin, de-Me-tangeretin and nevadensin (*Indian J Chem*, 1971, **9**, 189); 3 wogonins, isoscutellarein, apigenin and de-MeO-sudachitin (*ibid*, 1976, **14B**, 651); flavone (*Phytochemistry*, 1977, **16**, 399). Stembark, oleanonic aldehyde, sitosterol, erythrodiol & its -19 α- OH deriv. (*Planta Med*, 1977, **32**, 206).

G. jasminoides Ellis syn. G. florida auct. non Linn.

EtOH(50%) ext. of aerial parts, antivir. and spasmol. (*Indian J Exp Biol*, 1969, **7**, 250). Fruit, important component of several Chinese traditional med.; one such med. containing several plant products, used in chr. myelocytic leukemia (*in* Wagner & Wolff, 153; *in* Beal & Reinhard, 357).

Fruits, nonacosane, β-sitosterol and *d*-mannitol (*Yao Hsueh Hsueh Pao*, 1964, **11**, 342; *CA*, **61**, 8130c). Exts. of fruit, leaves and stalks, new iridoid glucd., gardenoside and geniposide; fruit, shanzhiside (*Tetrahedron Lett*, 1969, 2347; 1970, 3581); also genipin- 1-β-gentiobioside (*Chem Pharm Bull*, 1970, **18**, 1066); iridoid glucds., gardenoside, shaznhiside, Me-de-Ac- asperulosidate, geniposide and genipin gentiobioside (*Yakugaku Zasshi*, 1974, **94**, 577); gardoside and scandoside-Me-ester (*Phytochemistry*, 1974, **13**, 2219); iridoid glucds., 10-Ac-geniposide and picrocrocinic acid (*Chem Pharm Bull*, 1976, **24**, 2644).

Flower, essent. oil, constituents (*K"o Hsueh Fa Chan Yueh K'an*, 1979, **7**, 1036; *CA*, 1980, **92**, 124929d).

Geniposide—a laxt. constituent, biol. and chem. assay of compd. from fruits. Mech. of purg. action; fecal softening activity of crude drug from fruit mainly due to this iridoid glucd., though other iridoid glucds. also contributing factors; purg. activities of iridoid glucds. (*Planta Med*, 1974, **25**, 39; 219; 285).

*G. latifolia Ait.

Eng.–*Boxwood gardenia*; H.–*Papra*; Mar.–*Ghogari*; Tel.–*Pedda bikki.*

Young leaves pounded and applied to cattle wounds; also used in snakebite (*Econ Bot*, 1965, **19**, 242; 1970, **24**, 241).

Stembark, sitosterol, oleanolic, siaresinolic, spinosic acids and hederagenin (*Phytochemistry*, 1975, **14**, 307); triterp., 3- episiaresinolic acid (*Indian J Chem*, 1975, **13**, 747).

Found in Tamil Nadu and Karnataka.

G. resinifera Roth syn. *G. lucida* Roxb.

Gum-resin—as antisep. and stim. (*Bull Bot Surv India*, 1973, **15**, 17); carmin., stim. in dyspep. and anthelm. (*Bull Med Ethno Bot Res*, 1980, **1**, 120).

Indian essent.oils, chem., rev. covering physicochem. characteristics (*Perfum Essent Oil Rec*, 1967, **58**, 782); antimicrob. and anthelm. activity (*Indian Perfum*, 1979, **23**, 213).

Gum, str. of flavon. gardenin; gardenins A, B, C, D & E; gardenin A, de-Me-tangeretin, nevadensin and 2 wogonins; hexacosyl *p*-coumarate; wogonin deriv.; a flavone; other wogonin deriv. (*Indian J Chem*, 1968, **6**, 677; 1970, **8**, 398; 1972, **10**, 23; 1980, **19B**, 421; 1975, **13**, 785; *Phytochemistry*, 1977, **16**, 399; 1109).

G. turgida Roxb.; see **Ceriscoides turgida**

GARUGA (*Burseraceae*)

G. pinnata Roxb.

Leaf juice, astrin. (*J Econ Tax Bot*, 1981, **2**, 175).

Leaves, amentoflavone (*Indian J Chem*, 1978, **16B**, 846). Stembark gave +ve tests for steroid, terp., alk., flavon. and saponin (*Q J Crude Drug Res*, 1980, **18**, 77).

GAULTHERIA (*Ericaceae*)

G. fragrantissima Wall.

EtOH(50%) ext. of aerial parts, hypoten. (*Indian J Exp Biol*, 1971, **9**, 91).

Indian essent. oils, physicochem. characteristics, rev. (*Perfum Essent Oil Rec*,

1967, **58**, 782). Fresh leaves, essent. oil, 0.7-0.8%; containing Me-salicylate, 99.6% (*Indian J Pharm*, 1976, **38**, 56); from leaves from Karnataka plant, yield 1.25% [*J Res Indian Med*, 1978, **13**(3), 84].

Leaves also yield β-sitosterol, quercetin 3- galactoside and ursolic acid (*Indian J Pharm*, 1972, **34**, 125).

*G. procumbens Linn.,

Eng.–*Checkerberry; wintergreen.*

Essent. oil from plant or leaves used as rubft. and in perfumes (*Econ Bot*, 1966, **20**, 17).

Native of America, introduced into India.

GELONIUM (*Euphorbiaceae*)

See **SUREGADA**

GELSEMIUM (*Loganiaceae*)

*G. sempervirens (Linn.) St. Hil.

Mother tincture, antimicrob. (*Indian J Exp Biol*, 1977, **15**, 338).

Plant, alk. sempervirine, synth. (*J Chem Soc C*, 1970, 791); alks. 14-OH-gelsemicine; 1-MeO- & 21-oxo-gelsemine (*Monatsch Chem*, 1973, **104**, 99; 87; 1974, **105**, 1291; *CA*, **78**, 124788t; 124787s; 1975, **82**, 171270x).

Reported to occur in India.

GENDARUSSA (*Acanthaceae*)

G. vulgaris Nees syn. *Justicia gendarussa* Burm.

Leaves made into paste and applied on fractured or dislocated bones (*in* Jain, 142).

Roots yield β-sitosterol (*Indian J Chem*, 1969, **7**, 308). Leaves, β-sitosterol and an alk. [*J Res Indian Med*, 1974, **9**(1), 65].

GENIOSPORUM(*Lamiaceae*)

G. tenuifolium Merrill syn. *G. prostratum* Benth.

One of the constituents of drug for curing cold among children (*J Econ Tax Bot*, 1981, **2**, 188).

GENTIANA (*Gentianaceae*)

*G. argentea Royle
Kumaun–*Karu.*

Roots, tonic, stomch., febge. and in urinary disorders (*Indian Drugs*, 1976-77, **14**, 47).

Kumaun hills, U.P.

G. chirayita Roxb.; see **Swertia chirata**

G. detonsa Rottb.; see **Gentianopsis detonsa**

G. kurroo Royle
Plant, 6,7-di-MeO-coumarin (*Indian J Chem*, 1966, **4**, 457).

*G. lutea Linn.
Eng.–*Gentian, yellow gentian.*

Dried root-infusion, for lack of appetite and stomach disorders; powd. drug and tincture, similar action; former widely used in vet. med. as an appetiser, extremely weak febge. (Med. Plants, 117). Chewing of root for breaking smoking habit suggested (Herbal Med., 174).

Roots, bitter principles, volat. oil and abundance of sugar (Med. Plants, 117); gentiobiose (*J Org Chem*, 1964, **29**, 2079); alks. gentianine and gentialutine (*Acta Pol Pharm*, 1964, **21**, 265; *CA*, 1965, **62**, 13507d); bitter compds., rev. including gentiopicroside and amarogentine (*Pharm Weekbl*, 1966, **101**, 605; *CA*, 1967, **66**, 17024w); bitter constituents, gentiopicroside, amaroswertin, amarogentin & swertiamarin (*Phytochemistry*, 1974, **13**, 2819); bitter substances and essent. oil (*Herba Hung*, 1979, **18**, 311).

Gentiopicroside—glucd. of bitter taste, rev. (*Farumashia*, 1971, **7**, 172; *CA*, 1973, **79**, 50694f); bitter value of gentian constituents (*in* Wagner & Wolff, 152); as antiinflam. agent in carrageenin-induced foot oedema in rats (Jpn Kokai Tokyo Koho, 1979, 7926323; *CA*, **91**, 9485y). Estn. (*Yakugaku Zasshi*, 1979, **99**, 1047). Quant. detn. of bitter principles in root (*Planta Med*, 1980, **38**, 344; **40**, 55). Seasonal variation (*Q J Crude Drug Res*, 1981, **19**, 37).

Leaves, flavonic & xanthonic compds. (*An Fac Farm Porto*, 1966, **26**, 5; *CA*, 1968, **69**, 12907p; *Tetrahedron*, 1969, **25**, 1507; *Helv Chim Acta*, 1973, **56**, 284; 773; 3050); sepn. of xanthones and iridoid glycds. from plant (*ibid*, 1979, **62**, 2079); leaves, glucds. of isoorientin and isovitexin and β-amyrenol (*Planta Med Phytother*, 1974, **8**, 15; *CA*, **81**, 60953m).

Native of Europe and Asia minor; the drug (roots) imported into India.

G. moorcroftiana Wall. ex Griseb.; see **Gentianella moorcroftiana**

G. olivieri Griseb. syn. *G. dehurica* Fisch.

Flowers, oleanolic and ursolic acids (*Indian J Chem*, 1963, **1**, 409). Aerial parts, alks. (0.35-0.67%) gentianamine, gentianadine and gentianine; gentianamine, gentioflavine, oliverine and oliveridine; and gentiotibetine; oliveramine (*Khim Prir Soedin*, 1967, **3**, 182; 1969, **5**, 608; 1972, **8**, 350; 1973, **9**, 64; *CA*, **67**, 117007g; 1970, **73**, 84624z; **77**, 162012x; **78**, 159956y).

Gentianine—comparison of antiinflam. activity of alks.; gentianine (and also oliverine) more effective than gentianadine & gentianamine (*Farmakol Alkoloidov Serdech Glikozidov*, 1971, 146; *CA*, 1973, **78**, 79634b); gentianine (from *G. macrophylla* used in Chinese med.) effects on egg-white irritation "arthritis" in rats (*in* Beal & Reinhard, 382). Gentianine, CNS-depress., antiulcerogenic and inhibitory against gastric secretion in mice and rats (*Yakugaku Zasshi*, 1978, **98**, 1446). See also *Fagraea cochinchinensis.*

Roots, gentiopicroside; gentianine artefact (*Yakugaku Zasshi*, 1976, **96**, 362).

G. tenella Rottb.; see **Gentianella tenella**

GENTIANELLA (*Gentianaceae*)

*G. moorcroftiana Airy-Shaw syn. *Gentiana moorcroftiana* Wall. ex G. Don
Ladakh–*Chhumbi tikt.*

Plant decoct., in fever and as blood purifier. Flower ext., in nausea, giddiness, cough and cold (*J Econ Tax Bot*, 1982, **3**, 981). Phytochem. tests, folklore uses and pharmacognosy; used in Amchies system of med. in Ladakh region [*Nagarjun*, 1981-82, **25**, 4].

Northern parts of India, up to 6,000 m.

*G. tenella Borner syn. *Gentiana tenella* Rottb.

Eng.–*Tender gentian.*

Decoct. of leaves and stem given in fever (*J Econ Tax Bot*, 1982, **3**, 981). Plant flavons. (*Lloydia*, 1972, **35**, 290).

Jammu & Kashmir, Himachal Pradesh and Uttar Pradesh up to 4,600 m.

GENTIANOPSIS (*Gentianaceae*)

*G. detonsa (Rottb.) Ma syn. *Gentiana detonsa* Rottb.

Eng.–*Shaven-flowered gentian*; Ladakh–*Sheeti.*

Flower exts. check nausea, cough, headache and fever (*J Econ Tax Bot*, 1982, **3**, 981). Folklore uses, pharmacognostic studies and chem. tests; used in Amchies system of med. in Ladakh region [*Nagarjun*, 1981-82, **25**, 4].

Jammu & Kashmir and Himachal Pradesh up to 5,000 m.

GEOPHILA (*Rubiaceae*)

G. herbacea Kuntze syn. *G. reniformis* D. Don

In Samoa, plant used to treat diar. and intestinal disturbances (*Econ Bot*, 1974, **38**, 24).

GERANIUM(*Geraniaceae*)

G. mascatense Boiss. syn. *G. ocellatum* Camb.

EtOH(50%) ext. of plant, CNS depress. and hypoten. (*Indian J Exp Biol*, 1974, **12**, 512). Floral ext. inhibited germination of fungi (*Geobios*, 1980, **7**, 94).

G. nepalense Sweet

EtOH(50%) ext. of plant, hypoten. (*Indian J Exp Biol*, 1977, **15**, 208).

Plant, kaempferol 7-rhamnoside and kaempferitrin (*Shoyakugaku Zasshi*, 1972, **26**, 144; *CA*, 1973, **79**, 89454c). Hypoten.

compd., geraniin (Jpn Kokai, 1978, 7831687; *CA*, **89**, 30759j).

From var. *thumbergii*, isolation of gastrointestine- contracting choline-like substance, useful for treatment of gastrointestinal disorders such as gastroptosis (Jpn Kokai, 1976, 76144739; *CA*, 1977, **87**, 73365d).

Root tannin (*Bull RRL Jammu*, 1963, **1**, 136).

G. pratense Linn.

Leaves contain tannin, 12-20; and roots, 19-34% (*Cesk Farm*, 1965, **14**, 406; *CA*, 1966, **64**, 13087a). Exts. containing tannin compds., antibact.; preparation of med. active iodotannin from roots (*Tr Permsk Farm Inst*, 1967, No. 2, 63; 1969, No.3, 289; *CA*, 1969, **71**, 19791w; 1971, **75**, 40299j); w.-sol. flavon. compn., hypoten.; isokempferid and hexahydroflavone [*Eksp Med Morfol*, 1972, **11**(2), 45; *CA*, 1973, **78**, 23912y].

GERBERA (*Asteraceae*)

*C. gossypina (Royle) Beauv. syn. *G. lanuginosa* Benth. & Hook.f.

EtOH(50%) ext. of plant, spasmol. (*Indian J Exp Biol*, 1968, **6**, 232).

Plant, taraxerol & its OAc (*J Indian Chem Soc*, 1979, **56**, 326).

Western Himalayas; from Murrea to Kumaun up to 2,500 m.

G. piloselloides Cass.

Roots contain coumarin, piloselloidal, 3 acetophenones and chromenes (*Chem Ber*, 1975, **108**, 26).

GEUM (*Rosaceae*)

G. elatum Wall. ex G. Don

EtOH(50%) ext. of plant, abortif. (*Indian J Exp Biol*, 1980, **18**, 594).

G. roylei Wall. ex Bolle syn. *G. urbanum* auct. non Linn.

EtOH(50%) ext. of plant, CNS depress. (*Indian J Exp Biol*, 1974, **12**, 512).

Herb, germakranolides, cnicinolide, benedictinolide, benedictine and cnicin (*Naturwissenschaften*, 1965, **52**, 209).

Rhizomes contain gallic, ellagic, caffeic, chlorogenic, protocatechuic acids, catechin, triterps., etc. (*Sci Pharm*, 1964, **32**, 98; *CA*, **61**, 12330h); tannins (*Glas Hem Technol Bosne Hercegovine*, 1968, **16**, 113; *CA*, 1970, **72**, 63603f).

Transglycosylase activity in leaves and cotyledons [*Herba Hung*, 1966, **5**(2-3), 161; *CA*, 1968, **68**, 47065u]. Glucose transferase in roots, intramolecular transfer of glucose from the phenolic OH group to alc. OH in saligenin studied in detail (*Phytochemistry*, 1969, **8**, 1665). Modified method of isolation of glycd. gein (therapeutically important), on enzymic hydrolysis yielding eugenol and vicianose (a disaccharide of glucose and arabinose). Vicianosidase activity from roots and formation of glycds. in plant proved by *in vivo* experiments by infiltration of various phenolic compds. (*Planta Med*, 1970-71, **19**, 154; 1972, **22**, 93).

GINKGO (*Ginkgoaceae*)

*G. biloba Linn.

Leaves—standardized preparation containing procyanidin- flavon. mixt. (Tebonin) used in cardiovascular disorders; preparation used in patients suffering from Parkinson's disease, increased cerebral blood circulation (*Arzneim Forsch*, 1967, **17**, 491; *CA*, **67**, 52644r). Vasoactive drug (Ger. Offen., 1972, 2117429; *CA*, 1973, **78**, 47787n); ext., cosmetologically active (*Riv Ital Essenze Profumi Piante Off Aromi Saponi Cosmet Aerosol*, 1974, **56**, 13; *CA*, **81**, 126679x). 'Tanakan' (active principle of plant ext.), effective in induced cerebral ischemia in rats (*Therapie*, 1978, **33**, 651; *CA*, 1979, **90**, 115360t).

Nuts—against cancer in China (*Lloydia*, 1969, **32**, 188); seeds, insignificant carcinogenic activity (*in* Plant and Fungal Toxins, 262). Ext., antibact. against

Mycobacterium smegmatis(*Fitoterapia*, 1981, **52**, 129).

Chem. and pharmacol. of *G. biloba*, rev., 39 refs. [*Plant Med Phytother*, 1977, **11**(Special Issue), 189; *CA*, 1978, **88**, 31780a].

Leaves, shikimic acid; flavons. (*Bot Mag*, 1963, **76**, 391; *CA*, 1964, **61**, 12322h; *Naturwissenschaften*, 1965, **52**, 592; *Z Naturforsch*, 1965, **20B**, 1139; 1979, **34C**, 878); leaf flavonols, vasodilator in guinea-pigs and spasmol.; leaf constituents, rev., 23 refs.; phenolic components (*Arzneim Forsch*, 1966, **16**, 719; 1968, **18**, 537; 539).

Biflavonoids—of leaves, active in peripheral vasodilation and also exhibited antibradykinin activity (*Curr Sci*, 1970, **39**, 533); pharmacol., rev. 29 refs. (*J Indian Med Assoc*, 1970, **55**, 163). Sequoyitol and *d*-pinitol; biflavone, 1,5- MeO-bilobetin (*Phytochemistry*, 1972, **11**, 245; 1980, **19**, 1999).

Leaves, sesquiterp. bilobalide A (*Justus Liebigs Ann Chem*, 1969, **724**, 214; *J Am Chem Soc*, 1971, **93**, 3544); β-sitosterol (*Phytochemistry*, 1970, **9**, 1817).

Ginkgolides—diterps. from leaves and rootbark; ginkgolides A, B & C; ginkgolide A, extremely novel form of diterp.; root bark, also ginkgolide M (*Pure Appl Chem*, 1967, **14**, 89; *Chem Commun*, 1967, 259; *J Chem Soc C*, 1967, 2201; *Tetrahedron Lett*, 1967, 299); chem. of ginkgolides, rev., 18 refs. (*Kagaku To Seibutsu*, 1968, **6**, 628; *CA*, 1969, **70**, 38007r); with exts. containing bilobalide and ginkgolides A, B & C as main substances, significant increase of blood flow, in patients with cerebrovascular disease (*in* Beal & Reinhard, 259-60).

Fruit, pharmacol. of bilobol, compd. isolated from flesh (*Soul Uidae Chapchi*, 1964, **5**, 281; *CA*, 1966, **65**, 7861c). Phenolic toxic substances from fruit pulp; and sensitizers from seed (*Chem Pharm Bull*, 1968, **16**, 2282; *Phytochemistry*, 1975, **15**, 1959).

Ginnol identical with celidoniol (*An Quim*, 1969, **65**, 303; *CA*, **71**, 19499g). Antibact. fruits ext. contains anacardic acids, bilobols and cardanols (*Fitoterapia*, 1981, **52**, 129).

Plant constituent (*Hua Hsueh Hsueh Pao*, 1962, **28**, 52; *CA*, 1964, **60**, 1634a); sesquiterp.; bilobalide (*Justus Liebigs Ann Chem*, 1969, **724**, 214; *J Am Chem Soc*, 1971, **93**, 3544); sterols (*Lipids*, 1977, **12**, 511).

Heartwood, sesquiterp. bilobanone, str. (*Yakugaku Zasshi*, 1968, **88**, 562); others (*Chem Pharm Bull*, 1975, **23**, 1892). Constituents of pollen (*Shoyakugaku Zasshi*, 1980, **34**, 145).

Native of China, occasionally cultivated in Indian gardens, particularly on hills.

GIRARDINIA (*Urticaceae*)

G. diversifolia Friis syn. *G. heterophylla* Decne. var. *zeylanica* Hook.f.; *G. zeylanica* Decne.

Leaves contain pharmacol. active, 5-OH-tryptamine and histamine (*J Pharm Pharmacol*, 1964, **16**, 361); also Accholine (*Can J Physiol Pharmacol*, 1966, **44**, 621). Plant, β-sitosterol (*Indian J Chem*, 1973, **11**, 840).

GISEKIA (*Aizoaceae*)

G. pharnaceoides Linn.

EtOH(50%) ext. of plant; CNS depress. (*Indian J Exp Biol*, 1974, **12**, 512).

Plant contains triacontane, dotriacontane, myristone, sugars, etc. (*Phytochemistry*, 1972, **11**, 2883); flavons. (*Lloydia*, 1975, **38**, 346).

GIVOTIA (*Euphorbiaceae*)

*G. rottleriformis Griff.

Kan.–*Pumkki*; Mar.–*Polki*; Tam.–*Vendalai*; Tel.–*Tella puliki*.

EtOH(50%) ext. of stem bark, hypoten. (*Indian J Exp Biol*, 1974, **12**, 512).

Peninsular India.

GLEDITSIA (*Caesalpinaceae*)

G. sinensis Lamk

Leaves, flavons. (*Chem Pharm Bull*, 1977, **25**, 3408).

G. triacanthos Linn.

Pod, polyphenols (*Phytochemistry*, 1964, **3**, 263; *Ann Chem*, 1966, **691**, 181; *CA*, **64**, 15967c). Seed galactomannans; str. (*Ann Pharm Fr*, 1966, **24**, 69; *CA*, **65**, 4086e; *Carbohydr Res*, 1970, **15**, 291; *CA*, 1971, **74**, 20344t). Aq. dispersions of 2% plant polyhalosides (galactomannan), as hair softening and decrimping agent (Fr. Pat.,1971, 2067649; *CA*, 1973, **78**, 20125h). Triterp. glycds., triacanthoside A, B, C & D from pods; str. of C (*Khim Prir Soedin*, 1970, **6**, 482; 1972, **8**, 741; *CA*, **73**, 127740d; 1973, **78**, 108259r). See leaves also. Str. of major triterp. saponin, gleditsia C from fruit (*Planta Med*, 1980, **40**, 185).

Leaves, N-Me- β-Ph-Et-amine and tyramine (*Econ Bot*, 1966, **20**, 274); pharmacognosy [*Farmatsiya Sof*, 1969, **19**(6), 37;*CA*, 1970, **72**, 136320y]; alk., triacanthine, hydrocarbons and alcs. (*Pharmazie*, 1971, **26**, 493; *CA*, **75**, 126651e); saponin, and also from fruits, 4 saponins [*Farmatsiya Sof*, 1971, **21**(2), 34; *CA*, **75**, 137454u]. Leaves, flavons. (*Dokl Bolg Akad Nauk*, 1972, **25**, 71; *CA*, **77**, 72531m).

GLEICHENIA (*Gleicheniaceae*)

See **DICRANOPTERIS**

GLINUS (*Molluginaceae*)

G. lotoides Linn. syn. *Mollugo hirta* Thunb.; *M. lotoides* Kuntze

Plant—decoct. given in piles (*Bull Bot Surv India*, 1973, **15**, 17). EtOH(50%) ext., CNS depress. and diur. (*Indian J Exp Biol*, 1977, **15**, 208).

Whole plant yields γ- & β-sitosterol and oleanolic acid; sapogenin mollugogenol A & B; also C, E, F & D their constitutions (*J Indian Chem Soc*, 1973, **50**, 163; 1967, **44**, 454; 1969, **46**, 96; 98; 1061; *Tetrahedron*, 1969, **25**, 3301; *Indian J Chem*, 1970, **8**, 1042; 1975, **13**, 947; 1976, **14B**, 59).

Leaves, triterp. glycd., mollugocin A; new triterp. saponin from seeds, anthelm. (*J Indian Chem Soc*, 1976, **53**, 598;

Phytochemistry, 1976, **15**, 831; 1980, **19**, 1553).

G. oppositifolius DC. syn. *Mollugo oppositifolia* Linn.

EtOH(50%) ext. of plant, CNS depress. and diur. (*Indian J Exp Biol*, 1974, **12**, 512). Plant juice applied to rash and skin infections (*J Econ Tax Bot*, 1981, **2**, 180).

Plant contains spergulagenic acid and triterp. sapogenin, spergulagenin A; latter's constitution (*Tetrahedron*, 1966, **22**, 143; 1968, **24**, 1107; *Bull Nat Inst Sci India*, 1968, No. 37, 74; *Indian J Chem*, 1965, **3**, 283; 1964, **2**, 339; *J Indian Chem Soc*, 1966, **43**, 41; 1965, **42**, 137; 1967, **44**, 242).

Str. of spergulagenin A (*Tetrahedron Lett*, 1974, 1173; *Chem Pharm Bull*, 1975, **23**, 355; *Trans Bose Res Inst Calcutta*, 1977, **40**, 117; 1978, **41**, 95).

Roots contain mullugo glycd. A, α-spinasterol and β-sitosterol glucd. (*Phytochemistry*, 1971, **10**, 621); bis-nortriterp. sapogenol, spergulatriol (*Tetrahedron Lett*, 1976, 2327; *Chem Pharm Bull*, 1977, **25**, 2430); also spergulagenol (*Phytochemistry*, 1980, **19**, 1551).

GLIRICIDIA (*Fabaceae*)

G. sepium (Jack.) Walp. syn. *G. maculata* Steud.

Eng.–*Ration.*

In Panama, decoct. of leaves used in urticaria and rash. Also used in burns and erysepalas. Reported rodenticidal (*Q J Crude Drug Res*, 1979, **17**, 115).

Leaves, febge. (*Econ Bot*, 1970, **24**, 358). Ext. of leaf and stem, weak antimicrob. (*Lloydia*, 1972, **35**, 157). EtOH(50%) ext. of aerial parts, spasmol., CNS depress., diur. and antiinflam. (*Indian J Exp Biol*, 1977, **15**, 208).

Leaves yield ceryl alc., kaempferol rhamnoglucd.; also rhamnogalactoside (*Curr Sci*, 1966, **35**, 364; 1971, **40**, 106).

Heartwood, robinetin (*ibid*, 1973, **42**, 31); phenolic isoflav-3- one, sepiol; its

deriv. (*Tetrahedron Lett*, 1976, 1741; *J Agric Food Chem*, 1977, **25**, 723); flavons., gliricidin, sepinol, gliricidol and (–)-isomucronulatol (*Phytochemistry*, 1979, **18**, 1037).

GLOBBA (*Zingiberaceae*)

*G. marantina Linn.

Plant used as contracep. (*Planta Med*, 1973, **23**, 167).

Found in Khasi hills, Meghalaya.

*G. multiflora Wall.

Roots used against headache (*Bull Bot Surv India*, 1980, **22**, 165).

Distributed in Eastern Himalayas, Assam and Tripura.

GLOCHIDION (*Euphorbiaceae*)

*G. assamicum Hook.f.

EtOH(50%) ext. of plant, hypoglyc. (*Indian J Exp Biol*, 1980, **18**, 594).

Reported from Kheri, U.P.

*G. fagifolium Miq.

EtOH(50%) ext. of aerial parts, CNS depress. and hypoten. (*Indian J Exp Biol*, 1973, **11**, 43).

Reported from Sambalpur, Orissa.

*G. heyneanum Wall.

EtOH(50%) ext. of aerial parts, CNS depress., diur. and anticancer (*Indian J Exp Biol*, 1977, **15**, 208).

Found in Goalpara, Assam.

G. hohenackeri Bedd.

EtOH(50%) ext. of aerial parts, CNS depress., antivir., hypoten. and hypoglyc. (*Indian J Exp Biol*, 1968, **6**, 232).

Bark and roots contain triterps. 3-epilupeol, glochidone and glochidiol; str. of last two (*Tetrahedron*, 1966, 1513; *Bull Nat Inst Sci India*, 1968, No.37, 77).

*G. neilgherrense Wight

Kan.–*Banavara*; Nilgiris–*Henikay.*

EtOH(50%) ext. of aerial parts, hypoten. and diur. (*Indian J Exp Biol*, 1974, **12**, 512).

Common in Nilgiris above 2,500 m.

*G. sphaerogynum Kurz

EtOH(50%) ext. of aerial parts, CNS depress. and hypoten. (*Indian J Exp Biol*, 1977, **15**, 208).

Found at Goalpara, Assam.

*G. velutinum Wight

Kan.–*Salai-mara*; Mal.–*Kayara*; Mar.–*Paritza*; M.P.–*Koria*; Tam.–*Paniccavu*; P.–*Pundna*; U.P.–*Chamari*.

EtOH(50%) ext. of aerial parts, spasmol. and CNS depress. (*Indian J Exp Biol*, 1974, **12**, 512).

Found throughout India.

GLORIOSA (*Liliaceae*)

G. superba Linn.

Tubers—histological studies of gastrointestinal tract of rat after poisoning with tubers [*Ceylon J Med Sci*, 1967, **16**(1-2), 11]; root ext., no antiimplantation activity in albino rats (*Indian J Med Res*, 1970, **58**, 253). Tubers, abortif. (*Q J Crude Drug Res* 1972, **12**, 1922). Aq. ext. of root, ecbolic in animals and human [*J Res Indian Med*, 1972, **7**(2), 27; 1976, **11**(3), 34]. Paste, antid. in snake-bite (*Econ Bot*, 1978, **32**, 284). Root powd. given during rheum. fever (*J Econ Tax Bot*, 1981, **2**, 194).

Various plant parts used in spleen complaints, tumours erysipelas, sores and syphilis (*Econ Bot*, 1970, **24**, 241). EtOH(50%) ext. of plant, spasmol. and CNS depress. (*Indian J Exp Biol*, 1977, **15**, 208). Juice of leaves, piscic. (*Nagarjun*, 1979- 80, **23**, 177).

Root, source of colchicine; 0.23-0.3% (*Indian J Pharm*, 1967, **29**, 341); 7 new derivs. of alk. colchicine from tubers (*Chim Ind Milan*, 1967, **49**, 1304; *CA*, 1968, **68**, 87424s). Colchicine, chief alk., present in tubers, seeds and flowers, along with other colchicine derivs. [*Ceylon J Med Sci*, 1968, **17**(2), 1]. Seeds contain high levels of colchicine (*Curr Sci*, 1974, **43**, 87); neutral phenolic fraction of tubers of Indian and African origin, 24 alks. (*Planta Med*, 1975, **28**, 201). Tubers, sitosterol, its glucd., and β- & γ-lumicol-

chicines(*Indian J Chem*, 1976, **14B**, 908); also β-sitosterol, its glucd. and 2-OH-6-MeO benzoic acid (*J Inst Chem India*, 1980, **52**, 187).

Flowers contain luteolin, its glucd., N-formyl-de-Ac- colchicine, β-&γ-lumicolchicine, 3- de-Me-colchicine, its glucd. and 2-de-Me-colchicine (*Proc Nat Acad Sci India*, 1977, **47A**, 21).

GLOSSOCARDIA (*Asteraceae*)

G. bosvallia DC. syn. *G. linearifolia* Cass.

Essent. oil from plant, antimicrob. (*Planta Med*, 1979, **36**, 185); that from flowers, anthelm. (*Indian Perfum*, 1979, **23**, 210).

Constituents of essent. oil from plant (*J Sci Res Bhopal*, 1980, **2**, 37).

GLOSSOGYNE (*Asteraceae*)

G. bidens(Retz.) Alston syn. *G. pinnatifida* DC.

Plant used for relief in aching teeth (*Econ Bot*, 1965, **19**, 242); and in spleen complaints, syphilis, cholera, dysen., cough, male impotency, and failure of lactation (*ibid*, 1970, **24**, 241).

Essent. oil from plant, antibact. (*Indian Perfum*, 1978, **22**, 205).

GLYCINE (*Fabaceae*)

G. max Merrill syn. *G. soja* Sieb. & Zucc.; *G. hispida* Maxim; *Soja hispida* Moench Eng.–*Soybean.*

Oil—100ml dose decreased tendency to thrombosis in several days; linolenic acid, active constituent (*Nor Apotekerforen Tidsskr*,1964, **72**, 297; *CA*, **61**, 16684q). Ingredient in preparation for mastitis treatment in bovine udders (US Pat., 1965, 3222252; 1976, 3950554; *CA*, 1966, **64**, 6414g; **84**, 184933v); of compn. for treating fingernails and toenails (US, 1975, 3928561, *CA*, 1976, **84**, 111603v); for treatment of cholelithiasis (Jpn Kokai Tokyo Koho, 1980, 80130919; *CA*, 1981,**94**, 52982g).

Soybean—Unheated protein caused rickets in turkey poults (*Indian J Nutr Diet*, 1970, **7**, 113). Effect of protein diet on serum cholesterol and lipoprotein in healthy volunteers (*Am J Clin Nutr*, 1978, **31**, 1312; 1981, **34**, 1261; 1769). Soybean in treatment of type II hyperlipoproteinemia (*Schweiz Med Wochenschr*, 1979, **109**, 1852; *CA*, 1980, **92**, 57204y). Soymilk in treatment of acute diar. in infants[*J Nat Res Counc Thailand*, 1979, **12**(2), 75]. Soybean, nutrition and therapy, rev., 22 refs. (*Gygyszereszet*, 1967, **11**, 448; *CA*, 1968, **68**, 66157n); chem. & technol., 223 refs. (*Adv Cereal Sci Technol*, 1976, **1**, 325). Usefulness of biol. active factors for human, rev., 78 refs. (*J Am Oil Chem Soc*, 1979, **56**, 121); and atherosclerosis, rev., 38 refs. (*Atherosclerosis Berlin*, 1977, **4**, 445; *J Am Oil Chem Soc*, 1981, **58**, 416).

Seed ext. toxicity, trypsin inhibitory (*Arch Biochem Biophys*, 1966, **113**, 703); protease inhibitors; lipase inhibitor (*in* Liener, 10; 14-23); α-D- galactosidase-destroying blood-group B-antigens (*Eur J Biochem*, 1977, **77**, 419).

Bean ext., papain activator factor (*Biol Plant Acad Sci Bohemoslov*, 1964, **6**, 165; *CA*, 1966, **64**, 14510g); allantoinase, purification and properties (*Cereal Chem*. 1969, **46**, 656); β-amylase from defatted bean (Jpn Kokai, 1974, 7414685; *CA*, **81**, 45905z)

Bean agglutinin—lectin strongly aggregated human platelets (*Biochem Biophys Res Commun*, 1977, **75**, 200; *Yakugaku Zasshi*, 1979, **99**, 1141); agglutinins for neuraminidase-treated human erythrocytes (*Vox Sang*, 1964, **9**, 748). Preparation of mitogenic agent (*Ankara Univ Tip Fak Mecm*, 1968, **21**, 1025; *CA*, 1970, **72**, 76926p). Bacterial agglutinin (*Plant Physiol*, 1980, **66**, 847).

Saponins & sapogenins—sapogenins (*in* Liener, 163); chem. compn. (*Isr J Chem*, 1966, **2**, 246); soyasapogenol C & E (*J Chem Soc*, 1964, Suppl. 1, 5885; *Phytochemistry*, 1966, **5**, 799; 803); effect on animal growth (*J Sci Food Agric*, 1969,

20, 433); TLC (*J Am Oil Chem Soc*, 1970, **47**, 86); str. of 3 saponins (*Chem Pharm Bull*, 1974, **22**, 3010); in hulls, effect on hypocholesteremic action [*Lancet*, 1979, **1**(8109), 223].

Goitrogen—sepn. of thyroid-active fraction from unheated flours; in heated bean fraction; factors producing goitre in rats (*J Sci Food Agric*, 1972, **23**, 549; *J Food Sci*, 1980,**45**, 1179; *J Nutr Sci Vitaminol*, 1979, **25**, 309); purification and mode of action (*J Nutr*, 1973, **103**, 378); MeOH ext. of fat-free seed causes malignant thyroid (*in* Plant and Fungal Toxins, 263).

Antifung. principle from infected soybean (*Life Sci*, 1969, **7**, 1095). Aflatoxins of soybean, survey (*Cereal Chem*, 1969, **46**, 454). Detn. of aflatoxin B₁ [*Maslo-Zhir Promst*, 1974, (2), 13; *CA*, **80**, 119249e]; see also Bailey's Industrial Oil and Fat Products (*in* Swern, I, 386-87).Str.of phytoalexin (*Phytochemistry*, 1975, **14**, 1389).

Unsap. matter of oil—in compn. with that of avocado seed oil, for sclerosis of skin, pyorrhoea, etc.; with corticoids for eczema and infections; sterol-β- D-glucds. ext., haemostatic, vascular- stabilizing and antishock (Neth. Pat. Appl., 1966, 6601888; 1976, 7506328; Ger Offen, 1976, 2523284; *CA*, 1967, **66**, 5777n; 1977, **86**, 78684w; 1978, **88**, 11902p); in antilipaemic compn. (Brit. Pat., 1976, 1427253; *CA*, **85**, 51735f); sterols, cholesterol-lowering in patients with hypercholesteremia (*Atherosclerosis*, 1977, **28**, 325); effect on exp. arteriosclerosis (*Oyo Yakuri*, 1979, **18**, 291; *CA*, 1980, **92**, 141494a); antiplatelet activity of ST-2, an unsap. substance in oil(*Ketsueki To Myakkan*, 1980, **11**, 418; *CA*, 1981,**94**, 150081q); *in vitro*, stimulated *E. coli* (*Bull Soc Ital Biol Sper*, 1980, **56**, 2151; *CA*, 1981, **94**, 115102t).

Sterols and related compds.—triterps. and sterols (*J Am Oil Chem Soc*, 1966, **43**, 254); their sepn. (*Riv Ital Sostanze Grasse*, 1963, **40**, 660; *CA*, 1965, **62**, 8119f). Sterol detn. (*Fette Seifen Anstrichm*, 1972, **74**, 261; *CA*, **77**, 92733g; *Aust J Dairy Technol*, 1973, **28**, 135; *Kyushu Daigaku Nogakubu Gakugei Zasshi*, 1977, **32**, 21; *CA*, 1974, **80**, 11927u; 1978, **89**, 22487d).

Stigmasterol & β-sitosterol—both steroid drug precursors; soybean oil commercial source; obtained as by- products during extn. of natural vit. E from soybean oil extn. method; conversion to steroid drugs (*Trop Sci*, 1969, **11**, 196; Asolkar & Chadha, 132- 33; 140); their extn. (Markets Selected Med. Plants, 130).

Tocopherols—extn. (*J Am Oil Chem Soc*, 1964, **44**, 161; *Plant Med Phytother*, 1975, **9**, 224; *CA*, 1976, **84**, 86728n); oil, adequate vit. E (*J Am Diet Assoc*, 1975, **66**, 13).

Phospholipids—contain vit.Q (*Life Sci*, 1974, **15**, 1); vasopressor phospholipid in crude lecithin (*Lipids*, 1978, **13**, 468); phosphatides and blood lipids of primates (*J Food Prot*, 1979, **42**, 113); lecithin in compn. for hair oil (Eur. Pat. Appl. 1980, 19301; *CA*, 1981, **94**, 71275a).

Isoflavones—estrogenic, inhibit lipoxygenase activity, and exert an antihaemolytic effect on erythrocytes subjected to peroxidation, phenomenon in diet not clear (*in* Liener, 431), Estrogenic activity of soybean products (*J Agric Food Chem*, 1974, **22**, 806); hypolipidaemic activity (*Khim Farm Zh*, 1979, **13**, 58; *CA*, **90**, 179910e); isoflavones, 0.25% in defatted meal of which genistein (64%) and daidzin (23%); sepn. (*in* Liener, 431; *Phytochemistry*, 1973, **12**, 169; *J Chromatogr*, 1978, **150**,266); daidzin and genistin derivs. (*Agric Biol Chem*, 1979, **43**, 1415; 1980, **44**, 469).

Fat-free soybean alkylpyridine derivs. (*Yakugaku Zasshi*, 1964, **84**, 879). Leaves, fruit and stems contain alk. (*Q J Crude Drug Res*, 1980, **18**, 105).

Characteristics of oil (*Bangladesh J Agric*, 1979, **4**, 39; *CA*, 1981, **94**, 119702m).

G. labialis Linn. ; see **Teramnus labialis**

GLYCOSMIS (*Rutaceae*)

G. arborea (Roxb.) DC. syn. *G. pentaphylla* Correa

In homoeopathy, leaves used as antimal. tonic, and in biliary colic, worm-colic, diar. and dysen. (*Bull Bot Soc Bengal*, 1972, **26**, 25). EtOH(50%) ext. of aerial parts, spasmol. and diur. (*Indian J Exp Biol*, 1974, **12**, 512). Standardisation of homoeopathic mother tincture [*J Res Indian Med*, 1977, **12**(1), 1]. Claimed to cure throat cancer (*Bull Med Ethno Bot Res*, 1980, **1**, 447).

Root used in fever (*Bull Bot Surv India*, 1976, **18**, 161). Decoct. of crushed fruits and cumin seeds given in dysen. (*J Econ Tax Bot*, 1981, **2**, 67).

Stem and leaves contain alk. arborinine; leaves, also triterp., arborinone (*Indian J Chem*, 1969, **7**, 308; 1967, **5**, 523; 129).

Root bark contains alks. skimmianine,γ-fagarine and dictamine (*Trans Bose Res Inst Calcutta*, 1961, **24**, 121); alks., dictamine and skimmianine (*Sci Cult*, 1965, **31**, 529); glycozoline, chem. taxon.; str. (*Tetrahedron Lett*, 1966, 661; *Phytochemistry*, 1969, **8**, 769); carbazole deriv., glycozolidine; str. (*Sci Cult*, 1968, **32**, 181; *Indian J Chem*, 1972, **10**, 959; *Plant Biochem J*, 1974, **1**, 73); also 4 alks. including skimmianine (*Tetrahedron*, 1966, **22**, 3245).

Skimmianine—alk. from *Zanthoxylum* and others, extensive pharmacol.; sed. and hypothermic; skimmianine-iron complex, antimicrob. (*in* Wagner & Wolff, 119).

Flower heads, minor alk., glycophymine and amide glycomide; alk. str. (*Phytochemistry*, 1977, **16**, 2007; *Heterocycles*, 1979, **12**, 929; *CA*, **91**, 108128r). Quinolone alk., glycosolone (*Chem Ind Lond*, 1978, 272); minor alk., glycophymoline (*Phytochemistry*, 1979, **18**, 694).

Chem. of alk. arborine, rev., 20 ref.; chem. of quinozoline alks. including arborine, rev. (*Bull Calcutta Sch Trop Med*,

1963, **11**, 37; *J Inst Chem India*, 1967, **39**, 131). Toxicity of plant ext. and carbazole derivs. isolated from plant (*Curr Sci*, 1979, **48**, 344).

*G. mauritiana (Lamk) Tanaka syn. *G. pentaphylla* DC.

Gorakhpur–*Ban-nimbu*.

EtOH(50%) ext. of aerial parts, CNS depress. (*Indian J Exp Biol*, 1971, **9**, 91).

Root bark contains alks. skimmianine, γ-fagarine and dictamine (*Trans Bose Res Inst Calcutta*, 1961, **24**, 121). Chem. of alk. arborine, rev., 20 refs. (*Bull Calcutta Sch Trop Med*, 1963, **11**, 37).

Roots, β-sitosterol, glycozoline, glycozolidine, dictamnine, arborinine, skimmianine and 2 new alks. (*Phytochemistry*, 1980, **19**, 945).

Bark, alk. cardicine (*Taiwan Yao Hsueh Tsa Chih*, 1966, **18**, 33; *CA*, 1970, **72**, 136333e).

Leaves and stems, hentriacontane, hentriacontanol, vitexin, and friedelin (*Phytochemistry*, 1971, **10**, 2247).

Throughout the greater part of India.

GLYCYRRHIZA (*Fabaceae*)

G. glabra Linn.

Eng.–*Licorice*; *liquorice*.

Root—in China, as drug for strengthening muscle and bone, for increasing physical strength and for curing wounds (*in* Wagner & Wolff, 178); in peptic ulcer, useful; liquorice and other drugs; effect of various compn. [*East Pharm*, 1979, **26**(260), 79; *Indian Med Gazz*, 1979, **113**, 200; *Oyo Yakuri*, 1979, **18**, 469]. Effective in acute cases of conjunctivitis (*J Res Ayur Siddha*, 1980, **1**, 21); in hyperprolactinaemia [*Lancet*, 1979, 1(8111), 319]. Parameters for drug selection; quality [*Bull Fac Pharm Cairo Univ*, 1975, **14**(2), 41; *Gendai Toyo Igaku*, 1981, **2**, 46; 56; *CA*, **94**, 214408d-09e].

Constituent of Ayurvedic drug 'Madhuyasti' [*J Res Indian Med*, 1976, **11**(2), 45]; of drug 'Geriforte' (*Indian Drugs*, 1980-81, **18**, 346; *Rajasthan Med J*,

1980, **19**, 23); of Chinese drug for scleroderma; and pneum. (*Chinese Med J*, 1979, **92**, 427; 1981, **94**, 601); for local anaesthesia (*Planta Med*, 1979, **37**, 274); bark in drug for sterilization (*Econ Bot*, 1980, **32**, 273).

Root ext., estrogenic; contains among others β- sitosterol & stigmasterol (*Pharmazie*, 1970, **25**, 620; *CA*, 1971, **74**, 38764t; *Indian Drugs*, 1979-80, **17**, 145). Triterps. [*Fitoterapia*, 1979, **50**, 11;1967, **38**(4), 98; *CA*, 1968, **69**, 93590e]; major components, HPLC sepn. (*J Chromatogr*, 1979, **175**, 350). Chem. constituents of roots of several spp., rev., 73 refs. (*Taisha*, 1973, **10**, 619; *CA*, 1974, **81**, 101792n). Pharmacol., rev., 98 refs. (*Lyon Pharm*, 1976, **27**, 7; *CA*, **84**, 144362b); chem. compds., 54 refs.; chem. and pharmacol., 136 refs. (*Herba Pol*, 1981, **27**, 63; 1976, **22**, 312; *CA*, 1977, **87**, 144540c).

Deglycyrrhizinized liquorice (glycyrrhizin content less than 1%) used in treatment of peptic and duodenal ulcers; conflicting evidence (Markets Selected Med. Plants, 136).

Liquorice (root) contains glycyrrhizin, saponin and principal flavouring constituent; content varies according to variety and area of origin (*c.* 5.9 to 13.2%) and season; Chinese roots (*c.* 7%). Other constituents, triterps. Some minor saponins with analogous oleanane-type triterps. as aglycones, also isolated several flavon. glycds. including isoliquiritin, glucose up to 3.8%; sucrose, 2.4-6.5%; bitters, resins, mannite, etc. Sold in market as root (including stolons) peeled or unpeeled; solid liquorice ext. (blocks); sticks (from green root); and granulated (Markets Selected Med. Plants, 135).

Flavon. formonetin from roots (*Indian J Chem*, 1972, **10**, 128). Glycyrrhizin-free fraction of liquorice ext., FM 100, effective in gastric ulcer in rats; without side-effect such as oedema and hyperten., contains several isoflavons. (*in* Wagner & Wolff, 180, *Chem Pharm Bull*, 1978, **26**, 135; 141, 144); isoflavone glyzaglabrin (*Curr Sci*,

1977, **46**, 753); coumarins & isocoumarins (*Phytochemistry*, 1976, **15**, 352; 1182).

Glycyrrhizin—main principle, sweet tasting saponin, Ca and K salts of glycyrrhizinic acid which affords on acid hydrolysis, a oleanane-type triterp. glycyrrhetic (glycyrrhetinic) acid and 2 mols. of *D*-glucuronic acid (Markets Selected Med. Plants, 135). Possesses mineral corticoid-like action; retention of Na^+ and Cl^- and excretion of K^+. Noted as remedy for Addison's disease but pseudoaldosteronism caused by excess doses also reported. As antiinflam. saponin or its genin glycyrrhetic acid employed clinically in aphtha and other inflam. diseases, potentiating gluco-corticoid action. No direct hormonal activities but indirectly enhances mineralo-corticoid and gluco- corticoid activities. Saponin stimulates biosynth. of cholesterol in rat liver, however cholesterol in blood decreased by promotion of excretion of cholesterol by its metabolic effects.

Antigastric ulcer effect but with side effects (*in* Wagner & Wolff, 178-80); 'Glycram', a drug from roots containing glycyrrhizin, useful in neurocirculatory hypotension, clin. study (*Vrach Dalo*, 1967, **1**, 17; *BA*, 1968, **49**, 89163). Saponin antivir. against influenza type A infections in mouse tissue (*Tr Vses Nauch Issled Inst Lek Rast*, 1971, **14**, 204; *CA*, 1973, **78**, 155107z). Pharmacol. of glycyrrhizin (*Gifu Daigaku Igakubu Kiyo*, 1968, **15**, 792; 805; 810; *CA*, **68**, 94888v-90q); detn., TLC (quant.); HSLC; HPLC (also of glycyrrhetinic acid) (*Yakugaku Zasshi*, 1970, **90**, 497; 1976, **96**, 1035; 1488; 1981, **101**, 822; *Yakhak Hoe Chi*, 1981, **25**, 1; *CA*, **95**, 209736a).

Glycyrrhizin, amt. in roots and rhizomes (*Bot Zh*, 1963, **48**, 1332; *CA*, 1964, **60**, 9597d); extn. (Jpn Kokai, 1976, 7815406; 1978, 7808765; *CA*, 1978, **88**, 197637j; **89**, 117790m); from callus culture (US Pat., 1973, 37105121; *in* Beal & Reinhard, 482).

Sepn. and purification (Jpn Kokai Tokkyo Koho, 1980, 8013217; 1981, 8151500;

8186199; 8197298; *CA*, **93**, 31773d; **95**, 115956v-57w; 187607e).

Ammoniated glycyrrhizin as diabetic sweetner and as a taste corrigent in food and drug (Market Selected Med. Plants, 136).

Glycyrrhizic acid—active constituent of root. Pharmacol. of ammonium salts; preparation and med. uses (*Farmakol Toksikol Moscow*, 1964, **27**, 219; *CA*, **61**, 12506c; *Vopr Izuch Ispol's Solodki SSSR Akad Nauk SSSR*, 1966, 180; 167; 176; *CA*, 1968, **68**, 107868v; 113187p; 113291t; USSR Pat., 1969, 243780; *CA*, **71**, 74027b).

Detn. (*Arch Pharm Wein*, 1967, **300**, 717; *CA*, **67**, 114322v). Detn., spectrophotom colorim.; other methods; their comparison; HPLC [*Anal Chem*, 1964, **36**, 1871; *Farm Pol*, 1966, **22**, 35; *Farmatsiya Moscow*, 1967, **16**, 46; *Herba Hung*, 1966, **5**(2-3), 84; *Indian Drugs*, 1976- 77, **14**, 80; *An R Acad Farm*, 1980, **46**, 183; *Pharm Acta Helv*, 1976, **51**, 374; 1978, **53**, 46; *CA*, **65**, 12061a; **66**, 98551r; 1968, **68**, 25033a; 1981, **94**, 53030g; 1977, **87**, 122833r; **89**, 117936p].

Glycyrrhetic (glycyrrhetinic) acid— preparation (*Pharm Weekbl*, 1966, **101**, 661; *CA*, **65**, 15721h); estrogenic (*Egypt J Pharm Sci*, 1975, **16**, 245); isolation (Jpn, 1974, 7406093; *CA*, 1975, **82**, 86453c); preparatory method [*Khim Pharm Zh*, 1979, **13**(5), 97; *CA*, **91**, 71699z]; estn. (*Plant Med Phytother*, 1971, **5**, 214; *CA*, 1972, **76**, 56196e); see glycyrrhizin also. Synthesized carbenoxolone sodium prepared from acid, antiinflam. in treatment of gastric ulcers and claimed to help duodenal ulcer but conflicting evidence (*in* Plant and Fungal Toxins, 795).

Glycyrrhizinic acid (*Rastit Resur*, 1967, **3**, 262; *Sci Pharm*, 1973, **41**, 155; *CA*, 1968, **68**, 19446a; **79**, 70251n); HPLC (*Herba Pol*, 1981, **27**, 31).

GMELINA (*Verbenaceae*)

G. arborea Roxb.

Bark—EtOH(50%) ext.(also of wood of stem), hypoglyc. and antivir. (*Indian J Exp Biol*, 1968, **6**, 232). Decoct. given in stomach ailments; leaf infusion, carmin. (*Econ Bot*, 1980, **34**, 264).

Root—root bark improves thirst and relieves abdominal pain (*Q J Crude Drug Res*, 1970, **10**, 1555).

Plant—various parts used in swelling of throat, fever, dropsy, anasarca, spleen trouble, pain, colic, rheum., convuls., delirium, small pox, syphilis, sores, urticaria, dyspep., cholera, phthisis, broncht., asthma, diar., intoxication, haemor., septicaemia, gravel and rinderpest (*Econ Bot*, 1970, **24**, 241). In skeletal fracture (*Sri Lanka For*, 1980, **14**, 145).

Roots contain gmelinol. hentriacontanol-1, ceryl alc., *n*- octacosanol, β-sitosterol and a sesquiterp. (*Planta Med*, 1977, **32**, 71); cadinane type furanosesquiterp., gmelofuran (*Tetrahedron Lett*, 1978, 4719).

Leaves contain alk. (*Econ Bot*, 1969, **23**, 274); also luteolin (*Curr Sci*, 1967, **36**, 71); apigenin, quercetin, hentriacontanol and β-sitosterol(*Indian J Pharm*, 1970, **32**, 140); quercetogenin and other flavons. (*Phytochemistry*, 1979, **14**, 1135).

Heartwood, ceryl alc. and β-sitosterol; *n*- octacosanol and gmelinol (*Z Naturforsch*, 1970, **25B**, 270; 693). *n*-Hentriacontanol-1 (*J Indian Chem Soc*, 1971, **48**, 1175); and cluytyl ferulate; lignans, arboreol (*Indian J Chem*, 1971, **9**, 1027; 1972, **10**, 1120); gmelanone (*J Chem Soc Chem Commun*, 1974, 476); OH-lignans and other compds. (*Tetrahedron*, 1977, **33**, 133; 1975, **31**, 1277); 6"-bromoisoarboreol; lignan hemiacetal, gummidiol (*Tetrahedron Lett*, 1975, 4697; 1803).

G. asiatica Linn.

Fruits applied to forehead for relief from burning sensation in eyes and also to cool body (*J Econ Tax Bot*, 1981, **2**, 188).

EtOH(50%) ext. of aerial parts, anticancer (*Indian J Exp Biol*, 1980, **18**, 594).

Lignans, taxonomy of genus; leaves, quercetagenin and other flavons. (*Phytochemistry*, 1975, **14**, 824; 1135).

*G. philippensis Cham.

EtOH(50%) ext. of aerial parts, spasmol., diur. and anticancer (*Indian J Exp Biol*, 1980, **18**, 594).

Flowers contain kaempferol (*J Indian Chem Soc*, 1979, **56**, 944).

Grown in Indian gardens.

GNAPHALIUM (*Asteraceae*)

G. luteo-album Linn. syn. *G. affine* D. Don

Leaves, astrin. and in vulnerary troubles (*Indian Drugs*, 1976-77, **14**, 77).

Leaves contain luteolin glucd. (*Yakugaku Zasshi*, 1964, **84**, 895). Flowers, luteolin, its glucd. and a chalcone glucd., dehydro-*p*- asebotin; other flavons. (*Chem Pharm Bull*, 1974, **22**, 1800; *Agric Biol Chem*, 1975, **39**, 2239).

GNETUM (*Gnetaceae*)

G. montanum Markgraf syn. *G. scandens* Roxb.

Leaves, as piscic. (*Econ Bot*, 1970, **24**, 134).

*G. ula Brongn. non Karst.

Seed oil used in rheum.

EtOH(50%) ext. of aerial parts, spasmol. and hypoten. (*Indian J Exp Biol*, 1971, **9**, 91).

Plant contains bergenin and stilbene (*Phytochemistry*, 1981, **20**, 1455).

Found in evergreen forest of Western and Eastern Ghats up to 1,800 m.

GNIDIA (*Thymelaeaceae*)

G. glauca Gilg syn. *Lasiosiphon eriocephalus* Decne.

EtOH(50%) ext. of stem, antivir. (*Indian J Exp Biol*, 1968, **6**, 232).

Root bark, coumarin, lasicephalin; str. revision (*Chem Ind Lond*, 1971, 885; 1973,

792; *Indian J Chem*, 1974, **12**, 450); β-sitosterol (*ibid*, 1973, **11**, 840).

Leaves, coumarin, lasioerin (*Chem Ind Lond*, 1978, 954). Plant, coumarin glucd., erioside; also bicoumarin glycd., eriocephaloside (*Phytochemistry*, 1980, **19**, 1554; 1981, **20**, 2044); syringin, syringiresinol, genkwanin, its pyranoside β-sitosterol & its glucd. (*Planta Med*, 1981, **41**, 407).

GOMPHIA (*Ochnaceae*)

G. angusitifolia Vahl; see Ouratea angustifolia

GOMPHOSTEMMA (*Lamiaceae*)

*G. lucidum Wall.

Roots used in pneum. (Santapau & Henry, 73).

From Assam hills.

*G. parviflorum Wall.

EtOH(50%) ext. of plant, diur. (*Indian J Exp Biol*, 1977, **15**, 208).

Reported from Goalpara, Assam.

*G. wallichii Prain

Root ext. alongwith root ext. of *Coccinia grandis* given to stop frequent vomiting and headache (*Bull Bot Surv India*, 1980, **22**, 161).

Found in Meghalaya.

GOMPHRENA (*Amaranthaceae*)

*G. celosioides Mart.

EtOH(50%) ext. of plant, diur. (*Indian J Exp Biol*, 1977, **15**, 208).

Plant, ecdysterone (*Phytochemistry*, 1971, **10**, 2225).

More or less throughout India.

*G. globosa Linn.

Kan.–*Kemugonele.*

Virus infected leaves contain flavon., gomphrenol (*Phytochemistry*, 1978, **17**, 2138). EtOH ext., expect. in animals; flavone glycd. as active principle (*Yao Hsueh T'ung Pao*, 1981, **16**, 55; *CA*, **95**, 175615t).

Native of America, cultivated as an ornamental and has run wild.

GONATANTHUS (*Araceae*)

*G. pumilus (D.Don) Engl. & Krause

In China, herb used as antiasthmatic drug, its immunopharmacol. No marked direct bronchodilatory activity and no antiallergic action (*Acta Pharm Sin*, 1980, **15**, 7).

Subtropical Himalayas.

GONIOPTERIS (*Thelypteridaceae*)

G. prolifera Presl; see Ampelopteris prolifera

GORDONIA (*Theaceae*)

G. obtusa Wall. ex Wight & Arn.

Bark contains ellagic acid and coumarin (*Indian J Chem*, 1973, **11**, 840).

GOSSYPIUM (*Malvaceae*)

G. arboreum Linn.

Various plant parts used in earache, madness, convuls. and labour complaints (*Econ Bot*, 1970, **24**, 241). EtOH(50%) ext. of aerial parts, CNS depress. (*Indian J Exp Biol*, 1974, **12**, 512).

G. barbadense Linn.

Flowers, flavon. glucds. [*Dokl Akad Nauk Uzb SSR*, 1964, **21**(9), 30; *Khim Prir Soedin*, 1971, **7**, 142; *CA*, 1965, **62**, 9457d; **75**, 31270r; *Phytochemistry*, 1972, **11**, 1518]. Leaf polyphenolics (*Egypt J Chem*, 1974, **17**, 135).

Roots, antimicrob. terp.; infected plant contains naphthofuran precursors of sesquiterp. aldehydes (*Phytochemistry*, 1975, **14**, 1077; 1809).

Gossypol—in root bark along with β-sitosterol and α-amyrin (*J Afr Med Pl*, 1977, 17). Variation in content, in leaf, petiole, seed and bolls (*Sudan J Fd Sci Technol*, 1978, **10**, 37). Extn. (*Bull Fac Pharm Cairo Univ*, 1976, **15**, 341). See also under *G. herbaceum.*

G. herbaceum Linn.

Flowers used in uterine discharges (*Q J Crude Drug Res*, 1972, **12**, 1922).

Contracep. effects of alc. exts. in rats (*Contraception*, 1978, **18**, 191).

Antibact. activity of leaf ext. (*Geobios*, 1981, **8**, 277).

Gossypol—major pigment, dimeric naphthalene deriv., tautomeric, and active constituent of cotton seed and oil. Ranges of 0.68-2.36% gossypol in kernels of various cottonseed varieties grown in India reported (Murti & Acharya, 43-47, 59- 69). Its content (in domestic commercial glanded cotton seed kernels, 0.4 to 1.7%); a major obstacle to worldwide utilization of cottonseed protein as food for human being; glandless, gossypol-free cotton seed and a process for removal of glands during commercial processing of glanded seed by solvent extn. under development; highly reactive and responsible for reduction in nutritive quality of protein of cotton seed meal. Most free gossypol and a small amt. of bound one appear to be biol. active after ingestion; adverse effect counteracted by binding free gossypol during processing and by use of certain minerals, esp. Fe salts; also rev. of important studies including estn. (*in* Liener, 183-237). Oral toxicity of pigments in rats (*J Am Oil Chem Soc*, 1963, **40**, 14). Antivir. and cytotoxic (*J Pharm Sci*, 1975, **64**, 1073).

Removal of gossypol from oil (*Indian J Technol*, 1963, **1**, 435). Estn. of free gossypol in leaves and flower buds; also seed (*J Am Oil Chem Soc*, 1967, **44**, 267; 1968, **45**, 903); its content in cotton flower buds (*J Econ Entomol*, 1973, **66**, 327).Gossypol anal.,rev.,37 refs. (*J Assoc Off Anal Chem*, 1977, **60**, 252). Extn. of gossypol and oligosaccharides (*J Food Sci*, 1977, **42**, 1218). Detoxication of oilcake by removing gossypol, rev., 11 refs. [*Oils Oilseeds J*, 1976, **29**(2), 15]; release in fermentation of meal (*Indian J Exp Biol*, 1981, **19**, 574).

Gossypol from seed, root and stem; safe antifert. drug for males, clin. trials [*Reproduction*, 1981, **5**, 189; *Science*,

1981, **212**, 314; *Am Pharm NS*, 1981, **21**(11), 57]; related studies [*Lancet*, 1980, **1** (8173), 885]. Mech. of action (*IDMA Bull*, 1980 **11**, 229); mech. poorly understood. In an appropriate chem. form such as gossypol-polyvinyl pyrrolidone, safe spermic. in humans; also pharmacol. studies (*Contraception*, 1980, **21**, 183; 461; 1981, **24**, 203; 653; 97; *Acta Pharm Sin*, 1979, **14**, 662; *Biol Bull*, 1980, **159**, 467; 468; *Curr Sci*, 1981, **50**, 64).

Gossypol may cause hypokalemia and other effects; its effect on ATPase in rats (*Chin Med J*, 1980, **93**, 477; *Sci Sin*, 1981, **24**, 573). If oral administration is discontinued, fertility gradually recovers (*in* Beal & Reinhard, 365). Herbology in med., a plant product may get introduced in modern med. (*in* Plant and Fungal Toxins, 801-02).

Gossypol formation by cell suspension culture (*J Natl Prod*, 1981, **44**, 1).

G. hirsutum Linn.

Oil—checked rise in cholesterol level in human [*Med Zh Uzb*, 1964, (10),50;*CA*, 1965,**62**, 10907a]; beneficial in hypercholesterolemia and atherogenesis (*Circ Res*, 1966, **18**, 213). Ingredient of a compn. for mastitis treatment in bovine udders (US Pat., 1965, 3222252; *CA*, 1966, **64**, 6414g). Rats consuming crude cotton seed oil developed large thyroid and pituitary tumour (*J Nutr*, 1967, **91**, 55). Emulsion containing 15% oil, useful in hypovolemia in dogs (*Proc Soc Exp Biol Med*, 1967, **124**, 75).

Oil base material for injectable anaesthetic compn. (US Pat., 1965, 3216897;1966, 3253988; Belg., 1966, 670263; *CA*, **65**, 3679d; 10439a).

Ext. of seed coat, antifung. (*Geobios*, 1978, **5**, 49). Aq. sol. of ether ext. of stems, antibiot. against pathogenic bacteria and fungi [*Uzb Biol Zh*, 1972, **16**(2), 15].

Health hazards from cotton dust [*Arogya J Hlth Sci*, 1978, **4**(2), 84]. Effect of cotton dust and others on mucous membrane of upper respiratory tract, rev., 30 refs. (*Med Pr*, 1978, **29**, 65; *CA*, **89**,

1113p). Biol. active components in dust and other findings (*Proc Spec Sess Cotton Dust Res Beltwide Cotton Prod Res Confr*, 1977, 66; 1980, 10; 58; *CA*, **93**, 1631p; 1981, **94**, 77629k; 179843t).

Gas chromatogr. of unsap. matter of oil (*J Assoc Off Anal Chem*, 1966, **49**, 580); and anal. (*Pak J Biol Agric Sci*, 1966, **9**, 30; *CA*, 1967, **66**, 18032j). Characteristics of compds. from seeds and other parts, rev., 24 refs.; oral toxicity of pigments including gossypol (*J Am Oil Chem Soc*, 1979, **56**, 727; 1963, **40**, 14). See gossypol under *G. herbaceum.*

Essent. oil from bud, β-bisabolol (*J Org Chem*, 1968, **33**, 909); constituents (*Phytochemistry*, 1972, **11**, 2118; 1975, **14**, 2087). Steam volat. fraction, napthalenone deriv. (*J Org Chem*, 1976, **40**, 2958).

Flower buds, terp. hydrocarbons (*J Agric Food Chem*, 1965, **13**, 599; 1966, **14**, 332); sesquiterp. aldehyde *p*- hemigossypolone (*J Chem Soc Chem Commun*, 1976, 109). Insectic. sesquiterp., heliocide H_1, H_2; H_4 from glands of leaves and also bolls; H_3 (*Tetrahedron Lett*, 1977, 567; *J Agric Food Chem*, 1978, **26**, 115; *Phytochemistry*, 1978, **17**, 151); comparison of antibiot. activity of hemigossypolone, helicocide H_1 & H_2 (*J Econ Entomol*, 1978, **71**, 161).

Aflatoxins—detn. of aflatoxin B_1 in seed meal (*J Assoc Off Agric Chem*, 1965, **48**, 815; *CA*, 1966, **64**, 1267c); aflatoxins in hulls (*J Am Oil Chem Soc*, 1970, **47**, 5). Aflatoxins and *Aspergillus flavus* in Indian cotton seed (*Indian J Exp Biol*, 1971, **9**, 410); 2 major problems, occurrence of aflatoxins resulting from mold injection and presence of gossypol in cotton seed protein and overcoming them (*in* Swern, I, 362).

Seed oil rich in vit. E; contains tocopherol, 121.1mg/100g (*J Nutr*, 1963, **81**, 335; *CA*, 1964, **60**, 4700g; *Prikl Biokhim Mikrobiol*, 1974, **10**, 122). Sterol content of oil (*J Am Oil Chem Soc*, 1966, **43**, 168); sterols, (*c*.1.5%), mostly β-sitosterol; see also sitosterol in "Diosgenin and Other Steroid Drug Precursors" [*Aust J Dairy Technol*, 1973, **28**(3), 135; *CA*, 1974, **80**, 11927n; Asolkar & Chadha, 135-37; 140].

Total flavon. ext. from flower more effective than rutin in reducing capillary permeability [*Dokl Akad Nauk Uzb SSR*, 1969, **26**(10), 48; *CA*, 1971, **75**, 33583u]. Str. of hirsutrin from blossoms and isoquercetin from leaves (*Khim Prir Soedin*, 1970, **6**, 555; *CA*, 1971, **74**, 31932n).

Triterp. from cotton shrub (leaves) [*Uzb Khim Zh*, 1964, **8**(3), 43; *CA*, **61**, 15040e]. Antimicrob. terp. of gossypium from roots (*Phytochemistry*, 1975, **24**, 1071).

GOUANIA (*Rhamnaceae*)

*G. pepalensis Wall.

EtOH(50%) ext. of aerial parts, hypoten. and spasmol. (*Indian J Exp Biol*, 1971, **9**, 91).

Occurs in Baripada, Orissa.

GRACILARIA (*Rhodophyceae*)

G. lichenoides (Linn.) Harv.

Aq. ext. antihyperten.; contains prostaglandins (*Tetrahedron Lett*, 1979, 4505).

GRANGEA (*Asteraceae*)

G. maderaspatana Poir.

Leaves—infusion stomch. having deobstruent and antisp. (Uphof, 250). EtOH(50%) ext. of plant, spasmol., antifert. and hypoten. (*Indian J Exp Biol*, 1969, **7**, 250). Leaves given in hysteria (*J Econ Tax Bot*, 1980, **1**, 142).

Steroids, chondrillasterone and chondrillasterol (*Phytochemistry*, 1978, **17**, 2036). Diterp., strictic acid (*Indian J Chem*, 1979, **18B**, 529).

GRAPTOPHYLLUM (*Acanthaceae*)

G. pictum (Linn.) Griff. syn. *G. hortense* Nees; *Justicia picta* Linn.

Leaves and bark preparations used against tumours (*Lloydia*, 1967, **30**, 387).

GRATIOLA (*Scrophulariaceae*)

G. monniera Linn.; see **Bacopa monnieri**

GREVILLEA (*Proteaceae*)

G. robusta A. Cunn. ex R. Br.

EtOH(50%) ext. of aerial parts, spasmol., CNS depress. and diur. (*Indian J Exp Biol*, 1977, **15**, 208).

Leaves contain a phenol, robustol, str. (*Tetrahedron Lett*, 1970, 325); rutin, cinnamic acid derivs., etc. (*Aust J Chem*, 1973, **26**, 2257); arbutin derivs. (*Phytochemistry*, 1977, **16**, 793); flavon. (*Yunnan Chih Wu Yen Chiu*, 1979, **1**, 143; *CA*, **92**, 194469c). Phenolic constituents of wood and leaves (*Z Naturforsch*, 1980, **35C**, 344).

Wood contains grevillol (5-tridecyl-resorcinol) (*Aust J Chem*, 1965, **18**, 2015); also mono & bisnorstriatol (*Phytochemistry*, 1976, **15**, 1418).

GREWIA (*Tiliaceae*)

*G. abutilifolia Vent. ex Juss.

Root paste applied to abscesses (*Bull Med Ethno Bot Res*, 1980, **1**, 8).

Western Peninsula from Coorg to Malabar.

*G. elastica Royle

Ass.–*Man bijal*; H.–*Pharsia*, Oriya–*Mirgi chara*; P.–*Dhaman*.

EtOH(50%) ext. of stem bark, CNS depress. (*Indian J Exp Biol*, 1969, **7**, 250).

Sub-Himalayan tract up to 1,200m. Also in C. India and Western Ghats.

*G. emarginata Wight & Arn.

EtOH(50%) ext. of aerial parts, hypoten. (*Indian J Exp Biol*, 1974, **12**, 512).

Western Peninsula: Mysore, Pulney and Nilgiri hills.

G. hirsuta Vahl var. **helicterifolia** Parker

Plant—EtOH(50%) ext., antivir. and diur. (*Indian J Exp Biol*, 1971, **9**, 91; 1977, **15**, 208). Various plant parts used in headache, eye complaints, sores and cholera (*Econ Bot*, 1970, **24**, 241).

Root—applied to wounds (*Bull Bot Surv India*, 1973, **15**, 14; *Econ Bot*, 1978, **32**, 280); paste used in chest pain and rheum. pain (*Nagarjun*, 1980-81, **24**, 1).

*G. latifolia Mast.

EtOH(50%) ext. of aerial parts, CNS depress., hypoten. and antivir. (*Indian J Exp Biol*, 1969, **7**, 250).

Reported from Raipur. M.P.

G. microcos Linn.; see **Microcos paniculata**

*G. obtusa Wall.

EtOH(50%) ext. of aerial parts, spasmol. and hypoten. (*Indian J Exp Biol*, 1974, **12**, 512).

Found in Tamil Nadu.

*G. rothii DC. syn. *G. excelsa* Mast.

Root bark, lupeol and leucoanthocynidins (*Indian J Chem*, 1974, **12**, 1018).

Found in Eastern Himalayas.

*G. sapida Roxb.

Ass.–*phuhura*; B.–*Phalsa-tenga*.

Plant parts used in ulcerated tongue, colic, wounds, cholera and dysen.(*Econ Bot*, 1970, **24**, 241). EtOH(50%) ext. of roots, spermic., CNS depress. and anticancer (*Indian J Exp Biol*, 1980, **18**, 594).

Tropical Himalayas from Garhwal to Assam and in Kheri, U.P.

G. sclerophylla Roxb. ex G. Don

EtOH(50%) ext. of aerial parts, anticancer (*Indian J Exp Biol*, 1980, **18**, 594).

*G. serrulata DC.

EtOH(50%) ext. of aerial parts, antiinflam. (*Indian J Exp Biol*, 1977, **15**, 208).

Found in N-E India and Western Ghats.

G. subinaequalis DC. syn. *G. asiatica* auct. non Linn.

EtOH(50%) ext. of aerial parts, spasmol. and hypoten.; aq. ext. of stembark, antidiabetic (*Indian J Exp Biol*, 1971, **9**, 91; 1976, **14**, 196). Seed ext. and seed oil, antifert. activity (*Indian J Med Res*, 1971, **59**, 302; *Planta Med*, 1974, **26**, 391).

Bark contains taraxasterol, β-sitosterol and erythrodiol (*Curr Sci*, 1973, **42**, 820); lupeol, betulin, lupenone and friedelin; α-amyrin and heartwood, β-sitosterol (*J Indian Chem Soc*, 1975, **52**, 553; 1974, **51**, 830).

Flowers, δ - lactone of di-OH-hentriacontanoic acid (*Phytochemistry*, 1976, **15**, 1397); β- sitosterol and flavons.(*J Indian Chem Soc*, 1976, **53**, 623); and keto-alc., grewinol (*Lloydia*, 1976, **39**, 372).

Fruit pulp, flavons. and other constituents (*J Indian Chem Soc*, 1979, **56**, 649).

G. tenax Fiori syn. *G. populifolia* Vahl

Aq. ext. of stem and roots, antitumour (*Bull RRL Jammu*, 1962-63, **1**, 201). EtOH(50%) ext. of aerial parts, CNS depress. (*Indian J Exp Biol*, 1973, **11**, 43).

In Sudan, roots used in skin diseases; contain sterol, terp. and alk. (*Fitoterapia*, 1980, **51**, 143).

Stem bark contains triterps., β-sitosterol, etc. (*Indian J Chem*, 1979, **17B**, 537).

G. tiliaefolia Vahl

Plant used in fractures (*Sri Lanka For*, 1980, **14**, 145).

Triterps. of roots and bark (*Indian J Chem*, 1965, **3**, 237).

***G. tiliaefolia** Vahl var. **argentia** Burret.

EtOH(50%) ext. of aerial parts, CNS depress. and diur. (*Indian J Exp Biol*, 1977, **15**, 208).

Khandala, Maharashtra.

***G. tiliaefolia** Vahl var. **tiliaefolia** Vahl

EtOH(50%) ext. of stem bark, spermic and hypoten. (*Indian J Exp Biol*, 1977, **15**, 208).

Warangal, A.P.

***G. umbellifera** Bedd..

EtOH(50%) ext. of aerial parts, CNS depress., hypoten. and diur. (*Indian J Exp Biol*, 1974, **12**, 512).

Peninsular India.

G. villosa Willd.

Plant parts used in sores, wounds, cholera, dysen. and rinderpest (*Econ Bot*, 1970, **24**, 241). Stem ext., active in KB cell culture (*Fitoterapia*, 1981, **52**, 281).

In E. Africa, leaves used to reduce facial swelling and swollen eyes (*Econ Bot*, 1979, **33**, 50). In Sudan, roots used in skin diseases; contain sterol, terp. and alk. (*Fitoterapia*, 1980, **50**, 143).

GRISLEA (*Lythraceae*)

See WOODFORDIA

GUAIACUM (*Zygophyllaceae*)

G. officinale Linn.

Useful in correcting liver function (*Acta Phytother*, 1964, **11**, 141).

Heartwood, furoguaiacidin, a furanoid lignan (*Chem Ind Lond*, 1974, 77). Str. of enedione lignan, furoguaiaoxidin (*J Chem Soc Chem Commun*, 1975, 702).

GUAZUMA (*Sterculiaceae*)

G. ulmifolia Lamk syn. *G. tomentosa* Kunth

EtOH(50%) ext. of aerial parts, hypoten. (*Indian J Exp Biol*, 1974, **12**, 512).

Bark, pharmacol. (*J Pharm Pharmacol*, 1970, **22**, 116).

Bark contains friedelin, betulin and β-sitosterol (*Planta Med*, 1977, **32**, 247).

Leaves contain octacosanol and taraxerol-OAc [*J Res Indian Med*, 1976, **11**(1), 126]; friedelin-3-α -OAc, -3β-ol and β-sitosterol (*Curr Sci*, 1977, **46**, 776).

Plant, kaempferol glycds. (*Indian J Pharm*, 1977, **39**, 164). Constituents of heartwood (*Indian J Chem*, 1981, **20B**, 85; *J Indian Chem Soc*, 1981, **58**, 726).

GYMNEMA (*Asclepiadaceae*)

***G. hirsutum** Wight & Arn.

Various plant parts used in fever, dropsy, anasarca, colic, sores, chancre, syphilis, dysuria, orchitis, epididimitis or hydrocele, infant atrophy, stomach complaints, consumption, cough and broncht., neuralgia, pleur., pneum., male impotency, poor lactation, etc. (*Econ Bot*, 1970, **24**, 241).

Occurs in Bundelkhand, Bihar and Western Ghats.

G. sylvestre R.Br. ex Schult.

Leaves—ext., stim., cardiovascular, diur. and hypoglyc. Useful in glycosuria and has purg. action (*Acta Phytother*, 1972, **19**, 141). Alc. ext. of leaves, and stems, hypoglyc., extensive pharmacol.(*Indian J Med Res*, 1964, **52**, 200; *Bull Calcutta Sch Trop Med*, 1975, **23**, 6; *Indian J Pharm*, 1976, **38**, 161; *Indian J Pharmacol*, 1981, **13**, 99; *Indian J Exp Biol*, 1981, **19**, 715). Ext., *in vitro*, effective against diabetes; insulinotropic in rabbits (*Pak J Sci Res*, 1978, **30**, 65; *Orissa Vet J*, 1978, **12**, 147; *Pharmacol Res Commun*, 1981, **13**, 475); ingredient of antidiabetic preparation (*Maharashtra Med J*, 1981, **28**, 165).

Root and leaves used in stomach pain (*Econ Bot*, 1965, **19**, 243). EtOH(50%) ext. of aerial parts, spasmol. (*Indian J Exp Biol*, 1971, **9**, 91); plant used in skeletal fractures (*Sri Lanka For*, 1980, **14**, 145).

Leaves contain nonacosane, hentriacontane, tritriacontane and alc., conduritol A (*J Pharm Sci*, 1965, **54**, 1541); penta- OH-triterp., gymnestrogenin (*Helv Chim Acta*, 1968, **51**, 1235). Str. of gymnemagenin (*J Chem Soc Chem Commun*, 1968, 1681; *Helv Chim Acta*, 1969, **52**, 365).

Gymnemic acids—str. of gymnemic acid (*Helv Chim Acta*, 1967, **50**, 474); gymnemic acid A1 main component of gymnemic acid A of leaves, antisweet activity (*Life Sci*, 1969, **8**, 537); chem. and physical properties, antisaccharine principle of leaves (*J Agric Food Chem*, 1969, **17**, 704); major constituents, 3β-glucuronides of differently acylated gymnemagenins; str. of gymnemagenin (hexahydroxy-olean-12-ene) (*J Chem Soc Chem Commun*, 1968, 1681; *Helv Chim Acta*, 1969, **52**, 365); mixt. of 9 closely related acidic glycds., genins; chem. of gymnemagenin and gymnestrogenin (*J Pharm Sci*, 1970, **59**, 622; 1971, **60**, 190;

CA, **74**, 115832t). Derivs. of gymnemagenin from leaves (*J Chem Soc C*, 1970, 1823). Isolation and heterogeneity of A1(*J Agric Food Chem*, 1973, **21**, 899); acid & its derivs., *in vitro*, antivir. against influenza A2 virus (*J Pharm Sci*, 1974, **63**, 471); gymnemagenin, isolation [*J Inst Chem India*, 1981, **53**(Pt.IV), 155].

Plant bases choline, betaine, etc. (*J Pharm Sci*, 1967, **56**, 732).

Gymnamine, trace alk. from leaves (*Chem Ind Lond*, 1972, 537).

GYNOCARDIA (*Flacourtiaceae*)

G. odorata R. Br. syn. *Hydnocarpus odorata* Lindl.

Fruit pulp used as piscic. (*Econ Bot*, 1970, **24**, 34). EtOH(50%) ext. of aerial parts, spasmol., CNS depress. and diur. (*Indian J Exp Biol*, 1974, **12**, 512).

Plant contains glycd. gynocardin (*J Agric Food Chem*, 1969, **17**, 519).

GYNURA (*Asteraceae*)

G. crepidioides Benth.; see Crassocephalum crepidioides

GYROCARPUS (*Gyrocarpaceae*)

G. americanus Jacq. syn. *G. jacquinii* Gaertn.

Bark—in Tonga, drink taken for oedema after childbirth, and in treating stomachache and filariasis (*Econ Bot*, 1971, **25**, 440). EtOH(50%) ext., hypoten. (*Indian J Exp Biol*, 1973, **11**, 43).

Trunk bark contains alks., phaeanthine and pycnamine (Thesis, Andhra Univ., 1964; *Indian Sci Abstr*, 1965, **1**, 10220). Stem and fruit gave +ve test for alk. (*Lloydia*, 1972, **35**, 132).

HABENARIA (*Orchidaceae*)

*H. intermedia D. Don

Rhizomes, aphrodis., and tonic used in heart troubles (*Indian Drugs*, 1976-77, **14**, 47).

Found in Ranikhet, U.P.

HAEMANTHUS (*Amaryllidaceae*)

*H. albiflos Jacq.
Eng.–*Blood lilies.*
Aq.ext. of aerial parts, antimicrob. (*Nature Lond*, 1964, **202**, 825).
Bulb contains alks., lycorenine and tazettine (Wlth India, V, 1).
Cultivated in Indian gardens.

HAEMATOXYLON (*Mimosaceae*)

See **HAEMOTOXYLUM**

HAEMATOXYLUM (*Mimosaceae*)

H. campechianum Linn. syn. *Haematoxylon campechianum* Linn.
Eng.–*Logwood, peachwood, campeachy tree.*
Hematoxylin, constituent of heartwood, antiinflam. (*Planta Med*, 1977, **31**, 214).

HAGENIA (*Rosaceae*)

H. abyssinica (Bruce) Gmel. syn. *Brayera anthelmintica* Kunth
Eng.–*Flores koso.*
Leaves and flowers may prove useful in inducing abortion (*Econ Bot*, 1979, **33**, 29).
Leaves and flowers, flavonol. glycds. (*Arogya J Hlth Sci*, 1976, **2**, 140); 4 phloroglucinol derivs. (*Phytochemistry*, 1973, **12**, 2017).
Phloroglucinols—extracted from flowers, taeniafuge; basis for ethnopharmacol. (*in* Beal & Reinhard, 362-63); str. of phloroglucinols, kosotoxin and protokosin (*Acta Chem Scand*, 1974, **28B**, 1200; *Planta Med*, 1978, **34**, 153); HPLC sepn. of Ac-phloroglucinols (*J Chromatogr*, 1980, **188**, 213).

HAKEA (*Proteaceae*)

*H. saligna Knight
EtOH(50%) ext. of aerial parts, antivir., hypoten., CNS depress. and spasmol. (*Indian J Exp Biol*, 1974, **12**, 512).
Flowers, cyanogenic (Wlth India, V, 3).
Leaves, arbutin derivs. (*Phytochemistry*, 1977, **16**. 793); and resorcinol deriv., grevillol mono-Me ether & 2-C-Me-grevillol (*Indian J Chem*, 1977, **15B**, 1090). Wood, phenolic constituents (*Z Naturforsch*, 1980, **35C**, 344).
Cultivated as a hedge plant in Darjeeling and Nilgiris.

HALOXYLON (*Chenopodiaceae*)

H. recurvum Bunge ex Boiss.
Plant ash taken in stomach ulcers (*J Agric Trop Bot Appl*, 1966, **13**, 258).

H. salicornicum Bunge ex Boiss.
Plant alks., piperidine, aldotripiperideine, haloxine, halosaline and betaine (*Acta Pharm Suec*, 1967, **4**, 97; *CA*, **67**, 40992q); oil ext. of plant contains tyramine & its N-Me deriv. (*ibid*, 1968, **5**, 67; *CA*, **69**, 25045e). Plant, sterol compn. (*Egypt J Chem*, 1974, **17**, 869).

HAMELIA (*Rubiaceae*)

H. patens Jacq. syn. *H. erecta* Jacq.
Tea made from leaves given in fever and bloody diar. Root, purg. (*Econ Bot*, 1970, **24**, 359).
Plant parts, antineoplastic (*Rev Cubana Farm*, 1980, **14**, 311; 1981, **15**, 71).
Flowers, *d*-mannitol and cyanidin-3-rutinoside (*Phytochemistry*, 1971, **10**, 2125); ursolic acid, β-sitosterol & its glucd. (also in stems) (*Curr Sci*, 1973, **42**, 841); rutin, apigenin & its 7-glucuronide (*J Indian Chem Soc*, 1978, **55**, 623). Alk., isopteropodine (*Pharmazie*, 1977, **32**, 415; *CA*, **87**, 197237h); and stigmast-4-ene-3,6-dione (*ibid*, 1978, **33**, 82; *CA*, **88**, 186110f). Aerial parts, oxindole alks., palmirine and rumberine (*Tetrahedron Lett*, 1979, 3197); maruquine & isomaruquine (*An Quim Ser C*, 1980, **76**, 294; *CA*, 1981, **94**, 171040h); aerial parts yield 10 alks. pteropodine, isopteropodine, speciophylline, etc. [*Proc Conf Chem Biotechnol Biol Act Natl Prod*, 1st, 1981, **3**, 70; *CA*, 1982, **97**, 123894e].

HAMILTONIA (*Rubiaceae*)

See **SPERMADICTYON**

HAPLANTHUS (*Acanthaceae*)

H. tentaculatus Nees

Plant, flavanone glycd., haplanthin (*Indian J Chem*, 1976, **14B**, 644).

HAPLOPHRAGMA (*Bignoniaceae*)

*H. adenophyllum (Seem.) Dop syn. *Heterophragma adenophyllum* Seem.

Ass.–*Dhopa-paruli, ziron.*

EtOH(50%) ext. of aerial parts, antivir. and hypoten. (*Indian J Exp Biol*, 1971, **9**, 91).

Heartwood, lepachol and sitosterol (*Phytochemistry*, 1972, **11**, 1498). Pods, fixed oil, triterps. and other compds. (*Planta Med*, 1973, **23**, 125). Bark, *n*-hentriacontanol and β-sitosterol (*J Indian Chem Soc*, 1973, **50**, 561).

Found in forests of Assam and Andamans, and often cultivated in gardens.

HARDWICKIA (*Caesalpiniaceae*)

H. pinnata Roxb.; see **Kingiodendron pinnatum**

HARPEPHYLLUM (*Anacardiaceae*)

*H. caffrum Bernh. ex Krause

Eng.–*Kafir plum.*

In S. Africa, bark decoct. used as emetic and blood purifier (Wlth India, V, 8).

Leaves contain polyphenolics and flavons. (*Planta Med*, 1976, **29**, 129). Seed oil, dihydromalvalic acid (*J Am Oil Chem Soc*, 1981, **58**, 731).

Introduced into S. India.

HARPULLIA (*Sapindaceae*)

H. arborea (Blanco) Radlk.

Crushed bark applied on legs as a leech repellent (*J Econ Tax Bot*, 1981, **2**, 68).

HARTMANNIA (*Onagraceae*)

H. rosea G. Don; see **Oenothera rosea**

HEDERA (*Araliaceae*)

*H. colchica Koch
H.P.–*Kiraya.*
EtOH(50%) ext. of plant, antivir. (*Indian J Exp Biol*, 1971, **9**, 91).

Leaves, saponins, yielding on hydrolysis aglucones, oleanolic acid and hederagenin; triterps. oligoside, hederacolchiside E; & also D; Rutin (0.6%); minor glycds. (*Khim Prir Soedin*, 1968, **4**, 253; 1970, **6**, 484; 1980, **16**, 259; 1971, 7, 531; 1979, **15**, 236; *CA*, 1969, **70**, 35047t; 1971, **74**, 10352h; **93**, 66094k; **75**, 148518u; **91**, 189778c); triterps., antihypnotic in animals (*Soobshch Akad Nauk Gruz SSR*, 1971, **61**, 609; *CA*, **75**, 45630v); pharmacol. of saponins [*Zdravookhr Baloruss*, 1979, (4), 26; *CA*, **91**, 13911b].

Found in Himachal Pradesh.

H. nepalensis Koch syn. *H. helix* auct. non Linn.; *H. rhombea* Sieb. & Zucc.
Eng.–*Ivy.*

Various compns. used in cancer and induration of different kinds (*Lloydia*, 1967, **30**, 419). Usefulness of plant ext. in intoxication by irrit. gas (*Berufs Dermatosen*, 1972, **20**, 88; *CA*, **77**, 84142y); ext., antitumour, *in vivo* and *in vitro* against *Ehrlich ascites* (*Planta Med*, 1979, **36**, 150).

Berries—used as contracep. (*Planta Med*, 1973, **23**, 167). Toxic and pharmacodynamic action of seeds and berries, on rat (*Plant Med Phytother*, 1980, **14**, 221).

Leaves—decoct. used to kill lice in hair (*Nagarjun*, 1979-80, **23**, 177). In Italy, paste used as antirheum. and antineuralgic med. (*J Ethnopharmacol*, 1982, **6**, 165).

Extn. of antitussive, antisp. and antiinflam. triterp. mixt. from wood (Fr. M., 1968, 6330; *CA*, 1971, **74**, 91181b).

Whole plant yields alk. emetine (*Planta Med*, 1975, **27**, 127; *Egypt J Pharm Sci*, 1972, **13**, 321; *CA*, 1974, **81**, 169679m).

Anal. of plant, flowers and fruits, common compds. (*Herba Pol*, 1981, **27**, 303).

Leaves, extn. and str. of saponins (*Z Naturforsch*, 1965, **20B**, 708); 2 saponins, a saponoside and a lactone, fungistatic (*Bull Soc Pharm Marsille*, 1967, **15**, 279; *CA*, 1970, **72**, 54016q); saponins, antimicrob. (*Clujul Med*, 1978, **51**, 254).

Leaves also contain sesquiterps., β-elemene, elixene and germacrene B (*Chim Ind Milan*, 1970, **52**, 581; *CA*, **73**, 66750h); β-lectins, characteristics (*Aust J Plant Physiol*, 1978, **5**, 707); berries, saponins, molluscacidal (*Helv Chim Acta*, 1980, **63**, 606).

Hederasaponins—detn. (*Planta Med*, 1972, **21**, 29). α-Hederin, hederasaponins B & C (*Egypt J Pharm Sci*, 1974, **15**, 149; 179). 4 Triterp. saponins from stems (*Chem Pharm Bull*, 1978, **26**, 655). Saponins, antimicrob. (*Pharmazie*, 1978, **33**, 609; *CA*, **89**, 174385g). Antifung. activity of different plant constituents (*Ann Pharm Fr*, 1980, **38**, 545; *CA*, 1981, **95**, 125988w). Extn. of enriched saponins; hederasaponin C (4.7% of leaves) (*Fr. Demande*, 1981, 2459048; *CA*, **95**, 103302r).

α-& β-Hederins— α-hederin is 3-O[-*L*-rhamnopyranosyl (1 → 2)-α-*L*-arabinopyranoside] of hederagenin (3β, 23-di-OH-12-oleanen-28-oic acid) (Dictionary Org. Compds., II, 1992). Glycd(s)., intensely haemolytic but paradoxically haemolysis quicker and more complete with smaller than with higher concentrations. Irritant to alimentary canal, vasoconstrictor, hypoten. Hederin slows the heart and increases tonus and causes death by paralysis of respiration. For warm- blooded animals *c*.2-3 g/kg body wt., lethal; cold-blooded animals, less susceptible (Chopra *et al*, I, 444). α- & β-Hederins are intermediate glycds. of hederasaponins C & B respectively [B has CH_3 at 4 & C, CH_2OH group in triterp. molecule with sugars at 3 and 26 position (*CA* & Dictionary numbering differs)]; these two saponins provide disease resistance when ivy leaves get damaged by penetration of a parasite and undergo partial hydrolysis to α- & β-hederins with specific loss of sugars attached to 26-COOH, which are highly toxic to a range of fungi (α-hederin, at 50- 250μg/ ml), but not to *Pythium* and *Phytophthora* which have nonsterol membranes. Requirements for fungitoxicity lie in a degree of water solubility linked to active sites such as 26 free COOH group; if sugars at 3-position are lost, fungitoxicity completely disappears. Fungi, *Phyllosticta concentrica* and *Pestalotia macrospora* could grow in ivy leaves releasing a substance inhibitory to host enzyme system which converts hederasaponins to hederins (*in* Plant and Fungal Toxins, 752-53; *Z Pflanzenkr Pflanzenschutz*, 1973, **80**, 704; *CA*, 1974, **81**, 115189h); α-hederin, extn., and douvicidal, and antifung. activities (*Planta Med*, 1980, **39**, 234); see also extn. of enriched hederasaponins.

HEDYCHIUM (*Zingiberaceae*)

H. coronarium Koenig. ex Retz. syn. *H. flavum* Roxb.

In Hawaii, flowers and root used in foetid nostrils (*Econ Bot*, 1971, **25**, 245).

Essent.oil from rhizome, anthelm.; physicochem. characteristics; mild tranquillizer in male albino rats (*Indian J Pharm*, 1975, **37**, 143; 1976, **38**, 146; 1977, **39**, 58; *J Indian Chem Soc*, 1979, **56**, 941; *Indian J Pharmacol*, 1979, **11**, 147).

Rhizomes and leaves, phytochem. (*Egypt J Pharm Sci*, 1977, **18**, 465). Plant ext., antiinflam.; contains furanoid diterp. hedychenone (*Indian J Pharm Sci*, 1978, **40**, 227).

H. spicatum Buch.-Ham. ex Smith

Rhizome—drug hypoten. in dogs at low doses; lowers B.P. at high doses (*Nagarjun*, 1980-81, **24**, 7). EtOH(50%) ext., hypoglyc. and antiinflam. (*Indian J Exp Biol*, 1977, **15**, 208); useful in tropical pulmonary eosinophilia, clin. study (*Nagarjun*, 1979-80, **23**, 214).

Plant—alc. ext. of plant vasodilator, mild hypoten. and antisp. in animals [*J Res Indian Med*, 1974, **9**(2), 69]; insect repellent and used for preserving clothes (*Nagarjun*, 1979-80, **23**, 177). In Unani system, considered aphrodis. [*East Pharm*, 1980, **23**(272), 39].

Chem. of essent. oils, rev. (*Perfum Essent Oil Rec*, 1967, **58**, 782). Essent. oil from rhizomes, anthelm.; its physicochem. characteristics; mild tranquillizer in male albino rats (*Indian J Pharm*, 1975, **37**, 143; 1976, **38**, 146; 1977, **39**, 58; *Indian J Pharmacol*, 1979, **11**, 147). Rhizomes, essent. oil constituents (*Parfuem Kosmet*, 1979, **60**, 245); furanoid diterp., hedychenone & its 7-OH-deriv. (*Phytochemistry*, 1975, **14**, 1059; 1976, **15**, 827).

EtOH ext. of plant, antiinflam.; contains β- sitosterol & its glucd. (*Phytochemistry*, 1975, **14**, 578).

***H. spicatum** Buch.-Ham. ex Smith var. **acuminatum** Wall.

H.*–Haldu*.

EtOH(50%) ext. of plant, hypoten. and antiinflam. (*Indian J Exp Biol*, 1973, **11**, 43).

Chakrata, U.P.

HEDYOTIS (*Rubiaceae*)

H. auricularis Linn.; see **Oldenlandia auricularia**

H. biflora Wight & Arn.; see **Oldenlandia paniculata**

H. corymbosa (Linn.) Lamk; see **Oldenlandia corymbosa**

H. diffusa Willd. syn. *Oldenlandia diffusa* Roxb.

Formosan herb, antitumour against Ehrlich cancer cells in mice. Contains β-sitosterol and ursolic acid (*Taiwan Yao Hsueh Tsa Chih*, 1971, **23**, 4; *CA*, 1974, **80**, 124650h). Hexane ext. cytotoxic to both human and mouse cancer cells (*J Formosan Med Assoc*, 1979, **78**, 658). Herb, one of the constituents of Yunnan snakebite drug (*Acta Pharm Sin*, 1979, **14**, 557).

Plant, contains stigmasterol, γ-sitosterol and ursolic acid (*Aust J Chem*, 1964, **17**, 493); and oleanolic acid (*Yao Hsueh Hsueh Pao*, 1964, **11**, 809; *CA*, 1965, **62**, 96804b); β-sitosterol & its glucd. and *p*-coumaric acid (*ibid*, 1966, **13**, 181; *CA*, **65**, 7631b); anthraquinones [*Hua Hsueh*, 1979, (3), 60; *CA*, 1981, **94**, 1996g].

3 New iridoid glucds. from aerial parts; dried parts used as antiinflam. and antitumour drug (*Planta Med*, 1981, **43**, 28; *Arch Pharm Wein*, 1981, **314**, 831).

H. herbacea Linn. syn. *Oldenlandia herbacea* Roxb.

EtOH(50%) ext. of plant, diur. (*Indian J Exp Biol*, 1974, **12**, 512). Plant paste used in body pain (*J Econ Tax Bot*, 1981, **2**, 69).

H. scandens Roxb. syn. *Oldenlandia scandens* K. Schum.

EtOH(50%) of ext. of plant, diur. (*Indian J Exp Biol*, 1974, **12**, 512). Warm leaf paste applied on boils (*Bull Bot Surv India*, 1976, **18**, 166).

H. umbelata (Linn.) Lamk syn. *Oldenlandia umbellata* Linn.

Anthraquinone derivs. from plant (*Proc Soc Biol Chem India*, 1967, **26**, 46; *Leather Sci*, 1968, **15**, 49); also those from plant and roots; roots useful in haemoptysis [*J Res Indian Med*, 1972, **7**(3), 37].

HEDYSARUM (*Fabaceae*)

H. alhagi Linn.; see **Alhagi pseudalhagi**

H. gangeticum Linn.; see **Desmodium gangeticum**

H. purpureum Roxb.; see **Desmodium polycarpum**

H. triflorum Linn.; see **Desmodium triflorum**

H. tuberosum Roxb.; see **Pueraria tuberosa**

HEIMIA (Lythraceae)

*H. salicifolia Link syn. Nesaea salicifolia H.B.K.

Leaves—emetic, diur., laxt., vulnerary, antipyr., tonic, antisyp., diaphor. and astrin. Plant decoct. produces mild intoxication with amnesia and yellow vision.

Leaves contain bitter substance, nessin (Wlth India, VII, 18). Aerial parts, alks., lythrine, sinicuichine, heimine, sinine and cryogenine; str. (*Lloydia*, 1964, **27**, 15; 1965, **28**, 90); cryogenine decreased spontaneous motor activity, hypothermia, blepharoptosis and ataxia or analgesia; also antisp. (*Arch Int Pharmacodyn*, 1964, **150**, 220; *CA*, **61**, 15211f); nesodine and lyfoline; their strs. (*Lloydia*, 1965, **28**, 84; *Tetrahedron Lett*, 1966, 3641). Whole plant yields alks., lythrine and vertine; both diur. (US, 1965, 3184446; *CA*,**63**,2857h); preliminary pharmacol. of nesodine, cryogenine and other alks. (*Lloydia*, 1966, **29**, 348); str. of sinine (= lythridine) (*Tetrahedron Lett*, 1966, 5789); str. of sinicuichine (*Lloydia*, 1970, **33**, 483); str. of dehydrodecodine from herb (*Z Naturforsch*, 1971, **26B**, 970); minor alk., heimidine (OH-dihydrocryogenine) (*Lloydia*, 1971, **34**, 439); 2 stereoisomers of lythrine besides known alks. (*Phytochemistry*, 1975, **14**, 1883).

Young seedlings contain a Ph-quinoliziol (*Experientia*, 1974, **30**, 222); 2 Ph-quinolizidines (*Lloydia*, 1975, **38**, 477); also ester alks., de-MeO-abresoline & its 10-epi deriv. (*Phytochemistry*, 1978, **17**, 305).

Native of Mexico and Argentina and grown in Lloyd Botanic Garden, Darjeeling.

HELIANTHUS (Asteraceae)

H. annuus Linn.

Eng.-*Sunflower.*

Oil—polymeric fraction of oil, toxic and inhibits growth of animals. Administration for long period evoked fatty liver and granular dystrophy of kidney and heart [*Vopr Pitan*, 1964, **23**(2), 44; *CA*, **60**, 14900f]. Dietary lipids and arterial disease, rev., 112 refs. (*Sci Cult*, 1964, **30**, 70). Lowered blood cholesterol in human (*Eiyogaku Zasshi*, 1970, **28**, 194; *CA*, 1971, **75**, 60711r); retards intra-arterial occlusive thrombosis in rats (*Nutr Metab*, 1971, **13**, 140); extracted oil from dehulled seeds (dehulled as chlorogenic acid present in hulls interferes with lipid metabolism); reduced serum and hepatic cholesterol in healthy women (*Indian J Nutr Diet*, 1976, **13**, 371; 411). Effect of superheated oil on development of tumour in rats; increase in carcinogenesis [*Vopr Pitan*, 1971, **30**(1), 31; *Biol Nauki Moscow*, 1971, **14**(3), 61; *CA*; **75**, 3056g]. Effect in alloxan diabetic rabbits (*Atherosclerosis*, 1975, **22**, 349); on insulin dynamics in exogenous obesity, clin. study (*Ankara Univ Tip Fak Mecm*, 1974, **27**, 62;81; *CA*, 1976, **84**, 104237j; 104239k); on Freund's adjuvant- induced arthritis in rat (*J Pharm Pharmacol*, 1976, **28**, 533); on Ehrlich ascites tumour fluid lipoproteins (*J Lipid Res*, 1978, **19**, 457); caused weak platelet aggregation in rats, when fed for 1 yr. [*Rev Fr Corps Gras*, 1979, **26**(4), 171; *CA*, **91**, 69650h]. Useful in peptic ulcer, but consumption of oil by dogs led to total acidity [*Vopr Pitan*, 1972, **31**(3), 65; 1980, (1), 49]; dissolves gall stone, *in vitro* (*Herba Pol*, 1979, **25**, 293).

Oil, estrogenic properties, base material for skin rejuvenating compn. (*Sb Tr Inst Kosmetol*, 1968, 104; *CA*, 1970, **73**, 18447t; Fr. 1968, 1526966; *CA*, 1969, **71**, 42174f); in compn. for treating nails (US Pat., 1975, 3928561; *CA*, 1976, **84**, 111503v).

Seeds—given in snake-bite and flower heads, in lung trouble (*Econ Bot*, 1974, **28**, 316). Aflatoxin production in varieties (*Curr Sci*, 1974, **43**, 603).

Plant—growth inhibitor (in leaves and stems), annuithrin inhibitory of DNA/RNA synth. in cells of ascitic forms of Ehrlich carcinoma (*Phytochemistry*, 1981, **20**, 1883);ext., antibact. [*Med Surg*, 1965, **5**(2), 11]. Alc. ext., anticonvuls. (*C R Acad Bulg*

Sci, 1965, **18**, 691; *CA*, 1967, **48**, 2517).
Ext. reduced healing time of wounded skin
in exp. rats (*Indian J Med Res*, 1965, **53**,
539).

Polycyclic arom. hydrocarbons of un-
refined oil, most potent carcinogens known
to humans (*in* Plant and Fungal Toxins,
257); 3,4-benz(a)pyrene levels in oil (*Fette
Seifen Anstrichm*, 1969, **71**, 23; *CA*, **71**,
69447j; *Prikl Biokhim Mikrobiol*, 1970, **6**,
142; *Rev Fr Corps Gras*, 1970, **17**, 685;
CA, 1971, **74**, 75356g). Biol. effects of
unsap. fraction of oil (*Boll Soc Ital Biol
Sper*, 1980, **56**, 860; *CA*, **93**, 144179h).
Stigmasterol & β- sitosterol [*Maslo Zhir
Promst*, 1964, **30**(7), 11; *CA*, **61**, 12213e].
Triterps. and sterols [*J Am Oil Chem Soc*,
1966, **43**, 254; 1973, **50**, 300;
Phytochemistry, 1973, **12**, 1767; *Fette
Seifen Anstrichm*, 1973, **75**, 475; *CA*, 1974,
80, 13791k; *Rev Ital Sostanze Grasse*,
1974, **51**(2), 50; *CA*, **81**, 148446t; *Boll Lab
Chim Prov*, 1974, **25**(4), 37; *CA*, 1975, **82**,
29850f; *Sci Technol Alimenti*, 1974, **4**, 143;
CA, 1976, **85**, 107622m; *Glas Hem Drug
Beograd*, 1979, **44**, 619; *CA*, 1980, **93**,
24705e].

Seeds, level of carcinogenic hydrocarbons [*Vopr Onkol*, 1969, **15** (11), 85]. Seed
lecithin prevented hyperlipemia in rats
(*Herba Pol*, 1971, **17**, 404; *CA*, 1972, **77**,
43335v). Sterol glucds. (*Dokl Bolg Akad
Nauk*, 1974, **27**, 1387; *CA*, 1975, **82**,
121679e); flour, phenolic constituents (*J
Agric Food Chem*, 1975, **22**, 572);
hydrocarbons (*Phytochemistry*, 1975, **14**,
2726); a glucd. of chlorogenic acid [*Riv
Ital Sostanze Grasse*, 1978, **55**(5), 147; *CA*,
89, 213786k].

Flowers, glycds., haemolytic; sterols
and triterp. alc.; str. of glycds. of triterp.
acids (*Bull Acad Pol Sci Ser Sci Biol*, 1965,
13, 77; *CA*, **63**, 11249h; 1966, **14**, 645;
747; 1971, **19**, 179; *Rocz Chem*, 1967, **41**,
201; *CA*, **67**, 784s); str. of saponin, helian-
thoside C (*Khim Prir Soedin*, 1969, 129;
CA, **71**, 70889m).

Flowers, diterp. acid, trachyloban-19-
oic acid; receptacles, diterps.

(*Tetrahedron*, 1970, **26**, 5029; *An Quim*,
1979, **75**, 428; *CA*, **91**, 120388h). Petals,
neoxanthin (*Phytochemistry*, 1972, **11**,
3383). Flowers, ψ-taraxene derivs.,
heliantriol C & F; other heliantriols manilladiol and longispinogenin (*Pol J Chem*,
1979, **53**, 1071; 2465); essent. oil from
tubular corella, constituents (*Clujul Med*,
1979, **52**, 171); essence, as source of men-
thol (*Planta Med*, 1980, **39**, 272). Volat.
oil, sterols, etc. of flower heads (*Egypt J
Pharm Sci*, 1980, **21**, 83). Terps. chem. of
sunflowers, rev., 61 refs. [*Rev Latinoam
Quim*, 1981, **12**(2), 53; *CA*, **95**, 129271e].

Leaves, depsides (*Nature Lond*, 1966,
209, 80); triterp. alcs. from shoots
(*Phytochemistry*, 1971, **10**, 1946).

H. tuberosus Linn.

Eng.–*Jerusalem artichoke*.

Leaves, sesquiterp. lactone, heliangin
(*Tetrahedron*, 1966, **22**, 3137).

Flowers, leaves and stalks, essent. oil, β-
bisabolene (major); 42 compds. including
novel sesquiterp. helianthol A & B [*7th Int
Congr Essent Oils*, 1977, (Pub. 1979), **7**,
446; *CA*, 1980, **92**, 116234h].

Plant, new sesquiterp. alc. (*Parfum Cosmet Aromes*, 1980, Sp. Edn, 165). Leaves,
heliangin, de-Ac-viguiestenin and eriflorin
(*J Natl Prod*, 1981, **44**, 748).

Stem and leaves, +ve test for alk.
(*Lloydia*, 1974, **37**, 525). Chem. and
biochem. problems, rev., 12 refs [*Latv PSR
Zinat Akad Vestis*, 1976, (3), 77; *CA*, **85**,
17024p]. Derivs. of *ent*- atisirenic and *ent*-
kaurenic acids (*Phytochemistry*, 1980, **19**,
863).

HELICHRYSUM (*Asteraceae*).

*H. bracteatum Andrews

EtOH(50%) ext. of plant, spasmol. and
hypoten. (*Indian J Exp Biol*, 1971, **9**, 91).

Flavons. of different cultivars (*Planta
Med*, 1963, **11**, 325). Chalcone pigments
of yellow var. of flowers (*Arch Pharm*,
1965, **298**, 838; *CA*, 1966, **64**, 13015h).

Native of Australia, grown as ornamental.

HELICIA (*Proteaceae*)

*H. erratica Hook. f.

EtOH(50%) ext. of aerial parts, hypoten. (*Indian J Exp Biol*, 1980, **18**, 594).

Mawsynruam, Meghalaya.

HELICTERES (*Sterculiaceae*)

H. isora Linn.

EtOH(50%) ext. of aerial parts, spasmol. (*Indian J Exp Biol*, 1969, **7**, 250).

Roots used in cough and asthma; leaf paste, against skin ailments including eczema (*J Econ Tax Bot*, 1980, **1**, 139; 1981, **2**, 67).

Pods—fried and given to children to kill intestinal worms; decoct., in fever due to cold (*Bull Bot Surv India*, 1973, **15**, 14; 1980, **22**, 59); powd., in dysen. and vomiting; aq. ext. of seeds, in dysen. and in stomach pains (*Bull Med Ethno Bot Res*, 1980, **1**, 8; 318; *Econ Bot*, 1978, **32**, 280).

Seeds contain diosgenin (*Indian J Chem*, 1981, **20B**, 938).

HELINUS (*Rhamnaceae*)

*H. lanceolatus Brand.

EtOH(50%) ext. of aerial parts, CNS depress. and hypoten. (*Indian J Exp Biol*, 1973, **11**, 43).

Amarkantak, M.P.

HELIOTROPIUM (*Boraginaceae*)

*H. arborescens Linn. syn. *H. peruvianum* Linn.

Eng.–*Common heliotrope, cherry pie.*

Three alks. including lasiocarpine (*Bot Soc Quim Peru*, 1961, **27**, 161; *CA*, **61**, 15032a); roots contain cynoglossin (*Wlth India*, V, 31).

Native of Peru, grown as ornamental.

H. currassavicum Linn.

Plant contains lactone of δ-OH-hexanoic acid (*Experientia*, 1977, **33**, 707). Alks., heliotrine, its N- oxide, lasiocarpine and 7- angelylheliotridine; also β-sitosterol (*Indian J Chem*, 1977, **15B**, 494); coromandaline, heliovicine; and curas-

savine (*J Chem Soc Chem Commun*, 1978, 423; *Aust J Chem*, 1980, **33**, 1357).

H. elipticum Ledeb. syn. *H. eichwaldi* Steud. ex DC.

EtOH(50%) ext. of plant, hypoten. (*Indian J Exp Biol*, 1969, **7**, 250).

Veno-occlusive disease due to consumption of whole plant or seed, case report (*J Assoc Physns India*, 1978, **26**, 383).

Plant contains heliotrine-N-oxide (*Curr Sci*, 1966, **35**, 121); heliotrine, its 7-angelyl deriv., lasiocarpine & its N- oxide (*Indian J Chem*, 1975, **13**, 505). Alk. heliotropine (*Khim Prir Soedin*, 1976, 681; *CA*, 1977, **86**, 152617v). Seeds contain heliotrine, heliotridine, their 7-angelyl derivs. (*Indian J Pharm*, 1976, **38**, 156).

H. europaeum Linn. var. **lasiocarpum** Kazmi syn. *H. lasiocarpum* Fisch. & Mey.

Reproduction of chr. liver disease in dogs by feeding seeds [*Patol Fiziol Eksp Ter*, 1970, **14**(6), 41; *CA*, 1971, **74**, 74506u]. Plants as liver poisons, rev. covering toxicity data (*Int Symp Hepatotoxic*, 1973, 142; *CA*, 1975, **83**, 1555k).

Plant and seed oil, toxic; contain alks. heliotropine, heliotrine and lasicarpine [*Uzb Khim Zh*, 1965, **9**(3), 35; *CA*, **63**, 11884b]; alk. sepn. [*Med Promst SSSR*, 1965, **19**(4), 51; *CA*, **63**, 15159a].

H. indicum Linn.

Plant—used against inflam. of eyes (*Econ Bot*, 1970, **24**, 241); applied to boils, sores and insect-bite (*J Econ Tax Bot*, 1980, **1**, 143). Pharmacol. screening (*J Pharm Pharmacol*, 1978, **22**, 116).

Leaves—ext., antineoplastic (*Indian J Med Res*, 1968, **56**, 445; *Philipp J Sci*, 1967, **96**, 329); in Ghana, poultice for sores; cold infusion as enema for abdominal pain decoct. in convuls., used in gonor., erysipales and boils; also in diar. (*Ghana J Sci*, 1969, **9**, 119).

Aq. and alc. ext. of roots, oxytocic [*Rev Bras Farm*, 1968, **49**(2), 67; *CA*, **69**,

95034a]; roots, estradiol (high amt.) [*Bangladesh Med Res Counc Bull*, 1978, 4(2), 78].

Plant contains alks., indicine, Ac-indicine and indicinine (*J Chem Soc C*, 1967, 329); antitumour alk., indicine-N-oxide (*Lloydia*, 1976, **39**, 125). Aerial parts, alks., indicine, echinatine, supinine, heleurine, heliotrine, lasiocarpine, its N-oxide and unidentified base [*Bangladesh Pharm J*, 1976, **5**(3), 13; *CA*, 1977, **86**, 40191v]. Heliotrine, ganglion- blocking action (*Indian J Pharmacol*, 1981, **13**, 92). Whole plant, rapanone and lupeol (*Indian J Chem*, 1981, **20B**, 834).

H. ovalifolium Forsk.

Whole plant, retronecine and new alk., helifoline (*Phytochemistry*, 1981, **20**, 1991).

H. strigosum Willd.

Pyrrolizidine alk., strigosine (*J Chem Soc*, 1964, 1974).

HELLEBORUS (*Ranunculaceae*)

H. niger Linn.

Eng.–*Black hellebore, christmas rose.*

Plant—in compn. of a mouthwash containing aq. or alc. ext.; prevents infections and dental caries (Rom. 1978, 65014; *CA*, 1980, **92**, 64782p). Aq-alc. ext. in night cream (Rom. 1977, 62979; *CA*, 1980, **92**, 99452h); ext. in Romanian pharmaceutical compn. effective as antirheum. in rats (*Viata Med Rev Inf Pror Stiint Med*, 1979, **26**, 37; *CA*, 1980, **93**, 37046r).

Procedure to isolate steroidal glycd., hellebrigenin (Ger., 1964, 1176794; *CA*, 1965, **62**, 407b). Extn. of hellebrin from plant, compd. possesses cardiac activity (Ger. Offen, 1972, 2038110; *CA*, 1976, **76**, 13834m). Entire plant and esp. rhizome contains highly active glycds. that regulate cardiac rhythm, increase blood flow in arteries and have diur. action; should not be taken except under med. supervision. Drug (dried rhizomes) also contains a saponin and a volat. oil (Med. Plants, 54).

Stem, leaves, and flower, glycds; ranuncoside (*Planta Med*, 1973, **24**, 73; 1974, **25**, 376; **26**, 218); flavon. glycds. (*C R Congr Natl Soc Savantes Sect Sci*, 1974, **99**, 153; *CA*, 1976, **85**, 189226x).

Roots said to be available in druggists' shops; some plant specimens suitable for cultivation in gardens at high altitudes (Chopra *et al*, I, 109).

H. viridis Linn.

Eng.–*Green hellebore.*

Action similar to *H. niger*; poisonous (Med. Plants, 54).

Underground parts yield bufatetraenolide (*Planta Med*, 1973, **24**, 201). Principal sapogenin extn.; sapogenin ulcer- inhibiting and muscle-relaxing (Ger. Offen., 1976, 2519261; *CA*, 1977, **86**, 95984m).

HELMINTHOSTACHYS(*Ophioglossaceae*)

H. zeylanica (Linn.) Hook. syn. *H. dulcis* Kaulf.

Rhizome decoct. used in impotency. Leaf juice relieves tongue blisters (*Bull Med Ethno Bot Res*, 1980, **1**, 318).

Rhizome contains 4 flavons., ugonin A, B, C & D; their str. (*Chem Pharm Bull*, 1973, **21**, 1849; 1851; *CA*, 79, 113209z; 123663g); antipyr. and antiinflam. constituents of Chinese med., a mixt. of stigmasterol, fucosterol and dulcitol [*Hua Hsueh*, 1978, (1), 4; *CA*, 1980, **92**, 116322k].

HEMEROCALLIS (*Liliaceae*)

H. fulva Linn.

Root juice applied to cuts (*Bull Bot Surv India*, 1980, **22**, 161).

Stems and bulbs gave +ve test for alk. (*Proc West Va Acad Sci*, 1965, **37**, 143; *CA*, 1966, **65**, 4265f); alk., oxypinnatanine (*J S Afr Chem Inst*, 1976, **29**, 24; *CA*, 1977, **86**, 43992t).

HEMICYCLIA (*Euphorbiaceae*)

See **DRYPETES**

HEMIDESMUS (Periplocaceae)

H. indicus Schult.

Roots—pharmacognosy (*Indian J Pharm*, 1967, **27**, 35). Ayurvedic drug, 'Sariva', rev. and its diagnostic characters [*J Res Indian Med*, 1979, **14**(2), 67, 166]. Root juice given to children in tonsils (*Bull Med Ethno Bot Res*, 1980, **1**, 8). Aq. ext., bacteriostatic against *Mycobacterium leprae*; *p*-OMe salicylic aldehyde, active principle in ext. (*Lepr India*, 1981, **53**, 354).

Plant—used in abdominal tumours (*Lloydia*, 1967, **30**, 432). EtOH(50%) ext., antivir. (*Indian J Exp Biol*, 1968, **6**, 232). Used in skeletal fractures (*Sri Lanka For*, 1980, **14**, 145); antilithic (*Proc Indian Sci Congr*, 1981, IV, 156); ext., ingredient of drug for skin diseases (*J Sci Res Plants Med*, 1981, **2**, 101).

Roots, chem. of essent. oil, rev. (*Perfum Essent Oil Rec*, 1967, **58**, 782). Triterps. (*Phytochemistry*, 1973, **12**, 217).

Leaves, significant amt. of rutin (*ibid*, 1968, **7**, 1703). Steroids in cultured tissues and mature plant (*Z Pflanzenphysiol*, 1978, **89**, 401).

HEMIDICTYUM (Aspleniaceae)

H. ceterach Linn.; see Ceterach officinarum

HEMIONITIS (Hemionitidaceae)

*H. arifolia (Burm.) Moore

Eng.–*Male fern*; B.–*Chakulia*.

In Philippines, frond juice used in burns (Wlth India, V, 35); also used in ear-ache and as vermifuge [*J Res Indian Med*, 1974, **9**(4), 59].

Whole plant and rhizome ext., antibact. (*Econ Bot*, 1980, **34**, 284).

Plains and mountains of S. India up to 1,200m and in W. Bengal, Bihar and Orissa.

HEMIPHRAGMA (Scrophulariaceae)

*H. heterophyllum Wall.

EtOH(50%) ext. of plant, CNS depress. (*Indian J Exp Biol*, 1977, **15**, 208).

From Western Himalayas to Assam.

HERACLEUM (Apiaceae)

H. canescens Lindl.

Preliminary pharmacol. (*Indian J Exp Biol*, 1973, **11**, 43). Alc. ext. of root, pharmacol. active (*Perfum Essent Oil Res*, 1965, **56**, 217).

Roots, (from Kashmir), constituents and characteristics of essent. oil (*Riechst Aromen Koerperflegem*, 1964, **14**, 226; *CA*, **61**, 11842h).

Roots contain 9% coumarins (*in* Atal & Kapur, Med. Plants, 111).

H. lanatum Michx. syn. *H. candicans* Wall.; *H. nepalense* D. Don

EtOH(50%) ext. of plant, spasmol. (*Indian J Exp Biol*, 1968, **6**, 232).

Root essent. oil, constituents and characteristics (*Riechst Aromen*, 1963, **13**, 325; *CA*, 1965, **62**, 6336g).

Roots, furocoumarin, heraclenin (*Tetrahedron*, 1964, **20**, 87); and heraclenol (*Naturwissenschaften*, 1964, **51**, 537); imperatorin oxide (*Zh Obsch Khim*, 1965, **35**, 403; *CA*, **62**, 105071h); 8-geranoxypsoralen (*Tetrahedron*, 1966, **22**, 3221); xanthotoxin, xanthotoxol, sphondin, isoheraclenin and OMe-heraclenol; glucd., tert-O-β- glucosylheraclenol (*Indian J Chem*, 1970, **8**, 855; 1146); minor furocoumarins (*Indian J Chem*, 1971, **9**, 731); biocumarinyl deriv., candicanin (*Tetrahedron Lett*, 1971, 4221). Root and seed, coumarins; roots, diterp., candicopimaric acid (*Indian J Chem*, 1973, **11**, 410; 1097). Roots contain 4 coumarins including sphondin (*Phytochemistry*, 1975, **14**, 2533); also 4 known coumarins and β-sitosterol (*Yunnan Chih Wu Yen Chiu*, 1980, **2**, 224; *CA*, 1981, **94**, 2012y). Total coumarins, 9% (*in* Atal & Kapur, Med. Plants, 111).

Leaves, common furanocoumarins (*Phytochemistry*, 1970, **9**, 1145).

Xanthotoxin—8-MeO-psorelen; from roots (*Indian J Pharm*, 1975, **37**, 145); yield 2% from roots (*Res Ind*, 1970, **15**, 164); process for manufacture (*Annu Rep RRL Jammu*, 1975, 57); see also *Ammi majus*.

*H. pinnatum C.B. Clarke

Roots contain coumarins, 3%; can be used for commercial extn. of xanthotoxin (*in* Atal & Kapur, Med. Plants, 309).

Commonly found in Kashmir northwards up to 5,000 m.

H. wallichii DC.

Roots, coumarin; coumarins, and alk. cycleanine (*Phytochemistry*, 1975, **14**, 2533; 1976, **15**, 576).

HERITIERA (*Sterculiaceae*)

H. littoralis Dryand.

Eng.–*Looking glass tree.*

Shoot, tooth cleaners; fruits, tonic and stomach.; bark tannins (SEPASAT, 24).

*H. minor Lamk syn. *H. fomes* Buch.-Ham.

B., Oriya & Trade-*Sundri.*

EtOH(50%) ext. of aerial parts, hypoglyc. (*Indian J Exp Biol*, 1980, **18**, 594).

Leaves and bark, triacontanol, friedelin, taraxerol, β-amyrin and β-sitosterol (*J Indian Chem Soc*, 1978, **55**, 414).

Deltaic regions of Ganges, Brahmaputra and Mahanadi.

HERNANDIA (*Hernandiaceae*)

H. ovigera Linn. syn. *H. peltata* Meissn.

Leaf decoct. used in abdominal indurations (*Lloydia*, 1969, **32**, 250).

In Samoa, seed skin-irrit. Plant, ingredient in remedies for eye disease, stomchache and constip. Leaves and bark used for women taken ill after parturition. Bark, for boils and as laxt. (*Econ Bot*, 1974, **28**, 15).

Bark, 5 aporphine alks.; their identn. Trunk bark, hernandonine (*Tetrahedron Lett*, 1966, 1577; 4279; 1970, 3023). Alk., hernovine; str. of hernangerine; alks. of different plant parts from Bonin Islands (*Yakugaku Zasshi*, 1966, **86**, 763; 1143; 1972, **92**, 150); bark, thalicarpine (*Chem Pharm Bull*, 1967, **15**, 959).

Leaves, lignans, epiaschantin and epimagnolin; former piscic.(*Tetrahedron Lett*, 1973, 335).

Stem xylem, deoxypodophyllotoxin and alk. hernovine; constituents (*Taiwan Yao Hsueh Tsa Chih*, 1973, **25**, 8; *Proc Natl Sci Counc Part 2 Taiwan*, 1974, **7**, 185; *CA*, 1976, **84**, 102340n; 1977, **86**, 127150e).

Alks. and other root-bark constituents alk., oxothalicarpine (*J Chin Chem Soc Taipei*, 1976, **23**, 29; 1977, **24**, 91).

Seed, deoxypicropodophyllin and podorhizol (*Yakugaku Zasshi*, 1979, **99**, 674).

HERNIARIA (*Illecebraceae*)

H. glabra Linn.

Eng.–*Rupture wort.*

Dried flowering plant (as tisane), sed. in irritations of kidney calix and bladder; externally as application to wounds that are slow to heal (Med. Plants, 53).

Plant ext. contains compds. possessing spasmol. action, diur.; umbelliferone, herniarin, saponin, flavons., etc. (*Biul Inst Rosl Leczn*, 1963, **9**, 121; *CA*, 1964, **61**, 3570c). Leaves contain coumarins, flavons., anthraquinone glycd., saponin and alk. (*Rastit Resur*, 1967, **3**, 442; *CA*, 1968, **68**, 66392q). Herb contains 8 saponins (5.4-8.8%) (*Planta Med*, 1972, **21**, 29; 144). Variation of content of coumarins, saponins and flavons., on the location of plant grown (*Clujul Med*, 1977, **50**, 198). Herb ext. yields 2 flavon. glycds., 0.1-0.115; 2 coumarins, 0.012-0.013; and 8 triterp. saponins, 1.2-3.0% (with haemolytic action). Also contains rutoside; umbelliferone, herniarin (*ibid*, 1981, **54**, 73).

Herniarin— 7-MeO-2H-1-benzopyran-2-one, 9 Cl (7-MeO-coumarin, umbelliferone-Me-ether) (Dictionary Org. Compds., IV, 3692); relieves pains accompanying infections of bladder and kidneys; as diur. facilitates emission of Na and urea without increasing quantity of urine; readily decomposed (Med. Plants, 53).

H. hirsuta Linn.

Eng.–*Hairy rupture wort.*

Pharmacol. of exts.; compds. identical to those in *H. glabra* (*Biul Inst Rosl Leczn*, 1963, **9**, 121; *CA*, 1964, **61**, 3570c).

Aerial parts contain umbelliferone, scopoletin and herniarin (*Rastit Resur*, 1976, **12**, 411; *CA*, **85**, 174257j). Variation in the coumarin, saponin and flavon. contents with location (*Clujul Med*, 1977, **50**, 198).

HERPESTIS (*Scrophulariaceae*)

See **BACOPA**

HERPETOSPERMUM (*Cucurbitaceae*)

***H. pedunculosum** Baill.

EtOH(50%) ext. of aerial parts, spasmol. (*Indian J Exp Biol*, 1969, **7**, 250).

Temperate Himalayas and Assam.

HESPERIS (*Brassicaceae*)

***H. matronalis** Linn.

Eng.–*Sweet rocket.*

Saline exts. of seed agglutinate defibrinated rabbits blood (Wlth India, V, 41). Plant used in scirrhus indurations (*Lloydia*, 1969, **32**, 85).

Seeds contain cardenolides, corchoroside A, helveticoside and strophanthidin glucoboivinioside (*Diss Pharm*, 1965, **17**, 519; *CA*, 1966, **64**, 18029b); choline ester, hesperaline (*Arch Pharm Wein*, 1967, **300**, 176; *CA*, **66**, 102438d); isothiocyanate glucds. and their identn. (*Acta Pol Pharm*, 1969, **26**, 97; *CA*, **70**, 112328q); +ve test for alk. (*Lloydia*, 1974, **37**, 530).

Flower flavons. (*Diss Pharm Pharmacol*, 1971, **23**, 555; *CA*, 1972, **76**, 83555c).

Cultivated in hill gardens for its sweet-scented flowers.

HESPERTHUSA (*Rutaceae*)

H. alata Alston; see **Pleiospermum alatum**

H. crenulata Roem.; see **Naringi crenulata**

HETEROPHRAGMA (*Bignoniaceae*)

H. adenophyllum Seem.; see **Haplophragma adenophyllum**

H. quadriloculare (Roxb.) K. Schum. syn. *H. roxburghii* DC.

Roots prescribed as a drink in viper-bite (Chopra *et al*, II, 688).

EtOH(50%) ext. of aerial parts, antiprot. and hypoglyc. (*Indian J Exp Biol*, 1980, **18**, 594).

Leaf juice applied externally on toe-sores and chilblain (*Bull Med Ethno Bot Res*, 1980, **1**, 8).

Flowers contain hentriacontane and allantoin; fruit, allantoin; leaves, ursolic acid and sitosterol (*Phytochemistry*, 1972, **11**, 2349).

HETEROPOGON (*Poaceae*)

H. contortus Beauv. ex Roem. & Schult. syn. *Andropogon contortus* Linn.

Eng.–*Spear grass.*

Oil distilled from awns given in asthma; plant used in toothache, fever, atrophy, emaciation or cachexy, muscular pain, haemat., dysen. and scorpion sting (*Econ Bot*, 1965, **19**, 246; 1970, **24**, 241).

Grass, myo-inositol, galactinol and raffinose (*Aust J Chem*, 1972, **25**, 677).

HEVEA (*Euphorbiaceae*)

***H. brasiliensis** (H.B.K.) Muell. Arg.

Eng.–*Para rubber, caoutchouc tree.*

Oil of seed kernel, effective against houseflies and lice (Wlth India, V, 74).

Seeds, cyanoglucd., linamarin and enzyme, linase (Wlth India, V, 74; *Phytochemistry*, 1965, **4**, 89, 127).

Leaves, taraxerol (*Curr Sci*, 1966, **35**, 545); ubiquinones; flavons., vitexin & isovitexin (*Phytochemistry*, 1970, **9**, 2461; 1971, **10**, 2548); str. of heveaflavone (*Indian J Chem*, 1971, **9**, 895).

Latex, δ-tocotrienol (*Biochem J*, 1966, **100**, 138); 3 betaines, trigonelline, ergothioneine and hercynine; also ubiquinones; and a basic protein, hevamine (*Phytochemistry*, 1968, **7**, 109; 1970, **9**, 2461; 1976, **15**, 297).

Introduced into India, grown in plantations in S. India, Assam and Andamans.

HEYNEA (*Meliaceae*)

See TRICHILIA

HIBISCUS (*Malvaceae*)

H. abelmoschus Linn.; see Abelmoschus moschatus

H. cannabinus Linn.

Used in puerperal fever (*Econ Bot*, 1970, **24**, 241).

Leaves contain 5 flavon. glycds. including rutin and isoquercitrin; kaempferol deriv.; polyphenols; constituents (*Z Naturforsch*, 1964, **19B**, 857; *Khim Prir Soedin*, 1976, 257; 1979, 97; 219; *CA*, **85**, 59602f; **91**, 52705g; 171677j).

Sterols, triterp., etc. of leaves, seeds and fruits of Egyption plant (*Egypt J Chem*, 1976, **19**, 633; *(Indian J Chem*, 1975, **13**, 535). Plant contains Vit. B_6, 0.18 mg/100g edible portion (*Indian J Nutr Diet*, 1981, **18**, 9).

Flowers, myricetin glucd. (*Khim Prir Soedin*, 1976, 388; *CA*, **85**, 106650g); root polyphenols (*ibid*, 1979, 233; 1981, 394; *CA*, **91**, 171685k; **95**, 147134s).

Seed oil, analysis [*Proc Nat Acad Sci India*, 1974, **44A**(Pt 2), 113; *CA*, **83**, 128743a]. Seed hydrolytic enzymes (*Indian J Biochem Biophys*, 1977, **14**, 197).

H. esculentus Linn.; see Abelmoschus esculentus

H. ficulneus Linn.; see Abelmoschus ficulneus

H. furcatus Willd.

Plant used in fracture (*Sri Lanka For*, 1980, **14**, 145).

Petals, new flavon. glucd., hibiscatin, gossypin and gossypitrin (*Indian J Chem*, 1981, **20B**, 939).

*H. hirtus Linn.

EtOH(50%) ext. of plant, CNS depress. (*Indian J Exp Biol*, 1973, **11**, 43).

Reported from Hyderabad, A.P.

H. lampas Cav.; see Azanza lampas

*H. lobatus Kuntze

Plant used in debility and spermator. (*Nagarjun*, 1980-81, **24**, 263).

Shivpuri, M.P.

H. manihot Linn.; see Abelmoschus manihot

H. mutabilis Linn.

Flowers contain meratrin, quercimeratrin and other flavons. (*Curr Sci*, 1964, **33**, 112; *Phytochemistry*, 1971, **10**, 673).

Stems, flavon. glycd. of naringenin (*ibid*, 1979, **18**, 1766); and of eriodictyol (*Indian J Chem*, 1979, **17B**, 536).

H. rosa-sinensis Linn.

Flowers—emmen.; buds in treatment of vaginal and uterine discharges (*Q J Crude Drug Res*, 1972, **12**, 1922); ext., oral postcoital antifert. activity in female rats; and oral administration to rats affected spermatogenisis and endocrine function of testis (*Planta Med*, 1976, **26**, 151; 1977, **31**, 127); effect on estrous cycle in rat (*Probe*, 1978-79, **18**, 79); estrogenic (*Sci Cult*, 1980, **46**, 330); ingredient of antifert. drug, clin. trials (*J Sci Res Plants Med*, 1980, **1**, 41). Antifert. effect (*Curr Sci*, 1981, **50**, 360).

Flower ext., cytostatic and cytotoxic (*Indian J Exp Biol*, 1980, **18**, 1405); stalk applied to sore eyes; leaves and flowers on boils and to stop bleeding and in gonor.

(*Econ Bot*, 1974, **28**, 19). Flowers in menor. and root paste in cough (*J Econ Tax Bot*, 1981, **2**, 174).

Plant—ext., antiestrogenic in rats (*Experientia*, 1979, **35**, 1122; *Proc Indian Nat Sci Acad*, 1979,**45B**, 327). EtOH(50%) ext. of aerial parts, spasmol., CNS depress. and hypoten. (*Indian J Exp Biol*, 1969, **7**, 250). Various plant parts used in urinary complaints, consumption, dry cough, broncht. and menor. (*Econ Bot*, 1970, **24**, 241).

Leaves and stem bark used for abortion. In Samoa, roots and other parts used in remedies for gonor., vomiting of blood, and in stomach troubles (*ibid*, 1974, **28**, 19). Staminal column, diur. and used in kidney trouble (*Bull Med Ethno Bot Res*, 1980, **1**, 318). Alc. ext. of leaves antipyr., analg. and antiinflam. [*J Res Indian Med*, 1978, **13**(2), 58].

Leaves and stems yield taraxeryl-OAc and β-sitosterol (*Indian J Pharm*, 1971, **33**, 41). Flower flavons. (*Phytochemistry*, 1972, **11**, 1518).

H. sabdariffa Linn.

Seed oil., antimicrob. action (*Indian Drugs*, 1978-79, **16**, 147).

Unsap. matter of seed oil contains β-sitosterol (*J Chem UAR*, 1966, **9**, 127). Leaves, sitosterol- β-*D*-galactoside (*Phytochemistry*, 1975, **14**, 829). Seed sterols include ergosterol, 3.2% (*Planta Med*, 1979, **36**, 221).

Str. of hiviscin, pigment from calyx and bract (*Shokubutsugaku Zasshi*, 1969, **82**, 341; *CA*, 1970, **72**, 96801x). High concentration of hibiscic acid in flowers; flavon. and heterosides also present; succulent sepals and leaves recommended as antimicrob., anthelm. and hypoten. drug (*Planta Med Phytother*, 1971, **5**, 277; *CA*, 77, 16568s).

H. surattensis Linn.

Leaves used in intestinal disorders (*J Econ Tax Bot*, 1981, **2**, 67).

H. syriacus Linn.

Seeds contain acetylenic acid (*Chem Ind Lond*, 1965, 1840). Bark, 2 active antifung.

constituents; including canthin-6-one (*Yakugaku Zasshi*, 1978, **98**, 1508).

Constituent of essent. oil from buds and flowers (*J Agric Food Chem*, 1973, **21**, 1001).

H. tiliaceus Linn.

In Hawaii, buds used as laxt., in congested chest, childbirth and dry throat (*Econ Bot*, 1971, **25**, 245). Flowers used as antifert. agent (*Planta Med*, 1973, **23**, 167).

Bark and young leaves—used in treating skin disorders (*Econ Bot*, 1971, **25**, 441). In Samoa, leaves for gonor. and inner bark for pulmonary trouble. Leaves applied to wounds and inner bark also in intestinal pains and excessive menstrual discharge. Leaf in eye lotion (*Econ Bot*, 1974, **28**, 19). In New Guinea, leaves and bark sol., in cough [*South Pac Bull*, 1975, **25**(4), 32].

Plant—in Tonga, considered emmen., flowers emol. (*Econ Bot*, 1971, **25**, 441). Ext. of aerial parts, hypoglyc. (*Indian J Exp Biol*, 1980, **18**, 594). Used in skeletal fractures (*Sri Lanka For*, 1980, **14**, 145).

Heartwood contains sesquiterp. quinones, hibiscones A-D and hibiscoquinones, their strs. Roots of Brazilian plant, gossypol and mansonones D & F (*J Chem Soc Perkin Trans I*, 1980, 257).

H. trionum Linn.

Plant flavones (*Rev Med Targu-Mures*, 1966, **12**, 419; *CA*, 1967, **67**, 5666q).

H. vitifolius Linn.

Flowers contain hibifolin, a gossypetin glycd. (*Indian J Chem*, 1974, **12**, 890). A biflavon., gossypin from plant exhibited antiinflam. activity in rats equivalent to Phbutazone (*Indian J Pharmacol*, 1978, **10**, 277).

HIERACIUM (*Asteraceae*)

H. umbellatum Linn.

Aerial parts, apigenin, luteolin & its 7-β-*D*-glucopyranoside (*Khim Prir Soedin*, 1976, 660; *CA*, 1977, **86**, 86166n).

HIEROCHLOE (Poaceae)

H. odorata (Linn.) Beauv. syn. *H. borealis* Roem. & Schult.

Coumarin content of grass during vegetation (*Acta Pol Pharm*, 1973, **30**, 317; 1974, **31**, 233; *CA*, 1974, **80**, 6822t; 1975, **82**, 1926m).

HIPPEASTRUM (Amaryllidaceae)

H. equestre Herb.; see **Amaryllis belladonna**

HIPPOCRATEA (Hippocrateaceae)

H. indica Willd.; see **Reissantia indica**

*H. macrantha Korth.

EtOH(50%) ext. of aerial parts, spasmol., CNS depress., diur. and anticancer (*Indian J Exp Biol*, 1977, **15**, 208).

Reported from Goalpara, Assam.

HIPPOMANE (Euphorbiaceae)

H. mancinella Linn.

Choco Indians use latex as arrow poison (*Econ Bot*, 1970, **24**, 359). Latex ext., irrit. and cocarcinogenic; contains diterp. compds., (*Tetrahedron Lett*, 1975, 1587).

Leaves and twigs, w.-sol. ext., 8 compds. including 2 toxic, viz. hippomanins A & B; str. of hippomanin A (*Lloydia*, 1972, **35**, 470; 1977, **40**, 169; *Planta Med*, 1974, **25**, 166).

HIPPOPHAE (Elaeagnaceae)

H. rhamnoides Linn.

Plant—in Siberia, used in tumours (*Lloydia*, 1969, **32**, 154); in sunburn-preventing preparations; as emol. in prevention of eye region skin wrinkles; and other cosmetic preparations (Rom., 1977, 62981; 62719; 62718; 62716; 62720; 1978, 63708; *CA*, 1980, **92**, 99451g; 99459r; 99460j; 99461k; 99462m; 1979, **91**, 216683b).

Fruit (berries)—ext. in dry skin cream (Rom. Pat. 1978, 63707; *CA*, 1980, **92**, 28411h).

Plant, alks. harmol and harman (*Rozpr Wydz 3: Nauk Mat Przyr Gdansk Tow Nauk*, 1973, **8**, 137; *CA*, 1975, **82**, 54115c); polyphenols, extn. (*Khim Prir Soedin*, 1979, 854; *CA*, 1980, **93**, 41502d); quercetin and isorhamnetin (*Ssu-Ch'uan I Hsueh Yuan Hsueh Pao*, 1980, **11**, 174; *CA*, 1981, **94**, 171083z).

Berries, isorhamnitol; flavones (of leaves also) (*Farmacia Buc*, 1964, **12**, 655; 1967, **15**, 149; *Pharmazie*, 1966, **21**, 116; *CA*, 1965, **62**, 7587a; **67**, 41015k; **64**, 18031h); flavon. glycds.; (also 2 from leaves); flavons. (*Lloydia*, 1966, **29**, 225; *Izv Sib Otd Akad Nauk SSSR Ser Biol Nauk*, 1969, 116; *CA*, 1970, **73**, 73891h; *Rocz Chem*, 1971, **45**, 115; *CA*, **75**, 31210w; *Planta Med*, 1972, **22**, 418; *Khim Prir soedin*, 1978, 403; *CA*, **89**, 143362t).

Berries, terps. (*Farmacia Buc*, 1972, **20**, 659; *CA*, 1973, **79**, 15845j); ursolic acid; also from various plant parts; sterols of fruits and seeds (*Khim Prir Soedin*, 1975, 519; 1979, 868; 1981, 98; *CA*, **83**, 203756n; 1980, **93**, 22594u; **95**, 3376z).

Leaves, flavons.; isorhamnetin and astragalin (*Khim Prir Soedin*, 1975, 96; 1976, 97; 649; 663; 1977, 281; *CA*, **83**, 75365v; **85**, 30627g; 1977, **86**, 86160n; 136310j; **87**, 114616g). Bark, serotonin (*Zh Prikl Khim*, 1964, **37**, 2763).

H. rhamnoides Linn. ssp. **salisifolia** Sarvettaz syn. *H. salisifolia* D. Don

Bark paste used for wounds and ulcers [*J Res Indian Med*, 1973, **8**(1), 76]; ext., inhibitory in mouse fibrosarcoma (*Proc Indian Acad Sci*, 1962, **56B**, 1123).

Bark ext., tumour inhibitory; β-sitosterol and 2 alks. detected in ext. (*Indian J Pharm*, 1962, **24**, 165; 1970, **32**, 130).

HIPTAGE (Malpighiaceae)

H. benghalensis Kurz syn. *H. madablota* Gaertn.

EtOH(50%) ext. of aerial parts, CNS depress. and hypoten. (*Indian J Exp Biol*, 1971, **9**, 91).

Root bark, mangiferin (*J Pharm Sci*, 1968, **57**, 1039).

HODGSONIA (*Cucurbitaceae*)

*H. macrocarpa (Blume) Cogn. syn. *H. heteroclita* Hook. f. & Thoms.

Ass.–*Tapouguti*; B.–*Gular*; Lepcha–*Kathior-pat*; Lushai–*Khaum*.

Raw seed kernel, bitter oil used for med. purposes in Borneo. Fruits, hard bitter inedible flesh; but nut edible after roasting or baking (Wlth India, V, 103).

Eastern Himalayas, Assam and W. Bengal up to 2,000 m.

HOLARRHENA (*Apocynaceae*)

H. pubescens (Buch.-Ham.) Wall. ex DC. syn. *H. antidysenterica* (Roth) DC.

Bark—in dropsy and dysen. (*Indian For*, 1964, **90**, 50); pounded, used in stomach disorders (*Econ Bot*, 1965, **19**, 243); in abdominal and glandular tumours; seeds, for same purpose (*Lloydia*, 1967, **30**, 407); EtOH(50%) ext., hypoten. (*Indian J Exp Biol*, 1968, **6**, 232); paste applied in headache; decoct., in dysen. and fever; with powd. seeds, in bronch. fevers (*Bull Med Ethno Bot Res*, 1980, **1**, 8; 318; *J Econ Tax Bot*, 1981, **2**, 180); ingredient of herbal compn. for giardiasis (*Sachitra Ayurveda*, 1981-82, **34**, 401); useful in eczema (*J Res Ayur Sidha*, 1981, **2**, 109).

Plant—various parts in anaemia, spleen complaints, epilepsy, colic, labour complaints, spermator., constip., cold and dog-bite (*Econ Bot*, 1970, **24**, 241); ext., depress. on isolated frog's heart (*Bangladesh J Agric Sci*, 1975, **2**, 72; *BA*, **60**, 68195); rats, on feeding, produced liver lesions, and histopathology of lungs and kidneys (*J Ethnopharmacol*, 1981, **4**, 159).

Fruit—EtOH(50%) ext., antiprot., anticancer and hypoglyc. (*Indian J Exp Biol*, 1968, **6**, 232); seeds, astrin., febge., in diar. and intestinal worms (*Indian For*, 1964, **90**, 50); to regulate menstruation (*Q J Crude Drug Res*, 1972, **12**, 1922); see bark also.

Roots, given to cattle in disease in which tongue ejects out and gets swollen (*J Econ Tax Bot*, 1980, **1**, 142).

Bark, L-quebrachitol (*C R Acad Sci*, 1964, **258**, 2921); alks., dihydroisoconessimine and 3 α- aminoconan-5-ene (*Collect Czech Chem Commun*, 1964, **29**, 1591); base, kurcholessine (*Tetrahedron Lett*, 1964, 1659); 7α-OH-conessine and holonamine (*Ber*, 1964, **97**, 2316; *CA*, **61**, 12057a). In chr. amoebiasis, Bi-iodide compd. of total alks. given orally, compare favourably with emetine Bi-iodide (Chopra *et al*, I, 549). Standardisation of mother tincture [*J Res Indian Med*, 1979, **14**(1), 102]; triterp. and steroid (*Indian J Chem*, 1981, **20B**, 62).

Conessine—steroidal alk., antidysen. principle; estn. of alks.; assay of conessine in crude drug (*Indian J Pharm*, 1967, **29**, 3; 132); bark of 8 yr-old tree suitable for alk. production; contains 0.2% conessine (*Union Burma J Sci Technol*, 1969, **2**, 423); see also isolation, str., etc. (*in* Manske, VII, 320-26).

Leaves, alks. kurchiphylline, kurchiphyllamine, kurchaline, holadysine and holadysamine (*Bull Soc Chim Fr*, 1966, 1212); aminoglycosteroids, holantosines A & B; also C & D, and holarosine A (*Tetrahedron*, 1970, **26**, 1695; *Bull Soc Chim Fr*, 1971, 864); aminodeoxyglycosteroids, holarosine B, E & F (*Carbohydr Res*, 1972, **24**, 297; *CA*, 1973, **78**, 4474r); flavons. (*Indian J Exp Biol*, 1978, **16**, 516).

Root bark, holacetine; steroid formation in tissue culture (*Phytochemistry*, 1976, **15**, 1173; 681). Chem. and pharmacol., rev. [*Nagarjun*, 1980-81, **24**, 77; *Indian Med Gaz*, 1981, **115**(5), 179].

HOLCUS (*Poaceae*)

H. lanatus Linn.

Eng.–*Velvet grass*; *Yorkshire fog*.

Grass contains a CN glycd., causes poisoning when eaten (Wlth India, V, 107). Nondialyzable fraction of grass responsible for allergic bronch. asthma (*Minerva Pediat*, 1974, **26**, 452).

Triterp. and related compds. (*Yakugaku Zasshi*, 1970, **90**, 390; *Phytochemistry*, 1970, **9**, 2137).

Naturalized in India and found in Sikkim and Darjeeling up to 3,000 m.

HOLIGARNA (*Anacardiaceae*)

H. arnottiana Hook. f.

EtOH(50%) ext. of aerial parts, hypoten. (*Indian J Exp Biol*, 1974, **12**, 512).

Leaves, flavons., β-sitosterol and its glucd. (*Fitoterapia*, 1979, **50**, 265).

H. grahamii Hook. f.

EtOH(50%) ext. of aerial parts, spermic., hypoten. and diur. (*Indian J Exp Biol*, 1977, **15**, 208).

H. longifolia Buch.-Ham. ex Roxb.

Fruit, bark and sap used against indolent tumours (*Lloydia*, 1967, **30**, 394).

***H. nigra** Bourd.

EtOH(50%) ext. of aerial parts, CNS depress., hypoten. and diur. (*Indian J Exp Biol*, 1977, **15**, 208).

Found in evergreen forest of Kerala.

HOLMSKIOLDIA (*Verbenaceae*)

***H. sanguinea** Retz.

Eng.–*Parcel flowers, Chinese hat plant.* Ass.–*Manu-kataphul*; H.–*Kapni*; U.P.–*Rithoul.*

Aq. ext. of leaves, anticancer (*Philipp J Sci*, 1967, **96**, 393). EtOH(50%) ext. of aerial parts, CNS depress. and diur. (*Indian J Exp Biol*, 1977, **15**, 208).

From sub-tropical Himalayas, grown in gardens elsewhere for its orange-red flowers.

HOLOPTELEA (*Ulmaceae*)

H. integrifolia Planch.

Branches used as fish-poison (*Bull Med Ethno Bot Res*, 1980, **1**, 8). Stem bark paste and seeds in ringworm; former in scabies (*Bull Bot Surv India*, 1980, **22**, 59). Stem bark used externally and internally in rheum. (*Ancient Life Sci*, 1981-82, **1**, 117).

Bark, β-sitosterol (*Phytochemistry*, 1969, **8**, 791). Leaves, hexacosanol, octacosanol, β- sitosterol and β-amyrin; bark, friedelin and friedelan-3β-ol; heartwood, di-OH-olean-12-en-28- oic acid (*Planta Med*, 1974, **26**, 394; 1975, **27**, 290).

HOLOSTEMMA (*Asclepiadaceae*)

H. ada-kodien Schult. syn. *H. annulare* K. Schum.; *H. rheedianum* auct. non Spreng.

Bark, α-amyrin, lupeol and β-sitosterol (*J Sci Res Plants Med*, 1981, **2**, 76).

HOMALOMENA (*Araceae*)

H. aromatica Schott syn. *Calla aromatica* Roxb.

Useful in influenza; aroma of rhizome inhaled (*Bull Bot Surv India*, 1976, **18**, 166).

Rhizomes, essent. oil, chem. constituents and physicochem. properties (*Perfum Essent Oil Rec*, 1966, **57**, 421).

H. rubescens Kunth syn. *Calla rubescens* Roxb.

Rhizome, essent. oil, chem. constituents and physicochem. characteristics, rev. (*Perfum Essent Oil Rec*, 1967, **58**, 782).

HOMONOIA (*Euphorbiaceae*)

H. riparia Lour.

EtOH(50%) ext. of aerial parts, spasmol. (*Indian J Exp Biol*, 1969, 7, 250).

Root, unsap. matter, α-spinasteryl-OAc (*Indian Oil Soap J*, 1968-69, **34**, 179).

HOPEA (*Dipterocarpaceae*)

H. odorata Roxb.

Heartwood, hopeaphenol (*J Chem Soc*, 1965, 406).

***H. wightiana** Wall.

Kan.–*Nai-irupu*; Mal.–*Pongu*; Mar.–*Kavasi*; Tam.–*Ilapongu.*

EtOH(50%) ext. of aerial parts, CNS depress. and hypoten. (*Indian J Exp Biol*, 1974, **12**, 512).

Bark, β-sitosterol (*Indian J Chem*, 1969, **7**, 308).

Evergreen forests of W. coasts from Konkan southwards.

HOPPEA (*Gentianaceae*)

H. dichotoma Hayne ex Willd.

Plant glycd. hoppioside, hypoten. in dog; other pharmacol. studies (*Indian J Pharm*, 1976, **38**, 167). Plant, glycoxanthones and flavanone glycds., their str. (*Phytochemistry*, 1978, **17**, 2119).

HORDEUM (*Poaceae*)

H. vulgare Linn. syn. *H. sativum* Pers.
Eng.–*Barley.*

Seed—enriched barley meal, slightly hypoglyc. in human, hypocholesteremic in rats (*Eiye To Shokuryo*, 1966, **19**, 46; 1970, **23**, 426; *CA*, 65, 14190f; 1971, **74**, 96197w); mild estrogenic, ineffective in human (*Indian J Nutr Diet*, 1970, 7, 114). Effect on liver function in animals (*Can J Anim Sci*, 1975, **55**, 23).

Antibact. and antimycosidal barley ext. preparation (Ger. Offen., 1972, 2053182; *CA*, **77**, 52310k); ext., antifung. [*Environ India*, 1981, 4(I & II), 83].

Plant—straw of var. *hexastichon* contains antitumour substance (*J Antibiot Ser B*, 1966, **19**, 142). EtOH(50%) ext., antiprot. and antivir. (*Indian J Exp Biol*, 1968, **6**, 232). Used in cholera (*Econ Bot*, 1970, **24**, 241).

Seeds, ubiquinones (also in malt); ext., biflavon. proanthocyanidins (*Monatsschr Brau*, 1967, **20**, 7; 217; *CA*, 1968, **68**, 76936j; **69**, 27182x). Chrysoeriol (*Phytochemistry*, 1972, **11**, 1867); pearl barley, active components, useful as roborant, diur., etc. (Jpn Kokai, 1973, 7310212; *CA*, **78**, 164082q).

Barley grits contain pangamic acid (vit. B$_{15}$), 12mg/10g (*Z Lebensm Unters Forsch*, 1970, **143**, 411; *CA*, 1971, **74**, 75359k). Purification of barley-germ agglutinins (*Arch Int Physiol Biochem*, 1976, **84**, 617; *CA*, **85**, 175381g). Bioassay for biotin (*J Anim Sci*, 1978, **47**, 654). Flavon. sepn. from barley (*J Chromatogr*, 1981, **218**, 683).

Drying of grains with combustion gas increased content of carcinogenic hydrocarbons (*Tec Molitoria*, 1964, **15**, 137; *CA*, 1965, **62**, 16878h).

Plant, antifung. factor, identn.; compd., p- coumaroylagmatine (*Adv Chem Ser*, 1966, No.53, 80; *CA*, **65**, 6221b); seedlings, glycds. of hordatines A & B, as antifung. factors; their str. (*Tetrahedron Lett*, 1966, 2287; 2849); distribution of hordatines (*Phytochemistry*, 1978, **17**, 1093).

Pharmacol. of alk. hordenine and its deriv. (*Farmakol Alkalaidov Glikozidov*, 1967, 114; *CA*, 1969, **70**, 10233n). Volat. amino fraction, pyrrolidine (*J Inst Brew Lond*, 1970, **76**, 22).

Stem and leaves, flavones (*Agric Biol Chem*, 1973, **37**, 2663); cyanogenic glucd. from leaf ext. (*Phytochemistry*, 1979, **18**, 1515).

HORSFIELDIA (*Myristicaceae*)

H. irya Warb. syn. *Myristica irya* Gaertn.

Plant used in skeletal fractures (*Sri Lanka For*, 1980, **14**, 145).

Seeds contain *d*-asarinin and dodecanoylphloroglucinol (*Chem Pharm Bull*, 1972, **20**, 2278; *CA*, 1973, **78**, 19678y). Plant, chem. (*Asian Symp Med Pl Spices*, 1980, 79).

HOUTTUYNIA (*Saururaceae*)

H. cordata Thunb.
Eng.–*Tsi.*

Plant—in Chinese folk med., used as antimicrob., diur. and antitumour; contains quercitrin, Me-nonyl ketone and decanoyl acetaldehyde (*Pei I Hsueh Pao*, 1974, **6**, 75; *CA*, 1975, **83**, 152250h); ext., oral therapeutic agent for athlete's foot; also for treatment of rough skin; ext. with others, as tonic (Jpn Kokai, 1978, 7850313; Jpn Kokai Tokkyo Koho, 1979, 79145226; 1980, 80133317; *CA*, **89**, 95001a; 1980,

92, 135148z; 1981, **94**, 52986m). Drug ingredients of Chinese herbal med. for snake-bite (*Acta Pharm Sin*, 1979, **14**, 557).

Leaves—diur. and antiinflam. agents taken as therapeutic drink (Jpn Kokai Tokkyo Koho, 1981, 8197234; *CA*, **95**, 175787a); eaten for blood purification and applied to treat sores and boils (*Econ Bot*, 1981, **35**, 4).

Essent. oil—combination of volat. oil and trimethoprim, antagonistic to growth of drug-resistant clin. isolates [*Chung Ts'ao Yao*, 1981, **12**(4), 9; *CA*, **95**, 156432q].

Essent. oil from foliage, compn. (*Lloydia*, 1975, **38**, 92); chem. compn. of essent. oil of Chinese plant, different from that of Japanese (*Chih Wu Hsueh Pao*, 1979, **21**, 244; *CA*, 1980, **92**, 72695c); antimicrob. due to its constituent decanoyl acetaldehyde (*in* Beal & Reinhard, 378).

Aerial parts contain afzelin, hyperin, rutin, chlorogenic acid and β-sitosterol (*Shoyakugaku Zasshi*, 1978, **32**, 123; *CA*, 1979, **91**, 62628y).

HOVENIA (*Rhamnaceae*)

H. acerba Lindl. syn. *H. dulcis* auct. non Thunb.

Eng.–*Japanese raisin*.

Root bark contains 3 peptide alks., frangulanine, hovenine A & B (*Phytochemistry*, 1973, **12**, 2985).

Hovenosides—a saponin fraction from root, neuroleptic, myorelaxant, irrit., cardiovascular depress., vasodilator in animals (*Shoyakugaku Zasshi*, 1979, **33**, 103). Acid hydrolysis of hovenoside G (main saponin) afforded ebelin lactone (major sapogenin; artefact), glucose, arabinose and xylose; and jujubogenin (genuine) on Smith-de Mayo degradation (*Phytochemistry*, 1974, **13**, 2829); hovenosides G, D & I (*J Chem Soc Perkin Trans I*, 1978, 1289).

Leaves contain 10 saponins including 3 new (*ibid*, 1981, 1923).

HOYA (*Asclepiadaceae*)

H. carnosa R. Br.

Occurrence and biosynth. of cyclitols (*Phytochemistry*, 1966, **5**, 1091).

*H. globulosa Hook. f.

Mikir–*Mithanadai*; Nagaland *Thaihom*.

Leaf ash applied on dog-bite (*Bull Bot Surv India*, 1976, **18**, 166).

Mikir hills, Assam.

HUMBOLDTIA (*Caesalpinaceae*)

*H. brunonis Wall.

EtOH(50%) ext. of aerial parts, spermic. and CNS depress. (*Indian J Exp Biol*, 1977, **15**, 208).

Found in Western Ghats.

HUMULUS (*Cannabidaceae*)

H. lupulus Linn.

Eng.–*Hop*.

Hops—bracts and flowers of female plants forming a leafy conical inflorescence (strobilus) collected before fully mature; brown glandular hairs from bracts, more active; bitter principle and volat. oil, stimulate appetite, and is antibiot., regularises menses. Antibiot. activity of drug decreases rapidly with age (Med. Plants, 45). Hops, antisep. (*Bar'ba Poteryami Zhivotnovodstve Sb*, 1963, 183; *CA*, 1965, **62**, 11626g); chem. of constituents, 422 refs. (*Chem Rev*, 1967, **67**, 19). Sed. and hypnogenic effects, 141 refs. [*Schweiz Brau Rundsch*, 1967, **78**(4), 80; *CA*, **67**, 20115c]. But lupulone or hop ext., no sed. or hypnotic action, pharmacol. (*Arzneim Forsch*, 1967, **17**, 79; *CA*, **66**, 92374p). Alc. ext., effective spasmol. in animals (*Agressologie*, 1969, **10**, 105; *CA*, 1970, **72**, 41267x). Effect and toxicity on mice (*Sb Tr Inst Kosmetol*, 1968, 108; *CA*, 1970, **73**, 2162k). Active against *Bacillus subtilis* 168 (*Arch Mikrobiol*, 1973, **94**, 159; *CA*, 1974, **80**, 104426m). Med. properties and prospects of usage, 41 refs. (*Rastit Resur*, 1980, **45**, 1175). In

Romania, used as anthelm. (*Planta Med*, 1980, **39**, 257).

Estrogenic hops' ext. (contains estradiol), for cosmetics; in face creams; effective against dermatophytes; in skin preparations such as deodorants or soaps (USSR, 1968, 219112; 1973, 373085; *CA*, **69**, 80115d; **79**, 45795k; *Perfums Cosmet Savons Fr*, 1972, **2**, 555; *CA*, 1973, **78**, 62061q; USSR, 1973, 373085; *CA*, **79**, 45795k; Jpn Kokai, 1973, 7358115; 7358114; *CA*, 1974, **80**, 6907z - 08a; Ger. Offen., 1978, 2749274; *CA*, **89**, 11981j).

Chem. and pharm. of components (*Folia Pharm*, 1965, **5**, 653; *CA*, **63**, 1130f). Chem. rev., 169 refs. (*Brew Sci*, 1979, **1**, 279; *CA*, 1980, **92**, 179006f).

Hops, future prospects [*Brasserie*, 1969, **24**(264), 75; 78; *CA*, **71**, 48270]; developments in chem. and technology [*Mitt Versuchsstn Gaerungsgewerbe Wein*, 1969, **23**(4), 64; *CA*, **71**, 69310j]; rev., 12 refs. (*Tech Q Master Brew Assoc Am*, 1971, **8**, 112; *CA*, 1974, **81**, 10317g).

Essent. oil, chem. (*Kvasny Pruns*, 1969, **15**, 259; *CA*, 1970, **73**, 33851p); rev., 207 refs.[*J Inst Brew Lond*, 1981, **87**(2), 96]; thioester (*Tetrahedron Lett*, 1980, **21**, 1085); terp. Me-sulphide (*Chem Ind Lond*, 1980, 624). Soporific activity due to 2-Me-3-butene-2-ol in volat. fraction (*Z Naturforsch*, 1980, **35C**, 1096).

Bitter substances—extn.; iso-α & β-acids (lupulones), γ-acids (humulinones) and Δ-acids (hulupones) (US, 1967, 3320071; *CA*, **67**, 42586j). Lupulin sepn. (Fr., 1968, 1509697; *CA*, 1969, **70**, 40631h); 4-deoxyhumulones (*J Inst Brew Lond*, 1969, **75**, 32). Sepn. of sesquiterps, (*Phytochemistry*, 1969, **8**, 637). Extn. of iso- α-acids (Fr., 1969, 1560431; *CA*, 1970, **72**, 65402p); 2 isohumulinones; their sepn. (*J Chem Soc*, 1965, 1276; Belg., 1965, 658603; *CA*, 1966, **64**, 7329b); by ion- exchange (Brit. 1970, 1183669; *CA*, **73**, 33915n). Chem. & rev., 31 refs. [*Mitt Versuchsstn Gaerungsgewerbe Wien*, 1966, **20** (3-4), 36; *CA*, 1967, **66**, 45468n].

Lupoxes a & b (*An Soc Brew Chem Proc*, 1971, 265; *CA*, 1972, **76**, 111658y); and lupdoxes A & B (*Rep Res Lab Kirin Brew Co*, 1971, No.14, 71; *CA*, 1973, **78**, 159926p). Active against *Bacillus subtilis* 168 (*Arch Mikrobiol*, 1973, **94**, 159; *CA*, 1974, **80**, 104426m). Method and apparatus for recovering lupulin-rich products (Ger. Offen, 1977, 2613616; *CA*, **87**, 166016f). Methods for anal. of bitter substance [*Przem Ferment Rolny*, 1978, **22**(2), 3; *CA*, **89**, 127659q].

Polyphenols (*Collect Czech Chem Commun*, 1964, **29**, 1259; *Ann Sci Univ Besancon Bat*, 1963, No. 19, 21; 25; *CA*, 1964, **61**, 11001b; 13627b; *J Chem Soc*, 1964, 3816; *Ind Chin Belge*, 1963, **28**, 757; *CA*, 1964, **61**, 14950h; *J Chromatogr*, 1964, **16**, 130).

HUNNEMANNIA (*Papaveraceae*)

*H. fumariifolia Sweet

Eng.–*Mexican tulip poppy.*

Aerial parts and roots contain alks., hunnemanine, allocryptopine, protopine, chelerythrine, sanguinarine, chelilutine, chelirubine, coptisine, berberine and corysamine (*Collect Czech Chem Commun*, 1966, **31**, 1355). Top ext., antimicrob. (*Lloydia*, 1972, **35**, 157). Alk. fraction from roots, antimicrob. (*ibid*, 1978, **41**, 145).

Quaternary alks., cycloanoline (main alk. in aerial parts and roots), escholidine and alk. HF^3 (*Collect Czech Chem Commun*, 1980, **45**, 914). Petals of cultivar. *sunlite*, flavonol glycd. (*ibid*, 1973, **36**, 166).

Cultivated in Indian gardens at medium and high altitudes.

HUNTERIA (*Apocynaceae*)

H. legocii Livera syn. *H. corymbosa* Roxb.

Leaves alk., corymine (*Proc Chem Soc*, 1962, 298; *CA*, 1963, **58**, 3471h); Indian leaves, rhazine, but no corymine (*J Indian Chem Soc*, 1968, **45**, 853).

HURA (*Euphorbiaceae*)

H. crepitans Linn.

Seed ext., non-specific agglutinin properties with human blood (*Econ Bot,* 1960, **14**, 236).

Latex contains triterp. (*Phytochemistry,* 1963, **4**, 813); crepitin lectin (*Experientia,* 1969, **25**, 891).

Huratoxin — str. of piscic. constituent of sap (*Tetrahedron Lett,* 1971, 1141); piscic. activity 10-fold that of rotenone (*Agric Biol Chem,* 1971, **35**, 1084); tumour-promoting activity on mouse skin by daphnane ester (*in* Plant and Fungal Toxins, 268-70).

Seed lectin —purification of mitogenic proteins (*Biochem Biophys Commun,* 1979, **89**, 713). Mitogenic and hemagglutinin properties (*Biochem Biophys Acta,* 1980, **632**, 95); biol. properties (*Planta Med,* 1981, **41**, 344).

HYBANTHUS (*Violaceae*)

H. enneaspermus F. Muell. syn *Ionidium enneaspermum* DC.; *I. suffruticosum* Ging.

Roots, diur. (*J Econ Tax Bot,* 1980, **1,** 138). Dried powd. leaves used in asthma (*ibid,* 1981, **2,** 184).

Plant ext. contains alk. aurantiamide-OAc, β- sitosterol and isoarborinol (*Indian J Chem,* 1979, **17B**, 297).

HYDNOCARPUS (*Flacourtiaceae*)

H. alpina Wight

EtOH(50%) ext. of aerial parts, diur. (*Indian J Exp Biol,* 1977, **15**, 208).

H. anthelmintica Pierre

Source of non-drying oil used in leprosy. Seed monosaccharide and glycds., useful in leprosy (*Nippon Daigaku Yakugaku Kenkyu Hokoku,* 1974, **14,** 27; *CA,* 1976, **84**, 8877w).

H. kurzii (King) Warb. syn. *Taraktogenos kurzii* King

Oil of fresh ripe seeds, antileprotic (I.P., 1966, 113). In China and Argentina, oil

used against cancer (*Lloydia,* 1969, **32,** 180).

H. octandra Thw.

Bark contains xanthene, mangostin (*Phytochemistry,* 1973, **12**, 232); 6 triterps. (*Chem Ind Lond,* 1973, 790; *J Chem Soc Perkin Trans, I,* 1977, 418).

H. odorata Lindl.; see **Gynocardia odorata**

H. pentandra Oken syn. *H. laurifolia* Sleumer; *H. wightiana* Blume

Fruits, piscic. (*Econ Bot,* 1970, **24**, 134). Pericarp contains leucopelargonidin (*Curr Sci,* 1977, **40,** 187). Seed hulls, flavonolignan, hydnocarpin (*Tetrahedron Lett,* 1973, 3481); isohydnocarpin; 4 derivs. including MeO-hydnocarpin (*Indian J Chem,* 1974, **12,** 888; 993). Seed coat yields flavonolignans hydnowightin and neohydnocarpin (*Planta Med,* 1979, **37,** 79); flavonolignans (*Phytochemistry,* 1979, **18**, 506).

H. venenata Gaertn.

Bark, triterps. and sitosterol (*Phytochemistry,* 1977, **16**, 788).

HYDRANGEA (*Hydrangeaceae*)

*H. anomala D. Don. syn. *H. altissima* Wall.

Garhwal–*Kathmora*; Lepcha–*Semaklung.*

EtOH(50%) ext. of aerial parts, spasmol. and CNS depress. (*Indian J Exp Biol,* 1977, **15**, 208).

Himalayas, from Ravi eastwards to Assam up to 1,600-4,000 m.

H. aspera Buch.-Ham. ex D. Don ssp. **robusta** Mc-Clintock syn. *H. heteromalla* D. Don; *H. vestica* Wall.

EtOH(50%) ext. of aerial parts, CNS depress., spasmol., diur. and hypoten. (*Indian J Exp Biol,* 1974, **12**, 512).

Whole plant yields coumarins, umbelliferone, daphnetin-8-Me ether and fraxetin; leaves, sitosterol and ursolic acid (*J Indian Chem Soc,* 1975, **52**, 1222),

H. macrophylla (Thunb.) Ser. syn. *H. hortensis* Smith; *H. hortensia* DC.

Secoiridoid glucds., hydrangenosides A, B, C & D and other known iridoids from var. *macrophylla*; str. of hydrangenosides (*Tetrahedron Lett*, 1980, **21**, 1059; *Chem Pharm Bull*, 1981, **29**, 3421).

H. paniculata Sieb. var. **grandiflora** Sieb.

Mucous polysaccharide, paniculatan from inner bark (*Chem Pharm Bull*, 1976, **24**, 230).

HYDROCOTYLE (*Apiaceae*)

H. asiatica Linn.; see **Centella asiatica**

H. javanica Thunb.

Plant—EtOH(50%) ext., spermic. and spasmol. (*Indian J Exp Biol*, 1977, **15**, 208; 231). Fish poison (*Nagarjun*, 1979- 80, **23**, 177).

Plant, α-amyrin-OAc, lignoceric acid, stigmasterol & its glucd.; glucd. active principle (*Indian Drugs*, 1978- 79, **16**, 185).

H. sibthorpioides Lamk syn. *H. rotundifolia* Roxb.

Plant contains stigmasterol (*Indian J Chem*, 1975, **13**, 97).

HYDROLEA (*Hydrophyllaceae*)

H. zeylanica Vahl

EtOH(50%) ext. of plant, hypoglyc. and antiprot. (*Indian J Exp Biol*, 1968, **6**, 232). Leaves and paste used as poultice in callous ulcers (*Lloydia*, 1969, **32**, 251; (*J Econ Tax Bot*, 1980, **1**, 143).

HYDROPHYLAX (*Rubiaceae*)

*H. maritima Linn. f.

EtOH(50%) ext. of plant, spasmol. and hypoten. (*Indian J Exp Biol*, 1969, **7**, 250). Coastal regions of Western Peninsula.

HYGROPHILA (*Acanthaceae*)

H. auriculata Heine syn. *H. spinosa* T. Anders.; *Asteracantha longifolia* Nees

Plant—aq. ext. of herb ash, diur. in albino rats (*Indian J Med Res*, 1967, **55**, 714). EtOH(50%) ext., spasmol. and hypoten. Herb ingredient of indigenous drug 'Speman' having anabolic-cum-androgen-like activity in mice; also source of Ayurvedic drug 'Kokilaksha'; Unani drug, 'Talmakhana'; and Siddha drug 'Neermulli' [*Indian J Exp Biol*, 1968, **6**, 232; 1976, **14**, 170; *J Res Indian Med*, 1978, **13**(4), 69]. Used in cancer and tubercular fistula (*Econ Bot*, 1970, **24**, 241). Juice in anaemia (*Bull Bot Surv India*, 1976, **18**, 161). Leaves and roots alongwith flowers of *Stuea frondosa* taken in leucor. (*Nagarjun*, 1979-80, **23**, 217). Herb, necrotropic (antihepatotoxic) in dogs (*Cheiron*, 1981, **10**, 9).

Seeds, tonic and aphrodis. (*Econ Bot*, 1965, **19**, 244).

Aerial parts, alk. and sterols with pharmacol. of alk. fractions; essent. oil from whole plant, antibact.(*Indian J Pharm*, 1965, **27**, 109). Plant, lupeol, stigmasterol and hydrocarbons (*J Indian Chem Soc*, 1967, **44**, 82).

Seeds, sterols (*Indian J Pharm*, 1965, **27**, 18); oil characteristics; and compds. of unsap. matter (*Pak J Sci Ind Res*, 1967, **10**, 82).

Flowers contain apigenin glucuronide (*Indian J Pharm Sci*, 1981, **43**, 56).

Root pharmacognosy (*J Univ Poona Sci Technol*, 1981, No. 54, 211).

H. salicifolia Nees syn. *H. angustifolia* auct. non R.Br.

Leaf paste or juice used against tumour (*Lloydia*, 1967, **30**, 387).

HYMENOCALLIS (*Amaryllidaceae*)

H. littoralis (Jacq.) Salisb.

Plant ext. antivir. against *Coxsackie semliki* forest measles viruses (*Lloydia*, 1978, **41**, 463).

Flowers antifeedant (*Indian J Entomol*, 1980, **42**, 460).

Bulbs contain alks. (0.018% of wet wt. of bulb) including lycorine and tazettine; former inhibited feeding response of desert locusts (*Experientia*, 1980, **36**, 552).

Lycorine & some of its derivs., hypoten. (*in* Wagner & Wolff, 120).

HYMENODICTYON (*Rubiaceae*)

H. excelsum (Roxb.) Wall.

Bark—ext., antimicrob. (*Indian J Med Res*, 1961, **49**, 799). EtOH(50%) ext., hypoten. (*Indian J Exp Biol*, 1971, **9**, 91); decoct. in diar. (*Bull Med Ethno Bot Res*, 1980, **1**, 8).

Various plant parts used in burning sensation in chest, emaciation, carbuncle, sores, smallpox, atrophy and lactation complaints (*Econ Bot*, 1970, **24**, 241).

Roots contain several quinones (*J Chem Soc C*, 1971, 2001).

H. obovatum Wall.

Root and bark contain coumarin, aesculin; bark, scopoletin (*Indian J Chem*, 1965, **3**, 237; 1973, **11**, 840).

HYOSCYAMUS (*Solanaceae*)

*H. albus Linn.

Flower petals as one of the constituents, antinarcotic med. (Brit. 1967, ~~1096~~708; *CA*, 1968, **68**, 62681k).

Leaves and roots, alk. detn.[*Farmatsiya Sof*, 1968, **18**(2), 50; *CA* **69**, 10984f]. Alks., constituent of mixt. for treating lymphatic system (Ger. offen., 1971, 1963706; *CA*, **75**, 91299s).

Seeds available in Indian bazars; said to be imported from Middle East countries.

H. muticus Linn.

Plant contains alk., atropine or hyoscyamine, used as parasympatholytic & its sulphate, in eye ointment. Also contains alk., scopolamine (hyoscine) used as parasympatholytic and sed. (I.P. 1966, 52-55, 232, 233).

Leaves contain alk., 0.48% (*Ann Pharm Fr*, 1967, **25**, 59; *CA*, **67**, 8656x); alk. extn. (*Bull Fac Pharm Cairo Univ*, 1969, **8**, 205; *CA* 1970, **73**, 59241q). Aliphatic compds. from leaves and stems (*Phytochemistry*, 1981, **20**, 1315).

Cultivation of high alk. strain (*Indian J Pharm Sci*, 1979, **41**, 46).

H. niger Linn.

Eng.–*Henbane, hogbean, hyoscyamus.*

Leaves and flowering tops source of alk.; same as in *H. muticus* (I.P., 1966, 234-36). Tropine drugs of Pharmacopoeia Helvetica contained alk., 15-20 mg/100g (*Sci Pharm*, 1964, **32**, 136; *CA*, **61**, 14465f).

Total alks.—very similar to those of *Atropa belladonna*, but present in smaller amts.; action similar to belladonna but less drastic (Med. Plants, 138); harmful in eye compns. used by persons having glaucoma or excessive pressure within eye (*Fed Regist*, 1966, **31**, 6705; *CA*, **64**, 20413c); comparison of methods for detn. (*Pharm Zentralhalle Dtsch*, 1967, **106**, 357; *CA*, **67**, 51053k). Various plant parts contain hyoscyamine and hyoscine-N-oxides (*J Pharm Pharmacol*, 1973, **25** Suppl., 11p; *Phytochemistry*, 1975, **14**, 999); extn. by ion-exchange [*Indian Drugs Pharmac Ind*, 1973, **8**(3), 27]; from aerial parts (*Khim Prir Soedin*, 1977, 124; *CA*, **87**, 50201h); production in tissue culture (*Ann Bot Lond*, 1977, **41**, 943).

HYPECOUM (*Fumariaceae*)

H. leptocarpum Hook. f. & Thoms.

In Ladakh, herb used in stomachache (*Bull Med Ethno Bot Res*, 1980, **1**, 301).

HYPERICUM (*Hypericaceae*)

*H. cernnum Roxb.

Plant—EtOH(50%) ext., CNS depress. (*Indian J Exp Biol*, 1971, **9**, 91). Traditional uses and folklore in British Isles (*Econ Bot*, 1981, **35**, 289).

Crushed flowers used on wounds and boils (*Econ Bot*, 1971, **25**, 421).

Western temperate Himalayas, from Kumaun to Sirmur at 2,000- 3,000 m.

H. laxum Koidzumi syn. *H. japonicum* sensu Dyer non Thunb.

Beneficial for acute or chr. hepatitis due to total flavons. (*in* Beal & Reinhard, 376).

*H. mysorense Wight & Arn.

EtOH(50%) ext. of aerial parts, antifung., spasmol. and hypoten. (*Indian J Exp Biol*, 1974, **12**, 512).

Timber and roots contain 2,3-di-MeO-xanthone (*Phytochemistry*, 1979, **18**, 182).

From Konkan to Pulney hills at 1,200-2,000 m.

H. perforatum Linn.

Eng.–*(Perforated) St.-John's wort.*

Herb—spasmol., mild diur. and stimulates gastro-intestinal secretions esp. bile. Very pronounced cicatrising action on wounds, cuts and bruises (Med. Plants, 98); used in ulcers and abscesses in Europe, and in body pain; useful in goitre and, in treating bed sores in old people [*Acta Phytother*, 1971, **18**, 21; *Farm Zh*, 1972, **26**(6), 78; *BA*, 1973, **56**, 56516; *Fitoterapia*, 1979, **50**, 201].

Plant ext., antisep. (*Bor' ba Poteryami Zhivotnovodstv Sb*, 1963, 183; *CA*, 1965, **62**, 11626g); mother tincture, antimicrob. (*Indian J Exp Biol*, 1977, **15**, 338).

Plant, important ingredient of therapeutic compn. useful in rheum., angina pectoris, cardiac diseases, phlebitis, psoriasis, etc. (Belg. Pat., 1965, 654916; *CA*, 1966, **64**, 19329a); of aerosol cosmetics useful for development and firming of breasts (Fr., 1966, 1438314; *CA*, 1967, **66**, 22122f). Antibiot. compn. from plant, rev. (*Mikrobiol Zh Kiev*, 1969, **31**, 128; *CA*, **70**, 118006c). Hyperforate, ext. compn. from plant, inhibited lactic acid production by tumour slices in human brain (*Arzneim Forsch*, 1971, **21**, 1999; *CA*, 1972, **76**, 121509a).

Flowers—aq.ext. useful in care of sensitive skin (*Soap Perfum Cosmet*, 1967, **40**, 272; 276; 278).

Aerial parts, hyperin and quercetin [*Med Prom SSSR*, 1964, **18**(3), 41; *CA*, **61**, 8130b]; also rutin (*Anales Fac Quim Farm Univ Chile*, 1964, **16**, 133; *CA*, 1966, **64**, 13084f). Herb toxin, hypericin its str. and effect on animals (*Llyodia*, 1975, **38**, 68).

Flavons. from flowers, suppressed cocaine excitation in mice (*Biul Inst Roll Leczn*, 1964, **10**, 1; *CA*, 1965, **62**, 16819f). Bioflavons. possess vit. P activity [*Farmatsiya Sof*, 1965, **15**(2), 92; *CA*, **63**, 11250g]

Hypericin—hexa-OH-di-Me-naphthodi anthrone, red pigment on petals, leaves and stems of several *H.* spp. including *H. perforatum*, can be easily extracted from glandular spots with MeOH or EtOH. This dimeric compd. sensitizes cells of other organisms to wavelengths of light or sunlight; photooxidative or photodynamic compd., requiring presence of oxygen, acts as an oxogenous sensitizer for colourless cells which get injured or killed by visible light. Monomeric units of hypericins, not implicated in photosensitization. Nature of chromophore of bi-molecule and its absorption spectrum related to this unusual activity. Quercetin found in *Hypericum* can enhance or potentiate effects of hypericin. No disruption of animal liver function in hypericism suggesting photosensitization as primary and not secondary (*in* Plant and Fungal Toxins, 353-54; *in* Wagner & Wolff, 209).

H. uralum Buch.- Ham. ex.D. Don syn. *H. patulum* Thunb.

EtOH(50%) ext. of plant, spasmol. and diur. (*Indian J Exp Biol*, 1974, **12**, 512). Plant and seeds, astrin., anthelm. and diur., (*Indian Drugs*, 1976-77, **14**, 47).

HYPHAENE (*Aracaceae*)

*H. thebaica Mart.

Eng.–*Egyptian doum palm.*

Fruits—pounded nuts, for dressing of wounds (Uphof, 277). Aq. ext., stimulated contraction of frog heart, decreased B.P. in anaesthetized dog; contains alk. and glucd. (*Qual Plant Mater Veg*, 1972, **22**, 83).

Kernels, carbohydrate compn.; polysaccharide compn. (*Carbodydr Res*, 1967, **4**, 387; 1973, **27**, 447; *CA*, **79**, 75211j). Kernel and pollen grains, estrogen & estrone (*Phytochemistry*, 1973, **12**, 899).

Native of Egypt, cultivated in Indian gardens.

HYPOCHAERIS (*Asteraceae*)

H. glabra Linn.

Root affords sesquiterp. lactones & guaianolides (*Phytochemistry*, 1981, **20**, 2371).

HYPOXIS (*Hypoxidaceae*)

H. orchioides Kurz; see **Curculigo orchioides**

HYPSERPA (*Menispermaceae*)

*H. cuspidata (Wall.) Miers syn. *Limaçia cuspidata* Hook.f. & Thoms.

Plant contains 3 phenolic alks., limacine, limacusine and cuspidaline (*Tetrahedron Lett*, 1966, 4293); and their str. (*Yakugaku Zasshi*, 1967, **87**, 793).

Sikkim, Assam and Andhra Pradesh.

HYPTIS (*Lamiaceae*)

H. suaveolens (Linn). Poit.

Leaves—used in cancers and tumours (*Lloydia*, 1969, **32**, 265). Infusion taken in fever; applied in headache and to boils. In Ghana, steam from hot decoct. of shoot as a cure for malaria; and headache. Poultice used in curing wounds. Decoct. for piles and retention of pregnancy. Used as eye-lotion and nose-drop. Also used in colic and stomach-ache.

Plant—in Brazil, weed infusion, carmin. and as sudorific in catar. conditions; also used in colic and stomach-ache (*Ghana J Sci*, 1969, **9**, 119); juice applied during fever. It showed 100% antiimplantation activity in female rats (*Bull Med Ethno Bot Res*, 1980, **1**, 8; 408).

Plant phytoagglutinin responding to antigen A of human erythrocytes (*Izv Akad Nauk SSSR Ser Biol*, 1968, 59).

Essent. oil, antibact. (*Qual Plant Mater Veg*, 1971, **20**, 231; *Planta Med*, 1974, **26**, 196).

Essent. oil from leaves, twigs and flowers, constituents and characteristics, rev. (*Perfum Essent Oil Rec*, 1967, **58**, 782). Leaves and flowers, campesterol and

fucosterol; unsap. matter of leaves and floral parts showed antiimplantation activity in rats (*Indian Drugs*, 1981-82, **19**, 84; 127). Roots, β-sitosterol, oleanolic and α- peltoboykinolic acids (*J Natl Prod*, 1981, **44**, 735).

HYSSOPUS (*Lamiaceae*)

H. officinalis Linn.

Plant—dried flowering plant generally used as mild diur., spasmol. and resolutive in broncht.; culinary use as spice (Med. Plants, 131). Flowers contain volat. substances possessing bact. activity; aq. ext. prevents intestinal diseases in cattle (*Zemled Zhivotnovod Mold*, 1960, **6**, 69; *BA*, 1962, **40** 24852). Leaves, flowers and other parts used in various kinds of tumours and cancers (*Lloydia*, 1969, **32**, 265).

Essent. oil, Indian, chem., rev. (*Perfum Essent Oil Rec*, 1967 **58**, 782). Constituents of Egyptian oil; oil anthelm. against chicken worms (*Ascaridia galli*) and active against tuberculosis bacilli (*Egypt J Pharm Sci*, 1978, **19**, 177); chem. constituents of oil, CNS-toxic in large doses; also antimicrob. against buccal cavity bacteria. Essent. oil from plant, toxic to rats; pinocamphone & isopinocamphone toxic constitutents (*Med Leg Toxicol*, 1980, **23**, 9; *CA*, **93**, 20175j).

IBERIS (*Brassicaceae*)

I. amara Linn. syn. *I. coronaria* Hort.

Eng.- *Commmon annual rogkit, white candytuft, clown's mustard*.

EtOH(50%) ext. of seeds fungitoxic against *Helminthosporium oryzae* (*Nat Acad Sci Lett*, 1978, **1**, 287).

Alk., ibamarine, its str. (*Acta Chem Scand*, 1962, **16**, 649). Seeds, cucurbitacin K (*Arzneim Forsch*, 1963, **13**, 771; *CA*, 1966, **64**, 7037g); lectin with anti-M activity (*J Immunol*, 1969, **102**, 1295). Green parts, glucosinolates and cucurbitacin E & I (*Phytochemistry*, 1977, **16**, 1519).

ICHNOCARPUS (*Apocynaceae*)

I. frutescens R. Br.

Plant—in abdominal and glandular tumours (*Lloydia*, 1967, **30**, 407). EtOH(50%) ext., antivir.(*Indian J Exp Biol*, 1968, **6**, 232).

Various plant parts used in night blindness, bleeding of gums, ulcerated tongue, sores, enlargements of spleen, atrophy, emaciation of cachexy, convuls., cramps, delirium, icterus, pimples, measles, smallpox, ulcer, haemat., constip., cholera, dysen., cough, phthisis, broncht. and asthma (*Econ Bot*, 1970, **24**, 241). Root powd. used in skin eruptions (*Bull Bot Surv India*, 1973, **15**, 18). Leaf paste applied in headache and fever (*ibid*, 1980, **22**, 161).

Rev. on *Sariva*, 21 refs.; and identn. characteristics [*J Res Indian Med*, 1979, **14**(2), 69; 166].

Leaves, flavons. and phenolic acids, identn. (*Indian J Exp Biol*, 1978, **16**, 512); stem, new triterp. glycd. (*Phytochemistry*, 1980, **19**, 2053).

ILEX (*Aquifoliaceae*)

I. aquifolium Linn.

Plant—used in different kinds of tumours and cancers (*Lloydia*, 1967, **30**, 411). Effect of ext. on CNS in exp. animals (*Plant Med Phytother*, 1978, **12**, 248).

Leaves useful in influenza, broncht., pneum. and rheum. (Med. Plants, 91).

Leaves, theobromine detn. rev., also in stems (*Farm Vestn Ljubljana*, 1967, **18**, 9; *CA*, **67**, 120199b). Plant cutin and suberins, epoxyoctadecanoic acid; male and female flowers, triterps. and sterols (*Phytochemistry*, 1973, **12**, 1721; 1977, **16**, 139). Leaves, triterps. and sterols (*Planta Med*, 1978, **33**, 416).

Fruits, 27-(p-coumaroyloxy) ursolic acid (*Z Naturforsch*, 1980, **358**, 226); steroids, triterps., phenolic compds., etc. (*Z Pflanzenphysiol*, 1980,**19**, 1866).

*I. dipyrena Wall.

EtOH(50%) ext. of aerial parts, antiprot. (*Indian J Exp Biol*, 1973, **11**, 43).

Himalayas and hills of Assam.

*I. godajam Colebr.

In Indo-China, bark decoct. given in diar. and as diur. (Wlth India, V, 165).

Occurs in Himalayas and hills of Assam.

I. paraguariensis St. Hilaire syn. *I. paraguayensis* Hook.

Plant contains caffeoylquinic acid (*Ann Chim Rome*, 1963, **53**, 1315; *CA*, 1964, **61**, 6283c). Sepn. of caffeine (*Rev Fac Agron Univ Nac La Planta*, 1972, **48**, 1; *CA*, 1973, **78**, 109496c).

*I. vomitoria Ait. syn. *I. cassine* Walt. non Linn.

Eng.—*Cassena, yaupon.*

Leaf infusion as tonic; emetic in large doses (Wlth India, V, 165).

Native of N. America and cultivated in Indian gardens.

ILLICIUM (*Illiciaceae*)

I. anisatum Linn. syn. *I. religiosum* Sieb. & Zucc.

Fruit ext., antimicrob. (*Indian J Pharm*, 1968, **30**, 43).

Seed inhibited fungal growth (*Appl Environ Microbiol*, 1980, **39**, 818).

Fruit contains toxic substance shikimin besides shikiminic acid, shikimipicrin, etc. and an essent. oil; shikimin present in pericarp only and not in seed (Chopra *et al*, I, 121).

Essent. oil, characteristics and constituents (*J Philipp Pharm Assoc*, 1964, **50**, 361); constituents and their content variation w.r.t. place (*Can J Chem*, 1966, **44** 2461).Leaf oil, phenolic constituents (*Chem Pharm Bull*, 1978, **26**, 2671).

Str. of neoanisatin from seeds (*Tetrahedron Lett*, 1966, 4739). Str. of anisatin derivs., toxins of seeds (*Nippon Kagaku Zasshi*, 1966, **87**, 166; 171; *CA*, **65**, 15245g, h). Str. of toxic compds. from plant, rev., 17 refs. (***Kagaku To Kogyo***

Tokyo, 1968, **21**, 1136; *CA*, 1970, **72**, 98641u).

I. griffithii Hook. f. Thoms.

Fruits, poisonous (Santapau & Henry, 55).

*I. simonsii Maxim.

Arunachal Pradesh–*Munshing*.

EtOH(50%) ext. of aerial parts, CNS depress. and hypoten. (*Indian J Exp Biol*, 1974, **12**, 512).

Occurs in Arunachal Pradesh.

I. verum Hook.f.

Eng.–*Jute star, anise tree.*

Fruit, essent. oil constituents [*Dragoco Rep*, 1965, **12**(2), 27; *CA*, **63**, 428c]. Seeds contain *p*-OH-benzoic acid; fruits, flavon. glycds. (*Z Lebensm Unters Forsch*, 1980, **171**, 193; 1981, **173**, 288; *CA*, **93**, 202865s; **95**, 217683w).

IMPATIENS (*Balsaminaceae*)

*I. arguta Hook.f. & Thoms.

Sik.–*Rang-rang.*

EtOH(50%) ext. of plant, spasmol. (*Indian J Exp Biol*, 1980, **18**, 594).

Found in Eastern Himalayas.

I. balsamina Linn.

In Hawaii, plant used in ulcers (*Econ Bot*, 1971, **25**, 245). EtOH(50%) ext., anticancer (*Indian J Exp Biol*, 1980, **18**, 594).

Flowers, extn. of 2-OH -1,4-naptho-quinone (*Can J Biochem*, 1965, **43**, 293). Flavon. pigments of different plant parts (*Am J Bot*, 1966, **53**, 46). Seeds contain β-sitosterol (*J Oil Technol Assoc India*, 1973, **5**, 10).

*I. duthiei Hook.f.

EtOH(50%) ext. of plant, spasmol.; also spermic. (*Indian J Exp Biol*, 1969, **7**, 250; 1977, **15**, 231).

Occurs in Shimla, H.P.

*I. longipes Hook.f. & Thoms.

EtOH(50%) ext. of plant, spasmol. (*Indian J Exp Biol*, 1969, **7**, 250).

Darjeeling, W.Bengal.

*I. roylei Walp.

Roots eaten for cooling properties (*in* Atal & Kapur, Med. Plants, 522).

Temperate Western Himalayas.

*I. scabrida DC.

Kumaun–*Gul mendi.*

Plant, stim., astrin., used in cough, chest pain and muscular pains (*Indian Drugs*, 1976-77, **14**, 47).

Ranikhet hills of Kumaun, U.P.

IMPERATA (*Poaceae*)

I. cylindrica Rausch. syn. *I. arundinacea* Cyrill. var. *major* C.E. Hubbard ex Hubb. & Vaughan

Rhizome—in China, root and inflorescence used as diur., tonic, astrin. and antivir. Root also in fevers but not antipyr. (Watt & Breyer- Brandwikj, 474).

EtOH(50%) ext. of aerial parts, antivir. (*Indian J Exp Biol*, 1971, **9**, 91).

Plant, ingredient of Yunnan snake-bite drug (*Acta Pharm Sin*, 1979, **14**, 557).

Thai plant, tritcrp. arundoin and cylindrin; diur. property not confirmed (*Shoyakugaku Zasshi*, 1967, **21**, 65; *CA*, 1968, **69**, 54263f). Culms and blades, 7 triterp. Me-esters, str. detn. (*J Chem Soc D*, 1969, 601). Plant, serotonin (*Haksurwon Nonmunjip Cha'yon Kwahak P'yon*, 1975, **14**, 307; *CA*, 1976, **84**, 161804q).

INCARVILLEA (*Bignoniaceae*)

I. emodi (Lindl.) Chatterjee syn. *Amphicome emodi* Royle ex Lindl.

Roots, five alk. fractions and one steroid fraction and Rf of constituents (*Indian J Pharm*, 1966, **28**, 160); glycds. amphicoside and androsin (*Tetrahedron Lett*, 1971, 2839).

INDIGOFERA (*Fabaceae*)

*I. arborea Prain

Oriya- *Girlee.*

EtOH(50%) ext. of aerial parts, antiamphetaminic (*Indian J Exp Biol*, 1973, **11**, 43).

Koraput, Orissa.

I. astragalina DC. syn. *I. hirsuta* auct. non Linn.

Herb decoct. in cerebral disorders, diar. and stomch. (*Nagarjun*, 1980-81, **24**, 263). Phytochem. screening of plant (*An Fac Farm Univ Fed Pernambuce*, 1976, **16**,51; *CA*, 1978, **91**, 16730c).

I. cassioides Rottl. ex DC. syn. *I. pulchella* auct. non Roxb.

EtOH(50%) ext. of root, antivir. and spasmol. (*Indian J Exp Biol*, 1968, **6**, 232). Plant used in epilepsy, mucus in urine and in menor. (*Econ Bot*, 1970, **24**, 241).

*I. dosua Buch.- Ham. ex D. Don H.P.–*Kothu.*

EtOH(50%) ext. of aerial parts, hypoten. and spasmol. (*Indian J Exp Biol*, 1971, **9**, 91).

Found in Himachal Pradesh.

I. glandulosa Willd.

Antimicrob, activity *in vitro* of fixed oils from *I. glandulosa* and other Indian spp. (*Indian Drugs*, 1978-79, **16**, 144).

*I. heterantha Wall. ex Brandis syn.*I. gerardiana* Wall. ex Baker

EtOH(50%) ext. of aerial parts, anticancer; also pharmacol. (*Indian J Exp Biol*, 1968, **6**, 232; 1969, **7**, 250). Roots used in cough and muscular pains (*Indian Drugs*, 1976-77, **14**, 47); their juice in urinary disorders in animals (*Bull Med Ethno Bot Res*, 1980, **1**, 1).

Shimla, H. P. and Ranikhet, U.P.

I. linifolia (Linn. f.) Retz.

Antimicrob. action of fixed oil (*Indian Drugs*, 1978-79, **16**, 144).

Nonsap. matter of seeds, β-sitosterol [*Oils Oilseed J*, 1979, **31**(3), 21].

*I. mysorensis Rottl.

EtOH(50%) ext. of aerial parts, anticancer and diur. (*Indian J Exp Biol*, 1977, **15**, 208).

Tirupati, A. P.

I. oblongifolia Forsk. syn. *I. paucifolia* Del.

Plant useful in liver troubles, diar. and rheum. (*J Agric Trop Bot Appl*, 1966, **13**, 269). Roots boiled in milk taken as purg. (*J Econ Tax Bot*, 1981, **2**, 178).

I. spicata Forsk. syn. *I. enneaphylla* Linn.

Eng.–*Creeping or trailing indigo.*

Toxicity of dried plant to male albino rats (*Aust J Agric Res*, 1965, **16**, 713). Effect of plant ext. on rats (*Nature Lond*, 1967, **215**, 980). Toxic efect of seed on female rat (*J Pathol*, 1975, **117**, 195).

Clones containing 3-nitropropanoic acid highly toxic to chicks (*Crop Sci*, 1963, **3**, 415). Sepn. of endecaphyllins from toxic ext. (*J Pharm Sci*, 1965, **54** 1136). Seeds contain indospicine.

Indospicine — hepatotoxic amino acid, (*Nature Lond*, 1968, **217**, 354). Teratogenic factor causing cleft palate in pregnant rats (*Br J Exp Pathol*, 1970, **51**, 34P); str. and biol. studies (*Aust J Biol Sci*, 1970, **23**, 831). See also rev. (*in* Keeler *et al*, 581-83).

*I. subulata Vahl ex Poir.

EtOH(50%) ext. of aerial parts, hyperten. (*Indian J Exp Biol*, 1974, **12**, 512).

Coimbatore, T. N.

I. suffruticosa Mill. syn. *I. anil* var. *polyphylla* DC.

In Hawaii, plant used in rheum. pain, backache and womb (*Econ Bot*, 1971, **25**, 245).

Phytochem. screening of plant (*An Fac Farm Univ Fed Pernambuco*, 1976, **15**, 51; *CA*, 1979, **91**, 16730c). Plant contains a flavanone louisfieserone and β-sitosterol (*Planta Med*, 1978, **34**, 172).

I. tinctoria Linn.

Alc. ext. of aerial parts, antihepatotoxic against carbon tetrachloride induced hepatic injury in animals (*Indian J Exp Biol*, 1979, **17**, 685; 1981, **19**, 298). EtOH(50%) ext., hypoglyc. (*ibid*, 1980, **18**, 594). Root paste given in fever (*Bull Med Ethno Bot Res*, 1980, **1**, 8).

Antineoplastic action and toxicity of synth. indirubin, a component of plant (*Acta Pharm Sin*, 1981, **16**, 146).

I. trita Linn. f.

Fixed oil, antimicrob., *in vitro* (*Indian Drugs*, 1978-79, **16**, 144); possesses med. properties (Wlth India, V, 184).

INDONEESIELLA (*Acanthaceae*)

*I. echicides (Linn.) Sreem.

Plant, bitter tonic, used in fever and jaundice, also as adulterant or substitute for *kalmegha* [*J Res Indian Med*, 1973, **8**(2), 67].

Throughout greater part of India.

*I. intermedia Sreem.

Coimbatore–*Kobirithangi*.

Leaves and roots given in snake-bite (*J Econ Tax Bot*, 1981, **2**, 183).

Coimbatore and Cheyur, T.N.

INULA (*Asteraceae*)

*I. cappa DC.

EtOH(50%) ext of plant, anticancer (*Indian J Exp Biol*, 1980, **18**, 594).

Aerial parts, flavons. (*Phytochemistry*, 1979, **18**, 2003). Flower essent. oil, antibact. (*Indian Drugs*, 1981-82, **19**, 33).

Found in Eastern Himalayas.

*I. cuspidata C.B. Clarke

Antibact. activity of triterp⁵ of roots [*Indian Drugs Pharmac Ind*, 1977, **12**(3), 15].

Distributed throug..ˍ.ˈ India.

I. grandiflora Willd.

Plant contains biol. antisep. substance (*Bor'ba Poteryami Zhivotnovodstv Sb*, 1963, 183; *CA*, 1965, **62**, 11626h).

I. graveolens Desf.

Plant, sesquiterp. lactone, graveolide (*Gazz Chim Ital*, 1973, **103**, 239); new sesquiterp. lactones. Plant, ilicic acid; aerial parts, β-sitosterol and flavones (*Fitoterapia*, 1980, **51**, 161; 1979, **50**, 3; 251).

I. helenium Linn.

Dried rhizomes and roots, in lack of appetite, stomach trouble and as mild diur., contain volat. oil and resin (Med. Plants, 156).

In Europe, roots, as diaphor., expect. and in pulmonary disorders (*Acta Phytother*, 1971, **18**, 21; 1964, **11**, 111; 121).

Root ext., alantolactones (*Diss Pharm*, 1964, **16**, 547; *CA*, 1965, **62**, 12980f). Sesquiterp. lactones of roots (*Isr J Chem*, 1967, **5**, 23). Anthelm. action of ether ext. of roots; compds. (*Herba Pol*, 1967, **13**, 114; *CA*, 1968, **69**, 2064x). Roots, α & γ-sitosterol & its glucd. (*Diss Pharm Pharmacol*, 1969, **21**, 337; *CA*, 1970, **72**, 39750f). Essent. oil, helenin (*Herba Pol*, 1974, **20**, 349; *CA*, 1975, **83**, 120712u); damaradienol (*Rocz Chem*, 1975, **49**, 849; *CA*, **83**, 75401d).

Alantolactone(s)—relatively nontoxic to dogs; less toxic than santonin; strong anthelm. against ascaris (Chopra *et al*, 1, 496); detn. from root; also chloraminometric detn. [*Herba Pol*, 1966, **12**, 14; *CA*, **65**, 16790c; *Farmatsiya Sof*, 1971, **22**(5), 19; *CA*, 1972, **76**, 117546t]; allergic contact dermatitis in humans (*Phytochemistry*, 1976, **15**, 1573). Alantolactone & isoalantolactones, antimicrob. (*Rastit Resur*, 1977, **13**, 428); antidermatophytic (*Indian J Pharm Sci*, 1978, **40**, 129).

Aerial parts, scopoletin and umbelliferone (*Khim Prir Soedin*, 1976, 820; *CA*, 1977, **86**, 136307p); sesquiterp. lactones (*Phytochemistry*, 1978, **17**, 1165). Flavones. of inflorescence (*Herba Pol*, 1978, **24**, 107).

I. racemosa Hook.f.

Root—ext. antiinflam., antipyr. and antisp.; also hypoglyc. in rabbits [*J Res Indian Med*, 1976, **11**(3), 25; 1979, **14**(3 & 4), 159]. Aq. alc. ext., potent antiasthmic (*Q J Crude Drug Res*, 1980, **18**, 89).

Plant powd., hypolipid., clin. study (*Indian Drugs*, 1978-79, **16**, 141); also, anthelm. against earthworms and tapeworms (*Indian Perfum*, 1979, **23**, 208). Constituents of essent. oil from roots, rev. (*Perfum Essent Oil Rec*, 1967, **58**, 782); a germacranolide, inunolide (*Indian J Chem*, 1969, **7**, 310).

Root, alantolactones [*J Res Indian Med*, 1972, **7**(4), 39]; alc. ext. yields alantolactone, 0.7; isoalantolactone, 0.2 (both compds. antidermatophytic), β-sitosterol, 0.16 & its glucd., 0.4% (*Indian J Pharm Sci*, 1978, **40**, 129).

I. royleana DC.

Plant poisonous (Chopra *et al*, I, 496).

Roots yield royleanone, its OAc, 7-keto deriv., inuroyleanol and β-sitosterol (*Tetrahedron*, 1975, **34**, 1001); diterps. of roots (*Indian J Pharm*, 1976, **38**, 148). Essent. oil, chem. constituent (*J Indian Chem Soc*, 1978, **55**, 476); also new sesquiterp. lactone, 11,13-dihydroalantolactone and other known lactones (*Planta Med*, 1980, **38**, 282).

Amorphous base from plant reduces B.P., depresses respiration and relaxes muscles [*Res Bull (NS) Punjab Univ*, 1969, **111-14**, 1; *Q J Crude Drug Res*, 1970, **10**, 1555].

IONIDIUM (*Violaceae*)

See HYBANTHUS

IPHIGENIA (*Liliaceae*)

I. indica (Linn.) A. Gray

Colchicine ext. from plant, useful in damaged breast cancer tissues; and its amide more effective and less toxic in different tumours (*Chin Med J*, 1980, **93**, 191; 188).

IPOMOEA (*Convolvulaceae*)

I. alba Linn. syn. *I. bona-nox* Linn.; *Calonyction aculeatum* House

In Hawaii, plant used as laxt. (*Econ Bot*, 1971, **25**, 245). In Samoa, leaves used in filariasis, constip., boils and wounds; young shoots, as eye lotion (*ibid*, 1974, **28**, 11).

Seeds, alks., ipalbine and ipalbidine (*J Chem Soc D*, 1969, 709); kauranoic acids (*Tetrahedron Lett*, 1973, 789).

Leaves, calonyctin A (*Kexue Tongbao*, 1981, **26**, 806).

I. aquatica Forsk. syn. *I. reptans* Poir.

Flower juice dropped into inflammed eyes (*Econ Bot*, 1965, **19**, 243). EtOH(50%) ext. of plant, spasmol. (*Indian J Exp Biol*, 1969, **7**, 250). Buds applied to ringworms [*J Res Indian Med*, 1973, **8**(2), 67]. Plant juice, in liver complaints (*Bull Bot Surv India*, 1973, **15**, 19). In Andhra Pradesh, leaves in leprosy and fevers (*Bull Med Ethno Bot Res*, 1981, **2**, 85).

I. batatas (Linn.) Lamk

Eng.–*Sweet potato*.

Plant—in Philippines, as antidiabetic; in New Zealand, whole plant or its infusion, in cases of low fever and skin diseases.

Leaves—in Nyasaland, cooked in maize-soaked liquid to yield a lactag.; in Ghana, ground with salt applied to whitlow; good source of vit.B and C; unpleasant smell can be removed by drying, before cooking (*Trop Sci*, 1965, **7**, 56).

In Hawaii, bulb used in vomiting, asthma and constip. (*Econ Bot*, 1971, **25**, 45).

Tubers, hydrocyanic acid, 30 mg/100g, oxalic acid, 1.0% and phytic acid, 8% (*Indian J Nutr Diet*, 1970, **7**, 119). Phytosterols (*J Agric Food Chem*, 1977, **25**, 1222). Stem tips, indole-3-acetic acid (*Curr Sci*, 1968, **37**, 267).

Sweet potato capable of forming phytoalexins (stress metabolites) on mechanical injury, insect invasion, exogenous chemicals (such as $HgCl_2$) and microb. pathogens. Abnormal metabolites apparently have limited inhibitory effect against certain microb. pathogens but can render root unpalatable or even toxic to consuming animals.

Lung toxic, hepatotoxic, and nephrotoxic 2- & 3-substituted furans and related compds. occurring naturally, used as therapeutic agents; chem. of synthesized cogeners of these toxins studied. Lung toxic principles, of primary importance although hepatotoxic furans present in larger quant. in moldy sweet potatoes (*in* Plant and Fungal Toxins, 4-5).

Mold-damaged tubers—toxicity (*Nutr Rev*, 1973, **31**, 73); toxicity of novel sesquiterps. (*Food Cosmet Toxicol*, 1979, **17**, 353); synth. of 3-substituted; biogenesis of lung-toxic furans (*J Org Chem*, 1977, **42**, 108; *J Am Chem Soc*, 1977, **99**, 2302). Scopoletin (*Pharmazie*, 1981, **36**, 569). Hepatotoxic 3-substituted furanoterps. include ipomeamarone & its derivs., ipomeamaronol, myoporone, etc. Lung-toxic compds., 1,4-dioxy-1-(3-furyl) pentanes, 4-ipomeanol, etc. See sweet potato toxins and related toxic furans (*in* Plant and Fungal Toxins, 3-29).

4-Ipomeanol—most abundant and probably most responsible for lung toxicity (*in* Plant and Fungal Toxins, 23-29); responsible for fatal lung oedema of cattle; effect in bovine lung [*Chem Ind News*,1971, **49**(46), 25; *Vet Pathol*, 1978, **15**, 367]; isolation and characterization (*J Agric Food Chem*, 1972, **20**, 428); confirmation of str. by synth. (*Nature New Biol*, 1972, **236**, 158; *via* Plant and Fungal Toxins, 25, 35). Distribution, excretion, etc. in rat after i.p. administration; renal metabolism in mouse; *in vitro* studies (*Toxicol Appl Pharmacol*, 1975, **32**, 147; 1978, **45**, 229; *J Pharmacol Exp Ther*, 1978, **207**, 687); development of tolerance to pulmonary toxin, 4-ipomeanol (*Toxicology*, 1981, **19**, 85).

I. cairica Sweet var. **indica** Hook. f. syn. *I. palmata* Forsk.

Plant ext., analg. in rats (*Indian J Hosp Pharm*, 1978, **15**, 81). Petal ext., antifung. (*Geobios* 1981, **8**, 66); seed ext., active against dermatophytic fungi.

Leaves yield a mixt. of indole alks. ergosinine, ergocornine and ergocristine (*Indian Drugs*, 1979-80, **17**, 35; 70).

*I. carnosa R.Br.

EtOH(50%) ext. of plant, CNS depress. and hypoten. (*Indian J Exp Biol*, 1971, **9**, 91).

Kushalnagar, Karnataka.

I. coccinea Linn. syn. *Quamoclit coccinea* Moench

EtOH(50%) ext. of aerial parts, antiprot., hypoglyc. and anticancer (*Indian J Exp Biol*, 1968, **6**, 232).

Seed alk., elymoclavine (*Flora Jena*, 1963, **153**, 373; *CA*, 1968, **60**, 2043e).

I. cymosa Roem. & Schult.; see **Merremia umbellata**

I. dissecta Willd. syn. *I. coptica* (Linn.) Roth

Flowers, kaempferol & its glucd. (*J Indian Chem Soc*, 1980, **57**, 1247).

I. fistulosa Mart. ex Choisy syn. *I. carnea* auct. non Jacq.

Plant—ingestion produces haemolysis of blood in animals and causes death [*Indian Livestock*, 1963, **1**(3), 12; *Indian Farming*, 1966, **15**(10), 47]. EtOH(50%) ext. of aerial parts, CNS depress. (*Indian J Exp Biol*, 1971, **9**, 91). Ext., antimicrob. (*Fitoterapia*, 1980, **51**, 231).

Seed ext., antifung. [*Curr Sci*, 1975, **44**, 279; *Environ India*, 1981, **4**(I & II), 83]. Petal ext., antifung. (*Geobios*, 1981, **8**, 66).

Leaves yield resinous ester; contain glycds. of decanoic acids (*Phytochemistry*, 1965, **4**, 29); *n*-tritriacontane and marsilin (ester of 1-triacontanol and hexacosanoic acid), compd., sed. and anticonvuls. (*Indian J Chem*, 1974, **12**, 281); ergoline alks., agroclavine and α-dihydrolysergol (*Planta Med*, 1980, **40**, 328).

Leaves also contain triacontane and a triterp. saponin, ipamotocin (*Labdev*, 1964, **2**, 220); glycd. active on frog's heart, causing heart blockade immediately followed by rapid increase in rate and amplitude of heart beats; metal complexes of leaf protein, antimicrob. [*Indian Drugs Pharmac Ind*, 1978, **13**(3), 7; 1974, **14**(2), 23].

Stems, 1-triacontanol; roots, γ-sitosterol (*Indian J Chem*, 1974, **12**, 281); flowers, kaempferol and peonidin glucd. (*Planta Med*, 1980, **38**, 147).

I. gomezii C.B. Clarke; see **Merremia mamosa**

I. hederacea (Linn.) Jacq.

Seeds from Pakistan, alks. lysergol, chanolcavine, penniclavine, isopenniclavine and elymoclavine (*Leban Pharm J*, 1967, **9**, 93; *CA*, 1968, **69**, 99321q).

I. illustris Prain syn. *I. campanulata* auct. non Linn.

EtOH(50%) ext. of plant, hypoten. (*Indian J Exp Biol*, 1967, **7**, 250).

*I. leari Paxt.

Roots used by Mundas in dysen. (Wlth India, V, 254). EtOH(50%) ext. of plant, spasmol., hypoten. and anticancer (*Indian J Exp Biol*, 1967, **7**, 250).

Isolation of glycd. from plant, ipolearoside with anticancer activity against Walker carcinosarcoma 256 in rats (*Phytochemistry*, 1973, **12**, 2461).

Native of S. America, introduced into India and grown in gardens as ornamental.

I. mauritiana Jacq. syn. *I. digitata* auct. non Linn.

Ether sol. fraction of plant, hypoten. and muscle relaxant [*Vijnana Parishad Anusandhan Patrika*, 1965, 7(2-3), 85].

Tuber, β-sitosterol (*Indian J Appl Chem*, 1964, **27**, 155); constituents and pharmacol. of glycds.; glycd. paniculatin, active [*East Pharm*, 1969, 12(138), 53; *J Pharm Sci* 1969, **58**, 757].

*I. maxima G. Don ex Sweet syn. *I. sepiaria* Koenig ex Roxb. var. *stipulacea* C.B. Clarke
B.–Bankalmi.

EtOH(50%) ext. of aerial parts, diur. and hypoten. (*Indian J Exp Biol*, 1974, **12**, 512).

Ranghat, W.Bengal.

I. muricata Jacq. syn. *Calonyction muricatum* G. Don

Plant juice used to destroy bedbugs (*Nagarjun*, 1979-80, **23**, 177).

Seeds, glycd. muricatin; glycd. cardiac depress., spasmol. and hypoten. (*J Pharm Sci*, 1967, **56**, 771). Str. of muricatin (*Phytochemistry*, 1967, **6**, 735).

Seeds, alk. ipomine (*Tetrahedron*, 1977, **33**, 1733). Seed ext., alk. fraction, antimicrob. (*Acta Manilana Ser A*, 1978, **17**, 20; *CA*, 1979, **90**, 12204r). Str. revision for alk., ipomine (*Planta Med*, 1978, **34**, 93).

I. nil (Linn.) Roth syn. *I. hederacea* auct. non Jacq.

Seeds, purg. substitutes for *jalap* [*J Res Indian Med*, 1973, 8(2), 67]; toxicity in mice (*Nature Lond*, 1965, **207**, 302). Plant ext. hypoglyc. in rats [*Farm Zh Kiev*, 1964, 19(4), 52; *CA*, 1967, **66**, 1451e].

Seeds from Pakistan, alks. lysergol, chanolcavine, penniclavine, isopenniclavine and elymoclavine (*Leban Pharm J*, 1967, **9**, 93; *CA*, 1968, **69**, 99321q).

I. paniculata R. Br.

EtOH(50%) ext. of rhizome, antiamphetaminic (*Indian J Exp Biol*, 1973, **11**, 43).

Rhizomes, taraxerol-OAc and sitosterol (*Phytochemistry*, 1972, **11**, 2621).

I. pes-caprae (Linn.) Sweet syn. *I. biloba* Forsk.

Plant, flavons. (*Yakugaku Zasshi*, 1981, **101**, 482).

I. pes-tigridis Linn.

EtOH(50%) ext. of plant, spasmol. (*Indian J Exp Biol*, 1968, **6**, 232).

I. purga Hayne; see **Exogonium purga**

I. purpurea (Linn.) Roth

Toxicity of seeds (*Am J Hosp Pharm*, 1968, **25**, 88). Seed ext., antibact. (*Indian Drugs*, 1979-80, **17**, 239).

Seeds, alk. content (*Acta Pharm Jugosl*, 1971, **21**, 103; *CA*, 1972, **76**, 49894x); glycd., isopurpuroside (*Phytochemistry*, 1978, **17**, 451); new criodictyol glucd. and lupeol (*Indian J Pharm Sci*, 1981, **43**, 109).

I. quamoclit Linn. syn. *Quamoclit pennata* Bojer; *Q. vulgaris* Choisy

Plant used in ulcer and breast pain (*Econ Bot*, 1970, **24**, 241).

I. reniformis Choisy; see **Merremia gangetica**

*I. sagittata Lamk

EtOH(50%) ext. of aerial parts, CNS depress. (*Indian J Exp Biol*, 1971, **9**, 91). Lucknow, U.P.

I. sinuata Ort.; see **Merremia dissecta**

*I. staphylina Roem. & Sch.

Kan.–*Wagani.*

EtOH(50%) ext. of aerial parts, CNS depress. (*Indian J Exp Biol*, 1971, **9**, 91). Hassan and Mysore districts of Karnataka.

I. tricolor Cav. syn. *I. violacea* Linn.

Seeds—in Mexico as hallucinogens; chem. of active principles, rev. (*Bot Mus Leafl Harv Univ*, 1963, **20**, 194; 161; *CA*, 1964, **60**, 3945g; 5274f); Mexican drugs and their active principles, rev.; also pharmacol. rev. [*Planta Med*, 1964, **12**, 341; *Bull Narc*, 1971, **23**(1), 3]; ext., uterine stim. (*Am J Pharm*, 1965, **137**, 24; *CA*, **63**, 3307g); toxicity in mice (*Nature Lond*, 1965, **207**, 302).

Seeds contain elymoclavine & related compds., used as psychotomimetics (*Indian J Pharm*, 1963, **25**, 245); alks., chanoclavine, elimoclavine, peniclavine and isolysergic acid amide (*Farmacia Buc*, 1973, **21**, 719; *CA*, 1974, **81**, 87964m); chanoclavine-I (*Tetrahedron Lett*, 1977, 3137).

I. tridentata Roth.; see **Merremia tridentata**

I. turpethum R. Br.; see **Merremia turpethum**

I. vitifolia Sweet; see **Merremia vitifolia**

IRIS (*Iridaceae*)

I. decora Wall. syn. *I. nepalensis* D. Don

Rhizomes contain isoflavons., irigenin; irisolidone (*Indian J Chem*, 1963, **1**, 187; *J Org Chem*, 1965, **30**, 3561).

I. ensata Thunb.

Aerial parts, xanthose glycds. rev., 4 refs.; C-glycd. of apigenin; and phenolic acids (*Khim Prir Soedin*, 1974, 333; 1977, 116; 1979, 861; *CA*, 1975, **82**, 13927a; **87**, 50197m; 1980, **93**, 22591r).

Roots contain ceryl alc. (*Indian J Chem*, 1976, **14B**, 475).

I. germanica Linn. var. **florentiana** Dykes syn. *I. florentigna* Linn.

Plant—aq. ext., decreased smooth muscle activity, *in vivo* and had musculotropic spasmol. effect (*Trav Soc Pharm Montpellier*, 1971, **31**, 325; *CA*, 1972, **77**, 726f). In Ayurvedic med., ext. alongwith other plant ingredients used as oral contracep. (*Ancient Sci Life*, 1981-82, **1**, 72).

Rhizomes, isoflavons. irisolone; irilone (*Phytochemistry*, 1972, **11**, 3097; 1973, **12**, 734); tectoridin & homotectoridin (*Agric Biol Chem*, 1973, **37**, 145); benzophenone deriv.(*Phytochemistry*, 1974, **13**, 2894); and several other flavons.; isoflavons. and β-sitosterol, α- & β-amyrin (*Monatsh Chem*, 1973, **104**, 1394; *Fitoterapia*, 1980, **51**, 237).

Petals, C-glycosyl flavone, embinin (*Agric Biol Chem*, 1968, **32**, 537).

I. kumaonensis Wall. ex G. Don

EtOH(50%) ext. of plant, spasmol. and diur. (*Indian J Exp Biol*, 1977, **15**, 208).

Roots, isoflavons. (*Indian J Chem*, 1963, **1**, 230). Plant, iridin; iriskumaonin (*Phytochemistry*, 1972, **11**, 3097; 1978, **17**, 1441).

*I. pseudacorus Linn.

In Europe, astrin. in dysmen. and leucor. Acts as diur., stim. and used in hepatic disorders (*Acta Phytother*, 1971, **18**, 21).

Seed oil, irisquinone (*Chem Ind Lond*, 1975, 349); it may be mentioned here seeds of *I. pallasii* var. *chinensis*, whose active principle is irisquinone, have marked efficacy to cervix cancer U_{14} in mice, and also have inhibitory actions against liver cancer and lymphatic sarcoma, Ehrlich carcinoma (*in* Beal & Reinhard, 369).

Cultivated in Indian gardens for ornament.

ISATIS (*Brassicaceae*)

*I. tinctoria Linn.

Eng.–*Dyer's woad.*

Plant used for ulcers and other ailments (Wlth India, V, 271); and oedematous and malignant tumours (*Lloydia*, 1969, **32**, 85). Tryptanthrin from leaves, antimicrob. against dermatophytes (*Planta Med*, 1980, **38**, 275).

Seeds contain 3-butenyl isothiocyanate (Wlth India, V, 271); C- glycosyl flavon., isoscoparine (*Pharmazie*, 1980, **35**, 712; *CA*, 1981, **94**, 27433w).

Native of Western Tibet and Afghanistan, grown in Indian gardens.

ISCHAEMUM (*Poaceae*)

*I. muticum Linn.

Grass rich in vit. C; leaves as poultice for headache (Wlth India, V, 272).

Found in marshy and coastal regions of Karnataka and Kerala.

ISOPYRUM (*Ranunculaceae*)

I. anemonoides Kar. & Kir. syn. *I. thalictroides* Hook. f. & Thoms. non Linn.

Roots and rhizomes, alk., magnoflorine (*Planta Med*, 1966, **14**, 204); terterary nonphenolic bases (*Diss Pharm Pharmacol*, 1968, **20**, 303; *CA*, 1969, **70**, 44808u); 4-nonphenolic bisbenzylisoquinolines (*J Natl Prod*, 1981, **44**, 101); flavons., kaempferol and quercetin (*Ann Pharm Poznan*, 1967, **6**, 17; *CA*, 1969, **71**, 84489t).

ISOTOMA (*Campanuluceae*)

I. longiflora Presl; see **Laurentia longiflora**

ITEA (*Iteaceae*)

*I. chinensis Hook. & Arn.

Khasi–*Dieng-a-metrit, dieng-tem-sro.*

Fruit considered stomch. in China.

Khasi and Jaintia hills of Meghalaya at 3,000 m.

IXORA (*Rubiaceae*)

I. arborea Roxb. ex Smith syn. *I. parviflora* Vahl

Eng.–*Touchwood ixora.*

Plant used in dysuria and spider bite poisoning (*Econ Bot*, 1970, **24**, 241); EtOH(50%) ext. of aerial parts, antivir.; hypoten. and spasmol. (*Indian J Exp Biol*, 1971, **9**, 91; 1977, **15**, 208).

Leaves, ixoral and β-sitosterol (*Pak J Sci Ind Res*, 1968, **11**, 12; *CA*, **69**, 49795b.

*I. acuminata Roxb.

Ass.—*Thekeria.*

Root decoct., galact. (*Bull Bot Surv India*, 1976, **18**, 166).

Eastern Himalayas up to 800 m.

*I. brachiata Roxb.

EtOH(50%) ext. of aerial parts, hypoten. and diur. (*Indian J Exp Biol*, 1974, **12**, 612).

Reported from Gujarat.

*I. chinensis Lamk

In Philippines, infusion of fresh flowers in TB and haemor. Plant in urinary troubles in Malaysia; decoct. of root administered after childbirth (Wlth India, V, 277).

Leaves, sterols (*Aust J Chem*, 1968, **21**, 574); iridoid glucds., ixoroside, ixoside and geniposidic acid (*Phytochemistry*, 1975, **14**, 2647).

Native of China and Malaysia and grown in Indian gardens for its dense flowers.

I. coccinea Linn.

EtOH(50%) ext. of aerial parts, spermic. and CNS depress. (*Indian J Exp Biol*, 1977, **15**, 208).

*I. grandifolia Zoll. & Moritzi

Leaves administered to pregnant women to facilitate delivery; in Malaysia, infusion in stomach-ache (Wlth India, V, 277).

Andaman and Nicobar Islands.

*I. lobbii Loud.

Root poultice applied in headache; decoct. given before and after delivery, and in diar., in Malaysia (Wlth India, V, 277).

Grown in some Indian gardens.

I. nigricans R. Br. ex Wight & Arn.

EtOH(50%) ext. of aerial parts, antivir., spasmol. and CNS depress. (*Indian J Exp Biol*, 1971, **9**, 91).

*I. undulata Roxb.

EtOH(50%) ext. of aerial parts, anticancer and diur. (*Indian J Exp Biol*, 1980, **18**, 594).

24-parganas, W.Bengal.

JACARANDA (*Bignoniaceae*)

*J. mimosifolia D. Don syn. *J. acutifolia* auct. non Hunb. & Bonpl.; *J. ovalifolia* R. Br.

H.–*Nili gulmohar.*

Leaves contain volat. oil, poisonous to fish. Fruit, antisyphillitic, astrin., applied to buboes (Watt & Breyer- Brandwijk, 142).

Leaves, flavon. scutellarein & its 7-glucuronide; hydroquinone and triterps. (*Phytochemistry*, 1972, **11**, 1499; 1973, **12**, 220).

Capsules (fruits), β-sitosterol, ursolic acid and hentriacontane (*Pak J Sci Ind Res*, 1973, **16**, 178). Stem bark, lupenone and β-sitosterol (*Indian J Chem*, 1975, **13**, 869). Wood constituents (*J Indian Chem Soc*, 1979, **56**, 1269).

Cultivated in Indian gardens.

JAESCHKEA (*Gentianaceae*)

*J. gentianoides Kurz syn. *J. obligosperma Knobl.*

Ladakh –*Tikta.*

In Ladakh, whole plant used as blood purifier and in fever (*in* Atal & Kapur, Med. Plants, 523).

Herb contains gentisin, gentianose and alk., gentianine (*Nagarjun*, 1981-82, **25**, 4).

Kashmir and Western Himalayas.

JAMBOSA (*Myrtaceae*)

See SYZYGIUM

JASMINUM (*Oleaceae*)

*J. amplexicaule Buch.-Ham. ex G. Don Ass.–*Desipiri.*

Used in stomach ulcers (*in* Jain, 165).

Found in Assam.

J. angustifolium (Linn.) Willd.

Flowers, +ve test for indole (*Indian Perfum*, 1980, **24**, 46).

J. auriculatum Vahl

Leaf juice, useful in exp. wound healing [*Med Surg*, 1965, 5(1),27].

Leaves, lupeol; its epimer, hentriacontane and *n*- triacantanol, a triterp. jasminol, identified as lup-20-en-28- β-ol(*Curr Sci*, 1967, **36**, 233; *Experientia*, 1968, **24**, 421; 1970, **26**, 10);*d*-mannitol; volat. constituent, jasmone (*Indian J Appl Chem*, 1968, **31**, 240; 1970, **33**, 132).

*J. dispermum Wall.

EtOH(50%) ext. of aerial parts, anticancer and diur. (*Indian J Exp Biol*, 1980, **18**, 594).

Sub-Himalayan tract from Kashmir to Bhutan up to 3,200 m, and Khasi and Jaintia hills of Meghalaya.

J. humile Linn. syn. *J. bignoniaceum* Wall.; *J. chrysanthemum* Roxb.

Plant used to cure wens and hard lumps *Lloydia*, 1970, **33**, 302). Flowers, +ve test for flavons. (*ibid*, 1971, **34**, 99).

*J. laurifolium Roxb.

EtOH(50%) ext. of aerial parts, hypoten. (*Indian J Exp Biol*, 1973, **11**, 43).

Aka and Khasi hills of Meghalaya, and Lushai hills in Arunachal Pradesh.

*J. malabaricum Wight syn. *J. latifolium* Grah. non Roxb.

Kan.–*Dolle balli, tirgal*; Mar.–*Kundli, kusur, mogra, ranmogra.*

EtOH(50%) ext. of aerial parts, affects respiration (*Indian J Exp Biol*, 1971, **9**, 71).

Found in Western Ghats from Konkan southwards to Malabar, and in Nilgiris up to 1,600 m.

*J. mesnyi Hance syn. *J. primulinum* Hemsl.

Leaves, glucd., primulinoside (*C R Acad Sci*, 1965, **261**, 1757); bitter glucd., jasminin; its str. (*Nippon Kagaku Zasshi*, 1968, **89**, 62; *CA*, **68**, 112183x; *Tetrahedron*, 1970, **26**, 4561); ceryl alc., quercetin, rutin (0.58%), α-amyrin, ursolic acid and β-sitosterol (*Fitoterapia*, 1980, **51**, 197).

Grown as ornamental in Indian gardens.

J. multiflorum Andr. syn. *J. pubescens* Willd.

EtOH(50%) ext. of aerial parts, diur. (*Indian J Exp Biol*, 1974, **12**, 512). Boiled bark applied on burns (*Bull Med Ethno Bot Res*, 1980, **1**, 318).

J. officinale Linn.

EtOH(50%) ext. of aerial parts, hypoten. and anticancer (*Indian J Exp Biol*, 1968, **6**, 232). Flowers and leaf juice used in various kinds of tumours (*Lloydia*, 1970, **33**, 302). Shrub used in burns (*Khadi Gramodyog*, 1972-73, **19**, 274).

Pyridine and nicotinate derivs. (*Agric Biol Chem*, 1978, **42**, 1901).

Flowers, essent. oil extn. from high-yielding var. (*Indian Hort*, 1979, **24**, 20); +ve test for indole (*Indian Perfum*, 1980, **24**, 46).

*J. rigidum Zenk. non Thw.

EtOH(50%) ext. of aerial parts, anticancer (*Indian J Exp Biol*, 1977, **15**, 208).

Western Peninsula, plains, and hills up to 2,400 m.

J. sambac (Linn.) Ait.

Plant—causes dermatitis (*Indian J Med Res*, 1978, **68**, 650). EtOH(50%) ext. of aerial parts, CNS depress. and hypoten. (*Indian J Exp Biol*, 1973, **11**, 43).

Leaves—ext., antibact. [*Med Surg*, 1965, **5**(2), 11]; used against indolent and breast tumours (*Lloydia*, 1970, 1970, **33**, 303); as an ingredient of antiemmen. drug (*Econ Bot*, 1974, **28**, 22). Test for antibact. and antitumour activity (*Rev Cubana Farm*, 1980, **14**, 311; 1981, **15**, 71).

Dried flowers—ext. with tea leaves and Chinese pepper seed exts., antiperspirant (US 21973, 3743717; *CA*, **79**, 70094p).

Pyridine and nicotinate derivs. (*Agric Biol Chem*, 1978, **42**, 1901). Flowers, +ve test for indole (*Indian Perfum*, 1980, **24**, 46).

*J. undulatum Ker.

EtOH(50%) ext. of aerial parts, diur. (*Indian J Exp Biol*, 1974, **12**, 512).

Found in Goalpara, Assam.

JATEORHIZA (*Menispermaceae*)

J. palmata Miers syn. *J. calumba* Miers Eng.–*Calumba*.

Alk. ext. from roots, analg. and hypothermic effects in rats (*Garcia de Orta*, 1962, **10**, 339; *CA*, 1964, **61**, 13776h). Isolation of alks., palmatine, jateorrhizine, calumbamine, and calumbin (*Rev Port Farm*, 1964, **14**, 105; *CA*, **61**, 14466f). Root ext. antifung.; active alks. jatrorrhizine sulphate, palmatine iodide and columbine; palmarine and chasmanthine inactive (*Pharm Ztg*, 1968, **113**, 945; *CA*, **69**, 61517v). Roots contain alk., berberine and coptisine [*Shoyakugaku Zasshi*, 1971, **25**(2), 74; *CA*, 1972, **77**, 122005r]; also dimeric alks., protoberberine and bis-jatrorrhizine (*J Chem Soc Perkin Trans I*, 1972, 327).

Roots, bitter principle, palamarin (*J Chem Soc C*, 1966, 1482; Dictionary Org. Compds., IV, 4475). See also some aspects of chem. of diterp. bitter principles, rev. (*Planta Med*, 1966, **14**, 78).

JATROPHA (*Euphorbiaceae*)

J. curcas Linn.

Eng.–*Curcas nut, physic-nut tree, purging-nut tree.*

Seed & Seed oil—purg. more drastic than those of *Ricinus communis* (castor seed oil) and milder than those of *Croton tiglium* oil (Chopra *et al*, II, 793-94). Seed poisonous to human beings, cattle and swine; however two strains of this species, one with toxic seeds and other with nontoxic indistinguishable to eye. Symptoms of poisoning (Kingsbury, 191).

Seed used against warts and cancers (*Lloydia*, 1969, **32**, 167). Seeds, to promote hair growth; fruits, poisonous (*Econ Bot*, 1974, **28**, 14).

Seed cake—poisonous like seed, in addn. to usual irrit. symptoms, muscular twitching, deafness, impairment of sight and loss of memory observed (Chopra *et al*, II, 794).

Leaves—internally for jaundice; decoct., antidiar.; in stomach-ache and in cough (*Econ Bot*, 1970, **24**, 360; 438). A 10% aq. infusion, increased cardiac contraction in small doses (*Acta Med Philipp Ser 2*, 1974, **10**, 60). Used against warts and cancers. EtOH ext. of defatted leaves and twigs active *in vivo* and *in vitro* against P-388 lymphocytic leukemia; see also tumour-promoting antileukemic diterps. (*Lloydia*, 1969, **32**, 167; 1978, **41**, 161; 193-233).

Plant—used in whitlow, dropsy, anasarca, convuls., syphilis, neuralgia, pleur. and pneum. (*Econ Bot*, 1970, **24**, 241). EtOH(50%) ext. of aerial parts, CNS depress. and diur. (*Indian J Exp Biol*, 1977, **15**, 208). Preliminary pharmacol. (*Philipp J Sci*, 1978, **107**, 79). In Sri Lanka, used in fractures (*Sri Lanka For*, 1980, **14**, 145).

Stem bark in wound of animal bites (*Econ Bot*, 1971, **25**, 438); root bark in sores (*Bull Bot Surv India*, 1975, **16**, 20). Wood causes dermatitis (Behl *et al*, 129, 158).

Seeds, results of chem. investigation at variance and need confirmation (Kingsbury, 191); contain poisonous fixed oil (29- 40%), a toxalbumin, curcin.

Curcin—acrid, emet. and drastic principle appears to reside chiefly in embryo; if whole embryo be removed, 4 or 5 seeds may be used as a gentle and safe purg., does not influence blood carpuscles *in vitro* but damages blood vessels and acts in general like ricin from *Ricinus* seeds (Chopra *et al*, II, 794).

Seeds, dulcitol and β- sitosterol and glucd. Stem bark, β-amyrin, taraxerol and β- sitosterol (*Indian J Chem*, 1970, **8**, 1974).

Leaves, apigenin, vitexin & isovitexin (*Phytochemistry*, 1971, **10**, 2548); 2 new flavon. glycds. and a new dimer of a triterp. alc. (*Planta Med*, 1977, **31**, 274); constituents of leaves and twigs, α-amyrin, stigmasterol, stigmastenes, etc. (*Lloydia*, 1978, **41**, 161).

J. glandulifera Roxb.

Latex and leaf used in warts and tumours (*Lloydia*, 1969, **32**, 167).

Shrub contains pigment 3,3-di-Meacrylylshikonin (*Phytochemistry*, 1969, **8**, 1587); also pigment, isohexenylnaphthazarin; chem., biosynth., biol. and wound-healing properties (*Planta Med*, 1980, **38**, 193).

J. gossypifolia Linn.

Eng.–*Bellyache bush.*

Plant—similar to *J. multifolia* (Kingsbury, 192); cures tooth-ache; seed oil relieves body pain (*Econ Bot*, 1965, **19**, 245). Preliminary pharmacol. (*Indian J Exp Biol*, 1969, **7**, 250). Popular med. for cancer (*Lloydia*, 1969, **32**, 167).

Seeds, drastic purg., as potent as those of *J. curcas*.

Seed fatty oil used in indigenous med. as an external stim. in rheum. and paralytic affections; also in skin diseases. Seldom used internally although purg. Plant juice, acrid; root, purg. (Chopra *et al*, II, 795).

Dried residue of McOH ext. of fruit, molluscacidal (*Q J Crude Drug Res*, 1980, **18**, 141). Seed ext., active against storedgrain pest (*Indian J Agric Sci*, 1980, **50**, 637).

Jatrophone—tumour-inhibitor macrocyclic diterp. from roots; its str. and stereochem., antileukemic compd.; jatrophone and other electrophilic tumour inhibitors may act by selective alkylation of growth-regulatory biol. macromolecules, particularly of SH group (*J Am Chem Soc*, 1970, **92**, 4476; 1976, **98**,

2295). Diterp. jatropholones A & B from roots (*Tetrahedron Lett*, 1979, 979).

Bark, β-sitosterol (*J Indian Chem Soc*, 1964, **41**, 88). Leaf flavons.; root, stem and seeds, lignan, str. (*Phytochemistry* 1971, **10**, 1690; 1981, **20**, 2047).

J. multifida Linn.

Eng.–*Coral plant, physic nut.*

Yellow fruits poisonous to human beings particularly to children (Kingsbury, 192). Sap used in cancer (*Lloydia*, 1969, **32**, 167).

*J. podagrica Hook.

MeOH ext. of stem, antibact.

Tetra-Me-pyrazine—pharmacol. mech. of hypotens. action of alk.; alk. neuromuscular and cardiovascular; more pharmacol. investigations of alk. (*Planta Med*, 1980, **38**, 144; 235; 238; 281; 332, 1981, **42**, 223; **43**, 1).

Grown in Indian gardens for ornament.

*J. podagrica Hook. var. **elegans** Muell.-Arg.

Bark, alk. jatrophine (0.4% dry basis); toxic dose for guineapigs, 0.2g/kg body wt (Chopra *et al*, II, 795).

Grown in Indian gardens for ornament.

JOANNESIA (*Euphorbiaceae*)

*J. princeps Vell.

Seed oil called *Anda - assy*, used as purg. in vet. practice, four times more active than castor oil. Also used in skin diseases. Fruit and milky latex from bark used to stupefy fish (Wlth India, V, 298; Uphof, 289).

Bark yields essent. oil with strong odour of garlic and irritating repulsive taste; oil contains vesic. resin (Wlth India, V, 297).

Cultivated in Indian gardens.

JUGLANS (*Juglandaceae*)

J. regia Linn.

Eng.–*Walnut*

Bark—used against cancer (*Lloydia*, 1969, **32**, 261); paste for toe sores (*Econ Bot*, 1971, **25**, 418). Bark and leaves used as alter. and laxt.; in herpes, eczema and scrofula (*Acta Phytother*, 1971, **18**, 21); exts. useful in dentrifice for antisep., antibact., abrassive and tartar masking properties (*Pak J For*, 1971, **21**, 325); lactifuge; decoct. to stop mammery secretions, and in sore throat (*Khadi Gramodyog*, 1980-81, **27**, 401).

Leaves—used mostly dried. Stabilization of its bacteriostatic exts. (*Acta Pol Pharm*, 1964, **21**, 65; *CA*, 1965, **62**, 7592e). Used extensively in cancer (*Lloydia*, 1969, **32**, 261); as insectic. (*Econ Bot*, 1971, **25**, 418); also as contracep. drug (*Planta Med*, 1972, **23**, 167). In diabetes |*Farm Zh*, 1972, **27**(6), 78; *BA*, 1973, **56**, 56516|; it has only a weak action on diabetes. Tea taken internally in suppurations and skin eruptions; also as external application to these eruptions. Its action as vermifuge, uncertain (Med. Plants, 41). EtOH(50%) ext., CNS depress. and antivir. (*Indian J Exp Biol*, 1973, **11**, 43). Ext., toxic to tadpole larvae |*Environ India*, 1980, 3(I & II), 84|.

Fruit—nut, hull and oil extensively used in all kinds of tumours (*Lloydia*, 1969, **32**, 261); goitrogenic in rats (*Endocrinology*, 1970, **86**, 69). Production of active preparations from ripe fruit wall is complex and should be left to pharmacist (Med. Plants, 41). Kernel and its oil hypocholesteremic in rats (*Fats Oils Relat Food Prod Tehri Persp Symp*, 1976, 95; *CA*, 1978, **89**, 128243m). Unripe fruit, fish poison (*Nagarjun*, 1979-80, **23**, 177). Kernel, aphrodis.; green hull and unripe shell, antisyp., and vermifugal; oil useful against tapeworms and laxt. (*Khadi Gramodyog*, 1980-81, **27**, 401). Antibact. fluid from destructive distillation of shells (Indian Pat., 1974, 125090; *CA*, 1975, **82**, 1100n).

Stembark, β-sitosterol and betulin (*Khim Prir Soedin*, 1966, **2**, 291; *CA*, 1967, **66**, 487h); berberine (0.08%) |*Nat Appl Sci Bull*, 1974, **26**(2), 31|; flavon., sakuranetetin (*Yakugaku Zasshi*, 1965, **85**, 547; *Phytochemistry*, 1981, **20**, 869).

Leaves, glycosidases (*Bull Soc R Sci Liege*, 1966, **35**, 142; *CA*, **65**, 10859a). Polyphenolic complexes of leaves of *J. regia* and *J. niger*, highly antiinflam.; flavons. decreased B.P. in dogs. Leaves, hyperoside, juglanin (kaempherol- 3-arabinoside) and quercetin-3-α-L-arabinofuranoside (*Fenol' nye Soedin Ikh Biol Funkts Mater Vses Simp*, 1966, 95; *CA*, 1969, **71**, 19518m). Flavon. distribution in different parts (*Pharmazie*, 1969, **24**, 780; *CA*, 1970, **73**, 951t). Tannins, a little volat. oil, juglone (active in mycoses) hydrojuglone and other little known substances (Med. Plant, 41); constituents of volat. oil (*Rev chim Bucharest*, 1974, **25**, 242; *CA*, 1975, **82**, 82980z; *CA*, **77**, 111450f); anal. (*Rastit Resur*, 1980, **16**, 441).

Manufacture of antifung. and antibact. agent, curcumicidin from peels (Jpn, 1965, 14590; *CA*, 1966, **64**, 1910c). Unripe fruit, amino acid, citrulline (*Meiji Daigaku Nogakubu Kankyu Hokoku*, 1966, No. 20, 23; *CA*, 1968, **68**, 19552g). Fruit wall rich in vit. C. Action antiinflam. on mucosa and as general tonic (Med. Plants, 41). Estn. of F, Ca, Mg and P in nuts (*Indian J Med Res*, 1972, **60**, 1470). Sterols of nut oil (*Ann Bromatol*, 1978, **30**, 63; *CA*, **89**, 106147f).

Root bark, juglone, cyclotrijuglone, β-sitosterol (*Indian J Chem*, 1975, **13**, 749); also bisjuglone (*Phytochemistry*, 1978, **17**, 2042),

Juglone—active principle, 5-OH-1, 4-napthoquinone; present in green walnut shells and green parts of *J. regia* and *J. niger* (*Chem Pharm Bull*, 1967, **15**, 242; Med. Plants, 41); antifeedant to bark beetle, *Scolylus multistraitus* (*J Insect Physiol*, 1967, **13**, 1453); and from other spp. of *Juglans*; in some spp. of *Carya*. Wilting of plants growing near the walnut tree may be due to this quinone; also inhibits seedling growth and may even prove lethal; but not in every plant; it is possible that toxicity of walnut root leachates depends on soil conditions; toxic in poorly drained sites but not in well-drained sites.

Highly toxic to animals; and to earthworms when applied to soil; effects (*in* Plant and Fungal Toxins, 712-13; 715- 16). Antimicrob. [*Microbios Lett*,, 1977, **4**(15), 175; *CA*, 1978, **89**, 71511r]; antifung. (*J Agric Food Chem*, 1980, **28**, 340). Decreases tumour-growth rate in mice (*J Pharm Sci*, 1968, **57**, 1674); also found to exhibit tumour-promoting activity on female ICR/Ha swiss mouse skin, after a single subcarcinogenic dose of 1,2-di- Me-benzanthracene (*J Med Chem*, 1978, **21**, 26).

JUNCUS (*Juncaceae*)

J. effusus Linn. syn. *J. communis* Mey.

Leaf flavons., luteoline-7-glucd., diosmin and hesperidin (*C R Acad Sci Ser D*, 1966, **263**, 439). Aerial parts, phenolic constituents, effusol and juncusol (*Experientia*, 1980, **36**, 27). Juncusol (9, 10-dihydrophenanthrene), antimicrob. (*Life Sci*, 1981, **29**, 1977).

J. inflexus Linn. syn. *J. glaucus* Ehrh. ex Sibth.

Preliminary pharmacol. (*Indian J Exp Biol*, 1980, **18**, 594).

J. prismatocarpus R.Br.

EtOH(50%) ext. of plant, diur. (*Indian J Exp Biol*, 1980, **18**, 594).

JUNIPERUS (*Cupressaceae*)

*J. chinensis Linn.

Eng.–*Chinese juniper.*

Wood used for preparing cosmetics and as incense in China; yields an essent. oil similar to that of *J. virgiana* (Wlth India, V, 311).

Native of China and Japan; introduced into India.

J. communis Linn.

Eng.–*Common juniper, juniper.*

Berries—pharmacognosy (*Lok Sirovine*, 1968, **6**, 75; *CA*, 1971, **74**, 45566h). Ext., antiscabies (*Indian J Anim Sci*, 1969, **39**, 345); useful in psorptic mange in sheep

(*Indian J Vet*, 1969, **46**, 826); antifung. (*Indian J Anim Sci*, 1977, **47**, 226).

Berries and oil used in various kinds of tumours (*Lloyida*, 1970, **33**, 342): berries in mineral-plant drug for tumours (Fr. Demande, 1972, 2122318; *CA*, 1973, **78**, 102024p). Decoct. of berries with other plant ingredient given in diar. (*Econ Bot*, 1973, **27**, 266). Fruits, constituent of compn. for haemor. (Ger. Offen. 1975, 2337617; *CA*, **83**, 84846e).

Wood and bark ext., for short breath and to purify blood (*Econ Bot*, 1973, **27**, 266).

Fruits, cyclohexitol (*Khim Prir Soedin*, 1968, **4**, 277; *CA*, 1969, **70**, 88156j); Fruit terp., geijerone (*Helv Chim Acta*, 1972, **55**, 2429). Flavon. and other compds. (*Pol J Chem*, 1980, **54**, 213); umbelliferone, rutoside and isoquercetrin (*Rocz Akad Roln Poznaniu*, 1980, **117**, 61; *CA*, **93**, 201030d); ext. contains antiherpetic agents; purification, identn. and testing in primary human amnion cell cultures (*Drugs Exp Clin Res*, 1981, **7**, 69; 691; *CA*, **94**, 185478u; **95**, 200601v).

Essent. oil from fruit contains monoterp. (*Helv Chim Acta*, 1972, **55**, 2429; 1973, **56**, 1800); junionins (*J Chem Soc Chem Commun*, 1973, 746); diterp. acids including dimer of myrceocommunic acid (*An Quim*, 1973, **69**, 1065; *CA*, 1974, **81**, 74847a); β-elemen-7α-ol (*ibid*, 1977, **73**, 463; *CA*, **87**, 114688g).

Seeds, haemagglutinin with specific activity [*Univ Wyoming Agr Exp Sta (Laramie) Sci Monograph*, 1971, **24**, II, 1; *CA*, 1972, **76**, 70197n].

Needles, umbelliferone, rutin and other flavon. (*Diss Pharm Pharmacol*, 1966, **18**, 169; CA, **65**, 4262d); OMe-mucoinositol (*Phytochemistry*, 1972, **11**, 245).

Leaves, flavons. (*Rocz Chem*, 1977, **51**, 2131; *CA*, 1978, **88**, 101564j); 3 new diterp. acids (*Phytochemistry*, 1980, **19**, 1153).

J. polycarpos Koch syn. *J. excelsa* auct. non Bieb.; *J. macropoda* auct. non Bioss.

Fruit and resin used in ulcers and nasal polyps (*Lloydia*, 1970, **33**, 343). Essent. oil from berries, antifung. against keratinophylic microorganisms causing dermatophytic diseases in man (*Indian Drugs*, 1978-79, **16**, 43).

Berries, essent. oil, sugiol, 10-non-acosanol, β- sitosterol glucd., flavon. junipodin & its glycd., junipin (*Q J Crude Drug Res*, 1970, **10**, 1636); also hypolaetin glucd. (*Phytochemistry*, 1971, **10**, 434).

Leaf essent. oil, constituent (*Indian Perfum*, 1978, **22**, 182). Leaves, biflavons. (*Indian J Chem*, 1979, **17B**, 193); also biflavon. & flavon. glycds.; isoflavon. and stilbenes; 2 new isoflavons. junipegenin B & C (*Phytochemistry*, 1977, **16**, 1456; 1980, **19**, 1831; 1981, **20**, 341).

*J. procera Hochst.

Eng.–*East African cedar*.

Wood—fragrant and resistant to insect attack. It yields on steam-distillation an essent. oil similar to cedarwood oil from *J. virginiana* (Wlth India, V, 311).

Introduced into India in Nilgiris.

J. recurva Buch.-Ham. ex D. Don syn. *J. squamata* D. Don

Eng.–*Weeping blue juniper*.

Smoke from green wood, emet. (*Indian For*, 1970, **105**, 788). EtOH(50%) ext. of aerial parts, anticancer (*Indian J Exp Biol*, 1980, **18**, 594).

Plant, isocedrolic acid; 4-ketocedrol (*Experientia*, 1976, **32**, 827; 686). Sesquiterp. (*J Chin Chem Soc Taipei*, 1977, **24**, 141).

Leaves, biflavons., cupessuflavone & derivs. (*Phytochemistry*, 1973, **12**, 1494). Essent. oil from leaves and other spp., rev., 27 refs. (*Indian Perfum*, 1980, **24**, 57).

*J. virginiana Linn.

Eng. – *Juniper, red cedar; pencil cedar*.

Leaves, berries and branches, one of the constituent of lotion for regeneration of capillary glands (Fr. 1966, 1443889; *CA*,

1967, **66**, 108180k). Leaves used in warts and other excrescences (*Lloydia*, 1970, **33**, 345). Berries, a part of adjuvant for antitumour drug (Fr. Demande, 1972, 2129972; 1973, 2133521; *CA*, 1973, **78**, 140403u; 164090r).

Wood, twigs and fruits, as incence; wood yields 1-3% of volat. oil, known as Cedarwood oil in trade (Wlth India, V, 310).

Cedarwood oil—in insecticides., perfumary, soaps, liniments. etc.; also used as abortif; but in some cases, deaths reported due to its use (Wlth India, V, 310).

Alc. ext. of plant, podophyllotoxin, the tumour-inhibiting principle, active against sarcoma 180 in mice and human nasophyrynx carcinoma in cell culture (*J Pharm Sci*, 1965, **44**, 580). Cedarwood oil; characteristics and constituents, cedrene isomers (80%), cedrol(3-14%), etc.(Wlth India, V, 310). Trends in essent. oil chem. (*Perfum Flav*, 1980, **5**, 63).

Leaves, essent. oil constituents (*Can J Chem*, 1978, **46**, 3743).

Introduced into Indian gardens as ornamental.

*J. wallichiana Hook.f. syn. *J. pseudo-sabina* Hook.f. non Fisch. & Mey.

Eng.–*Black juniper*; H.–*Bhil*; Sik.– *Techokpo*.

Various var. of herb extensively used in all types of tumours and cancers (*Lloydia*, 1970, **33**, 343).

Essent. oil, antimicrob. (*Prikl Biokhim Mikrobiol*, 1977, **13**, 185). Leaves, coumarins, siderin, coumarsabin & MeO-coumarsabin (*Phytochemistry*, 1981, **20**, 2778). Flavons. of needles (*Khim Prir Soedin*, 1981, 799).

Essent. oil from berries, mono-, di- & sesquiterp. (*An Quim*, 1978, **74**, 680; 1093; *CA*, 1979, **91**, 74741t; **89**, 160110b).

Temperate Himalayas up to 6,000 m.

JURINEA (*Asteraceae*)

J. dolomiaea Boiss. syn. *J. macrocephala* DC.; *Dolomiaea macrocephala* DC.

Arom. oil from roots, in gout and rheum. (*Indian For*, 1961, **87**, 104; *Indian J Hort*, 1979, **36**, 336).

JUSSIAEA (*Onagraceae*)

See **LUDWIGIA**

JUSTICIA (*Acanthaceae*)

J. betonica Linn.

Preliminary pharmacol. (*Indian J Exp Biol*, 1971, **9**, 91).

J. ecbolium Linn.; see **Ecbolium viride**

J. gendarussa Burm.; see **Gendarussa vulgaris**

J. picta Linn.; see **Graptophyllum pictum**

J. procumbens Linn. syn. *Rostellularia procumbens* Nees

Leaves, essent. oil, antifung. (*Flavour Ind*, 1972, **2**, 484). Justicidins A & B (major), diphyllin and lignan neojusticin; last compd. fish-killing (*Chem Pharm Bull*, 1970, **18**, 862). Plant, 1-MeO-2,3-naphthalide lignans, justicidins C & D (*Tetrahedron Lett*, 1970, 923); var. *leucantha*, 6 lignans including justicidin A & B, neojusticin A & B, diphyllin and taiwanin E (*Tetrahedron*, 1970, **26**, 4301). Var. *simplex*, flowers contain peonidin glucd. (*Vijnana Parishad Anusandhan Patrika*, 1978, **21**, 177).

*J. prostrata Gamble

Plant lignan, retrochinensin (*J Chem Soc Chem Commun*, 1979, 165); prostalidins A, B & C; prostalidin A, antidepress. in mice and rats (*Chem Ind Lond*, 1979, 854).

Gangetic plains, Jammu & Kashmir and S. India.

*J. purpurea Linn. var. **vahlii** C.B. Clarke syn. *J. diffusa* Willd.

Root, remedy for madness (Wlth India, V, 313).

Found in Bihar and Western Ghats.

J. simplex D. Don; see **Rostellularia mollissima**

*J. tranque-bariensis Linn. f.
Tam.–*Sivanarvembu*.
Leaves—juice cooling and aper. Given for small-pox in children; bruised leaves applied to contusions (Wlth India, V, 313).
Found in Karnataka.

*J. vasculosa Wall.
Leaves, for inflam. (Wlth India, V, 313).
Found in Sibsagar, Assam and Khasi hills, Meghalaya at 800-2,000 m.

KAEMPFERIA (*Zingiberaceae*)

K. galanga Linn.
Eng.–*Black thorn*.
Plant used as hallucinogen (*Science*, 1969, **163**, 245). Rhizome essent. oil, antifung. (*Flavour Ind*, 1971, **2**, 484).
Leaves and flowers, total flavons. having antiphl., vit. P activity, etc. (*Farmakol Toksikol Moscow*, 1969, **32**, 438).
Root, Et-*p*-MeO-*trans*-cinnamate, main compd. [*Duoc Hoc*, 1979, (5), 9; *CA*, 1980, **93**, 22612y].

K. rotunda Linn.
Tubers, crotepoxide, (*Indian J Chem*, 1970, **8**, 468).

KALANCHOE (*Crassulaceae*)

K. integra (Medic.) Kuntze syn. *K. spathulata* DC.
EtOH(50%) ext. of plant, hypoten. and anticancer (*Indian J Exp Biol*, 1971, **9**, 91).
Leaves, ext., LD$_{50}$ studies, nontoxic in animals (*Indian J Pharmacol*, 1979, **11**, 301). Aq. ext. of leaves, toxicity study in sheep (*Indian J Anim Sci*, 1981, **51**, 522).
Flowers, triterps. and sterols; leaves and flowers, flavon. glycds. (*Phytochemistry*, 1976, **15**, 1999; 1981, **20**, 530).

K. laciniata DC. syn. *Cotyledon laciniata* Roxb.
Leaves —antisep. Applied to bite of insects. Juice given in dysen. and phthisis. In Malaysia, as poultice for cough and cold;

in lotions for smallpox (Wlth India, V, 315).
Various plant parts used in fever, urticaria, dyspep., broncht. and asthma (*Econ Bot*, 1970, **24**, 241).
EtOH(50%) ext. of plant, CNS depress. (*Indian J Exp Biol*, 1977, **15**, 208).

K. pinnata Pers. syn. *Bryophyllum calycinum* Salisb.; *B. pinnatum* Kurz

Leaves —juice of succulent ones used in burns (*Bull Bot Surv India*, 1976, **18**, 161). In Assam, mixed with those of *Aegle marmelos* given in blood and amoebic dysen. (*Bull Med Ethno Bot Res*, 1980, **1**, 447); eaten to control diabetes (*Ethnomedicine*, 1980, **6**, 139).
Plant exts. (also of leaves), antifung. (*Geobios*, 1978, **5**, 49; *Acta Bot Indica*, 1979, **7**, 147); antilithic (*Proc Indian Sci Congr*, 1981, III, 156).
Leaves yield glycds. of quercetin and kaempferol (*Planta Med*, 1971, **20**, 368); and fumaric acid (*Indian J Pharm*, 1972, **34**, 20); phenolic components (*Planta Med*, 1973, **23**, 149).
Cellular sap., flavon. (*Khim Prir Soedin*, 1969, **5**, 597; *CA*, 1970, **73**, 84621w). Plant ext. contains in its unsap. matter, *n*-alkane (*n*-hentriacontane and *n*- triacontane, major); *n*-alkanol; α - & β-amyrin and sitosterol (*Phytochemistry*, 1972, **11**, 1500).

KALLSTROEMIA (*Zygophyllaceae*)

*K. pubescens (G. Don) Dandy
In Ghana, used in constip. (Fl. Bhagalpur, 88). Plant as new source for diosgenin; anal. of plant parts (*J Inst Chem India*, 1976, **48**, 170).
Diosgenin — weed, a possible commercial source of diosgenin, a steroid drug precursor (Asolkar & Chadha, 51); extn. procedure (Indian Pat, 1976, 139136; *CA*, 1980, **92**, 91186d); enzymatic transformation of glycds. (*J Chem Res*, 1980, No. 1, 64). Cultivation and variation in content (*Indian Drugs*, 1980-81, **18**, 431). Weed as

diosgenin-yielding crop (*Indian J Pharm Sci*, 1981, **43**, 172).

W. Bengal.

KANDELIA (*Rhizophoraceae*)

K. rheedii Wight & Arn. syn. *K. candel* (Linn.) Druce

Stems, 2,6-di-MeO-benzoquinone (*Phytochemistry*, 1976, **15**, 2028).

KAYEA (*Clusiaceae*)

See **MESUA**

KERRIA (*Rosaceae*)

***K. japonica DC.**

Eng.–*Japanese rose.*

Leaves and roots contain small amt. of HCN (Wlth India, V, 317). Leaves, rich in ascorbic acid (200mg/100g).

Plant contains flavon. glycd., pectolinaroside (*C R Acad Sci Ser D*, 1970, **270**, 2710).

Native of Japan, cultivated in Indian gardens for ornament.

KHAYA (*Meliaceae*)

***K. senegalensis** A. Juss.

Eng.–*Senegal khaya, African mahogany.*

Bark, astrin., bitter tonic, antipyr., antimal., anthelm., cmmcn., used in liverfluke of cattle.

Flowers, in gastric disorder, syphilis.

EtOH(50%) ext. of aerial parts, diur. (*Indian J Exp Biol*, 1977, **15**, 208).

Bark alk. calicendrine (Watt & Breyer-Brandwijk, 745). Timber and bark, angolensate derivs.; bark, limonoids (*J Chem Soc Chem Commun*, 1967, 790; 1969, 58). Gum polysaccharides (*ibid*, 1970, 365).

Grown in Calcutta gardens.

KICKXIA (*Scrophulariaceae*)

K. ramosissima (Wall.) Janch. syn. *Linaria ramosissima* Wall.

Aq. ext. of aerial parts, hypoglyc. in rabbit (*in* Atal & Kapoor, Med. Plants, 593).

KIGELIA (*Bignoniaceae*)

K. pinnata DC.

Eng.–*Sausage tree*; H.–*Jhar phanoos.*

Fruit, cytostatic compd. (Ger. Offen, 1974, 2417071; *CA*, 1975, **82**, 9065v). Fruits and leaves, flavons. (*Fitoterapia*, 1981, **52**, 189).

Bark, β-sitosterol; ferulic acid (*Indian J Chem*, 1969, **7**, 308; 1971, **9**, 611); also lapachol, stigmasterol and 6-MeO-mellein (*Phytochemistry*, 1971, **10**, 1603).

Roots, isocoumarin, 6-MeO-mellein; wood, naphthoquinone and lignan (*Indian J Chem*, 1970, **8**, 851; *Phytochemistry*, 1981, **20**, 2271); root heartwood yields octacosanol, lapachol, kigelin, rhodamine B, stigmasterol & β-sitosterol (*J Indian Chem Soc*, 1981, **58**, 825).

KINGIODENDRON (*Caesalpiniaceae*)

K. pinnatum (Roxb.) Harms syn. *Hardwickia pinnata* Roxb.

Oleoresin from tree, used in sores of elephant (Wlth India, V, 320).

Oleoresin contains monoterps. and diterps., viz. hardwickiic, kolavic, kolavenic acids, and kolavenol (*Tetrahedron Lett*, 1964, 3751); also kolavelool; kolavonic and kolavenolic acids (*Tetrahedron*, 1979, **35**, 985; 2301).

Essent. oil from resin, physicochem. constants and constituents (*Perfum Essent Oil Rec*, 1967, **58**, 782).

KIRGANELIA (*Euphorbiaceae*)

K. reticulata (Poir.) Baill. syn. *Phyllanthus reticulatus* Poir.

EtOH(50%) of aerial parts, antiprot., antivir., spasmol. and hypoten. (*Indian J Exp Biol*, 1968, **6**, 232).

Leaves contain friedelin, its 3 derivs., glochidonol and. β-sitosterol; stems, friedelin, betulinic acid and β-sitosterol (*Phytochemistry*, 1976, **15**, 797). Roots, triterps., β-sitosterol, etc. (*J Indian Chem Soc*, 1981, **58**, 102).

KLEINHOVIA (*Sterculiaceae*)

K. hospita Linn.

In Samoa, bark used to treat wounds. Leaves and bark, poisonous (*Econ Bot*, 1974, **28**, 27).

KNEMA (*Myristicaceae*)

*K. attenuata (Wall.) Warb. syn. *Myristica attenuata* Wall.

Preliminary pharmacol. (*Indian J Exp Biol*, 1973, **11**, 43).

Bark contains lignan, attenuol (*Experientia*, 1978, **34**, 422; *Tetrahedron*, 1979, **35**, 1665).

From Western Ghats, S. Kanara southwards in evergreen forests.

*K. linifolia (Roxb.) Warb.

Juice of leaves mixed with stem juice of *Spatholobus roxburghii* taken in dysen. (*Bull Bot Surv India*, 1980, **22**, 161).

Found in W. Bengal, Arunachal Pradesh and Assam hills.

KNOXIA (*Rubiaceae*)

*K. sumatrensis (Retz.) DC. syn. *K. corymbosa* auct. non Willd.

EtOH(50%) ext. of plant, diur. (*Indian J Exp Biol*, 1977, **15**, 208).

Shrub yields ursolic acid, β-sitosterol and an oily residue (*J Indian Chem Soc*, 1969, **46**, 301).

Tirupati, A.P.

KOCHIA (*Chenopodiaceae*)

*K. prostrata Schrad.

Tincture made from EtOH ext. of plant, antiinflam. in rats; other pharmacol. investigation (*Farmakol Alkaloidov Glikozidov*, 1967, 178; *CA*, 1969, **70**, 56096y).

Found in Western Himalayas in dry regions of Kunawar and Zanskar.

K. scoparia Schrad.

Preliminary screening for antitumour activity (*Shoyakugaku Zasshi*, 1979, **33**, 95).

Herb ext., campesterol (50% of unsap. matter) (*Yakhak Hoeji*, 1969, **13**, 144; *CA*, 1971, **75**, 40312h). Micro detn. of seed saponin; sapogenin, oleanolic acid (*J Agric Food Chem*, 1973, **21**, 232). Aerial parts, 4 alks.; including harman and harmine (*Lloydia*, 1978, **41**, 289; *Acta Pol Pharm*, 1965, **22**, 181; 1978, **35**, 497; *CA*, **63**, 18643f; 1979, **90**, 148489v).

*K. trichophylla Voss

Eng.–*Summer cypress, fire bush.*

EtOH(50%) ext. of plant, CNS depress. (*Indian J Exp Biol*, **11**, 43).

Plant, hentriacontane and hentriacontanol (*Indian J Chem*, 1966, **4**, 545; *Indian J Appl Chem*, 1970, **33**, 261).

Cultivated in Indian gardens.

KOELPINIA (*Asteraceae*)

*K. linearis Pall.

Ladakh–*Nodar.*

Plant used in rheum. (*in* Atal & Kapur, Med. Plants, 523).

Leaf coumarins, cichorin, esculin and esculetin (*Khim Prir Soedin*, 1976, 537; *CA*, **85**, 174266m).

Reported from Punjab and Kashmir.

KOELZELLA (*Apiaceae*)

*K. pabularia (Lindl.) Hiroe

Fruits and roots, med. (Santapau & Henry, 91).

Found in Kashmir.

KOKOONA (*Celastraceae*)

K. zeylanica Thw.

Inner bark, triterps., friedelane, kokoononol, kokoondiol and kokoonol (*J Chem Soc Chem Commun*, 1979, 434); also zeylanol, zeylanonol & zeylandiol; zeylasterone from outer stem bark; kokzeylanol and kokzeylanonol (*Tetrahedron Lett*, 1979, 1727; 1980, **21**, 4749; 1981, **22**, 1425).

KOPSIA (*Apocynaceae*)

K. fruticosa DC.
Eng.–*Pink kopsia.*
EtOH(50%) ext. of root, hypoten. and diur. (*Indian J Exp Biol*, 1980, **18**, 594).
Str. of indole alk. kopsine from leaves and bark (*Symp Phytochem Proc Meeting Univ Hong Kong*, 1961, 27; *CA*, 1964, **61**, 16109h). Leaves, alks. fruticosine and fruticosamine (*J Chem Soc C*, 1967, 813). Stem bark, β- amyrin, its-OAc and γ-sitosterol (*J Indian Chem Soc*, 1968, **45**, 962). Leaves, flavons. and phenolic acids (*Indian J Exp Biol*, 1978, **16**, 512).

KORTHALSELLA (*Viscaceae*)

*K. japonica (Thunb.) Engl.
Presence of toxic proteins reported (*Acta Pharm Suec*, 1981, **18**, 179; *CA*, **95**, 55848z).
From Himalayas, Assam hills and Western Ghats.

KRAMERIA (*Krameriaceae*)

*K. argentea Mart.
Eng.–*Brazilian* or *para rhatany.*
Roots —useful astrin. in diar., haemorrhoides, etc. Also as hemostatic and tonic, in mouth washes and in gargles; contain *c.* 10% tannins (Hocking, 120).
Brazilian species, used as a substitute for Peruvian rhatany in India.

K. triandra Ruiz. & Pav.
Extn. of tannin, as possible antitumour agent (*J Pharm Sci*, 1969, **58**, 839). History of med. uses of roots, rev., 30 refs. (*Dtsch Apoth Ztg*, 1981, **121**, 46).

Roots, 2 phenols; may be useful in sun protection compn. (*Planta Med*, 1981, **42**, 144).

KYDIA (*Malvaceae*)

K. calycina Roxb.
EtOH(50%) ext. of leaves, CNS depress. and hypoten. Stem bark ext. potentiates barbiturate (*Indian J Exp Biol*, 1969, **7**, 250). Leaf paste used in body pain (*Bull Bot Surv India*, 1973, **15**, 14).
Root paste applied on oedema (*Bull Med Ethno Bot Res*, 1980, **1**, 8). Root, as fabge. and in rheum. (*J Econ Tax Bot*, 1981, **2**, 174).
Stems and roots contain hibiscone C, hibiscoquinone B and a new quinone (*Proc Indian Sci Congr*, 1980, III, 73).

KYLLINGA (*Cyperaceae*)

K. brevifolia Rottb. syn. *Cyperus brevifolius* Hassk.
Herb decoct. given in constip. and dysen. (*Nagarjun*, 1980- 81, **24**, 240; 242). In China, herb used for treatment of chyluria; contains vitexin and an unidentified flavon. (*Chung Ts'ao Yao*, 1980, **11**, 342; *CA*, 1981, **94**, 71290w).

K. nemoralis Dandy ex Hutchin. syn. *K. monocephala* Rottb.
Plant used in tumours and icterus (*Econ Bot*, 1970, **24**, 241).
Tubers contain enterokinase inhibitors (*J Biosci*, 1981, **3**, 371).

K. tenuifolia Steud. syn.*K. triceps* Rottb.; *Cyperus triceps* (Rottb.) Endl.
Roots used in liver disorders (*J Econ Tax Bot*, 1980, **1**, 145). Plant, in diabetes (Hocking, 120).

INDEX OF LANGUAGE, REGIONAL & TRADE NAMES

A

Absinthe (Eng.)	92
Aden-cha-kanher (Mar.)	22
Ad samerwo (G.)	53
African blue lily (Eng.)	28
African cape aloe (Eng.)	49
African mahogany (Eng.)	383
Agarwood (Eng.)	80
Aggai (H.)	274
Agrimony (Eng.)	32
Ailanto (Eng.)	33
Ajbar (Kash.)	126
Akee apple (Eng.)	127
Alligator apple (Eng.)	28,71
Alligator pepper (Eng.)	28
Aloewood (Eng.)	80
Alyce clover (Eng.)	54
Amari (Ass. & Trade)	59
Ambrette plant (Eng.)	2
American aloe (Eng.)	29
American beauty berry (Eng.)	155
American jute (Eng.)	7
American maiden hair fern (Eng.)	24
American sumac (Eng.)	151
Amli (Garhwal)	126
Angelica (Eng.)	70
Angel's trumpet (Eng.)	143
Anise tree (Eng.)	367
Annatto (Eng.)	126
Arecanut (Eng.)	84
Areca palm (Eng.)	84
Arnato (Eng.)	126
Arnica (Eng.)	91
Arruttuvarai (Mal.)	308
Artichoke (Eng.)	252
Asana (Mar.)	141
Ashgourd (Eng.)	119
Ash-leaved maple (Eng.)	14
Asparagus (Eng.)	100
Asparagus fern (Eng.)	100
Assam indigo (Eng.)	114
Assam rubber (Eng.)	314

Assam rum (Eng.)	114
Athalanghi (Tam.)	315
Attak (Mar.)	316
Auk (H.)	157
Australian blackwood (Eng.)	9
Australian christmas orchid (Eng.)	153

B

Badar (Kash.)	2
Bael tree (Eng.)	26
Baen (B.)	108
Bagali (Oriya)	303
Baloon vine (Eng.)	170
Bamora (H.)	119
Banakhor (P.)	82
Banavara (Kan.)	329
Banderhulla (B.)	285
Bangra (H.)	152
Bankalmi (B.)	372
Bankapas (B.)	1
Ban-nimbu (Gorakhpur)	333
Baobab tree (Eng.)	22
Bara garri (Kumaun)	33
Baragoran (B.)	193
Bara heloch (Ass.)	79
Barbodos aloe (Eng.)	46
Barley (Eng.)	358
Baro-nirkhut (Garo)	88
Barubutsali (Tel.)	206
Basaka (Ladakh)	189
Bat-soh-pila (Khasi)	67
Baunra (H.)	308
Bearberry (Eng.)	83
Beebread (Eng.)	133
Beele-Isie cress (Eng.)	115
Beet root (Eng.)	123
Begger lice (Eng.)	123
Bejli (Ass.)	114
Bel (G.)	173
Belladonna, Indian (Eng.)	104
Belladonna lily (Eng.)	55
Bellyache bush (Eng.)	377

Bell/yellow bauhinia (Eng.)	117
Bengal cardamom (Eng.)	59
Bengal gram (Eng.)	200
Bengal quince (Eng.)	26
Bergamot orange (Eng.)	208
Bet (Ass.)	153
Betelnut palm (Eng.)	84
Bhabar (H.& B.)	303
Bhedra (Jaunsar)	33
Bhil (H.)	381
Bhoy samerwo (G.)	54
Bhubi (Tripura)	112
Bhui tad (Mar.)	21
Bhumlati (Ass.)	188
Bhuter-chira (B.)	182
Bidhuli (Ass.)	114
Bigarade orange (Eng.)	208
Bilimbi (Eng.)	108
Birbut (Mundari)	54
Birch-leaved acalypha (Eng.)	12
Birch tree (Eng.)	123
Bird chilli (Eng.)	169
Bird of paradise (Eng.)	151
Bird's nest fern (Eng.)	102
Birkapas (B.)	1
Bir-manthan (Santal)	106
Bir-rambara (Mundari)	106
Bir-yambiri (Mundari)	147
Bisalballi (Kan.)	141
Bishop weed (Eng.)	56
Bishop wood (Eng.)	125
Biskachu (B.)	224
Bitter apple (Eng.)	207
Bitter orange (Eng.)	208
Bitter winter cress (Eng.)	115
Biyonihaputa (Ass.)	182
Black berry lily (Eng.)	119
Black currant tree (Eng.)	77
Black hellebore (Eng.)	349
Black juniper (Eng.)	381
Black maidenhair fern (Eng.)	25
Black mangrove (Eng.)	25
Black spleen/wort (Eng.)	101
Black thorn (Eng.)	382
Black/true mustard (Eng.)	138
Black wattle (Eng.)	9
Bleeng (Lepcha)	114
Blood flower (Eng.)	99
Blood lilies (Eng.)	342
Blue pimpernell (Eng.)	62
Bocho tupuri (Mundari)	130
Bol-simbal (Garo)	83
Bombay aloe (Eng.)	29
Bondvel (Mar.)	87
Bonohandi (Oriya)	297
Borage (Eng.)	133
Bor atlah bar (Ass. & B.)	314
Borpat (Ass.)	34
Botya gingaru (Kumaun)	33
Box elder (Eng.)	14
Box grass (Eng.)	182
Boxwood gardenia (Eng.)	324
Brab tree (Eng.)	133
Bracteated birthwort (Eng.)	88
Brank (Eng.)	310
Brazilian/para rhatany (Eng.)	385
Breadfruit (Eng.)	97
Brown/Indian mustard (Eng.)	136
Brussel sprouts (Eng.)	139
Buddhist bauhinia (Eng.)	117
Bughanan's mango (Eng.)	145
Bugloss (Eng.)	64
Bukangda (Mikir)	114
Bullock's heart (Eng.)	72
Bundum (Bihar)	297
Bung-fung (B.)	296
Burr marigold (Eng.)	124
Butterfly tree (Eng.)	117
Button tree (Eng.)	73,74

C

Cabbage (Eng.)	139
Cabbage angelin tree (Eng.)	65
Cakri (H.P.)	174
Calamus (Eng.)	18
Calcutta cane (Eng.)	114
Calico flower (Eng.)	90
Californian poppy (Eng.)	301
Calumba (Eng.)	376
Camel thorn (Eng.)	39
Campanilla (Eng.)	40
Campeachy tree (Eng.)	342
Camphor plant (Eng.)	22
Canary-bird bush (Eng.)	237
Candlenut tree (Eng.)	39
Cannabis (Eng.)	163
Cantala (Eng.)	29

Caoutchouc tree (Eng.)	352	Chinese gooseberry (Eng.)	21
Cape belladonna (Eng.)	55	Chinese hat plant (Eng.)	357
Cape forget-me not (Eng.)	64	Chinese juniper (Eng.)	379
Caper (Eng.)	167	Chinese laurel (Eng.)	76
Caraway (Eng.)	174	Chinese mustard (Eng.)	136
Cardamom (Eng.)	289	Chinese rice-flower (Eng.)	31
Caroa bean tree (Eng.)	192	Chinese trumpet creeper (Eng.)	161
Carob (Eng.)	192	Chinese water chestnut (Eng.)	289
Carrot (Eng.)	262	Chipli (Nepal)	79
Cashewnut (Eng.)	60	Chirchitta (H. & P.)	124
Cassena (Eng.)	366	Chiru (Tam.)	193
Cassie flower (Eng.)	8	Chitundi (Kan.)	204
Catmint (Eng.)	217	Chives (Eng.)	45
Cauliflower (Eng.)	138	Chobolaksinriube (Miri)	13
Cayenne pepper (Eng.)	169	Chomrik (Lepcha)	118
Cedarwood (Eng.)	187	Chorlanta (B.)	199
Celery (Eng.)	78,136	Chor pushi (H.P.)	124
Century plant (Eng.)	29	Chota-chirayata (H.)	293
Ceylon cinnamon (Eng.)	204	Chota-goale (B.)	187
Chaara paruppu (Mal.)	145	Christmas rose (Eng.)	349
Chagukadukhuan (Nagaland)	56	Chur-chur (B.)	176
Chahalubor (Mikir)	56	Cinna attatotai (Tam.)	23
Chak (Mikir)	114	Cinnamom (Eng.)	204
Chakko (Meghalaya)	181	Citron (Eng.)	209
Chakulia (B.)	350	Clown's mustard (Eng.)	365
Chakwa (B.)	73	Coastal cypress (Eng.)	156
Chamari (U.P.)	330	Cobra-lily/flower (Eng.)	88
Chamaria (Garhwal)	96	Cocklebur (Eng.)	32
Champari (Mar.)	316	Cocks-foot-grass (Eng.)	256
Charandalai (Tam.)	122	Collavan (Tam.)	259
Chavukku (Tam.)	9	Colosynth (Eng.)	207
Chavuri (Kan.)	146	Colza (Eng.)	136
Checkerberry (Eng.)	324	Common annual rogkit (Eng.)	365
Chenille plant (Eng.)	13	Common bamboo of Bengal (Eng.)	114
Cheria astalotakam (Mal.)	23	Common buckwheat (Eng.)	310
Cherimolia (Eng.)	70	Common columbine (Eng.)	80
Cherimoyer (Eng.)	70	Common hare's ear (Eng.)	147
Cherry pie (Eng.)	348	Common heliotrope (Eng.)	348
Cheruka (Mal.)	141	Common juniper (Eng.)	379
Chhamolja (Garo)	79	Common wattle (Eng.)	8
Chhota gingaru (Jaunsar)	33	Coral plant (Eng.)	378
Chhota hansraj (Pachmarhi hills)	195	Coral red wood (Eng.)	22
Chhumbi tikt (Ladakh)	325	Coriander (Eng.)	232
Chicory (Eng.)	201	Corn cockle (Eng.)	32
Chile pine (Eng.)	82	Couch grass (Eng.)	32
Chilli (Eng.)	169	Country mallow (Eng.)	6
China cassia (Eng.)	203	Cow parsley (Eng.)	76
Chinese cabbage (Eng.)	135	Crab's-eye (Eng.)	3
Chinese dye tree (Eng.)	126	Creat (Eng.)	65

Creeping indigo (Eng.) 368
Cross-vine (Eng.) 125
Crow killer (Eng.) 62
Cucumber (Eng.) 243
Cucumber tree (Eng.) 108
Cuddapah almond (Eng.) 145
Culcutta cane (Eng.) 114
Cumin (Eng.) 244
Curacao aloe (Eng.) 46
Curcas nut (Eng.) 376
Cury kale (Eng.) 138
Custard apple (Eng.) 72
Cutch tree (Eng.) 7
Cycads (Eng.) 249

D

Dabi (H.) 150
Dalne-katus (B.) 181
Damiyu-arong (Mikir) 112
Dandaro (G.) 12
Dandiyase (Kan.) 297
Danwa (Jaunsar) 33
Daom (Lepcha) 14
Dasmori (Mar.) 290
Davana (Kan., Mar. & Tam.) 95
Davanamu (Tel.) 95
Deadly nightshade (Eng.) 104
Dehra (Kondh) 73
Deobans (H.) 114
Desert date (Eng.) 112
Desert rose (Eng.) 22
Desipiri (Ass.) 375
Deura (H.) 308
Devil's tree (Eng.) 51
Dhakta dhampta (Mar.) 54
Dhaman (P.) 339
Dhau (G.) 74
Dhaunkara (H., G. & Rajasthan) 74
Dhauria (Rajasthan) 73
Dhingsong (Khasi) 299
Dhopa-paruli (Ass.) 343
Dhungaria phool (Sik.) 29
Diang-chao (Khasi) 34
Dieng-a-metrit (Khasi) 374
Diengauro-la-pyrno (Ass.) 263
Dieng-chhang (Khasi) 27
Dieng-la-phynia (Ass.) 263
Dieng-sohjaphon (Ass.) 119

Dieng-tem-sro (Khasi) 374
Dill (Eng.) 67
Dindiga tree (Eng.) 74
Dita bark tree (Eng.) 51
Divi-divi plant (Eng.) 151
Doda-da (Andaman) 116
Dog flower (Eng.) 77
Dog funnel (Eng.) 74
Dog grass (Eng.) 32
Dojuka (Garo) 112
Dola (Khasi) 27
Dolle balli (Kan.) 375
Dom (Lepcha) 14
Double chamomile (Eng.) 74
Dragon mugwort (Eng.) 93
Drakspose (Ladakh) 125
Dudhi (Mundari) 54
Durpa tandar (U.P) 126
Durumbihir (Mundari) 125
Dwarf aloe (Eng.) 29
Dwarf or common ragweed (Eng.) 56
Dwarf white bauhinia (Eng.) 116
Dyer's woad (Eng.) 374

E

Early winter cress (Eng.) 115
East African cedar (Eng.) 380
East-African laburnum (Eng.) 159
Easter-lily vine (Eng.) 118
East-Himalayan fir (Eng.) 3
Ebony (Eng.) 278
Egyptian doum palm (Eng.) 364
Egyptian garlic (Eng.) 43
Elephant creeper (Eng.) 87
Elephant-root yam (Eng.) 59
Elephant's lime tree (Eng.) 194
Endive (Eng.) 200
Ergot (Eng.) 212
Estragon (Eng.) 93
European ash (Eng.) 318
European beech (Eng.) 311

F

Fatfati (Mar.) 227
Feathery coconut palm (Eng.) 85
Feijoa (Eng.) 13
Fennel (Eng.) 317
Fetid bugbane (Eng.) 202

Field mustard (Eng.)   140
Fire bush (Eng.)   384
Flores koso (Eng.)   342
Flos adonis (Eng.)   25
French mulberry (Eng.)   155
Frog leaf (Eng.)   136
Fu (Nagaland)   148

G

Gaadar (G.)   54
Gadugu thumma (Tel.)   10
Galappa palm (Eng.)   22
Gandephul (B.)   193
Ganguli (Bihar)   297
Gaozaban (Trade)   64
Gargela (H.)   130
Garlic (Eng.)   43
Garlic mustard (Eng.)   40
Garlic wort (Eng.)   40
Garuda pakshini (Oriya)   283
Gatharu (Tel.)   193
Gaurkarsi (Oriya)   141
Gentian (Eng.)   325
Geranium tree (Eng.)   117
Ghatti tree (Eng.)   74
Ghogari (Mar.)   324
Giant-bamboo reed (Eng.)   98
Giant taro (Eng.)   46
Girlee (Oriya)   367
Goat's beard (Eng.)   98
Goat weed (Eng.)   30
Goat's horn mangrove (Eng.)   25
Gobbusoppu (Kan.)   129
Golden trumpet (Eng.)   40
Golden tussel (Eng.)   159
Golden wattle (Eng.)   11
Goose grass (Eng.)   321
Goparmowa (Kumaun)   293
Gorabnurey (H.)   67
Gora-hasel (Kondh)   73
Goran (H.)   193
Gortah (Oriya)   193
Goyalo (Rajasthan)   196
Grains of paradise (Eng.)   28
Grapefruit (Eng.)   210
Greater ammi (Eng.)   56
Greater galangal (Eng.)   50
Green amaranth (Eng.)   54

Green ebony persimmon (Eng.)   277
Green hellebore (Eng.)   349
Green pigweed (Eng.)   55
Green wattle (Eng.)   8
Green or wild amaranth (Eng.)   55
Groundnut (Eng.)   80
Guar (Eng.)   248
Gudda (Kan.)   316
Gular (B.)   356
Gul-inilam (H.)   132
Gul mendi (Kumaun)   367
Gum arabic tree (Eng.)   11
Gumbo (Eng.)   1
Guttikuncha (Tel.)   152
Gyesa (Lepcha)   299

H

Hairy rupture.wort (Eng.)   352
Haldu (H.)   345
Hangarian brome (Eng.)   142
Hangerian pumpkin (Eng.)   244
Han sampige (Kan.)   316
Hantige (Kan.)   21
Hanumaanaphala (Kan.)   70
Hanumaanaphalamuchettu(tree)(Tel.)   70
Hard sola (Eng.)   27
Hare's ear (Eng.)   146
Harinhara (B.)   141
Harkamoli (Oriya)   13
Hathethazori (H.)   127
Hawthorn (Eng.)   235
Heartseed (Eng.)   170
Hedge garlic (Eng.)   40
Hedge mustard (Eng.)   115
Hemlock (Eng.)   227
Hemp-nettle (Eng.)   321
Henbane (Eng.)   363
Henikay (Nilgiris)   329
Herald's trumpet (Eng.)   118
Hill mahua (Eng.)   34
Hill mango (Eng.)   225
Himalayan boxwood tree (Eng.)   150
Himalayan chestnut (Eng.)   28
Himalayan desert candle (Eng.)   296
Himalayan maple (Eng.)   14
Hinchang (Nagaland)   216
Hogbean (Eng.)   363
Hollyhock (Eng.)   38

Honeyplant (Eng.) 57
Hooirjo (B.) 118
Hop (Eng.) 359
Horse chestnut tree (Eng.) 27
Horseradish (Eng.) 90
Horsetail (Eng.) 296
Huluni (Kan. & Tam.) 308
Hungarian pumpkin (Eng.) 244
Huring kuru (Mundari) 130
Huring sargujia.ba (Mundari) 124
Hyoscyamus (Eng.) 363

I

Ikuhia (Ass.) 27
Ilapongu (Tam.) 357
Illinda (Tel.) 277
Inchane (G.) 12
Indian acalypha (Eng.) 12
Indian alder (Eng.) 46
Indian aloe (Eng.) 46
Indian birch (Eng.) 123
Indian birthwort (Eng.) 88
Indian butter tree (Eng.) 34
Indian chestnut (Eng.) 181
Indian colza (Eng.) 140
Indian dill (Eng.) 68
Indian gooseberry (Eng.) 291
Indian hemp (Eng.) 163
Indian horse chestnut (Eng.) 28
Indian lavender tree (Eng.) 147
Indian lilac (Eng.) 108
Indian liquorice (Eng.) 3
Indian mallow (Eng.) 7
Indian oak (Eng.) 115
Indian olibanum tree (Eng.) 134
Indian rubber tree (Eng.) 314
Indian silver fir (Eng.) 3
Indian snowberry (Eng.) 140
Indian spinach (Eng.) 116
Indian squill (Eng.) 282
Indian wormwood (Eng.) 95
Ipecac (Eng.) 191
Ire rubber (Eng.) 320
Itwari (Rajasthan) 7
Ivy (Eng.) 343

J

Jackbean (Eng.) 162
Jackfruit tree (Eng.) 97
Jafarabad aloe (Eng.) 46
Jajew (Khasi) 118
Ja-lenag-kren (Khasi) 145
Jali (Meghalaya) 235
Jalpaiguri cardamom (Eng.) 59
Jangli adua (H.) 187
Jangli bhendi (Mar.) 1
Jangli gazar (Kash.) 194
Japanese raisin (Eng.) 359
Japanese rose (Eng.) 159, 383
Japanese wind-flower (Eng.) 67
Javanese wool plant (Eng.) 27
Jequirity (Eng.) 3
Jerusalem artichoke (Eng.) 347
Jerusalem oak (Eng.) 196
Jew's mallow (Eng.) 231
Jhar phanoos (H.) 383
Jimson weed (Eng.) 261
Jinjok (Garo) 87
Jowa (B. & Tripura) 114
Juniper (Eng.) 379,380
Jute plant (Eng.) 230
Jute star (Eng.) 367

K

Kaaduthogari (Kan.) 106
Kabashi (B.) 14
Kachi grass (Bangalore) 251
Kadivalasoppu (Kan.) 77
Kafir plum (Eng.) 343
Kagli (Kan.) 8
Kainjli (Jaunsar) 14
Kakandan (Tam.) 144
Kakolisag (Eng.) 283
Kakrai (H.) 7
Kala zira (H.) 146
Kalet (Lepcha) 288
Kalizewar (P.) 147
Kaman-bi (Lakhimpur) 27
Kamchal (Ass. & Meghalaya) 118
Kamvakkunai (Tam.) 277
Kanana kanda (Sans.) 59
Kanbher (Mar.) 13
Kandyeo-pam (Lepcha) 18
Kangiabel (H.) 141
Kankara (B.) 144
Kannali (Mal.) 8

Kantali (G.)	1
Kapni (H.)	357
Karangli (Tam.)	8
Karanja (Mar. & H.)	173,265
Kardahi (Mar.)	74
Kardal/kardor (Mar.)	64
Karnadi (Mar.)	7
Karu (Kumaun)	325
Kasili (Mar.)	7
Kat (Eng.)	183
Kataphal (H.)	112
Kath (Eng.)	183
Kathior-pat (Lepcha)	356
Kathmora (Garhwal)	361
Kattuchena (Mal.)	59
Kattukalrmei (Tam.)	59
Kattupurvaracu (Tam.)	315
Kattuthuvarei (Tam.)	106
Kauri buti (H.P.)	34
Kavasi (Mar.)	357
Kayara (Mal.)	330
Kekar (Oriya)	144
Kempu jali (Kan.)	8
Kemugonele (Kan.)	336
Khaki weed (Eng.)	53
Khaksha (Garhwal)	130
Khaja (H.)	141
Khanpa (Ladakh)	94
Khato-palak (Rajasthan)	292
Khaum (Lushai)	356
Khella (Eng.)	57
Khempasibaphang (Cachar)	79
Khokaray (Oriya)	175
Khoree (Kash.)	82
Khum (Manipur)	114
Kikra (P.)	33
Kilansadu (Mal.)	151
Kiluvai (Tel.)	225
Kiraya (H.P.)	343
Kirci (H.)	175
Kiwi fruit (Eng.)	21
Knol-khol (Eng.)	139
Kobirithangi (Coimbatore)	369
Kochi grass (Bangalore)	
Kochomah (Ass.)	18
Kodaivelom (Tam.)	10
Kohlrabi (Tam.)	139
Koinine (Ass.)	143
Kondamavu (Kan.)	225

Konden (Santal)	297
Koria (M.P.)	330
Kothu (H.P.)	368
Kundja (Garhwal)	96
Kundli (Mar.)	375
Kurunfan (Mal.)	21
Kurungan (Tam.)	21
Kusur (Mar.)	375

L

Lady of the night (Eng.)	144
Lady's bedstraw (Eng.)	321
Lady's finger (Eng.)	1
Lady's mantle (Eng.)	38
Lagos silk rubber (Eng.)	320
Lajauri (Oraon)	125
Lalchini (H.)	59
Lalee (B.)	59
Lal khair (Mar.)	8
Lamb's tail (Eng.)	74
Lampa (H.)	199
Lampati (Trade)	285
Large or greater cardamom (Eng.)	59
Latkania (Delhi)	161
Leek (Eng.)	43
Lemon (Eng.)	209
Lemon grass (Eng.)	251
Lemon verbena (Eng.)	49
Leopard lily (Eng.)	119
Lesser galangal (Eng.)	50
Lesser/small quking grass (Eng.)	141
Lesser spear grass (Eng.)	199
Leteku (Ass.)	112
Letka (B.)	112
Levant/fish berry (Eng.)	62
Licorice/Liquorice (Eng.)	333
Lily-of-the-valley (Eng.)	228
Lime (Eng.)	208
Lion's foot (Eng.)	38
Lipstick tree (Eng.)	126
Livid-flowered birthwort (Eng.)	90
Locust bean (Eng.)	192
Logwood (Eng.)	342
Lombopullu (Mal.)	135
Looking glass tree (Eng.)	351
Love-lies bleeding (Eng.)	54
Luncliara (Mundari)	118

M

Macassar kernels (Eng.)	142
Mada (Tel.)	108
Madagascar orange ball tree (Eng.)	146
Madagascar periwinkle (Eng.)	184
Madar (H.)	157
Madarwood (Eng.)	92
Mad-dog weed (Eng.)	40
Magha latenga (Oriya)	124
Magnonette vine (Eng.)	74
Maiden hair fern (Eng.)	24
Maka (Mar.)	152
Makla (B.)	114
Makor (Mal.)	114
Malabans (H.)	114
Malabar catmint (Eng.)	70
Malabar nightshade (Eng.)	116
Malabar nut (Eng.)	23
Malacca eagle wood (Eng.)	80
Malaikonnel (Tam.)	21
Male fern (Eng.)	350
Maloti (Oriya)	28
Manaca (Eng.)	144
Man bijal (Ass.)	339
Mandania (B. & H.)	21
Mandarin orange (Eng.)	210
Mandiara (Kumaun)	299
Mangosteen (Eng.)	322
Man-lata (B.)	193
Manu-kataphul (Ass.)	357
Marabale (Kan.)	13
Maraneli (Mar.)	13
Marang (Mundari)	152
Margosa tree (Eng.)	108
Marigold (Eng.)	153
Marijuana (Eng.)	163
Marnil (Kash.)	25
Marsh mallow (Eng.)	53
Masa (H.)	146
Match-stick tree (Eng.)	51
Matta-ara (H.)	76
Mauritius hemp (Eng.)	320
Mauritius hullu (Kan.)	135
Mauritius papeda (Eng.)	209
Mayweed (Eng.)	74
Meadow fescue (Eng.)	312
Meleguetta pepper (Eng.)	28
Mexican poppy (Eng.)	85
Mexican tulip poppy (Eng.)	360
Mikrum-rik (Lepcha)	60
Milfoil (Eng.)	14
Mirgi chara (Oriya)	339
Mithanadai (Mikir)	359
Mogra (Mar.)	375
Moka or mocha aloes (Eng.)	49
Moktok (Manipur)	112
Monkey-apple (Eng.)	71
Monkey bread tree (Eng.)	22
Monkey jack (Eng.)	98
Monkeynut (Eng.)	80
Monkey puzzle (Eng.)	82
Monkey turmeric (Eng.)	126
Moonworf (Eng.)	135
Moorukonda (Tel.)	13
Morinda (H.)	2
Mouhilika (Ass.)	141
Mountain ebony (Eng.)	117
Mountain fleece (Eng.)	126
Mountain soursop (Eng.)	71
Mountain spinach (Eng.)	104
Mountain tobacco (Eng.)	91
Mukkutikorei (Tam.)	146
Mundani (B. & H.)	21
Munshing (Arunachal Pradesh)	367
Murligidda (Kan.)	145
Mushre katus (B.)	182
Musk mallow (Eng.)	2
Muskmelon (Eng.)	243
Myriya (B.)	27
Mysore thorn (Eng.)	151

N

Naga birch (Eng.)	123
Nahalbeli (Oriya)	204
Nai-irupu (Kan.)	357
Nalbila (H.)	204
Namappoondu (Tam.)	54
Nardul (B.)	135
Naria (B.)	27
Nari jatanriba (Mundari)	53
Narubotuku (Tel.)	297
Nagro-head (Eng.)	72
Nauri lupu era (Mundari)	27
Neem tree (Eng.)	108
Nepal cardamom (Eng.)	59
Nepalese alder (Eng.)	46

Nepal trumpet flower (Eng.) 118
Netharhat (Bihar) 283
New Zealand banana (Eng.) 13
Night jesmine (Eng.) 194
Nili gulmohar (H.) 375
Nilmar (Kash.) 25
Ninai (Mar.) 277
Ningal (Tam.) 315
Nirdipul (Tam.) 135
Nirijappe (Kan.) 259
Niroli (Mal.) 315
Nodar (Ladakh) 384
Non-kung (Lepcha) 288
Nunnera (Tam.) 73

O

Oats (Eng.) 107
Okra (Eng.) 1
Old maid (Eng.) 184
Ondodi (Oriya) 277
Onion (Eng.) 41
Orache (Eng.) 104
Orange (Eng.) 210
Orange eye butterfly (Eng.) 145
Orchid tree (Eng.) 117
Ote jetang (Mundri) 129
Oyster bay pine (Eng.) 156

P

Paalamalle (Tel.) 28
Padh (Khasi) 102
Pak-choi (Eng.) 136
Pakhanbed (H.) 122
Pakkan chatta (Oraon) 118
Palmyra palm (Eng.) 133
Paludar (P.) 2
Paniccavu (Tam.) 330
Pansi(a) (Bihar, Kan. & Oriya) 73
Paper mulberry (Eng.) 142
Papra (H.) 324
Paprika (Eng.) 168
Para rubber tree (Eng.) 352
Parcel flowers (Eng.) 357
Paritza (Mar.) 330
Paruduppai (Tam.) 297
Pashanabheda (Sans.) 122
Pasomasi (Ass.) 293
Pati (H.) 96

Pay moostey (Tam.) 87
Peachwood (Eng.) 342
Peacock's tail (Eng.) 21
Peanut (Eng.) 80
Pedda bikki (Tel.) 324
Pedda sara (Tel.) 145
Pencil cedar (Eng.) 380
Persian manna plant (Eng.) 39
Petsai (Eng.) 136
Phalsa-tenga (B.) 339
Pharsia (H.) 339
Pheasant's eye (Eng.) 25
Phuhura (Ass.) 339
Physic-nut tree (Eng.) 376
Pig weed (Eng.) 54
Pinang palm (Eng.) 84
Pindroow fir (Eng.) 2
Pineapple (Eng.) 63
Pineapple guava (Eng.) 13
Pinguin (Eng.) 141
Pink kopsia (Eng.) 385
Pink powderpuff (Eng.) 154
Pink/Red cedar shingle-tree (Eng.) 21
Piri kecho ara (Mundari) 131
Pissu mar (H.P.) 130
Pitraj (B.) 59
Piyala (H.) 145
Poinsettia (Eng.) 306
Polki (Mar.) 328
Pond-apple (Eng.) 71
Pongu (Mal.) 357
Porcupine papeda (Eng.) 209
Pottuvarai (Tam.) 278
Prarie grass (Eng.) 142
Prickly-chaff flower (Eng.) 15
Prickly custard apple (Eng.) 71
Prickly poppy (Eng.) 85
Prostrate amaranth (Eng.) 54
Pu (P.) 27
Pulladi (Tam.) 268
Pumkki (Kan.) 328
Pumpkin (Eng.) 244
Pundna (P.) 330
Purging-nut (tree) (Eng.) 376
Purple convolvulus (Eng.) 87
Purple-stalked dragon (Eng.) 59
Putharaval (Mal.) 77
Putike (Tel.) 259
Putthigadi (Tel.) 199

Q

Quarter vine (Eng.)	125
Queen of the shores (Eng.)	116
Queen palm (Eng.)	85
Quince (Eng.)	251

R

Ragha (H.)	2
Rai (P.)	2
Rain tree (Eng.)	144
Raman-bih (Ass.)	27
Rampat (Ass.)	114
Rang-rang (Sik.)	367
Ran mogra (Mar.)	375
Rape (Eng.)	136,140
Ratanjot (Trade)	91
Ration (Eng.)	329
Rattle snake fern (Eng.)	135
Red amaranth (Eng.)	54
Red bed tree (Eng.)	22
Red cedar (Eng.)	380
Red chinchona (Trade)	202
Red cutch (Trade)	8
Red hot cat-tail (Eng.)	13
Red pepper (Eng.)	169
Red periwinkle (Eng.)	184
Red root amaranth (Eng.)	54
Red/yellow cinchona (Eng.)	202
Reskunsemar (Ladakh)	197
Rhodes grass (Eng.)	197
Ribbon grass (Eng.)	99
Risakuhi (Mundari)	136
Rithoul (U.P.)	357
Rockweed (Eng.)	319
Roman chamomile (Eng.)	74
Roman wormwood (Eng.)	56
Roucou (Eng.)	126
Rough green pigweed (Eng.)	54
Rudanti (H.)	103
Rudrawanti (H.)	103
Rulthlu (Lushai)	83
Rum (Ass.)	114
Rupture wort (Eng.)	351

S

Sabai (H. & B.)	303
Sacking tree (Eng.)	76
Safflower (Eng.)	174
Saffron tree (Eng.)	126
Salai-mara (Kan.)	330
Salamander tree (Eng.)	76
Samara kokadi (G.)	124
Samboo (Ladakh)	236
Samrali (H.P.)	130
Sandra (Tel.)	8
Sangkenrop (Khasi)	27
Saptarangi (H.)	176
Sarala-devadaaru (Tel.)	122
Saraparuppu (Tam.)	145
Sarivan (H.)	268
Sarlok-asing (Abor)	27
Sarpabuti (J. & K.)	147
Saseni (Ass.)	308
Sathi (Ladakh)	135
Sausage tree (Eng.)	383
Savoy cabbage (Eng.)	140
Scarlet pimpernel (Eng.)	62
Scurvy cress (Eng.)	115
Seemai velam pattai (Tam.)	8
Sema-klung (Lepcha)	361
Semaphone plant (Eng.)	268
Senegal khaya (Eng.)	383
Seville orange (Eng.)	208
Shallot (Eng.)	40
Shanipillu (Tam.)	135
Shankhpushpi (H.)	195,229
Shaven-flowered gentian (Eng.)	326
Sheeti (Ladakh)	326
Shena (Mal.)	59
Shiah-tyngkhwari (Khasi)	13
Shine jeerige (Kan.)	146
Shola (H.)	27
Silk cotton tree (Eng.)	132
Silpano (Dharchula)	122
Silpil (P.)	147
Silver fern (Eng.)	195
Silver fir (Eng.)	2
Silver wattle (Eng.)	8
Sisal (Eng.)	29
Sivamalli (S.)	116
Sivanarvembu (Tam.)	382
Smooth broom grass (Eng.)	142
Snake's head (Eng.)	318
Snake-lily (Eng.)	88
Snapdragon (Eng.)	77
Soan pura (Mundari)	128

Sohkha (Meghalaya)	283	Tambreswari (P.)	230
Soh-pen (Ass.)	297	Tamsir-arong (Manipur)	79
Sonooya (Eng.)	72	Tangamasing (Miri)	182
Sontul (Lushai)	79	Tapouguti (Ass.)	356
Sour/bitter orange (Eng.)	208	Tarragon (Eng.)	93
Soursop (Eng.)	71	Tassel flower (Eng.)	54
Sowa (Eng.)	68	Techokpo (Sik.)	381
Soybean (Eng.)	330	Teisu (Nagaland)	118
Spangyankarpo (Ladakh)	192	Telegraph plant (Eng.)	268
Spanish bamboo-reed (Eng.)	98	Tella puliki (Tel.)	328
Spanish chestnut (Eng.)	181	Tender gentian (Eng.)	326
Spanish needles (Eng.)	123	Teri pods (Eng.)	151
Spanish pellitory (Eng.)	61	Terragon (Eng.)	93
Spear grass (Eng.)	352	Thaihom (Nagaland)	359
Spengyankarpo (Ladakh)	192	Thale cress (Eng.)	80
Spiny bamboo (Eng.)	114	Tharbal (H.)	119
Spiny pigweed (Eng.)	55	Thar-ki-haldi (H.)	233
Spiny or thorny amaranth (Eng.)	55	Thekeria (Ass.)	374
Spreading pigweed (Eng.)	54	Thera (Ass.)	285
Squirrel corn (Eng.)	269	Thomson's aster (Eng.)	102
St. gapukokandan (Tam.)	144	Thorn apple (Eng.)	261
Stickle wort (Eng.)	32	Three-lobed butterburr (Eng.)	124
St. John's wort (Eng.)	364	Thuddaponna (Tel.)	144
Stogzil (Ladakh)	233	Tikoni-borua (Ass.)	150
St. Thomas tree (Eng.)	117	Tikta (Ladakh)	375
Sucotrine aloe (Eng.)	49	Til (Ladakh)	101
Sugar apple (Eng.)	72	Timarrakh (P.)	293
Sugarbeet (Eng.)	122	Tiny (Lushai)	114
Summer cypress (Eng.)	384	Tiokra-molli (Nagaland)	145
Summer lilac (Eng.)	145	Tirgal (Kan.)	375
Sundri (B., Oriya & Trade)	351	Tooth-pick ammi/fruit (Eng.)	57
Sunflower (Eng.)	346	Touchwood ixora (Eng.)	374
Surata (M.P.)	280	Trailing amaranth (Eng.)	54
Swamp mahogany (Eng.)	302	Trailing indigo (Eng.)	368
Sweet flag-root/sedge (Eng.)	18	Tree of heaven (Eng.)	33,34
Sweet melon (Eng.)	243	Trincomalle wood (Eng.)	122
Sweet orange (Eng.)	210	True cinnamon (Eng.)	204
Sweet pepper (Eng.)	168	Trumpet vine (Eng.)	161
Sweet potato (Eng.)	370	Tsi (Eng.)	358
Sweet rocket (Eng.)	352	Tunga (H.)	235
Sweet-scented bedstraw (Eng.)	321	Tung oil tree (Eng.)	38
Sweetsop (Eng.)	72	Turnip (Eng.)	140
Sweet sultan (Eng.)	55	Tuttiri (Tam.)	199
Sweet vernal grass (Eng.)	75		
Sweet william (Eng.)	269		

T

U

		Uganballi (Kan.)	87
		Umbhu (Ladakh)	146
Tall/false oat-grass (Eng.)	92	U-mei-tong-krong (Meghalaya)	141

Upaniya jhar (Kumaun)   130
Upas tree (Eng.)   76
Usipag (Ass.)   1

V

Valiakuppameni (Mal.)   13
Val muriccha (Mal.)   315
Vangvathus (Lushai)   16
Varuda (Tel.)   144
Vasaka (Eng.)   23
Vattattali (Mal.)   13
Vegetable mercury (Eng.)   144
Vellaimandarai (Tam.)   116
Vellarai (Tam.)   293
Vellum-matti (Tam.)   261
Velutthamandarom (Mal.)   116
Velvet grass (Eng.)   356
Velvet plant (Eng.)   235
Vendalai (Tam.)   328
Venkandan (Tam.)   108
Venus hair (Eng.)   25
Vernapata (Kumaun)   64
Vine (Eng.)   233
Vine-leaved anemone (Eng.)   67
Vishaphale (Kan.)   21
Vomban (Lushai)   127

W

Wagani (Kan.)   373
Walking maiden hair fern (Eng.)   24
Wall flower (Eng.)   195
Wall-rue (Eng.)   102
Walnut (Eng.)   378
Water hemlock (Eng.)   201
Water leaf (Eng.)   136
Watermelon (Eng.)   207
Water-plantain (Eng.)   40
Wati (Garo)   114
Weeping ash (Eng.)   318
Weeping blue juniper (Eng.)   380
West-Himalayan alder (Eng.)   46
West Himalayan high-level fir (Eng.)   3

West-Himalayan low-level fir (Eng.)   2
West Indian ipecacuanha (Eng.)   99
White butterfly bush (Eng.)   146
White candytuft (Eng.)   365
White maiden hair (Eng.)   102
White sapota (Eng.)   176
White weed (Eng.)   30
White wild musk mallow (Eng.)   1
Wild basil (Eng.)   153
Wild blite (Eng.)   54
Wild carrot (Eng.)   194
Wild chamomile (Eng.)   74
Wild jack (Eng.)   98
Wild mustard (Eng.)   215
Wild oat (Eng.)   106
Wild pineapple (Eng.)   141
Wild strawberry (Eng.)   318
Wild wistaria (Eng.)   132
Willow leaved jesmine (Eng.)   194
Wintergreen (Eng.)   324
Wood oil tree (Eng.)   39
Woolly foxglove (Eng.)   271
Woolly morning glory (Eng.)   87
Wormseed (Eng.)   94
Wormwood (Eng.)   92

Y

Yali (Lepcha)   14
Yarrow (Eng.)   14
Yatli kung (Lepcha)   14
Yaupon (Eng.)   366
Yellow chinchona (Trade)   202
Yellow gentian (Eng.)   325
Yellow rocket (Eng.)   115
Ylang-ylang (Eng.)   161
Yorkshire fog (Eng.)   356

Z

Zanzibar aloe (Eng.)   49
Zergul (H.)   153
Ziron (Ass.)   343

INDEX OF ACTIVE PRINCIPLES AND OTHER IMPORTANT COMPOUNDS

[Unlike in the text, here full names of radicals, acetyl (Ac–), butyl (Bu–),ethyl (Et–), methyl (Me–), methoxy or oxymethyl (MeO–), oxy (O–), acetate or acetoxy (–OAc), hydroxy (–OH), phenyl (Ph–), propyl (Pr–), etc., have been used in compound names. Dagger (†) denotes active principle including disease-causing ones; bold page number, activity or description].

A

Abrasine	4
†Abrin(s)	4,5,6
†Absinthin	**93**
Acamelin	9
Acanthicifoline	13
Acetovanillone	286
†1′-Acetoxychavivol acetate	**50**
†1′-Acetoxyeugenol acetate	**50**
Acetylamarolide	33
Acetylbarlerin	115
7α-Acetyldihydronomilin	170
†Acetylshikonin	**91**
16-Acetylstrospeside	22
Achilleine	15
Achillicin	15
†Achyranthine	**16**
Acolongifloroside K	17
Aconine	17
†*trans*-Aconitic acid	20,142
ψ-Aconitine	17,18
†Acorenone B	**269**
Acospectoside A,B & C	17
Acrovestone	20
Actein	202
Actinea	202
†Adifoline	**25**
Adonitoxin	25
Aegelenine	26
†Aegeline	**26**
†Aescin	**28**
Affinisine	51
†Aflatoxins 81,82,84,107,221,232,331,**338**	
†Aflatoxin B₁	**81,82**,84
Agave saponins I-IX	29
Agrimols A,B,D & E	32
†Agrimonolide	**32**
Agrimophol	32
†Agroclavine	212,**371**
†Agropyrene	32

Agrostenin (Githagin)	33
†Ailanthinone	**34**
Ailantholide	34
Ailantone	33,34
Ajacine	228
Ajaconine	227
Ajacusine	228
†Ajmalicine (Raubasine)	183,184,**186**
Ajmalizine, see Ajmalicine	
Akuammicine	52
ψ-Akuammicine	52
Akummidine	52
ψ-Akuammigine	52
Al 60	36
Alamarine	36
Alangamide	36
Alangicine	35
Alangimarckine	36
Alangimaridine	36
Alangimarine	36
†Alantolactone	369,**370**
Albasipidin	283
Aldotripiperideine	342
Alkanin-β,β′- dimethylacrylate, see arnebin-1	
Alaknin mono acetate, see arnebin-3	
Allamandicin	40
†Allamandin	**40**
Allamdin	40
Allantoin	33,286,288,352
†Allicin	**43,44,45**
†Alliin	45,125
†Allisatin	**44**
†Allithiamine	**45**
†Allitin	**45**
Allocryptonine	86
Allocryptopine	86,269, 360
α- & β-Allocryptopine	300
l-Alloelaeocarpiline	289
†Allohimachalol	**188**
†Allyl alcohol	**42**

Allyl isothiocyanate	139	Antirrhinoside	77
†Allyl persulphide	**312**	†Apigenin	**29**
†Allyl propyl disulphide	**41,42**	†Apigenin 7,4′-dimethoxy ether	**65**
†Alocutin A	**47**	†Apiol	**68**,69
Alocutin B	48	†Apoatropine	**105**
Aloenin	48	Apohyoscine	285
†Aloin	**48**,49	Aposcopolamine	143
†Aloinoside B	**49**	Arborine	332
†Alomicin	**49**	Arborinine	332,333
Alstonine	184,187	†Arbutin	**83**
Alstophylline	51	Arctiopicrin	83
†Alstovenine	**52**	†Arecaidine	**84**,85
Δ^3-Alstovenine	52	†Arecoline	**84**,85
Amabiline	254	†Aristolic acid	**89**
Amarogentin	325	†Aristolochic acid	88,**89**,90
Amarolide	33	Aristolochine	89
Amaroswertin	325	Arnebin-1 & -3(Alkanin β,β-	
Ambiguine	228	dimethylacrylate & Alkanin	
†Ambrosic acid	**56**	monoacetate)	91
3α-Aminoconan-5-ene	356	†Arnebin I & III	**91**
†α-Amino-β-methylaminopropionic		†Artemisiifolin	**56**
acid	**250**	Artemisin	95
(−)-α-Amino propiophenone, see		†Artemisinin	**93**
Cathinone		†β-Asarone	19,**20**,21
†Ammidin, see Imperatorin		γ-Asarone	152
†Ammoidin, see Xanthotoxin		†Asarones	**20**
†Anacrotine (Crotalaburnine)	238,240	†Asclepin	**99**
†Anacyclin	**62**	†Asiatic acid	**190**
Anagyrine	303	†Asiaticoside	**190**
Analobine	73	†L-Asparaginase	**168**
†Ancistrocladidine	64,65	†Asparagusic acid	**100**
Ancistrocladinine	64,**65**	†Asperuloside	134,**321**
Ancistrocladine	64,65	Asperulosidic acid	134
Ancistrocladisine	64,65	†Aspidinol	**283**
†Ancistrodine	**65**	Asteglasine A	199
Ancistroquinone	65	†Astragalin	**278**
†Andrographolide	**66**	Atalantolide	103
7-Angelylheliotridine	348	Atalaphyllidine	103
Anhydroalstonatine	52	Atalaphylline	103
Anisatin	366	Atherospermine	71,72
Ankorine	36	Atidine	18
Anodendrosides A,B₁ & B₂, E₁,E₂,F,G	73	Atisine	18
Anomurine	72	†Atropine	104,**105**,260-61,363
†Anonaine	71,**72**,73	†Atylosol	**106**
Anthranoyllycoctonine	264	†Aucubin	**106**,145
†Antialloside	**76**	Aurantiamide acetate	361
†α- & †β-Antiarin	76	†Auriculoside	**7**
†Antiogoside	**76**	Avadhridine	264
†Antioside	**76**	†Avenacine A & B	**107**

Chondrillasterone	338	Colchamine	222
Chonemorphine	197	†Colchicine	**88,222,330**
Chrysarobin	65	†Coleforsin	**223**
†Chrysoeriol-7-O-β-D-		†ColosideA(α-Elaterin2-d-	
glucopyranosidyl-(2→1)- D-		glucopyranoside)	**207**
apiofuranoside	258	†Coleonol, see Forskolin	
†Chrysophanic acid	177,**180**	Collutine	222
†Chrysophanic acid-9-anthrone	**180**	Columbamine	63,121
Chukrasins A-D & F	200	Columbine	376
†Chymopapain C	**172**	Colycotomine	11
Cicerin	200	Compenoside	161
Cichoriin	201	Conamine	320
†Cicutine	**201**	†Concanavaline A	**162**
Cicutol	201	Condelphine	264
†Cicutoxin	**201**	†Conessine	320,356
Cimicifugoside	202	γ-Coniceine	227
†Cinchonine	**203**	†Coniferin	**113**
†Cinchophyllamine	202	†Coniine	**227**
Cinerin I & II	198	†Convallatoxin	76,**228**
†Cinnacassiol C₁	**203**	†Convallatoxol	76,**228**
Cinnamaldehyde	203	Convalloside	76,228
†Cinncassiol D₁,D₂ & D₃	**203**	Coptisine	86,319,360,376
†Cinnzeylanine	**204**	Corchoral	230
†Cinnzeylanol	**204**	†Corchoroside A	**231,352**
†Cirantin	**208**	Corchoside C	230
Cissamine	206	†Cordacin	**283**
†Cissampareine	**206**	Cordifoline	25
†Citral	209,**251**,252	Coreximine	72
Citrullonol	207	(−)-Coreximine	233
†Clausmarins A & B	**212**	Corlumine	233
†Clavicepamine	**212**	Coromandaline	348
†Clavine	**212**	†Coronaridine	185,187,**298**
†Cleistanthin	**214**	Corydine	73
Clitorin	192	Corygovanine	233
†Cnicin	189,**205**,327	Corymine	360
Cnicinolide	327	Corysamine	360
†Cocaine	**300**	†Costic acid	**305**
Coccoline	218	†p-Coumaric acid	**90**
Coccolinine	218	†p-Coumaroylagmatine	**358**
Cocculidine	218	Cotinine	172,194
Cocculine	218	Crinidine	237
Cocculitine	218	Crinosine	237
Coccuvine	218	Croalbidine	237
Coclaurine	72,218	Croalbinecine	237
Cocsoline	219	Croburhine	238
Cocsuline	219	Crotalaburnine, see Anacrotine	
†Cocsulinine	**219**	Crotalarine	238
†Codeine	**223**	Crotastriatine	239
†Coixenolide	**222**	Crotaverrine	240

Crotoflorine 240
Crotsparinine 240
†Cryogenine **346**
†Cryptocaryalactone **241**
Cryptopine 86,319
†Cryptopleurine 90,**130**
†Cucurbitacin B 243,286
†Cucurbitacin Q1 **243**
Cucurbitacin E 62
Cucurbitacins B,D,E,I,L & R;C-E, L &
   R; E, G-I, E & I,K; 62; 286; 207,
     241,356
†Cucurrbitin **244**
†Curassavicin **99**
Curassavine 348
Curcin 377
†Curcumicidin **379**
†Curcumin **247**
†Curcuminoid **248**
†Curcumol **246**
†curdione **246**
l-Curine 206
†dl-Curine dimethiodide **206**
Cuspidaline 365
†Cycasin **249**
†Cyclamin **250**
Cuscohygrine 105,261,300
Cycleandrine 250
Cycleanhomine chloride 250
Cycleanine 206,351
Cycleanorine 250
Cycleapeltine 250
Cycloanoline 360
Cyclobuxine D 150
(–) Cyclobuxupaline C 150
Cyclomicrobuxinine, see Buxtauine
(+)-Cyclopapilosine D 150
β-Cycloprethrosin 198
Cycloprotobuxine C 150
Cyclovirobuxine D 150
†Cymarin 25,76,**182**
†Cymarol 76,**182**
†Cynarin **253**
†Cynaropicrin 253
Cynaustine 254
Cynaustraline 254
Cystisine 303
Cytisine 132

D

Daidzin **332**
Dalbin 257
Dalbinol 257
Dalpanol 257
Daphnetoxin 258
Daphylloside 134
†Daturalactone **261**
6-Deacetylnimbin 110
†Decanoyl acetaldehyde **358**
Dehydrobufontenine 98
Dehydrocheilanthifoline 319
Dehydrodecodine 346
13,18-Dehydroexcelsin 34
13, 18-Dehydroglaucarubol-15-
   isovalerate 34
Dehydroelatericin B (Cucurbitacin L) 207
†Dehydroevodiamine **304**
Dehydroprotoemetine 36
Delcoside 227
Delcosine 227
Delnudine 264
Delsoline 227
Demethooxyabresoline 346
Demethoxykanugin 266
Demethylalstophylline 51
3-Demethylcolchicine 330
†Demethylhomopterocarpin **162**
De-N-methylorientaline 300
Demethylpsychotrine 35,36
O-Demethylpurpureine 72
Denudatine 264
10-Deoxyadifoline 25
10-Deoxycordifoline 25
6-Deoxyharpagide 321
12-Deoxy-16-hydroxyphorbol 114
†12-Deoxy-5β-hydroxyphorbol-13-
   myristate **114**
12-Deoxyphorbol 114
Deoxyphorbol acetate 195,307
†12-Deoxyphorbol esters **306**
Deoxypicropodophyllin 351
Deoxypodophyllotoxin 351
Deoxytubulosine 36
Deoxyvasicinone 24
Desglucocheirotoxin 76
Desoxy-16-buxidienine 150
Desmodol 182-83

Dhurrin	133	Echinatine	304,349
Diacetyl-ψ-aconitine	17	Echinopsine	287
†Diallyl disulphide	**45**	Echitamine	52
†Diallyl thiosulphonate	**43**	Echitoserpidine	52
†Diallyl trisulphide	**45**	Echitoserpine	52
Dicentrine	206˙	Echitovenaldine	52
†α-Dichroine	**270**	Echitovenidine	52
Dictamnine	270,332,333	19-epi-(+)-Echitoveniline	52
Difucohexaacetate	319	(–)-Echitoveniline	52
†Digitaloids	**304**	Echitovenine	52
Digitogenin	194	Ehretinine	287
Digitonin	273	Elaeocarpidine	289
Digitoxigenin	118	dl-Elaeocarpine	289
Digitoxigenin-α-L-rhamnoside	76	†Elaeodendroside A	**181**
†Digitoxin	**272**,273	†Elaedendradiol B	**181**
†Digoxin	**272**,273	Elatericin A & B	286
F-Dihydroatisine	18	Elatericin B (Cucurbitacin I)	207
3β-Dihydrocadambine	75	Elaterin (Cucurbitacin E)	207 ˙
Dihydroergotoxine, see Hydergine		α-Elaterin	286
Dihydrosoconessimine	356	α-Elaterin2-d-glucopyranoside, see	
†Dihydroparthenolide	**56**	Coloside A	
†Dihydrosamidin	**58**	Elatine	264
†Dihydrovindolinine	**185**	Elaterin glucoside	207
†Dillapiol	67,**68**,69	Eldeline	264
3,4-Dimethoxy-w-(2-		Eleagnine	98
piperidyl)acetyphenone	130	Elemanolide lactone	191
Nb-Dimethylechitamine	52	†Elephtopin	**289**
2,6-Dimethoxyquinone	33	†Elymoclavine	371,372,**373**
†N′,N′-Dimethylhistamine	176	†Embelin	**291**
N,N-Dimethyllindacarpine	233	†Emetine	36,**191**,343
Dimethyltryptamine	11	†Emiline	**292**
N,N-Dimethyltryptamine	182,267-68	Enhydrin	294
N,N-Dimethyltryptamine		Enicoflavine	293
methohydroxide	98	†Entanin	293
N,N-Dimethyltryptophan	300	†Ephedrine	183,**294,295**
Diomelquinone A	278	†d-Ephedrine	295
†Diosbulbins	**275**	†ψ-Ephedrine	**294**,295
Dioscorine	277	†Ephedroxane	**294**
Diosgenin	29,113,234,**276-77**	d-Epialloelaeocarpiline	289
†Diospyrol	**278**	16-Epialstovenine	53
5, 22-Dioxokopsane	53	†Epiaschantin	**351**
Durantosides	285	†l-Epicatechin	**61**,236
†Dysobinin	**286**	†4-Epidioscorine	**277**
		16-Epivenenatine	53
E		Erbidine	299
		Ergine	87
β-Ecdysone	196	Ergocornine	**213**,371
Ecdysteroids	35	Ergocristine	**213**,371
Ecdysterone	16,17	Ergokryptine	**213**

†Ergolines 87,**213**
Ergometrine 87
Ergonorine 142
Ergosinine 371
Ergosterol 354
†Ergosterol peroxide 63
†Ergotamine 32,142,**213**
Ergothioneine 32,353
†Ergotoxine 142,**213**
†Erucic acid **137**
Erysimoside 267
Erysodine 299,300
Erysodinophorine 299
†Erysoline **170**
Erysonine 300
Erysophinophorine 299
Erysophorine 299
Erysopine 300
Erysotramidine 299
Erysotrine 299,300
Erysotyrine 300
Erysovine 299,300
Erythlaurine 218
Erythrabine 299
Erythraline 300
Erythramide 218
Erythrartine 300
Erythrascine 299
Erythratidine 299
Erythrinine 300
Erythrocentaurine 293
Erythroculine 218
Escholidine 360
Escholine 301
Escholinine 301
Eschscholtzine 301
Esculetin 201
Esculin 201
†Estragole **93**
†(24S)-Ethylcholesta-5,22,25-triene-
  3β-ol **216**
†Ethyl-p-methylcinnamate **248**
Euatroside 304
Eucalyptin 302
Eugenol 203,204
†Eupatoriopicrin **304**
†Euphorinin **306**
†Euphoscopin A **306**
†Euphoscopin B **306**

Eupolauridine, see Canangine
Eurcomalactone 308
Evobioside 267
Evodiamine 303
Evolitrine 20
†Evolvine **308**
†Evomonoside 76,**173**
Excelsin 34

F

γ-Fagarine 197,270,332,333
Fagomine 310
Falconitine 17
†Febrifugine **269**
Feretoside 134
†Ficin **313**
Filicin 284
Filixic acid 283
†Flavaspidic acid **283**,284
†Flemichapparins A-C **316**
†Formononetin **200**
N-Formylchonemorphine 197
†Forskolin (Coleonol) **223**
†Frugoside **99**
Fruticosamine 385
Fruticosine 385
Fumaramine 319
†Fumaric acid 168
Fumaridine 319,320
Fumarilicine 319
Fumariline 319
Fumaritine 319,320
Funtumafrine C 197
Furoguaiacidin 340

G

†Gaillardin 320
Galioside 321
Galiridoside 321
Gallicin 95
Galucine 50
Gardenoside 323
Gardoside 323
†Gedunin **170**
Genipin gentiobioside 323
†Geniposide **323**
Geniposidic acid 374
Genistein **332**

Genisteine	255	**H**	
Gentialutine	325		
Gentianadine	325	Halosaline	342
†Gentianine	**311,325**,375	Haloxine	342
Gentiobiose	325	Hamatine	65
Gentiocrucine	293	Hamayne	237
†Gentiopicroside	**325**	Harman	288,355,384
Gentiotibetine	325	Harmine	384
†Geranin	**326**	Harmol	288,355
†Ginkgolide A,B,C & M	**327**	Harpagide	321
Githagin, see Agrostenin		Hayatidine	206
Glaucarubol	34	†Hayatine (*dl*-Bebeerine)	**205**,206
†Glaucarubol-15-isovalerate	**34**	Hayatinine	206
Glaucescenine	259	Hecogenin	29,**30**,320
†Gllaucarbuninone	**34**	Hederacolchiside D & E	343
Glaucarubin	34	Hederagenin	128
Glaucescine	259	Hederasaponins B & C	344
Glaucine	73	†α- & β-Hederins	**344**
†Glaziovine	**72**	Hedychenone	344,345
Gleditsia C	328	Heimidine	364
Glucosinolates	138,139,140	Heimine	346
Gluroside	321	Heleurine	349
Glycophymine	332	Helianthol A & B	347
Glycophymoline	332	Helianthoside C	347
Glycosolone	332	Helifoline	349
Glycozolidine	332	†Heliocide H_1-H_4	**338**
Glycozoline	332,333	†Heliosin	**306**
†Glycyrrhetic acid	**334**	Heliotridine	346
†Glycyrrhetinic acid	**334**	†Heliotrine	348,**349**
†Glyrrhizic acid	**334**	Heliotrine N-oxide	348
†Glycyrrhizin	333,**334**	Heliotropine	348
Goitrin	138,139	Heliovicine	348
†Gossypin	353,**354**	†Hellebrin	**349**
Gossypitrin	296	Helminthosporin	179
†Gossypol	111,**336**,354	Helveticoside	267,352
Govadine	233	Heptaphylline	211,212
Govanine	233	Heptazolidine	211
Gramine	98,268	Heptazoline	211
†Granilin	**173**	Hercynine	353
†Guggulusterol-I,-II,-III	**229**	Hernandonine	351
†Guttiferin	**322**	Hernangerine	351
†γ-Guttiferin	**322**	†Herniarin	351,**352**
†αGuttiferin	**322**	Hernovine	351
†β-Guttiferin	**322**	†Hersaponin	**112**
†X-Guttiferin	**323**	†Hesperidin	**208**,209,210
Guvacine	84	Heteratisine	18
Gymnamine	341	Heterophyllidine	18
†Gymnemic acids	**341**	Heterophylline	18
		Heterophyllisine	18

Heteroside	62
Hetidine	18
Hetisine	18
Hetisinone	18
Heyneanine	298
†Heyneatine	**298**
Hibiscones A-D	354
Hibiscone C	385
Hibiscoquinone B	385
†Higenamine	**73**
†Himachalol	**188**
Hippomanins A & B	355
†Histamine	**328**
Holacetine	356
Holadysamine	356
Holadysine	356
Holonamine	356
α- & β-Homochelidonines	301
Honghelina	22
Hongheloside A	22
Hopeanine	144
†Hoppioside	**358**
†Hordenine	39,166,267,268,296, **358**
†Hovenosides	**359**
Hulupones	360
Humulinones	360
Hunnemanine	360
†Huratoxin	**361**
†Hydergine (Dihydroergotoxine)	**213**
Hydrangenosides A-D	362
†p-Hydroxyacetophenone	**96**
1-Hydroxyacridone	131
†2-Hydroxyarctiin	**174**
1-Hydroxycanthine-6-one	33
7α-Hydroxyconessine	356
4-(2-Hydroxyethyl)-5-vinylnicotinic acid lactone	310
14-Hydroxygelsemicine	324
†Hydroxyisonobilin	**75**
Hydroxylupanine	255
†16α-Hydroxy-3-ketoisomultiflorene	**77**
1-Hydroxy-7-methoxyacridone	131
8-Hydroxy-5-methoxypsoralen	69
1-Hydroxy-N-methylacridone	131
†5-Hydroxytryptamine	**328**
†Hypoxanthine-9-L-arabinofuranoside	**132**
†Hyoscine (Scopolamine)	104,**105**, 143,260,261-62,285,363
Hyoscine-N-oxide	363
†Hyoscyamine	104,105,143,260, 261-62,285,**363**
l-Hyoscyamine	260
Hypaphorine	4,267,268,299,300
Hypericin	364
†Hyperin	**306**
Hyperoside	32,236,306
†Hypoglycin A & B	127,**128**
I	
Ibamarine	365
Ibogamine	298
Imperatorin (Ammidin)	56,57,69
†Imperialine	**318**
Indaconitine	17,18
Indicine	349
†Indicine N-oxide	**349**
Indicinine	349
†Indirubin	**368**
Indizoline	211
†Indospicine	**368**
ψ-Indoxyl voacangine	298
Inokosterone	16,17
Insularine	206
Inulin	62
Inunolide	369
†Integerrimine	**238**
Ionidine	301
Ipalbidine	370
Ipalbine	370
Ipecoside	191
†Ipolearoside	**372**
Ipomeamarone	371
Ipomeamaronol	371
†4-Ipomeanol	**371**
Ipomine	372
Irehdiamines A & B	320
†Irisquinone	**373**
Isabelin	56
†Isoalantolactone	**370**
Isoatisine	18
Isocephaeline	36
Isochaksine	176
d-Isochondrodendrine	206
Isococculine	218
†Isocorydine	72,73,**218**,233
Isocrotsparinine	240
Isodictamnine	270

Isodihydrocadambine	75	†Karanjin	**266**
†Isofebrifugine	**269**	Kashmirine	319
†Isoflavones	**332**	†Khellin	**58**
†Isofraxidin	**197**	Kokusginine	20
epi-Isoelaeocarpiline	289	Kopsine	385
Isoergine	87	Kopsinine	52
Isoguvacine	84	Koptisine	301
†Isohexenylnaphthazarin	**377**	Kosamine	142
Isoimperatorin	69	†Kosmoside	**142**
Isoliquiritin	333	Kosotoxin	342
Isolysergic acid amide	87	Kurchaline	356
Isomaculosidine	270	Kurchiphyllamine	356
†Isomorellin	**322**	Kurchiphylline	356
†Isoneomorellin	**322**		
Isopenniclavine	372		
†Isophyllum A-E	**157**	**L**	
Isopimpinellin	56,57,69,78,79	Lactucin	201
Isopinocamphone	365	Lactucopicrin	201
Isopteropodine	342	Lamarchinine	36
Isosenkirkine	240	†Lanatosides A,B,C	**273**
Isositsirikine	184	Lanuginosine	73
l-α-Isosparteine	255	†Lapachol	**108**
Isotalatizidine	264	Lappoconitine	18,264
Isotetrandrin	250	Lasiocarpine	348,349
†Isothankuniside	**190**	Laudanidine	241
Isotriglochinin	46	Laurifine	218
Isotubulosine	35,176	Laurifinine	218
†Isovoacristine	298	†Laurifoline	**218**
Ixoroside	374	Laurifonine	218
Ixoside	374	Laurolitsine	203
		Lauroscholtzine	301
J		Lawsone	56
		†Lebbekanin A-H	**37**
†Jacareubin	**157**	†Lebbekanin E	**37**
Japindine	197	†Lemoran	**209**
Jasminin	376	†Leucodelphinidin	**294**
Jasminol	375	†Leurocolombine	**184**
Jasmolin I & II	198	Leurosidine-Nb-oxide	185
Jateorrhizine	121, 376	†Leurosine	183,184,**185**,**187**
Jatrarrhizine	233	Limacine	250,365
†Jatrophone	**377**	Limacusine	365
†Juglone	**175,379**	†d-Limonene	**245**
†Juncusol	**379**	Limonin	208,209,210,211,303,304
Junipodin	380	†Linalool acetate	**197**
Justicidins A-D	381	Linamarin	8,353
		Linarin	188,205
K		†Liriodenine	**71,72,73**
		Lochnericine	183
†Kaempferol-4'-O-glucoside	**306**	†Lochnerine	**185**
Kanugin	266		

†Lochnerinine 183
Loganin 184
Lotaustralin 8
β-Lumicolchicine 330
γ-Lumicolchicine 330
Lupulones 360
Luteicine 222
Luteidine 222
Luteine 222
Lycaconitine 264
Lycorenine 342
†Lycorine 237,246,362
ψ-Lycorine 55
Lyfoline 346
Lysergic acid 212
Lysergic acid amide 87
Lysergol 372
Lythridine, see Sinine
†Lythrine 346

M

Macralstonidine 51
†Macralstonine 51
Macrocarpamine 51
Macrocasalhine 51
Macrosalhine 51
†Madecassic acid 190
†Madecassoside 190
Madegascaric acid 190
Madurensine 237
†Magnoflorine 63,88,121,159,218,264,374
†Majudin, see Bergapten
†Malayoside 76
Manaceine 144
†Manacine 144
†Mangiferin 166,248,356
†Mangostins 322
Marckidine 35
Marckine 35
†Margaspidin 284
†Marsilin 371
Maruquine 342
Matairesinol monoglucoside 174
Matrine 303
N-Mecephaeline 36
Medicagol 200
†Meliantriol 110
Menismine 206

†Mercapto-L-cysteines 44
Metaloidine 143
Methoxsalen 57
(+)-Methoxyarmepavine 73
Methoxyatheroline 72
(+)-4"-Methoxycurine 206
Methoxydauricine 225
(−)-11-Methoxyechitovenedine 52
1-Methoxygelsemine 324
†p-Methoxysalicyclic aldehyde 350
Methylazoxymethanol 249,250
N-Methylbicycloatalaphylline 103
†2-Methyl-3-butene-2-ol 360
†Methylcatalpol 145
N-Methylcephaeline 36
†N-Methylcrotsparine 240
Methylcycaconitine 264
†S-Methyl-L-cysteine sulfoxide 139,140
†Methyl disulphide 42
l-Methylenepyrrolizidine 238
†N-Methylflindersine 170
Methyllycaconine 264
Methyl-4-methoxy-β-carboline-1-car-
     boxylate 33
N-Methylmorpholine 179
4-Methyl-2,6-napthyridine 77
8-N-Methylornithine 105
†Methylsinapate 136
Nb-Methyltetrahydroharman 267
†N-Methyltyramine 208,267
N-Methyltyrosine 65
Mexicanolide 170
†Mezerein 258
Michelalbine, see Norushinunine
Microphyllone 173
Minovincinine 52
Mithaconitine 17
†Mollugocin A 328
†Monocrotaline 238,239
Monospermine 149
Montanin 114
†Morellin 322
Mucronatine 239
Mucronatinine 239
†Muricatin 372
Murrayacine 211
Murrayanine 211
Myoporone 371
Myosmine 172,194

Myrtucommulone A 155

N

Nadurensine 239
Nantenine 181
†Naphthopyrone **223**
Narceimine 319
Narcissin 193
Nareline 52
†Neojusticin **381**
†Neomorellin 322,**323**
Neopulchellidine 320
Neoquassin 33
†Nesodine **346**
Nessin 346
Nicotine 11,12,172,194,285
Nilgirine 239
†Nimbidin **111**
Nimbin 110
†Nimbiol **111**
Nimbolide 110
Nimbolin A & B 110
†Nitrobergapten **57**
3-Nitropropanoic acid 368
†Nobiletin **208**,210,211
†*trans*-2-Nonenal **262**
Noracronycine 131
Norchelerythrine 86
Norcorydine 73
Norephedrine 183
Norgalucine 50
Norisocorydine 73
Norlaureline 73
Nornicotine 194
N-Nororientaline 299
Norpallidine 320
Norpseudoephedrine 183
Norpurpureine 72
Norsanguinarine 86
Norsinoacutine 240
Nortropine 285
Norushinunine (Michelalbine) 71,72,73
Nurlumidine 319

O

Obacunone 209,210,211
Ochratoxin 81
Odorine 31

Odorinol 31
†Odoroside G & H **173**
Oleandrigenin 118
Oleandrin 118
†Oligomeric procyanidins **236**
Oligoside 343
†Olitoriside **231**
Oliveramine 325
Oliveridine 325
Oliverine 325
Orientaline 241
Othosenine 292
†Ouabain **17,231**
†Oxoglaucine 72
21-Oxoleurosine 185
†Oxopurpureine **72**
1,8-Oxotetrahydropalmatine 63
Oxothalicarpine 351
Oxoushinsunine 72,73
Oxyacanthine 120,121
Oxyberberine 121
Oxypinnatanine 349
Oxysanguinarine 319
Oxysparteine 255

P

Palamarin 376
†Palasonin **149**
Palmarine 376
Palmatine 63,121,376
Palmatisine 17
Palmirine 342
Palmitone 203
†12-O-Palmitoyl-16-hydroxyphorbol-
13-acetate **39**
†Paniculatin **372**
†Papain **172**
Papainase 205
†Paraquine **194**
Pareirine 206
Parfumidine 319
Parfumine 319
†Pellitorine **62**
Pendine 219
Penduline 219
Pendulinine 219
Penniclavine 87,372,373
†Pericalline **184,298**

Pericyclivine 185
†Peripalloside 76
†Pcriplocymarin 182
Periplogenin 76,299
Perloline 312
Phaeanthine 341
†Phenyldehyde 313
†2-Phenylethylisothiocyanate 138,139
†1-Phenylhepta-1,3,5-triyne 124
1-Phenyl-1,2,propanedione 183
Phlorin 119
†Phloroglucide 284
†Phloroglucinols 342
Phloroglucinol triacetate 319
Phorbol-12,13-diesters 241
†Phorbol 12-tiglate 13-decanoate 241
Phyllantidine 292
Phyllantine 292
†Phyllemblin 292
†Phytosterin B 124
†Phytosterolin 313,315
Picralinal 52
Picralstonine 51
†Picrinine 51,52
Picrocrocinic acid 323
†Pimara-8(14),15-dien-19 oic acid 82
†Pinguinain 141
Pinocamphone 365
Pinselin, see Cassiollin
Piperidine 342
†Podophyllotoxin 381
Polypodine B 196
Powelline 237
Prazerigenin 277
Precasine 4
Precatorine 4
Precocenes 1 & 2 30
Preskimmianine 270
†Proazulenes 15
†Proceranin A 38
Proceric acid 37
Proresiniferatoxin 307
Proscillaridin A 282
†Prostalidin A 381
Prostalidins A-C 381
†Protoanemonin 214
Protoberberine 376
Protokosin 342
†Protopine 86,233,269,301,319,320,360

†Prunfelsamidine 144
†Psilostachyin 56
Psoralen 26,103,208,318
Psyochotrine 35,36
Pteropodine 342
†Puchiin 289
Pulchellidine 320
Pulchellin B,C,E & F 320
†Punarnavoside 132
Punarnavine 1 & 2 132
Punicic acid 280
Putranjivic acid 284
Putranjivosides A-D 284
Pycnamine 341
†Pyrethrin I & II 198
†Pyrethroids 198
Pyrethrol 198
Pyrethrosin 198

Q

Quassin 33
Quercetin 43
Quercetrin 265
Questin 180
†Quinchophyllamine 202
†Quinchophylline 202
†Quinidine 202
†Quinine 202,203
Quinone 202

R

Rapanone 84
Raubasine, see Ajmalicine
Rauwolscine 183
Reserpine 52,53
Resiniferatoxin 307
†Reticuline 71-73,203,218,241
Retronecine 349
Retusine 239
Rhazine 52,360
Rhodamine B 383
†Rhodexin B 242
Rhodoxanthin 296
Ricin 5,6
†Robustaol A 302
Roemerine 73
Rohitukin 78
Rotenoid 265

Rotenone 239
Roxburghiline 31
†Rubrosterone **17**
Rudrakine 289
Rumerine 342
Rutacridone 131
†Rutaecarpine **303**
Rutaevin 209,304
Rutamarine 131,
†Rutin 8,11,15,21,26,28,100,117,
118,131,134,145,147,168,240,**310**,343,350
Rutinoside 270

S

†Saikosaponins (Saikosides) a-f 146,**147**
†Saikosides, see Saikosaponins
Salanin 110
Salicilic acid 321
Salsolidine 39,267,268
dl-Salsoline 36
†Samidin **58**
†Sanguinarine **86**,301,319,360
†Santonin **94**,95
†β-Santonin **95**
ψ-Santonin 95
†Sativin I & II **45**
Scholarine 52
†Scoparone **96**
†Scopolamine, see Hyoscine
†Scordine **45**
Scordinine A & B 45
Scordinine A₁,A₂ & B 45
Scormine 45
Secologanic acid 184
†Sedanenolide **78**
Sempervirine 324
Senecionine 238
†Sennoside A 177,178,181
†Sennoside C **177**
Serpentine 187
Severine 103
†Shatavarin IV **101**
Shazhiside 323
Shikimin 366
Shikimipicrin 366
Shinjulactone B 33
†Sieversinin **96**
Sinalbin 136,138

Sinapine 136,137,140
Sinapin thiocyanate 136
Sinicuichine 346
Sinigrin 136,138
Sinine (Lythridine) 346
β-Sitosterol 33,**332**
†Skimmianine 26,197,**332**,333
Solanidine 169
Solanine 169
Solasonin 194
Somalin 22
Sophoranol 303
†Sparsiflorine **240**
†Sparteine **255**
Speciophylline 342
†Spectabiline **17**,239
Stachydrine 15,167,300
S-l-Stachydrine 268
Stepharine 72,279
†5-Stigmastene-3β,7α-diol **63**
Stigmasterol **332**
†Strictamine **52**
Strigosine 349
†Strophalloside **76**,299
Strophanthidin 76,267,299
Strophanthidin glucoboivinioside 352
Strophanthidine tetroside 25
g-Strophathin 17
k-Strophanthins 17
k-Strophanthins-B 25
†Strophanthin-K **231**
β-Stylopine 269
(−)-Stylopine 233
†Sucapigraveol **79**
†Sulphoraphane **170**
Supinine 304,349
Swertiamarin 325
†Swertisioside **293**
†Synephrine 208,**303**

T

Tabersonine 185
†Tangeretin **208**,210,211
†Tanghinoside **192**
†Tannic acid **160**
Taxifolin 188
Taxiphyllin 114
Tazettine 55,342,362

Tectoquinone 281
†Tetrahydroalstonine 184,185,**187**
†Δ⁹-*tras*-Tetrahydrocannabinol **164,165**
dl-Tetrahydrocoptisine 319
(±)-Tetrahydroglazievine 240
Tetrahydroharman 288
Tetrahydropalmitine 121
†5,7,3′,4′-Tetrahydroxyflavan-3-ol **310**
†2,4,3′,5′-Tetrahydroxystilbene **98**
N,N′-Tetramethylholarrhimine 320
†Tetramethylpyrazine **378**
†Tetrandrine **250**
†*d*-Tetrandrine **250**
†*dl*-Tetrandrine **250**
Thalicarpine 351
†Theobromine 160,161,**221**,366
†Theophylline **160,221**
Theveside 192
†Thevetin B **192**
Theviridoside 192
†Thiopropanal-S-oxide **42**
†6α-Tigloyloxychaparrin **34**
†α-Tigloyloxychaparrinone **34**
Tigogenin 30,194,234,320
Tigonin 193
Tingenone 304
Tinyatoxin 195
Tombozine 184
Tricin-5-O-glucoside 205
Trifucol nona acetate 319
Triglochinin 46,290
Trigonelline 4,13,15,54,268,353
Trilobine 218
Trimethoxygallamide 52
†1,3,7-Trimethylxanthine **221**
†Triolein **143**
†*n*-Tritriacontane **77**
Tropine 144,260,261,285
ψ-Tropine 260
Tryptamine 267
†Tryptanthrin 114,**374**
†Tubaic acid **265**
†β-Tubaic acid **265**
Tubotaicoine 52
Tubulosine 35,36
ψ-Twistane 320
Tyramine 267,268,342

U

Umbellatine 121
†Usaramine 237,**238**,239
Uscharidin 158
Uscharin 158
†Uzarigenin **99**
†Uzarin **99**

V

Vakatidine 17
Vakatisine 17
Vakatisinine 17
Vakognavine 17
Valeroidine 285
Valtropine 285
Vanillin 181
†Vasakin **23**
†Vasicine 23,24
Vasicinine 23
†Vsasicinol **24**
†Vasicinone 23,**24**
Vasicol 24
Venalstonidine 52
Venalstonine 52,184
†Venenatine **52**
Veneserpine 52
Venoterpine 36,52,183
Venoxidine 52
Veratrine 228
Veratroyl-ψ-aconine 17,18
Verbenalin (Cornin) 119
†Vertine **346**
†Villalstonine **51**
†Vinamidine **184**
†Vinblastine (Vinleukoblastine) **185**
Vincaline I & II 184
Vincamine 184
Vincapusine 183
Vincarine 184
Vincarodine 184
Vincathicine 184
Vincoline 184
†Vincristine [(vin)leurocristine] **185**
Vincubine 184
†Vindesine **185**
†Vindoline **183**,184,185
†Vindolinine **185**
Vindorosine 183

Vinervine	184	†Wuchuyine	**304**
Vinleukoblastine, see Vinblastine			
Vinleurocristine, see Vincristine		**X**	
Vinoterpine	183		
Vinsedicine	185	†Xanthochymol	**323**
Vinsedine	185	Xanthorin	179
†5-Vinyl-2-oxazolidinethione (Vinyl		†Xanthotoxin (Ammoidin)	56,57,79,103,
thiooxazolidone, 5-Vinyl- OZT)	**138**		131,350
5-Vinyl-OZT, see 5-Vinyl-2-		†Xanthotoxol	57,**69**
oxazolidinethione		†Xylitol	**172**
Vinyl thiooxazolidone, see 5-Vinyl-2-		Xylocarpin	170
oxazolidinethione		†Xylomollin	**170**
†Visnadin	**58**	(−)-Xylopine	73
†Vitamin U	**244**		
†Vitexin	**91**	**Y**	
Voacristine hydroxyindolnine	298		
Vocangine	298	Yamogenin	113
†Vulgarin	97	Yatanine	142
		Yatanoside	142
W		†Yatansin	**143**
		Yejuhua lactone	199
Wallinchoside	118	δ-Yohimbine	184
Weldolactone	287	Yuccanin	194